MW00603649

Diabetic Neuropathy: Clinical Management, Second Edition

CONTEMPORARY DIABETES

ARISTIDIS VEVES, MD, DSc
SERIES EDITOR

Diabetic Neuropathy: *Clinical Management, Second Edition*, edited by *Aristidis Veves, MD, DSC, and Rayaz A. Malik, MBChB, PhD, 2007*
The Diabetic Foot*, Second Edition*, edited by *Aristidis Veves, MD, DSC, John M. Giurini, DPM, and Frank W. LoGerfo, MD, 2006*
The Diabetic Kidney, edited by *PEDRO CORTES, MD, AND CARL ERIK MOGENSEN, MD, 2006*
Obesity and Diabetes, edited by *Christos S. Mantzoros, MD, 2006*

Diabetic Neuropathy

Clinical Management, Second Edition

Edited by

Aristidis Veves, MD, DSc

Beth Israel Deaconess Medical Center
Harvard Medical School
Boston, MA

and

Rayaz A. Malik, MBChB, PhD

Manchester Royal Infirmary
and University of Manchester,
Manchester, UK

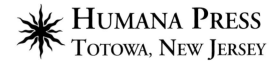
Humana Press
Totowa, New Jersey

999 Riverview Drive, Suite 208
Totowa, New Jersey 07512

www.humanapress.com

Production Editor: Michele Seugling

Cover Illustration: Figure 3, Chapter 17, by Michael Polydefkis, "Punch Skin Biopsy in Diabetic Neuropathy."

Cover design by Karen Schulz

For additional copies, pricing for bulk purchases, and/or information about other Humana titles, contact Humana at the above address or at any of the following numbers: Tel.: 973-256-1699; Fax: 973-256-8341, E-mail: orders@humanapr.com; or visit our Website: www.humanapress.com

This publication is printed on acid-free paper. ∞

ANSI Z39.48-1984 (American National Standards Institute) Permanence of Paper for Printed Library Materials.

Printed in the United States of America. 10 9 8 7 6 5 4 3 2 1

e-ISBN 978-1-59745-311-0

Library of Congress Control Number: 2007932486

To my wife Maria and my son George.

— Aristidis Veves

To my wife Robina and beautiful daughters: Imaan, Hana and Ayesha.

— Rayaz A. Malik

Preface

It has been almost a decade since the first edition of *Clinical Management of Diabetic Neuropathy* was published. Since then, all societies have seen an explosion in obesity and diabetes. As a result, there is also an explosion in long-term diabetes complications, including diabetic neuropathy. Diabetic neuropathy therefore remains a major health problem that has not only serious consequences for the patient but also carries a significant financial burden for the health care-providing organizations of every society.

Another change that has taken place since the last edition is the accumulation of considerable data that has drastically expanded our knowledge regarding the pathophysiology and natural history of the disease. Unfortunately, this expansion in our knowledge has not been accompanied by success in treating diabetic neuropathy. Thus, considerable clinical research efforts that employed various therapeutic modalities, including aldose reductase inhibitors, nerve growth factor, and PKC beta inhibitors, failed to provide positive results and are currently not expected to gain approval for clinical use.

For *Diabetic Neuropathy: Clinical Management, Second Edition,* we have made every effort to reflect the above changes. We have included new chapters that focus more detail on the pathophysiology of the disease, and we have also expanded the sections regarding the diagnosis and the management of the various presentations of diabetic neuropathy. We feel very fortunate that we were able to recruit all leading authorities in their respective fields, and we believe that this has tremendously increased the quality of this edition. We therefore hope that this edition will be helpful not only to the practicing clinicians but also to researchers who would like to examine this condition in more detail.

We would like to sincerely thank all of the contributors to *Diabetic Neuropathy: Clinical Management, Second Edition*, as it is their hard work that has resulted in this successful textbook. We would like also to thank Humana Press for their trust in our abilities and all of their help in accomplishing this project.

Aristidis Veves, *MD, DSc*
Rayaz A. Malik, *MBChB, PhD*

List of Color Images

The images listed below appear in the color insert within the text.

Contents

Contributors

Misha-Miroslav Backonja • *Department of Neurology, School of Medicine and Public Health, University of Wisconsin—Madison, Madison, WI*

Geert Jan Biessels • *Department of Neurology of the Rudolf Magnus Institute for Neuroscience, University Medical Centre, Utrecht, The Netherlands*

Andrew J. M. Boulton • *Department of Medicine, Manchester Royal Infirmary, Manchester, UK*

Edward J. Boyko • *VA Puget Sound Healthcare System, Seattle, WA*

Rebecca C. Burnand • *Faculty of Life Sciences, University of Manchester, Manchester, UK*

Nigel A. Calcutt • *Department of Pathology, University of California San Diego, La Jolla, CA*

Antonella Caselli • *Microcirculation Lab, Beth Israel Deaconess Medical Center, Harvard Medical School, Boston, MA*

Sookja K. Chung • *Department of Anatomy, The University of Hong Kong, Hong Kong, SAR China*

Stephen S. Chung • *Department of Physiology, The University of Hong Kong, Hong Kong, SAR China*

Rita M. Cowell • *Department of Psychiatry and Behavioral Neurobiology, University of Alabama at Birmingham, Birmingham, AL*

Andrew G. Demaine • *Molecular Medicine Research Group, Peninsula Medical School, Plymouth, UK*

Eva L. Feldman • *Department of Neurology, University of Michigan, Ann Arbor, MI*

Roy Freeman • *Autonomic Lab, Beth Israel Deaconess Medical Center, Boston MA*

John W. Griffin • *Department of Neurology, The Johns Hopkins Hospital, Baltimore, MD*

Corinne G. Jolivalt • *Department of Pathology, University of California San Diego, La Jolla, CA*

Hideki Kamiya • *Department of Pathology, Wayne State University, Detroit, MI*

Phillip A. Low • *Department of Neurology, Mayo Clinic, Rochester, MN*

Thomas E. Lyons • *Division of Podiatric Medicine and Surgery, Harvard Medical School, Beth Israel Deaconess Medical Center, Boston, MA*

Juan-R. Malagelada • *Digestive System Research Unit, Hospital General Vall d'Hebron, Autonomous University of Barcelona, Barcelona, Spain*

Rayaz A. Malik • *Division of Cardiovascular Medicine, University of Manchester, Manchester, UK*

Justin McArthur • *Department of Neurology, The Johns Hopkins Hospital, Baltimore, MD*

Andrew P. Mizisin • *Department of Pathology, University of California San Diego, La Jolla, CA*

Irina G. Obrosova • *Pennington Biomedical Research Center, Louisiana State University, Baton Rouge, LA*

Henri Pharson • *Department of Internal Medicine, Strelitz Diabetes Institutes, Eastern Virginia Medical School, Norfolk, VA*

Gary L. Pittenger • *Department of Internal Medicine, Strelitz Diabetes Institutes, Eastern Virginia Medical School, Norfolk, VA*

Michael Polydefkis • *Department of Neurology, The Johns Hopkins Hospital, Baltimore, MD*

Sally A. Price • *Faculty of Life Sciences, University of Manchester, Manchester, UK*

James W. Russell • *Department of Neurology, University of Maryland, Baltimore, MD*

Gérard Said • *Service de Neurologie and Laboratoire Louis Ranvier, Hopital de Bicetre, Assistance Publique-Hopitaux de Paris and Universite Paris-sud, Paris, France*

Anders A. F. Sima • *Departments of Pathology and Neurology and The Morris Hood Comprehensive Diabetes Centre, Wayne State University, Detroit, MI*

Nalini Singh • *VA Puget Sound Health Care System, Seattle, WA*

Vladimir Skljarevski • *Lilly Research Laboratories, Indianapolis, IN*

Martin J. Stevens • *Division of Medical Sciences, University of Birmingham, Birmingham, UK*

Christian Stief • *LMU University of Munich Hospital, Clinic for Urology, Munich, Germany*

Goran Sundkvist • *Department of Endocrinology, University of Lund, Malmo University Hospital, Sweden*

Solomon Tesfaye • *Diabetes Research Unit, Royal Hallamshire Hospital, Sheffield, UK*

David R. Tomlinson • *Faculty of Life Sciences, University of Manchester, Manchester, UK*

Jagdeesh Ullal • *Department of Internal Medicine, Strelitz Diabetes Institutes, Eastern Virginia Medical School, Norfolk, VA*

Aristidis Veves • *Microcirculation Lab, Beth Israel Deaconess Medical Center, Harvard Medical School, Boston, MA*

Aaron I. Vinik • *Department of Internal Medicine, Strelitz Diabetes Institutes, Eastern Virginia Medical School, Norfolk, VA*

Stephanie Wheeler • *VA Puget Sound Health Care System, Seattle, WA*

Bingmei Yang • *Molecular Medicine Research Group, Peninsula Medical School, Plymouth, UK*

Weixian Zhang • *Department of Pathology, Wayne State University, Detroit, MI*

Dan Ziegler • *German Diabetes Center, Leibniz Center at the Heinrich Heine University, Institute for Clinical Diabetes, Düsseldorf, Germany*

Douglas W. Zochodne • *Department of Clinical Neurosciences, Foothills Medical Center, University of Calgary, Alberta, Canada*

1
Historical Aspects of Diabetic Neuropathies

Vladimir Skljarevski, MD

SUMMARY

Ancient records of diabetes generally contain no reference to its complications involving the nervous system. A few rare exceptions describing autonomic and painful neuropathies are all coming from the Orient. It was not until the 18th century that Western physicians started studying diabetes and its complications. Eventually, the works of the 19th century (de Calvi, Pavy) clearly established the link between diabetes mellitus and diabetic neuropathies. The epochal discovery of insulin in 1921 triggered a wide interest and more systematic approach to research of diabetic complications, leading to S. Fagerberger's conclusion that many of them share the underlying microvascular pathology.

Key Words: History; diabetes; neuropathy; complications.

INTRODUCTION

The history of diabetic complications, including neuropathies, cannot be separated from the one of diabetes itself. Ancient texts describing what is believed to be diabetes mellitus represent clinical records of polyuric states associated with increased thirst, muscle wasting, and premature death. In these early texts, neuropathic elements of the clinical picture of diabetes can be found extremely rarely. It was not until the 18th century that neuropathy became recognized as a common complication of diabetes and the subject of scientific interest and systematic studies. The epochal discovery of insulin opened a whole new chapter in the history of diabetes and diabetic neuropathies. However, everyone will agree that the problem of diabetic complications, although extensively studied, is far from being solved.

THE ANCIENT PERIOD

The first ever record of diabetes appears to be the papyrus named after the Egyptologist Ebers, who found it in an ancient grave in Thebes. It is written in hieroglyphs. The exact time of its writing is unknown, but most estimates date it around 1550 BC. It contains descriptions of a number of diseases including a polyuric state resembling diabetes, which was to be treated with a decoction of bones, wheat, grain, grit, green lead, and earth *(1)*. The term "diabetes" was first used by Aretaeus of Kappadokia in the 2nd century AD. It comes from the Greek prefix "dia" and the word "betes" meaning "to pass through" and "a water tube," respectively *(2)*. Ancient Greeks and Romans alike saw diabetes as a disease of the kidneys. "Diabetes is a dreadful affliction, not very frequent

From: *Contemporary Diabetes: Diabetic Neuropathy: Clinical Management, Second Edition*
Edited by: A. Veves and R. Malik © Humana Press Inc., Totowa, NJ

among men, being a melting down of the flesh and limbs into urine. The patients never stop making water and the flow is incessant, like the opening of aqueducts. Life is short, unpleasant and painful, thirst unquenchable, drinking excessive, and disproportionate to the large quantity of urine, for yet more urine is passed. One cannot stop them either from drinking or making water. If for a while they abstain from drinking, their mouths become parched and their bodies dry; the viscera seem scorched up, the patients are affected by nausea, restlessness, and a burning thirst, and within a short time, they expire *(1)*."

It was not noticed until the 5th century AD that, at that time, rare condition of polyuria was associated with sweet-tasting urine. Chen Chuan in China named it "hsiao kho ping," and made a note that the urine of the diseased is sweet and attracts dogs. He recommended abstinence from wine, salt, and sex as treatment *(1,3)*. At about the same time Indian physician Susruta wrote in Sanskrit that the urine of patients is like "madhumeha," i.e., tastes like honey, feels sticky to the touch, and strongly attracts ants *(1,4)*. His treatment recommendation is colorfully summarized in the following words: "A kind of gelatinous substance (silajatu) is secreted from the sides of the mountains when they have become heated by the rays of the sun in the months of Jyaishitha and Ashadha. It cures the body and enables the user to witness a hundred summers on earth" *(5)*.

Susruta may deserve credit for what seems to be the very first record of symptoms attributable to diabetic neuropathy: "Their premonitory symptoms are—feeling of burning in the palms and soles, body (skin) becoming unctuous and slimy and feel heavy, urine is sweet, bad in smell, and white in color, and profound thirst… Complications (upadrava) include diarrhea, constipation, and fainting" *(6)*. Susruta also made a very important observation that the disease affects two types of people: the older, heavier ones and the thin who did not survive long. All other known early records that most likely represent a description of some form of diabetic neuropathy come from the Orient. Persian philosopher and physician Ibn Sina, known as Avicenna (980–1037 AD) in the West, described diabetes in his famous "El-Kanun." He observed gangrene and the "collapse of sexual function" as complications of diabetes *(4)*. The same manifestation of autonomic neuropathy was recorded in ancient Japanese text containing a detailed description of the "water-drinking illness" (mizu nomi yami) as suffered by nobleman Fujiwara No Michinaga from the Heian Era *(7,8)*.

THE MIDDLE AGES

During the Middle Ages, a number of writers made mention of diabetes, but not its neurological complications. Interestingly, none of them spoke of the sweet properties of urine either, and it was not until well into the 17th century when Thomas Willis recalled attention to it. Another century had passed before Dobson, in 1775, showed that the taste of diabetic urine depended on sugar, which he demonstrated by evaporating the urine and producing the sugar in crystals *(9)*. The Middle Ages should also be remembered by the most poetic description of the diabetes-associated copious flow of urine ever. It was made by the English poet and physician Sir Richard Blackmore in 1727. "…as when the Treasures of Snow collected in Winter on the Alpine Hills, and dissolved and thawed by the first hot Days of the returning Spring, flow down in Torrents through the abrupt Channels, and overspread the Vales with a sudden Inundation" *(10)*.

DIABETIC NEUROPATHY IN WESTERN MEDICINE

John Rollo, a surgeon of the British Royal Artillery, was systematically studying diabetes. He was probably the first person to use the adjective mellitus (from the Latin and Greek roots for "honey") to distinguish the condition from the similar one but without glycosuria (in Latin, insipidus means tasteless). He was the first one to recommend a diet low in carbohydrates as a treatment for diabetes. Rollo summarized his therapeutic experience with diabetes in a book published in 1798 *(11)*. His detailed clinical observations include symptoms consistent with diabetic autonomic neuropathy. "His skin is dry. His face flushed. He is frequently sick, and throws up matter of a viscid nature, and of bitterish, and sweetish taste. After eating he has a pain of his stomach, which continues often half an hour… He makes much urine, 10–12 pints in the 24 hours, to the voiding of which he has urgent propensities peculiarly distressing to him, and constantly dribbling" *(11)*.

Despite his remarkable insight into the nature of diabetes, John Rollo failed to acknowledge a direct link between diabetes and the nervous system. This was not the case with Marchal de Calvi who, in 1864, correctly identified that relationship *(12)*. The works generated at the end of the 19th century had definitively established the concept of peripheral neuropathy as a complication of diabetes. In 1884, Althaus confirmed the findings of de Calvi and emphasized the nocturnal character of pain *(13)*. In that same year, Bouchard pointed to the fact that the knee-jerks are frequently absent in cases of diabetes *(14)*. A few years later, Ross and Bury systematically studied reflexes in 50 patients with diabetes *(15)*. Frederick William Pavy, in his address to the Section of Medicine of the British Medical Association, provided a classical description of neuropathic signs and symptoms associated with diabetes, acknowledging the link between them. His description included "heavy legs, numb feet, lightning pain and deep-seated pain in feet, hyperaesthesia, muscle tenderness, and impairment of patellar tendon reflexes" *(16)*. Pavy also made a point that occurrence of neuropathic symptoms may precede that of clinical diabetes *(16,17)*.

Davies Pryce, a resident surgeon of Nottingham Dispensary, deserves credit for providing the first report on macro- and microscopic changes in peripheral nerves of diabetic patients and suggesting a connection between "diabetic neuritis and perforating foot ulcers" *(18)*. "It will be seen that a good many of the causes which have been believed to produce perforating ulcers and peripheral neuritis were also present—i.e., cold, alcohol, diabetes, vascular disease, and continued pressure. It is probable that all these played a part in the causation of the disease but I would venture to assign considerable share to diabetes and vascular disease" *(18)*.

Layden proposed the first clinical classification of diabetic neuropathies as follows:

1. Hyperesthetic or neuralgic form;
2. Motor or paralytic form; and
3. Ataxic or pseudotabetic form *(19)*.

By the end of the 19th century, the awareness of diabetic neuropathy was sufficient enough to enable Purdy to conclude: "It is rare to meet with a case of diabetes in which there is not more or less nervous disturbance" *(20)*. Charcot brilliantly summarized clinical features of diabetic peripheral neuropathy *(21)*. "He complains about flashing pain existing for 18 months which wakes him up at night. The pain is occurring five and six times a day, followed by hyperaesthesiae. He also has pins and needles in the legs which prevent him from feeling the nature of the floor. He always feels too hot or too cold in his feet. On physical examination there is complete absence of patellar reflexes, Rhomberg's signs very positive, pupillary reflexes absolutely normal for light and accommodation" *(22)*. Scientific interest in diabetic neuropathies witnessed during late 19th century led to initiation of animal experiments in this field. Auche from Bordeaux, France published the results of his experiments with injecting sugar into the nerves of guinea pigs. He concluded that diabetic neuropathy was a vaso-motor problem, but that the sugar itself did not play an important role in the pathophysiology of the disease *(23)*.

THE MODERN ERA

Banting's epochal discovery of insulin in 1921 changed not only the world of diabetes, but also the history of medicine *(24)*. The postinsulin era brought a surge of research activities related to diabetic neuropathies. Several authors, including Jordan and Broch, observed a common dissociation between neuropathic symptoms and objective signs of disease *(25,26)*. Wayne Rundles from the University of Michigan published a review of 125 cases of diabetic neuropathy. His observations created a basis for the suggestion that development of neuropathy is dependent on the degree of glycemic control *(27)*. The work of Rundles, along with that of Root, significantly contributed to the understanding of diabetic autonomic neuropathy *(28)*. Garland provided a description of the predominantly proximal, often transient, painful neuropathy not accompanied by sensory disturbances. He named the condition diabetic amyotrophy *(29,30)*. Stainess and Downie, in the early sixties, started using quantitative sensory testing and nerve conduction studies in neuropathy research *(31,32)*.

In 1959, Sven-Erik Fagerberg from Göteborg, on thoroughly studying 356 cases of diabetes, proposed an association among diabetic neuropathy, retinopathy, and nephropathy. In approx 50% of the cases, he performed microscopic analysis of peripheral nerves and discovered substantial abnormalities in the nerve microvasculature, especially prominent in those with clinical signs of neuropathy. By combining epidemiological and pathological evidence, Fagerberg proposed the theory that diabetic neuropathy, retinopathy, and nephropathy share an underlying microvascular pathology *(33)*. In the arena of diabetic neuropathies, the end of the 20th century will be remembered as the period of large clinical trials testing potential therapeutic agents. So far none of the agents tested, with the exception of insulin, have as both safe and capable of altering the course of diabetic neuropathy *(34)*. Therefore, the race continues.

REFERENCES

1. Pickup JC, Williams G (eds.). The history of diabetes mellitus, in *Textbook of Diabetes*. Blackwell Science, Oxford, 1997, pp. 23–30.
2. Papaspyros NS. The history of diabetes mellitus, 2nd ed. Thieme, Stuttgart, 1964. Reprinted in *Textbook of Diabetes*. Blackwell Science, Oxford, 1997, 1.3p.
3. Gwei-Djen L, Needham J. Records of diseases in ancient China. *Am J Chin Med* 1976; 4:3–16.
4. Grossman A (ed.). Clinical endocrinology, in *Notes on the history of endocrinology*, Blackwell Sciences Publications, Oxford, 1992, pp. 1040–1943.
5. Kaviraj Kunja Lal Bhishagratna (ed.). An English Translation of The Sushruta Samhita, Calcuta, 1911, pp. 28–29.
6. Murthy KRS, translator. Ilustrated Susruta Samhita. (Sutrasthana and Nidana Sthana). Chaukhambha Orientalia, Varanasi, India, 2000, p. 106.

7. Kiple KF (ed.). The Cambridge World History of Human Disease. Cambridge University Press, Cambridge, 1995, pp. 353–354.
8. Hurst GC. Michinaga's Madalies. *Monumenta Nipponica* 1979;34:101–112.
9. Purdy CW. Diabetes—its causes, symptoms and treatment. (Davis FA, ed.), Philadelphia, PA, 1890, pp. 76–78.
10. Gottlieb SH. What's in a name?—your healthy heart. The water siphon disease. ADA 2002. www.findarticles.com/p/articles/mi_0817/is_12_55/ai_94590378. Last accessed January 17, 2005.
11. Rollo J. Cases of the diabetes mellitus with the results of the trials of certain acids. (Dilly C, ed.), London, 1798.
12. De Calvi M. Recherches sur les accidents diabetiques. (Asselin P, ed.), Paris, 1864.
13. Althaus J. Ueber Sklerose des Rückenmarkes. Otto Wigand, Leipzig, 1884, pp. 169–171.
14. Bouchard C. Sur la perte des reflexes tendineux dans le diabète sucré. *Progrès méd* 1884;12:819.
15. Ross J, Bury J. On peripheral neuritis. A treatise. Charles Griffin Ltd., London, 1893, pp. 361–372.
16. Pavy FW. Introductory address to the discussion on the clinical aspects of glycosuria. *Lancet* 1885;2:1085–1087.
17. Pavy FW. Physiology of the Carbohydrates; The application as food and relation to diabetes. J&A Churchill, London, 1894.
18. Pryce TD. Perforating ulcers of both feet associated with diabetes and ataxic symptoms. *Lancet* 1887;2:11–12.
19. Layden E. Die Entzundung der peripheren Nerven. Deut Militar Zaitsch. 1887;17:49.
20. Purdy CW. Diabetes—its causes, symptoms and treatment. (Davis FA, ed.), Philadelphia, PA, 1890.
21. Charcot JM. Sur un cas de paraplegie diabetique. *Arch Neurol* 1890;19:305–335.
22. Charcot JM. Sur un cas de paraplegie diabetique. *Arch Neurol* 1890;19:305–335. Reprinted in JD Ward, Historical aspects of diabetic peripheral neuropathy, in *Diabetic Neuropathy* (Boulton AJM, ed.), Aventis, Bridgewater, NJ, 2001, pp. 6–15.
23. Auche MB. Des alterations des nerfs peripheriques chez les diabetiques. *Arch Med Exp Anat Pathol* 1890;2:635–676.
24. Banting FG, Best CH. The internal secretion of the pancreas. *J Lab Clin Med* 1922; 7:256–271.
25. Jordan WR. Neuritic manifestations in diabetes mellitus. *Arch Int Med* 1936;57:307.
26. Broch OJ, Kløvstad O. Polyneuritis in diabetes mellitus. *Acta Med Scandinav* 1947;127:514.
27. Rundles RW. Diabetic neuropathy: General review with report of 125 cases. Medicine, Baltimore, MD. 1945;24:111–160.
28. Root HF. The nervous system and diabetes, in *The treatment of diabetes mellitus*, 10 ed. (Joslin EP, ed.), Lea & Febiger, Philadelphia, PA, 1959, 483p.
29. Garland H. Diabetic amyoptrophy. *Brit M J* 1955;2:1287.
30. Garland H. Neurological Complications of diabetes mellitus: Clinical aspects. *Proc R Soc Med* 1960;53:137.
31. Steiness I. Diabetic neuropathy. Vibration sense and abnormal tendon reflexes in diabetics. *Acta Med Scand* 1963;394:1–91.
32. Downie AW, Newell DJ. Sensory nerve conduction in patients with diabetes mellitus and controls. *Neurology* 1961;11:876–882.
33. Fagerberg S-E. Diabetic neuropathy: A clinical and histological study on the significance of vascular affections. *Acta Med Scand* 1959;164(Suppl 345):1–97.
34. Diabetes Control and Complications Trial Research Group. The effect of intensive treatment of diabetes on the development and progression of long-term complications in insulin dependent diabetes mellitus. *N Engl J Med* 1993;329(14):977–986.

2
The Epidemiology of Diabetic Neuropathy

Stephanie Wheeler, MD, MPH, Nalini Singh, MD, and Edward J. Boyko, MD, MPH

SUMMARY

Peripheral neuropathy is a devastating complication of diabetes mellitus because of the debilitating symptoms it causes or associated higher risk of other complications, in particular those involving the lower extremity. This chapter will review the prevalence, incidence, and risk factors for different types of diabetic neuropathy. There are seven major types of diabetic neuropathy: (1) distal symmetric polyneuropathy, (2) autonomic neuropathy, (3) nerve entrapment syndromes, (4) proximal asymmetric mononeuropathy (also known as diabetic amyotrophy), (5) truncal radiculopathy, (6) cranial mononeuropathy, and (7) chronic inflammatory demyelinating polyradiculopathy (CIDP). This chapter will focus mainly on the first two types of neuropathy, but will review the available data on the epidemiology of the other types of neuropathy. Cross-sectional or case–control studies conducted in a population-based sample (such as a defined community or health plan enrollment) were considered for this chapter based on review of Medline citations using the keywords "epidemiology," "diabetes," and "neuropathy" from 1966 to February 2005 review of bibliographies of the articles obtained from the Medline search for relevant citations, and review of the authors' files. Clinic-based cross-sectional or case–control studies have not been considered except in the case of rare conditions, for which no other data exists. All prospective studies, and some randomized controlled trials, were considered. Of the five community-based cross-sectional studies reviewed of subjects with type 2 diabetes that presented data on risk factors for neuropathy, three reported a higher prevalence of this outcome with longer diabetes duration and higher glycosylated hemoglobin, and two found neuropathy prevalence correlated with age and height. Only three community-based cross-sectional studies addressed neuropathy prevalence in subjects with type 1 diabetes in association with risk factors. Two of these investigations reported a correlation between diabetes duration and neuropathy prevalence. No other significant risk factor was reported by more than one community-based study done with subjects with type 1 diabetes. Prospective research on the risk of distal symmetric polyneuropathy confirms its relationship to poorer glycemic control as reflected by fasting plasma glucose or hemoglobin A1c (HbA1c) at baseline. Four prospective studies reported duration of diabetes as a risk factor for neuropathy, three reported smoking as a risk factor, two reported age and two reported baseline coronary artery disease as risk factors for neuropathy. The literature on risk factors for diabetic autonomic neuropathy can be characterized as smaller in size and less consistent in comparison with that available for distal symmetric polyneuropathy. The only risk factor reported in more than one study was female gender, found to be associated with higher risk by two authors. There have been no prospective population-based studies

From: *Contemporary Diabetes: Diabetic Neuropathy: Clinical Management, Second Edition*
Edited by: A. Veves and R. Malik © Humana Press Inc., Totowa, NJ

of diabetic amyotrophy and mononeuropathies in subjects with diabetes. However, some prevalence figures for these types of neuropathy can be derived from a few cross-sectional studies, which are described in the chapter. CIDP is a relatively new diagnosis. In 1991, the American Academy of Neurology defined diagnostic clinical and electrophysiological criteria for CIDP. All studies on CIDP are cross-sectional and clinic-based.

Key Words: Diabetic neuropathy; diabetes; epidemiology; incidence; prevalence; risk factors.

INTRODUCTION

Peripheral neuropathy is a devastating complication of diabetes mellitus (DM) because of the debilitating symptoms it causes or associated higher risk of other complications, in particular those involving the lower extremity. The epidemiology of diabetic neuropathy is not as well understood in comparison with other complications of this metabolic disorder, including retinal, renal, and coronary artery disease. Different peripheral nerves may be damaged through a variety of pathological processes as described in other chapters of this book. This chapter will review the prevalence, incidence, and risk factors for different types of diabetic neuropathy. The natural history of diabetic neuropathy will be briefly described regarding foot complications.

There are seven major types of diabetic neuropathy:

1. Distal symmetric polyneuropathy.
2. Autonomic neuropathy.
3. Nerve entrapment syndromes.
4. Proximal asymmetric mononeuropathy (also known as diabetic amyotrophy).
5. Truncal radiculopathy.
6. Cranial mononeuropathy.
7. Chronic inflammatory demyelinating polyradiculopathy (CIDP).

This chapter will focus mainly on the first two types of neuropathy, but will review the available data on the epidemiology of the other types of neuropathy. With the exception of nerve entrapment syndromes these remaining types occur infrequently.

EPIDEMIOLOGICAL PRINCIPLES RELEVANT TO THE STUDY OF DIABETIC NEUROPATHY

In order to understand published research on the epidemiology of diabetic neuropathy, certain principles of epidemiological study design must be taken into consideration. These principles guided these authors in the selection of relevant citations and data presentation. Cross-sectional or case–control studies conducted in a population-based sample (such as a defined community or health plan enrollment) were considered for this chapter based on review of Medline citations using the keywords "epidemiology," "diabetes," and "neuropathy" from 1966 to February 2005 review of bibliographies of the articles obtained from the Medline search for relevant citations, and review of the authors' files. Clinic-based cross-sectional or case–control studies have not been considered except in the case of rare conditions for which no other data exists, because of the potential problem of selection bias associated with these study designs *(1)*. All prospective studies, and some randomized controlled trials, were considered. Prospective research is less likely to be biased because of differences in probability of subject selection based on disease (neuropathy) and risk factor presence. Prospective research is a stronger study design in inferring the possibility of causation, because the presence of risk factors may be determined before neuropathy onset.

The problem of measurement error in the assessment of the presence or absence of diabetic neuropathy is well recognized. Nerve conduction velocity, arguably the most objective and accurate test available for the diagnosis of this complication, is known to sometimes result in erroneous classification. For example, nerve conduction velocity may be normal in diabetic subjects with symptoms of distal symmetric polyneuropathy *(2)*. This misclassification problem is even more problematic when a test result is used to formulate a clinical plan for an individual patient, in comparison with epidemiological analysis where population statistics are the result of interest. When misclassification of neuropathy or risk factor status occurs nondifferentially (randomly), the net result is bias of any observed difference toward the null value *(1)*. Therefore observed differences found in an epidemiological analysis of risk factors for diabetic neuropathy validly reflect potential causative factors for this complication, but probably underestimate the magnitude of the risk increase. Epidemiological studies may draw valid conclusions regarding risk factors for diabetic neuropathy even if the techniques used to measure neuropathy and the potential risk factor are known to be inaccurate.

DISTAL SYMMETRIC POLYNEUROPATHY—PREVALENCE AND RISK FACTORS (CROSS-SECTIONAL RESEARCH)

Dyck et al. *(3)* examined the prevalence of neuropathy among all clinically diagnosed diabetic subjects who resided in Rochester, Minnesota. Only 380 of 870 eligible subjects (44%) agreed to participate, possibly because of concern about the lengthy neurodiagnostic study protocol. Neuropathy was defined if two criteria were satisfied:

1. Abnormal nerve conduction in more than one nerve or abnormal test of autonomic function (low heart rate variation in response to breathing or the Valsalva maneuver).
2. Neuropathic symptom or sign or abnormal quantitative sensory testing.

Median duration of diabetes was 14.5 years for subjects with type 1 diabetes and 8.1 years for subjects with type 2 diabetes. Although the prevalence of neuropathy was high (Table 1), most subjects with neuropathy were asymptomatic (about 71%).

A community-based study in San Luis Valley, Colorado, measured prevalence of neuropathy in a bi-ethnic (Hispanic and Anglo) population *(4,5)*. Neuropathy was defined if two of three criteria were satisfied:

1. Neuropathic discomfort in feet and legs.
2. Abnormal Achilles tendon reflexes.
3. Inability to feel an iced tuning fork on the dorsum of the foot (test of thermal sensation).

Subjects with type 2 diabetes had the highest prevalence of neuropathy, whereas subjects with IGT defined according to World Health Organization criteria had prevalence about midway between normal glucose tolerance (NGT) and type 2 diabetes (Table 1). No subjects with type 1 diabetes were included in this study. Significantly higher prevalence of neuropathy was found in relation to greater age, diabetes duration, glycosylated hemoglobin, male gender, and insulin use. Factors not associated with neuropathy prevalence included blood pressure, height, smoking, previous alcohol use, ankle-arm index, and serum cholesterol, lipid, and lipoprotein levels.

Table 1
Distal Symmetric Polyneuropathy: Prevalence, Incidence, and Risk Factors From Cross-Sectional Research Studies

Reference	Subjects	Prevalence	Significant risk factors	Odds ratio (95% CI)
3	100 type 1 diabetes, 259 type 2 diabetes	54%	Not reported	–
		45%	–	–
4	277 type 2 diabetes, 89 IGT, 496 NGT	27%	Age (5 year increase)	1.2 (1–1.4)
		11%	Male gender	2.2 (1.2–4.1)
		4%	Diabetes duration (5 year increase)	1.3 (1–1.6)
			Glycosylated hemoglobin (2.5% increase)	1.3 (1–1.8)
			Insulin use	2.7 (1.4–5.2)
6	363 type 1 diabetes	34%	Diabetes duration, 10 year increase	1.2 (1.1–1.2)
			Glycosylated hemoglobin (1% increase)	1.4 (1.2–1.7)
			HDL cholesterol (0.13 m*M*) decrease	1.2 (1.1–1.3)
			Current smoking	2.2 (1.3–3.8)
			Any macrovascular disease	2.3 (1–5.4)
10	2405 DM, 20,037 non-DM	30% type 1 diabetes, 38% type 2 diabetes	Diabetes duration	Not reported
			Hypertension	Not reported
			Poor glucose control	Not reported
11	1084 DM	14%	Age at diagnosis	Not reported
			Diabetes duration	Not reported
			Plasma creatinine	Not reported
			Insulin dose	Not reported
			Orthostatic blood pressure fall	Not reported
12	1077 (20% type 1 diabetes, 80% type 2 diabetes)	17%	Type 1 diabetes	–
			Height (1 cm increase)	1.06 (1–1.13)
			Retinopathy	9 (7.7–10.3)
			Type 2 diabetes	
			Height (1 cm increase)	1.06 (1.03–1.08)

(Continued)

Table 1 *(Continued)*

Reference	Subjects	Prevalence	Significant risk factors	Odds ratio (95% CI)
			Age (1 year increase)	1.02 (1–1.05)
			Alcohol "units"per week (1 unit increase)	1.03 (1–1.05)
			HbA1c (1% increase)	1.2 (1.1–1.4)
			Retinopathy	2.1 (1.7–2.6)
13	375 DM (78% type 1 diabetes)	[a]	Type 1 diabetes	–
			Age	Not reported
			Diabetes duration	Not reported
			Type 2 diabetes	–
			Height	Not reported
14	137 type 2 diabetes, 139 nondiabetic controls	53–63%, depending on the test	Not reported	–
15	2451 non-DM, 419 DM	13.3% non-DM, 28.5% DM	Age	Not reported
			Ethnicity	Not reported
			Diabetes	Not reported

[a]Not reported, because all persons with diabetes were not included in this survey

The Pittsburgh epidemiology of diabetes complications study included 363 subjects with type 1 diabetes more than 18 years of age in a defined community (Allegheny County, PA) *(6–8)*. Two of three of the following criteria had to be satisfied to fulfill the definition of neuropathy:

1. Abnormal sensory or motor signs on clinical examination.
2. Neuropathic symptoms.
3. Abnormal tendon reflexes.

Overall neuropathy prevalence was 34% (18% in 19–29 year olds, and 58% in those 30 years of age or older) (Table 1). Higher prevalence of neuropathy was associated with longer diabetes duration, higher glycosylated hemoglobin, lower HDL-cholesterol, smoking, and presence of peripheral vascular, coronary artery, or cerebrovascular disease (Table 1). Another analysis of the Pittsburgh population explored the association between physical activity and distal symmetric polyneuropathy among 628 subjects with type 1 diabetes between 8 and 48 years of age *(9)*. Male subjects who reported higher historical levels of leisure time physical activity (adjusted for diabetes duration, age, and current activity levels) had a significantly lower prevalence of neuropathy. No association between historical levels of physical activity and neuropathy prevalence was seen in females.

Data from the US National Health Interview Survey were used to generate neuropathy prevalence statistics on a nationwide sample of diabetic subjects with diabetes *(10)*. A total of 2405 self-reported subjects with diabetes and 20,037 self-reported subjects without diabetes were surveyed for the presence of symptoms of neuropathy in the extremities (numbness, pain, decreased hot or cold sensation). Prevalence of symptoms was more than three times greater in subjects with diabetes vs subjects without diabetes (Table 1). Among subjects with type 2 diabetes, higher prevalence of symptoms was associated with longer diabetes duration, hypertension, and self-reported frequent high blood glucose, whereas age, gender, height, insulin treatment, and smoking were unrelated to this outcome.

A population-based survey in Western Australia included 1084 diabetic subjects with diabetes, estimated to be 70% of the total that resided in this geographical area *(11)*. Sensory neuropathy was defined as a bilateral reduction in pinprick sensation in the feet during a sensory examination performed by endocrinologists. Neuropathy was found in 14% of subjects, and was related to greater age at diabetes diagnosis, diabetes duration, plasma creatinine, insulin dose, and orthostatic blood pressure difference (Table 1).

In a survey of 10 general practices in an English community, 1077 subjects with diabetes were identified and screened for neuropathy *(12)*. Two of the following five criteria fulfilled the definition of neuropathy:

1. Neuropathic foot symptoms.
2. Loss of light touch sensation.
3. Impaired pinprick sensation.
4. Absent ankle jerk reflexes.
5. Vibration perception threshold greater than 97.5% of an age-standardized value.

A total of 16.8% of subjects with diabetes fulfilled these criteria, in comparison with 750 non-diabetic subjects controls drawn from the same general practices. Risk factors associated with higher neuropathy prevalence are shown in Table 1.

A survey of subjects with diabetes in a defined community in Sweden yielded 375 subjects between the ages of 15–50 with diabetes (78% type 1 diabetes) *(13)*. A vibrameter was used to assess vibration threshold and pain sensation was evaluated with application of an electric current to the foot. Among subjects with type 1 diabetes, neuropathy presence was associated with greater age, diabetes duration, and height, although the association with height disappeared in multivariate analysis after adjustment for gender. Among subjects with type 2 diabetes, neuropathy was associated with greater height only.

A survey of subjects with type 2 diabetes in a Dutch community revealed a high prevalence of neuropathy, but also found that a substantial proportion of subjects without diabetes also tested positive for neuropathy, probably because the high median age of the population (70 years) *(14)*. Proportion of subjects with diabetes and control subjects with abnormal results by test is as follows: temperature 63% vs 49%, vibration (128 Hz tuning fork) 53% vs 33%, and absent tendon reflexes 62% vs 21%. Analysis of risk factors for neuropathy was not performed.

The 1999–2000 National Health and Nutrition Examination Survey (NHANES) *(15)* examined 2873 men and women aged >40 years, and included 419 people with diabetes. Peripheral neuropathy was assessed using self-reported symptoms and by testing foot sensation with the 5.07 gauge Semmes-Weinstein nylon monofilament. The plantar surface of the foot was tested for sensation at three sites on each foot. Peripheral neuropathy was defined as >1 insensate area(s). The overall prevalence of peripheral neuropathy was 14.8%, among whom over three-fourths were asymptomatic. Among individuals without diabetes, the prevalence of peripheral neuropathy was 13.3% (95% confidence interval [CI] 11.4–15.3), of whom only 2.3% were symptomatic. The prevalence among those with diabetes was 28.5% (95% CI 22–35.1%), among whom 10.9% were symptomatic. The prevalence of peripheral neuropathy increased steeply with age and was higher in non-Hispanic blacks, Mexican Americans, and people with diabetes.

Another community-based study that was conducted in two municipalities in Sicily will be mentioned but not discussed in detail, because only subjects who responded affirmatively to questions regarding the presence of symptoms of neuropathy were evaluated further by a neurologist *(16)*. This method likely led to considerable underascertainment of neuropathy prevalence.

Although not community-based, two other cross-sectional studies are worthy of mention because of their large sample sizes and, in one case, multinational composition. The EURODIAB IDDM Complications Study examined prevalence of neuropathy, defined if two or more of the following were present: symptoms, absence of two or more ankle or knee reflexes, abnormal vibration perception threshold, and abnormal autonomic function (postural systolic blood pressure fall of 30 mmHg or more or loss of heart rate variability as demonstrated by an R-R ratio <1) *(17)*. The factors positively correlated with neuropathy prevalence were age, diabetes duration, HbA1c, weight, current smoking, severe ketoacidosis, macroalbuminuria, and retinopathy. The UK Prospective Diabetes Study examined the association between neuropathy and potential risk factors among newly diagnosed subjects with type 2 diabetes. Neuropathy was defined as absence of both ankle reflexes or both knee reflexes, or mean biosthesiometer reading from both great toes of 25 V or greater. A cross-sectional report on 2337 subjects at the onset of the study found 5% of subjects had absent ankle or knee reflexes and 7% had abnormal biosthesiometer readings *(18)*. Neuropathy was significantly related to the presence of smooth or hairless skin, but unrelated to HbA1c, fasting plasma glucose, smoking, serum lipid and lipoprotein levels, and the albumin:creatinine ratio.

Of the five community-based cross-sectional studies reviewed of subjects with type 2 diabetes that presented data on risk factors for neuropathy, three reported a higher prevalence of this outcome with longer diabetes duration and higher glycosylated hemoglobin, and two found neuropathy prevalence correlated with age and height. The remaining risk factors reported were not reproduced by other investigators. The 1999–2000 NHANES study did not determine which type of diabetes the patient reported, so it is not possible to determine an association between diabetes type and risk factors. Only three community-based cross-sectional studies addressed neuropathy prevalence in subjects with type 1 diabetes in association with risk factors. Two of these investigations reported a correlation between diabetes duration and neuropathy prevalence. No other significant risk factor was reported by more than one community-based study done with subjects with type 1 diabetes. Cross-sectional research affirms the importance of intensity and duration of hyperglycemia as potential risk factors for neuropathy, but also suggests other possible etiologies, as shown in Table 1.

DISTAL SYMMETRIC POLYNEUROPATHY—INCIDENCE AND RISK FACTORS (PROSPECTIVE RESEARCH)

The most important epidemiological study performed to date is the Diabetes Control and Complications Trial (DCCT). Although designed to answer a therapeutic question, this trial provides much valuable information regarding the incidence of diabetic neuropathy

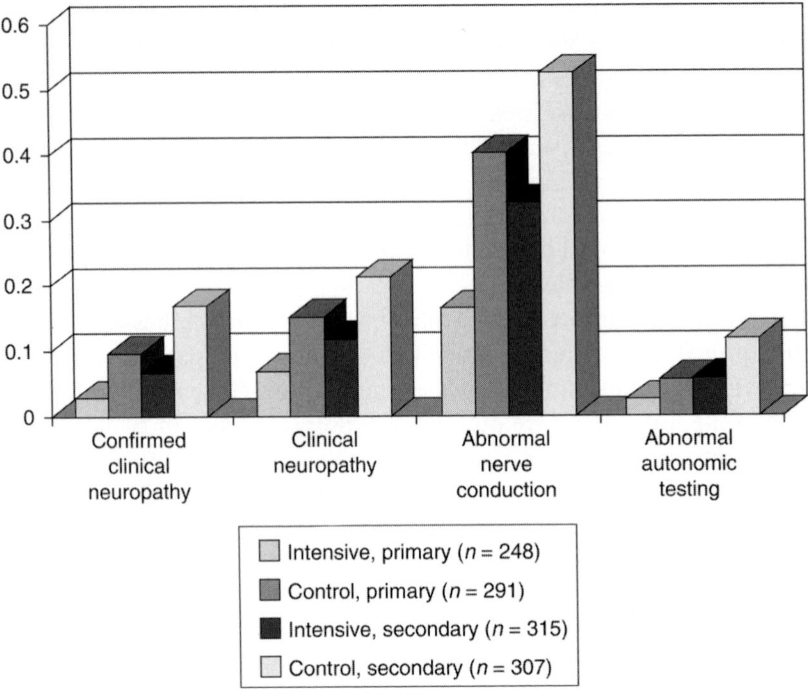

Fig. 1. Cumulative incidence of neuropathy after 5 years of follow-up in intensively treated and control subjects enrolled in the diabetes control and complications trial. Definitions of neuropathy and primary and secondary cohorts are provided in the text. Intensive treatment consisted of three or more insulin injections per day or an insulin pump, in comparison with two injections of insulin daily in the control group.

and its relation to glycemic control. This clinical trial included 1161 subjects with type 1 diabetes who were followed for 5 years for the development and progression of neuropathy. Subjects were randomized to intensive or control treatment groups, after being initially divided into a primary (diabetes for 5 years or less, no microalbuminuria, no retinopathy) or secondary prevention (diabetes for 15 years or less, moderate or less nonproliferative retinopathy, urinary albumin excretion less than 200 mg per 24 hour) subgroups, depending on the presence of end point complications at baseline. Clinical neuropathy was defined as two of the three following conditions: (1) neuropathic symptoms; (2) sensory deficit to light touch, position, temperature, or pinprick; and (3) abnormal deep tendon reflexes. Confirmed clinical neuropathy was defined as an abnormal clinical exam plus either abnormal nerve conduction in two or more nerves or abnormal response to autonomic testing. After 5 years of follow-up, the cumulative incidence of clinical neuropathy, confirmed clinical neuropathy, and abnormal nerve conduction was lower in the intensively treated vs control groups, irrespective of presence of complications at baseline (Fig. 1). Among controls, the cumulative incidence of clinical neuropathy was 15–21%, depending on presence of baseline complications. Cumulative incidence of abnormal nerve conduction was very high among controls (40–52%). These data demonstrate the crucial role of hyperglycemia in the development of distal symmetric polyneuropathy, but also suggest that neuropathy will continue to develop even in intensively treated subjects exposed to milder degrees of hyperglycemia.

The UK Prospective Diabetes Study (UKPDS) *(19)*, a randomized intervention trial of intensive vs conventional diabetes treatment, enrolled 3867 subjects with newly diagnosed type 2 diabetes, with a median follow-up of 10 years. Neuropathy was defined as loss of both ankle or both knee reflexes or vibration sensation measured with a biosthesiometer having a mean reading from both great toes of 25 V or more. At baseline 11.8% of subjects assigned intensive therapy, and 11.4% of subject's assigned conventional therapy had an abnormal biosthesiometer reading. After 12 years follow-up, on average, there was no difference in the proportion of subjects with peripheral neuropathy between the intensive and conventional treatment arms. Absent ankle reflexes were found in 35% of subjects in the intensive treatment group and in 37% in the conventional group ($p = 0.60$). Absent knee reflexes were found in 11% of subjects in the intensive treatment group and 12% in the conventional treatment arm ($p = 0.42$). Biosthesiometer readings were abnormal in 30.2% of the intensive treatment group and 32.8% in the conventional treatment group ($p = 0.42$).

The European Diabetes Prospective Complications Study identified risk factors for the development of distal symmetric polyneuropathy in 1172 subjects with type 1 DM in 31 centers throughout Europe *(20)*. The subjects were assessed for neuropathy at baseline and again an average of 7.3 years later. Neuropathy was defined if the patient had two or more of the four measures: the presence of one or more symptoms such as numbness or burning in the feet, the absence of two or more reflexes of the ankle or knee tendons, a vibration-perception threshold measured by biothesiometer that was abnormal for the patient's age, and abnormal autonomic function (loss of heart rate variability with an R-R ratio of less than 1.04, postural hypotension with a fall in systolic blood pressure of 20 mmHg or more, or both). "Pure" peripheral neuropathy was defined as distal neuropathy without autonomic symptoms or abnormal autonomic–function tests. At follow-up, 23.5% of the subjects had developed neuropathy. After adjusting for complications of diabetes, which included urinary albumin excretion rate, retinopathy and cardiovascular disease, the risk factors for incident diabetic neuropathy were duration of diabetes in years (Odds ratio [OR] 1.25, 95% CI 1.03–1.51), current glycosylated hemoglobin per % of hemoglobin (OR 1.64, 95% CI 1.33–2.03), change in glycosylated hemoglobin value during follow-up period (OR 1.44, 95% CI 1.17–1.77), body-mass index (OR 1.20, 95% CI 1.01–1.43), and smoking (OR 1.68, 95% CI 1.20–2.36). The presence of cardiovascular disease at baseline was independently associated with a higher incidence of neuropathy (OR 2.12, 95% CI 1.16–3.86).

The Epidemiology of Diabetes Complications *(21)* Study followed 453 subjects with type 1 diabetes who were free of neuropathy at baseline, for an average of 5.3 years. Diabetic peripheral neuropathy was defined as the presence of two or more of the following: sensory, motor or autonomic symptoms, sensory and/or motor signs, and/or absent tendon reflexes. A total of 68 subjects (15%) developed diabetic peripheral neuropathy by the end of follow-up, giving an incidence rate of 2.8 per 100 person-years. Risk factors identified at baseline for incident symmetric polyneuropathy in a Cox proportional hazards model included (Hazard Ratio, 95% CI): type 1 diabetes duration, per 1 SD increase 1.82 (1.41–2.33); height, per 1 SD increase 2.04 (1.57–2.66); glycohemoglobin, per 1 SD increase 1.64 (1.27–2.11); smoking, yes or no 1.73 (1.06–2.82); and hypertension, yes or no 4.10 (2.33–7.24).

Several other prospective studies were designed to specifically define the incidence of and risk factors for diabetic neuropathy. Of 288 veterans with diabetes but no neuropathy, 20% developed neuropathy after 2 years of follow-up *(22)*. Neuropathy was defined as insensitivity to the 5.07 monofilament at one or more of nine sites on either foot. Risk factors for incident neuropathy in multivariate logistic regression analysis included (OR, 95%CI): height, 2.5 cm increase 1.2 (1.1–1.4); previous foot ulcer 2.1 (1–4.1); age, 1 year increase 1.04 (1–1.08); glycohemoglobin, 1% increase 1.2 (1–1.3); CAGE alcohol score *(23)*, four questions answered positively vs none 7 (1.7–29); current smoking 0.2 (0.1–0.7); and serum albumin level adjusted for serum creatinine, 1 mg per dL increase 0.3 (0.1–0.8).

The Rochester Diabetic Neuropathy Study *(24)* invited all the subjects with diabetes that lived within the geographical confines of Rochester, Minnesota to participate. The study reported on 264 subjects, 97 with type 1 diabetes and 149 with type 2 diabetes, who were followed for a mean of 6.9 years. Although this study is prospective, incidence of neuropathy was not evaluated. Severity of neuropathy was the outcome studied. Neuropathy was defined using the neuropathy impairment score of lower limbs plus 7 tests. These tests included vibration testing at the toes, heart rate variation with deep breathing, and nerve conduction studies of the lower extremity motor and sensory nerves. There was a 36.4% prevalence of at least one nerve conduction abnormality in two or more nerves. Only 9.5% of these subjects were symptomatic. Higher mean glycohemoglobin, duration of diabetes, and type 1 vs type 2 diabetes were associated with the severity of diabetic peripheral neuropathy. However, the authors did not adjust for baseline severity of neuropathy.

Another investigation followed 231 subjects with type 2 diabetes, who were free from distal symmetric neuropathy at baseline, for a mean follow-up period of 4.7 years to assess risk factors and incidence of this outcome *(25)*. Distal symmetric neuropathy was defined as described previously for the San Luis Valley cross-sectional study. Incidence of this outcome was 6.1 per 100 person-years (95% CI 4.7–7.8). In a logistic regression model that included age, duration of type 2 diabetes, insulin treatment, glycohemoglobin, smoking, Hispanic ethnicity, gender, history of myocardial infarction, and angina, the following factors were independently related to neuropathy incidence: Duration of type 2 diabetes (5 year increase) (OR 1.3, 95% CI 1–1.6); current smoking (OR 2.2, 95% CI 1–4.7), and history of myocardial infarction (OR 3.5, 95% CI 1.2–9.7). Insulin treatment (OR 2, 95% CI 0.9–4.4) and female gender (OR 1.7, 95% CI 0.9–3.3) were associated with neuropathy incidence at borderline statistical significance.

Data from a cohort of subjects with type 1 diabetes seen within 1 year of diagnosis at Children's Hospital of Pittsburgh were analyzed after four years of follow-up to assess the incidence of neuropathy in relation to baseline glycemic control, defined as poor (glycosylated hemoglobin 11% or greater, $n = 220$) or fair (less than 11%, $n = 438$) *(26)*. Distal symmetric polyneuropathy was defined as presence of two of three criteria: neuropathic symptoms, decreased or absent tendon reflexes, or signs of sensory loss. Four year cumulative incidence of this outcome in this cohort of subjects with a mean age of 28 years, all of whom were diagnosed before age 17, was 13%, with an approx threefold higher risk in poor vs fair control groups (RR 3.2, $p < 0.001$).

Finnish subjects with newly diagnosed type 2 diabetes ($n = 133$) were followed for 10 years for the development of peripheral neuropathy defined on the basis of nerve conduction velocity and clinical symptoms *(27)*. At baseline, 4.5% of subjects had polyneuropathy, whereas after 10 years of follow-up this proportion increased to 20.9%. Higher cumulative incidence of neuropathy was related to higher baseline fasting plasma glucose, lower fasting serum insulin, and lower serum insulin one and two hours following a 75 g oral glucose load. Baseline age, smoking, alcohol use, serum lipid values, urinary albumin excretion, and use of antihypertensive medication were unrelated to incidence of polyneuropathy after 10 years.

A sample of 444 younger onset (diagnosed with diabetes before 30 years of age and taking insulin) and 406 older onset diabetic subjects without neuropathy from an 11 county area in Wisconsin were followed for up to 10 years for the development of self-reported loss of tactile sensation or temperature sensitivity *(28)*. Higher glycosylated hemoglobin was related to higher incidence of symptomatic neuropathy, even after adjustment for age, duration of diabetes, and gender in a multivariate model.

The only other prospective study of risk factors for diabetic neuropathy that enrolled more than 100 subjects compared baseline measures of HbA1c, age, diabetes duration, and height in relation to change in thermal, vibration, and monofilament perception of the feet more than two years of follow-up in 201 medical clinic subjects with type 2 diabetes (30% African–American, 67% Hispanic) *(29)*. Subjects were divided into an upper fiftieth percentile change for all sensory tests vs those with change less than the fiftieth percentile for all tests. The comparisons of baseline measures by this classification did not show significant differences for any potential risk factor.

Four other small prospective studies have been performed on risk factors for diabetic neuropathy. A cohort of subjects with type 1 diabetes ($n = 96$) enrolled in a randomized control trial of intensive glucose control was followed for development of neuropathy defined as two or more abnormal lower extremity nerve conduction velocities or abnormal vibration or thermal sensation *(30)*. No association was found between baseline HbA1c and incidence of neuropathy over 5 years of follow-up, although higher HbA1c during follow-up was significantly related to this outcome, except for change in vibration sensation, which was related to diabetes duration only. In another cohort of subjects with type 1 diabetes, 77 subjects ages 25–34 years without clinical neuropathy at baseline were followed for 2 years for the development of clinically overt neuropathy (as previously defined for the Pittsburgh Epidemiology of Diabetes Complications Study) *(31)*. Nephropathy (defined as an albumin excretion rate greater than 200 μg per min on at least 2 of 3 occasions) and higher vibration perception threshold at baseline independently predicted the development of neuropathy, which occurred in 9% of subjects. Change in vibration sensation was measured over five years in a cohort of 71 newly diagnosed subjects with type 2 diabetes *(32)*. Mean fasting blood glucose over the 5-year period, male gender, age, and body mass index positively correlated with change in vibration sensation threshold. A study of 32 newly diagnosed subjects with type 1 diabetes followed for 5 years found poorer glucose control (HbA1c of 8.3% or greater) related to diminished nerve conduction and decreased thermal (but not vibration) sensation *(33)*.

One large cohort study is worthy of mention for historical purposes. Pirart followed 4400 subjects with diabetes in a Belgian clinic for the development of complications between 1947 and 1973 *(34)*. The cumulative incidence of neuropathy was 50% after 25 years of follow-up, and was found to occur more frequently in subjects with poorer glucose control by urine and blood testing. Although the sample size of this study is impressive, its methodology is compromised by a vague definition of neuropathy and outdated methods for measurement of glycemic control.

Prospective research on the risk of distal symmetric polyneuropathy confirms its relationship to poorer glycemic control as reflected by fasting plasma glucose or HbA1c at baseline, as reported by nine of the eleven largest (more than 100 subjects) and two smaller (less than 100 subjects) cohort studies. Four prospective studies reported duration of diabetes as a risk factor for neuropathy, three reported smoking as a risk factor, two reported age, and two reported baseline coronary artery disease as risk factors for neuropathy. The following potential risk factors were reported in one prospective study: male gender, height, increase in body-mass index, nephropathy, high CAGE alcohol use score, low serum albumin level, insulin treatment, nonsmoking, and fasting and stimulated serum insulin levels. However, another prospective study produced contradictory results by finding female gender and current smoking associated with neuropathy *(25)*. Whether these discrepant results arise from differences in neuropathy definition, dissimilar patient populations, or both, cannot be determined at the current time.

PREVALENCE, INCIDENCE, AND RISK OF AUTONOMIC NEUROPATHY

Diabetic autonomic neuropathy has been the subject of fewer research investigations in comparison with distal symmetric polyneuropathy. The Framingham Heart Study performed a cross-sectional evaluation of the 1919 people from the Framingham Offspring Study who had ambulatory electrocardiographic recordings available *(35)*. Subjects were categorized according to normal fasting blood glucose (<110 mg per dL), impaired fasting blood glucose (>110 and <126 mg per dL), or DM (fasting blood glucose >126 mg per dL and/or the use of insulin or an oral hypoglycemic agent). Autonomic neuropathy was defined by a time domain variable, the standard deviation of normal RR intervals, and three frequency domain variables (low frequency [LF 0.04–0.15 Hz], high frequency [HF 0.15–0.40 Hz] and the LF:HF ratio). The authors adjusted for age, sex, body-mass index, heart rate, systolic and diastolic blood pressure, hypertension treatment, cardiac medications, cigarette smoking, and coffee and alcohol consumption in multivariable regression analysis. It was found heart rate variability was decreased in subjects with diabetes, in comparison with subjects with normal fasting glucose. The subjects with impaired fasting glucose had decreased heart rate variability intermediate between those with diabetes and those with normal fasting glucose. In a community-based cross-sectional study of 168 subjects with type 1 diabetes, abnormal autonomic function, as measured by the expiratory:inspiratory (E:I) ratio and the mean circular resultant, was associated with female gender, high LDL-cholesterol, and hypertension *(36)*. In addition, abnormal E:I ratio was related to low HDL-cholesterol, whereas abnormal mean circular resultant was associated with higher serum triglycerides. Definitions for abnormal E:I ratio or mean circular resultant were not provided in this publication.

Several prospective studies of autonomic neuropathy risk have been reported. The DCCT found mixed results regarding the association between intensive glucose control and 5 years cumulative incidence of autonomic neuropathy defined as R–R variation with breathing less than 15 per minute, Valsalva ratio less than 15 with R–R variation with breathing less than 20 per minute, or orthostatic blood pressure drop of 10 mmHg or more with a blunted catecholamine response (Fig. 1) *(37)*. Greater R–R variation with breathing was seen with intensive treatment in the primary prevention cohort only at the end of follow-up, whereas Valsalva ratio did not differ by intensive treatment in either cohort. A Finnish cohort of 133 newly diagnosed subjects with type 2 diabetes was followed for 10 years for the development of parasympathetic neuropathy defined as an E:I ratio of 1.10 or lower, and sympathetic neuropathy, defined as an orthostatic systolic blood pressure decline of 30 mmHg or more *(38)*. At baseline, 4.9% of subjects with type 2 diabetes had parasympathetic neuropathy, although apparently none had sympathetic neuropathy. After 10 years of follow-up, rates of these neuropathies were 65 and 24.4%, respectively. In a stepwise logistic regression model that considered as independent variables age, gender, body mass index, systolic blood pressure, fasting plasma insulin and glucose, and ischemic ECG changes, only fasting plasma insulin (OR 3.1, 95% CI 1.3–7.6) and female gender (OR 3.4, 95% CI 1.2–9.8) were independently and significantly related to cumulative incidence of parasympathetic neuropathy. In a similar logistic model for sympathetic neuropathy cumulative incidence that considered all these factors plus use of diuretic medication, only diuretic use entered the model at $p < 0.05$ (OR 2.9, 95% CI 1–8.2). The previously mentioned Stockholm clinical trial followed 96 subjects with type 2 diabetes for changes in autonomic function as measured by respiratory sinus arrhythmia, Valsalva maneuver, and orthostatic blood pressure fall *(30)*. Baseline HbA1c was unrelated to change in autonomic function, but HbA1c during 5 years of follow-up was significantly related to this outcome. The remaining prospective study was small in size ($n = 32$ subjects with type 1 diabetes), and found poorer glucose control (HbA1c > 8.3%) related to diminished heart rate variability at rest and during deep breathing over five years of follow-up *(33)*.

The UK Prospective Diabetes Study evaluated the heart-rate response to deep breathing as one of the surrogate end points *(19)*. There was no difference between the intensive and conventional diabetes treatment groups after 12 years of follow-up. However, the median basal heart rate was 69.8 beats per minute (IQR 62.5–78.9) in the intensively treated group in comparison with 74.4 beats per minute (IQR 65.2–83.3) in the conventional group ($p < 0.001$).

The Steno-2 Study *(39)* randomized 160 subjects with type 2 diabetes with microalbuminuria to conventional treatment or to intensive, multifactorial treatment which provided a stepwise implementation of behavior modification and pharmacological therapy that targeted hyperglycemia, hypertension dyslipidemia, and microalbuminuria, along with secondary prevention of cardiovascular disease with aspirin. Subjects were followed for a mean of 7.8 years. Autonomic neuropathy was defined as heart rate variation on deep breathing. R–R variation higher than 6 beats per minute was considered normal, 4–6 was considered impaired, and less than 4 to have absent variation. Orthostatic hypotension was defined as a drop in systolic blood pressure of 25 mmHg or more. At baseline, 27% of these subjects with microalbuminuria had autonomic neuropathy. Autonomic neuropathy progressed in 43 subjects (53%) in the conventional treatment group and in 24 subjects (30%) in the intensive-therapy group. The hazard ratio was 0.37 (95% CI 0.18–0.79).

The literature on risk factors for diabetic autonomic neuropathy can be characterized as smaller in size and less consistent in comparison with that available for distal symmetric polyneuropathy. The only risk factor reported in more than one study was female gender, found to be associated with higher risk by two authors. The absence of a consistent relationship between glucose control and autonomic neuropathy risk raises the possibility that the course of this complication is set soon after diabetes develops and is not amenable to change thereafter, or that available research, including the DCCT, may have been statistically underpowered for the detection of this association.

DIABETIC AMYOTROPHY AND MONONEUROPATHIES IN PERSONS WITH DIABETES

There have been no prospective, population-based studies of diabetic amyotrophy and mononeuropathies in subjects with diabetes. However, some prevalence figures for these types of neuropathy can be derived from a few cross-sectional studies. In a cross-sectional survey based in Rochester, Minnesota, asymptomatic carpal tunnel syndrome (CTS) was found in 22% of those with type 1 diabetes and 29% of those with type 2 diabetes, whereas the corresponding prevalence for symptomatic cases was 11% and 6%, respectively *(40)*. Ulnar and femoral cutaneous entrapment was found in 2% of type 1 diabetes and 1% of type 2 diabetes subjects. Cranial mononeuropathy and truncal radiculopathy were not observed in the Rochester population, whereas proximal asymmetric polyneuropathy was identified in 1% of type 1 diabetes and type 2 diabetes subjects *(40)*. No incidence data were available for any of these types of neuropathy.

In a cross-sectional, hospital-based study, O'Hare et al. *(41)* studied the presence of various types of neuropathy (by interview assessment) in 800 consecutive subjects with diabetes (336 type 1, 464 type 2) treated at one diabetes center and 100 subjects without diabetes attending an otolaryngology clinic. The prevalence of neuropathy in subjects with diabetes was 22.9%. Less common types included amyotrophy (total prevalence: 0.8%), oculomotor neuropathy (0.1%), peroneal neuropathy (0.1%), and truncal neuropathy (0.1%). Risk factors for neuropathy in type 1 diabetes were age (56.7 ± 15 years in subjects with neuropathy vs 44.9 ± 18 years in those without neuropathy, $p < 0.001$) and duration of diabetes (17 ± 10 years in subjects with neuropathy vs 13 ± 9 years in those without neuropathy, $p < 0.001$). In type 2 diabetes, age was also associated with neuropathy (64.2 ± 9 years in subjects with neuropathy vs 60 ± 12 years in those without neuropathy, $p < 0.002$). Unlike previous epidemiological studies, the O'Hare study documented the presence of various types of neuropathy, in addition to diabetic peripheral neuropathy, in a large group of subjects with diabetes. However, the interview assessment of sensory neuropathy was likely to be insensitive, and the study was neither prospective nor population-based.

Another cross-sectional study assessed the presence of median mononeuropathy (MM) in 414 subjects with diabetes and mild neuropathy enrolled in a randomized controlled treatment trial of tolrestat vs placebo *(42)*. MM was defined by criteria from nerve conduction studies and was differentiated from CTS, a diagnosis based on history, physical exam, and electrophysiological findings. The prevalence of MM was 23%, and it was associated with longer duration of diabetes in both type 1 (22.5 years in subjects with MM vs 16 in those without MM, $p = 0.003$) and type 2 diabetes (8.8 years in subjects with MM vs 7.0 years in those without MM, $p = 0.034$). In type 2 diabetes, height and body mass index were also predictors of MM. The inclusion of subjects with mild neuropathy already enrolled in a treatment trial creates selection bias. A fourth cross-sectional study of CTS included 470 subjects from a diabetes clinic, a neurology clinic, and community volunteers *(43)*. Fifty-two had neither diabetes nor neuropathy, 81 had diabetes without neuropathy, and 337 had diabetes and neuropathy. The prevalence of CTS, determined by clinical evaluation using accepted criteria, was 2% in subjects without diabetes, 14% in patient with diabetes without neuropathy, and 30% in subjects with diabetes and polyneuropathy. CTS was linked to a longer duration of diabetes (14 ± 12.5 years in those with neuropathy vs 10.8 ± 10.7 years in those without neuropathy). This study was one of few that examined the point prevalence of CTS in subjects with diabetes, and like the one previously described, suggests that MM and CTS are common in people with diabetes, especially in those with diabetic peripheral neuropathy. However, since these studies are neither prospective nor population-based, these results may be biased and cannot be extrapolated to the general diabetic population.

Case–control studies have addressed whether diabetes is a significant risk factor for CTS. In the earliest study, 156 cases were identified from the population by self-report ($n = 28$) and from neurology clinic ($n = 128$), and controls were 476 subjects without CTS from the community *(44)*. The diagnosis of CTS was confirmed by neurophysiological testing. Significant independent risk factors were height (per 1 cm) (OR = 0.9), frequent wrist activities (OR = 1.1), leg varicosities in men (OR = 9.8), menopause in the previous year (OR = 2.3), and hysterectomy (OR = 1.8). In order to examine the effect of selection bias, risk factor analysis was repeated for the 28 cases derived from the population (rather than clinic) and yielded similar results. The low diabetes prevalence in cases (2.6%) and controls (3.7%) resulted in lower power and precluded any conclusion about diabetes as a risk factor. Three other case–control studies concluded that diabetes is a risk factor for CTS. In one large retrospective case–control study of enrollees of New Jersey Medicare or Medicaid programs during a 3-year period, 627 people who underwent open or endoscopic CTS procedures were selected as cases, and 3740 controls were frequency-matched by age and gender with the cases *(45)*. Risk factors were inflammatory arthritis (OR 3.1, 95% CI 2.2–4.2), corticosteroid use (OR 1.6, 95% CI 1.2–2.1, DM (OR 1.4, 95% CI 1.2–1.8), female sex (OR 1.6, 95% CI 1.3–2), and hemodialysis (OR 9, 95% CI 4.2–19.6). Although this study did have a large sample size, it suffers from several limitations: retrospective study design; selection bias (subjects who underwent surgery may have had more severe CTS); potentially inaccurate case ascertainment (clinical conditions were defined by diagnostic codes and prescriptions, not by chart review); and a failure to adjust for obesity, which may causally influence the association between diabetes and CTS.

Two more recent case–control studies also suggest that diabetes may be risk factor for CTS but again have limited validity because of similar weaknesses in study design to those already described (*46,47*). In the first, both cases and controls were drawn from hospitals and clinics, and controls included subjects with upper limb symptoms who did not meet electrophysiological criteria for CTS *(46)*. In the second, cases were subjects who had undergone a CTS procedure, and controls were seen for general reconstructive surgery or presented with acute hand symptoms to a plastic surgeon *(47)*. Of note, one major strength of the first study was that it did present the results of both multivariable analysis (in which diabetes was a significant risk factor with CTS) and stratified analysis using obesity as a stratifying factor *(46)*. After adjusting for obesity, diabetes was no longer a significant risk factor.

CHRONIC INFLAMMATORY DEMYLINATING POLYRADICULOPATHY (CIDP) IN PERSONS WITH DIABETES

CIDP is a relatively new diagnosis. In 1991, the American Academy of Neurology defined diagnostic clinical and electrophysiological criteria for CIDP *(48)*. All studies on CIDP are cross-sectional and clinic-based. In one study, cases were requested by letter from neurologists in four Thames health regions in southeast England *(49)*. The personal case series of two investigators were also included. The subjects' clinical data were reviewed to confirm the diagnosis of CIDP by standard diagnostic criteria established by an ad hoc subcommittee. The degree of certainty of the diagnosis was classified as definite, probable, possible, or suggestive. Population statistics were obtained from the Office of Population Censuses and Survey. The prevalence of definite and probable CIDP in the Southeast Thames region was 1/100,000. In this study, case ascertainment may have been affected by the fact that reported cases were excluded if there was no available confirmatory data. In addition, authors noted that a tertiary referral center in one of the four Thames health regions had a special focus on inflammatory neuropathy *(49)*. In a second similar study, cases and relevant clinical data were requested from all 94 neurologists in New South Wales, and 84% responded. Population data was derived from the Australian national census *(50)*. The crude prevalence of CIDP in New South Wales was 1.9/100,000. And the crude annual incidence was 0.15/100,000 *(50)*.

One large cross-sectional study examined the possible association between diabetes and CIDP. Among 1127 subjects seen in an electrophysiology lab over a 14 month period, 189 subjects (16.8%) had diabetes *(51)*. The prevalence of CIDP (diagnostic criteria modified from the American Academy of Neurology in 1991) was 16.9% in subjects with diabetes and 1.8% in subjects without diabetes (OR 11.04, 95% CI 6.1–21.8, $p < 0.001$). There was no difference in the prevalence of CIDP in type 1 and type 2 diabetes (26.7% vs 16.1%, $p = 0.49$). This study demonstrated selection bias because subjects referred to the electrophysiological laboratory tended to have more severe neuropathy and possibly a greater likelihood of CIDP. In order to determine which clinical manifestations are linked to types of neuropathy other than diabetic polyneuropathy, Lozeron et al. *(52)* examined and performed nerve conduction studies on 100 consecutive subjects with diabetes with symptomatic neuropathy referred to one neurology center over 3.25 years. The prevalence of CIDP (by clinical presentation and nerve conduction studies) was 9%. The sample size of this case series was small, and the results reflect selection bias and cannot be generalized to the whole diabetic population.

NEUROPATHY AS A RISK FACTOR FOR DIABETIC FOOT ULCER

A key factor in the pathogenesis of diabetic foot complications is the loss of protective sensation because of advanced neuropathy. Two case–control studies and four prospective studies demonstrate a higher risk of foot ulcer in association with sensory lower limb neuropathy as measured with the 5.07 monofilament or the biothesiometer. The earlier of the two case–control studies addressed whether neuropathy and vasculopathy were risk factors for foot ulceration in 46 subjects with diabetes and foot ulcers and 322 control subjects in a general medicine clinic *(53)*. Neuropathy was assessed by vibratory, monofilament, and ankle tendon reflex testing. Ankle-arm blood pressure indices and transcutaneous oxygen pressure (TcPO2) on the dorsal foot were used to assess the presence of peripheral vascular disease. In multivariable logistic regression analysis, absence of Achilles tendon reflexes (adjusted OR 6.48, 95% CI 2.37–18.06), abnormal 5.07 monofilament test (adjusted OR 18.42, 95% CI 3.83–88.47), and TcPO2 < 30 mmHg (adjusted OR 57.87, 95% CI 5.08–658.96) were significant risk factors for foot ulceration *(53)*.

In the second case–control study, 225 age-matched subjects with diabetes were enrolled sequentially at several clinics in one large diabetes center *(54)*. Seventy-six cases had existing foot ulceration or recently healed foot ulceration, and 149 controls without ulceration were also recruited. Neuropathy, defined as a vibration perception threshold > 25 volts measured with a biothesiometer, was the most significant risk factor for foot ulceration (OR 15.2). Other risk factors included history of amputation (OR 10); elevated plantar pressure (> 65 N per cm^2, OR 5.9); > one subjective symptom of neuropathy (OR 5.1); hallux rigidus, hallus valgus, or toe deformity (OR 3.3); poor diabetes control (OR 3.2); longer duration of diabetes (OR 3), and male sex (OR 2.7). This study was thorough in its assessment of all risk factors documented in previous studies. However, the clinic-based study population was not a random sample, and it was not prospective (Table 2).

In the earliest of the four prospective studies, diabetic American Indians (n = 356) with impaired foot sensation to the 5.07 monofilament had a 9.9 fold increase in risk of incident foot ulcer over a mean of 2.7 years of follow-up *(55)*. Higher vibration perception threshold (>25 V) as measured with a biothesiometer was associated with a nearly sevenfold increase in foot ulcer risk among 469 diabetic subjects followed for at least 3 years *(56)*. In the third prospective study, two hundred forty-eight subjects from three large diabetic foot centers were screened for neuropathy using the Neuropathy Symptom Score, the Neuropathy Disability Score, the biothesiometer, and the 5.07 monofilament *(57)*. Over 30 months, risk factors for foot ulcers were a Neuropathy Disability Score ≥ 5 (RR 3.1. 95% CI1.3–7.6), a VPT ≥ 25 V (RR 3.4, 95% CI 1.7–6.8), abnormal 5.07 monofilament test (RR 2.4, 95% CI 1.1–5.3), and a plantar foot pressure ≥6 kg per cm^2 (RR 2.0, 95% CI 1.2–3.3). Recruiting consecutive subjects was less likely to yield a healthy population. Also, it is not clear how closely subjects were followed for the development and treatment of new ulcers.

The largest of these prospective cohort studies followed 749 subjects with diabetes enrolled in a VA general medicine clinic for an average of 3.7 years *(58)*. At baseline the subjects underwent a very thorough evaluation of multiple potential risk factors. Case ascertainment bias was minimized by regular surveillance of subjects by study personnel and as needed assessments of newly developed foot lesions by study staff. Potential bias owing to loss to follow-up was minimized, and, on completion, data was available for 77% of

Table 2
Epidemiological Studies of Neuropathy as a Risk Factor for Foot Ulceration

Reference	Type of study	Population	Screening tool for neuropathy	Follow-up time	Risk factors	Odds ratio or relative risk ratio (95% CI)
53	Case–control study	46 subjects w/DM and foot ulcers, 322 controls at general medicine clinic	Monofilament, biothesiometer, Achilles tendon reflexes	N/A	Absence of Achilles tendon reflexes (adjusted abnormal 5.07 monofilament test TcPO2 <30 mmHg)	6.48 (2.37–18.06) 18.42 (3.83–88.47) 57.87 (5.08–658.96)
54	Case–control study	225 age-matched subjects w/DM followed at one large diabetes center: 76 cases w/existing foot ulceration or history of foot ulceration, 149 controls from other clinics, not a random sample	Biothesiometer	N/A	Loss of protective sensation (VPT > 25 V)	15.2
					History of amputation	10
					Elevated plantar pressure >65 N per cm^2	5.9
					≥1 subjective symptom of neuropathy	5.1
					Hallux rigidus, hallus valgus, toe deformity	3.3
					Poor diabetes control	3.2
					Duration of diabetes >10 year	3
					Male sex	2.7
55	Prospective cohort study	356 American Indians w/DM followed in primary care setting	5.07 monofilament	32 months	Insensitivity to 5.07 monofilament	9.9 (4.8–21)

56	Prospective cohort study	469 consecutive pts seen in DM center and foot clinic	Biothesiometer	3 years	VPT > 25 V	6.82 (2.75–16.92)
57	Multicenter prospective cohort study	248 subjects from three large diabetic foot centers	Neuropathy symptom score Neuropathy disability score Biothesiometer 5.07 monofilament	30 months	High neuropathy disability score (≥5)	3.1 (1.3–7.6)
					High VPT (≥25 V)	3.4 (1.7–6.8)
					High SWF (≥5.07)	2.4 (1.1–5.3)
					High foot pressure (≥6 kg per cm^2)	2 (1.2–3.3)
58	Prospective cohort study	749 pts w/DM enrolled in a VA general medicine clinic w/o a foot ulcer	5.07 monofilament	3.7 years	Foot insensitivity to monofilament	2.2 (1.5–3.1)
					Past history of amputation	2.8 (1.8–4.3)
					Past history of foot ulcer	1.6 (1.2–2.3)
					Insulin use	1.6 (1.1–2.2)
					Charcot deformity	3.5 (1.2–9.9)
					15 mmHg higher dorsal foot transcutaneous PO_2	0.8 (0.7–0.9)
					20 kg higher body weight	1.2 (1.1–1.4)
					0.3 high ankle-arm index	0.8 (0.7–1)
					Poor vision	0.9 (1.4–2.6)
					13 mmHg orthostatic BP fall	1.2 (1.1–1.5)

VPT, vibration pressure threshold; SWF, Semmes-Weinstein monofilament; TcPO2, transcutaneous oxygen pressure.

subjects enrolled. Independent risk factors for foot ulceration included foot insensitivity to the 5.07 monofilament (RR 2.2, 95% CI 1.5–3.1), past history of amputation (RR 2.8, 95% CI 1.8–4.3), past history of foot ulceration (RR 1.6, 95% CI 1.2–2.3), insulin use (RR 1.6, 95% CI1.1–2.2), Charcot deformity (RR 3.5, 95% CI 1.2–9.9), 15 mmHg lower dorsal foot transcutaneous PO_2 (RR 0.8, 95% CI 0.7–0.9), 20 kg higher body weight (RR 1.2, 95% CI 1.1–1.4), 0.3 higher ankle-arm index (RR 0.8, 95% CI 0.7–1), poor vision (RR 0.9, 95% CI 1.4–2.6), and 13 mmHg orthostatic BP fall (RR 1.2, 95% CI 1.1–1.5) *(58)*. This study and others emphasized the importance of screening for loss of protective sensation in daily clinical practice in order to identify those subjects at risk who require intensive education and other interventions in order to prevent foot ulceration.

TYPE 1 DM VS TYPE 2 DM

There is very little data for a direct comparison of the incidence and prevalence of neuropathy in the two major types of diabetes. Comparison between studies is very difficult because of the different methods used for defining neuropathy. The DCCT, which studied subjects with type 1 diabetes, showed after 5 years follow-up that abnormal nerve conduction in at least two nerves occurred in 15–30% of subjects that were tightly controlled, and in 40–52% of controls *(37)*. In the UKPDS, which studied subjects with type 2 diabetes, after 6 years follow-up, biosthesiometer readings in both toes were abnormal in 19% of intensively treated subjects and in 21% of conventionally treated controls *(19)*. These two studies cannot be directly compared because the methods of defining neuropathy, and the time intervals at which results were described, are both different. However, the frequency with which the control subjects in the DCCT trial developed abnormal nerve conduction is striking. Broadly speaking, it is possible that tight control may have a greater effect on reducing incidence of diabetic neuropathy in type 1 diabetes compared with type 2 diabetes.

IS IMPAIRED GLUCOSE TOLERANCE A RISK FACTOR FOR DIABETIC NEUROPATHY?

The San Luis Valley Diabetes Study demonstrated a higher prevalence of distal sensory neuropathy among subjects with IGT in comparison with NGT (11.2% vs 3.5%) *(4)*. This finding was not supported in a study of 51 Swedish subjects with persistent IGT for 12 to 15 years who were in comparison with 62 age-matched nondiabetic controls *(59)*. Nerve conduction velocities did not significantly differ between the IGT and the NGT groups. Abnormal heart rate variation with breathing was more common in IGT vs NGT subjects (29% vs 8%, $p < 0.01$), suggesting that IGT may increase the risk of developing autonomic neuropathy. The Framingham Heart Study found that heart rate variability was lower in subjects with impaired fasting glucose, in comparison with subjects with normal fasting glucose, but this result was not statistically significant after adjusting for clinical variables *(35)*. Whether IGT increases risk of diabetic sensory or autonomic neuropathy cannot be determined from available data.

IMPLICATIONS FOR FUTURE EPIDEMIOLOGICAL RESEARCH

Research on the epidemiology of diabetic neuropathy is at an earlier stage in comparison with other diabetic complications. Considerable advances would occur in this field if standardized definitions were developed and used in multiple investigations, although care should be taken to avoid protocols that would be burdensome to study participants, because these would increase the likelihood of bias because of unacceptably low participation rates. Also, measurement methods should be used which easily translate into clinical practice. Important potential confounding variables must be considered in future studies, including alcohol consumption in particular, height, and possibly nutritional factors as well. Further investigation of the association between hyperlipidemia and risk of neuropathy is warranted to examine the possibility that this complication may have, in part, a macrovascular etiology. Prospective studies of large cohorts of diabetic subjects would likely yield the best quality information concerning potential causative risk factors for diabetic neuropathy. Because of the low frequency of occurrence of diabetic focal neuropathies, the case–control approach would be best suited to identify risk factors for these outcomes. One can hope that these efforts will lead to better methods to prevent this difficult to manage complication of DM.

REFERENCES

1. Rothman KJ. *Modern Epidemiology*. Boston: Little, Brown & Co., 1996.
2. Oh, S. *Clinical Electromyography*. Baltimore, MD: University Park, 1984.
3. Dyck PJ, Kratz KM, Lehman JL, et al. The Rochester Diabetic Neuropathy Study: design, criteria for types of neuropathy, selection bias, and reproducibility of neuropathic tests. *Neurology* 1991;41:799–807.
4. Franklin GM, Kahn LB, Baxter J, Marshall JA, Hamman RF. Sensory neuropathy in non-insulin-dependent diabetes mellitus. *Am J Epidemiol* 1990;131:633–643.
5. Franklin GM, Shetterly SM, Cohen JA, Baxter J, Hamman RF. Risk factors for distal symmetric neuorpathy in NIDDM. *Diabetes Care* 1994;17:1172–1177.
6. Maser RE, Steenkiste AR, Dorman JS, et al. Epidemiological correlates of diabetic neuropathy. Report from Pittsburgh Epidemiology of Diabetes Complications Study. *Diabetes* 1989;38:1456–1461.
7. Maser RE, NielsenVK, Bass EB, et al. Measuring diabetic neuropathy. Assesssment and comparison of clincial examination and quantitative sensory testing. *Diabetes Care* 1989;12:270–275.
8. Orchard TJ, Dorman JS, Master RE, et al. Factors associated with avoidance of severe complications after 25 yr of IDDM. Pittsburgh Epidemiology of Diabetes Complications Study I. *Diabetes Care* 1990;13(7):741–747.
9. Kriska AM, Laporte RE, Patrick SL, Kuller LH, Orchard TJ. The association of physical activity and diabetic complications in indiviuals with insulin-dependent diabetes mellitus: the Epidemiology of Diabetes Complications Study—VII. *J Clin Epidemiol* 1991;44: 1207–1214.
10. Harris M, Eastman R, Cowie C. Symptoms of sensory neuropathy in adults with NIDDM in the US population. *Diabetes Care* 1993;16:1446–1552.
11. Knuiman MW, Welborn T, McCann VJ, Stanton KG, Constable IJ. Prevalance of diabetic complications in relation to risk factors. *Diabetes* 1986;35:1332–1339.
12. Walters DP, Gatling W, Mullee MA, Hill RD. The prevalence of diabetic distal sensory neuropathy in an English community. *Diabet Med* 1992;9:349–353.
13. Bergenheim T, Borssen B, Lithner F. Sensory thresholds for vibration, perception, and pain in diabetic patients aged 15–50 years. *Diabetes Res Clin Practice* 1992;16:47–52.
14. Verhoeven S, van Ballegooie E, Casparie AF. Impact of late complications in Type 2 diabetes in a Dutch population. *Diabet Med* 1991;8:435–438.

15. Gregg EW, Sorlie P, Paulose-Ram R, et al. Prevalence of lower-extremity disease in the US adult population >40 years of age with and without diabetes. *Diabetes Care* 2004;27:1591–1597.
16. Savettieri G, Rocca WA, Salemi G, et al. Prevalence of diabetic neuropathy with somatic symptoms: a door-to-door survey in two Sicilian municipalities. Sicilian Neuro-Epidemiologic Study (SNES) Group. *Neurology* 1993;43:1115–1120.
17. Tesfaye S, Stevens LK, Stephenson JM, et al. Prevalence of diabetic peripheral neuropathy and its relation to glycaemic control and potential risk factors: the EURODIAB IDDM Complications Study. *Diabetolgia* 1996;39:1377–1384.
18. Anonymous, UK Prospective Diabetes Study 6. Complications in newly diagnosed type 2 diabetic patients and their association with different clinical and biochemical risk factors. *Diabetes Res* 1990;13:1–11.
19. Anonymous, Intensive blood-glucose control with sulphonylureas or insulin compared with conventional treatment and risk of complications in patients with type 2 diabetes (UKPDS 33). *Lancet* 1998;352(9131):837–853.
20. Tesfaye S, Chaturvedi N, Eaton SE, et al. Vascular risk factors and diabetic neuropathy. *N Engl J Med* 2005;352:341–350.
21. Forrest KY, Maser RE, Pambianco G, Becker DJ, Orchard TJ. Hypertension as a risk factor for diabetic neuropathy. A prospective study. *Diabetes* 1997;46:665–670.
22. Adler AI, Boyko EJ, Ahroni JH, Stensel V, Forsberg RC, Smith DG. Risk factors for diabetic peripheral sensory neuropathy: results of the Seattle prospective diabetic foot study. *Diabetes Care* 1997;20:1162–1167.
23. Ewing JA. Detecting alcoholism: the CAGE questionnaire. *JAMA* 1984;252:1905–1907.
24. Dyck PJ, Davies JL, Wison DM, Service FJ, Melton LJ III, O'Brien PC. Risk factors for severity of diabetic polyneuropathy. Intensive longitudinal assessment of the Rochester Diabetic Neuropathy Study cohort. *Diabetes Care* 1999;22:1479–1486.
25. Sands ML, Shetterly SM, Franklin GM, Hamman RF. Incidence of distal symmetric (sensory) neuropathy in NIDDM. *Diabetes Care* 1997;20:322–329.
26. Loyd CE, Becker D, Ellis D, Orchard TJ. Incidence of complications in insulin dependent diabetes mellitus: a survival analysis. *Am J Epidemiol* 1996;143:431–441.
27. Partanen J, Niskanen L, Lehtinen J, Mersvaala E, Siitonen O, Uusitupa M. Natural history of peripheral neuropathy in patients with non-insulin-dependent diabetes mellitus. *N Engl J Med* 1995;333:89–94.
28. Klein R, Klein BE, Moss SE. Relation of glycemic control to diabetic microvascular complications in diabetes mellitus. *Ann Intern Med* 1996;124(1 pt 2):90–96.
29. Sosenko JM, Kato M, Soto R, Bild DE. A prospective study of sensory neuropathy in patients with Type 2 diabetes. Diabet Med 1993;10:110–114.
30. Reichard P. Risk factors for progression of microvascular complications in the Stockholm Diabetes Intervention Study (SDIS). *Diabetes Res Clin Practice* 1992;16:151–156.
31. Maser RE, Becker DJ, Drash AL, et al. Pittsburgh Epidemiology of Diabetes Complications Study. Measuring diabetic neuropathy follow-up study results. *Diabetes Care* 1992;15: 525–527.
32. Hillson RM, Hockaday T, Newton DJ. Hyperglycemia is one correlate of deterioration in vibration sense during the 5 years after diagnosis of Type 2 (non-insulin-dependent) diabetes. *Diabetolgia* 1984;26:122–126.
33. Ziegler D, Mayer P, Muhlen H, Gries FA. The natural history of somatosensory and autonomic nerve dysfunction in relation to glycemic control during the first five years after the diagnosis of type 1 (insulin-dependent) diabetes mellitus. *Diabetolgia* 1991;34: 822–829.
34. Pirart J. Diabetes mellitus and its degenerative complications: a prospective study of 4,400 patients observed between 1947 and 1973. *Diabetes Care* 1978;1:168–188.

35. Singh JP, Larson M, O'donnell CJ, et al. Association of hyperglycemia with reduced heart rate variability (The Framingham Heart Study). *Am J Cardiol* 2000;86:309–312.
36. Maser RE, Pfeifer M, Dorman JS, Kuller LH, Becker DJ, Orchard TJ. Diabetic autonomic neuropathy and cardiovascular risk. Pittsburgh Epidemiology of Diabetes Complications Study III. *Arch Intern Med* 1990;150:1218–1222.
37. Group, T.D.C.a.C.T.E.o.D.I.a.C.R. The effect of intensive diabetes therapy on the development and progression of neuropathy. *Ann Intern Med* 1995;122:561–568.
38. Toyry JP, Niskanen LK, Mantysaari MJ, Lansimies EA, Uusitupa MIJ. Occurrence, predictors, and clinical significance of autonomic neuropathy in NIDDM. Ten year follow-up from diagnosis. *Diabetes Care* 1996;45:308–315.
39. Gaede P, Vedel P, Larsen N, Jensen G, Parving HH, Pedersen O. Multifactorial intervention and cardiovascular disease in patients with type 2 diabetes. *N Engl J Med* 2003;348: 383–393.
40. Dyck PJ, Kratz KM, Karnes JL, et al. The prevalence by staged severity of various types of diabetic neuropathy, retinopathy, and nephropathy in a population-based cohort: the Rochester Diabetic Neuropathy Study. *Neurology* 1993;43(4):817–824.
41. O'Hare JA, Abuaisha F, Geoghegan M. Prevalence and forms of neuropathic morbidity in 800 diabetics. *Ir J Med Sci* 1994;163(3):132–135.
42. Albers JW, Brown MB, Sima AA, Greene DA. Frequency of median mononeuropathy in patients with mild diabetic neuropathy in the early diabetes intervention trial (EDIT). Tolrestat Study Group For Edit (Early Diabetes Intervention Trial). *Muscle Nerve* 1996;19(2):140–146.
43. Perkins BA, Olaleye D, Bril V. Carpal tunnel syndrome in patients with diabetic polyneuropathy. *Diabetes Care* 2002;25(3):565–569.
44. de Krom MC, Kester AD, Knipschild PG, Spaans F. Risk factors for carpal tunnel syndrome. *Am J Epidemiol* 1990;132(6):1102–1110.
45. Solomon DH, Katz JN, Bohn R, Mogun H, Avorn J. Nonoccupational risk factors for carpal tunnel syndrome. *J Gen Intern Med* 1999;14:310–314.
46. Becker J, Nora DB, Gomes I, et al. An evaluation of gender, obesity, age and diabetes mellitus as risk factors for carpal tunnel syndrome. *Clin Neurophysiol* 2002;113(9):1429–1434.
47. Karpitskaya, Y, Novak CB, Mackinnon SE. Prevalence of smoking, obesity, diabetes mellitus, and thyroid disease in patients with carpal tunnel syndrome. *Ann Plast Surg* 2002;48(3): 269–273.
48. Research criteria for diagnosis of chronic inflammatory demyelinating polyneuropathy (CIDP). Report from an Ad Hoc Subcommittee of the American Academy of Neurology AIDS Task Force. *Neurology* 1991;41(5):617–618.
49. Lunn MP, Manji H, Choudhary PP, Hughes RA, Thomas PK. Chronic inflammatory demyelinating polyradiculoneuropathy: a prevalence study in south east England. *J Neurol Neurosurg Psychiatry* 1999;66(5):677–680.
50. McLeod JG, Pollard JD, Macaskill P, Mohamed A, Spring P, Khurana V. Prevalence of chronic inflammatory demyelinating polyneuropathy in New South Wales, Australia. *Ann Neurol* 1999;46(6):910–913.
51. Sharma KR, Cross J, Farronay O, et al. Demyelinating neuropathy in diabetes mellitus. *Arch Neurol* 2002;59(5):758–765.
52. Lozeron P, Nahum L, Lacroix C, Ropert A, Guglielmi JM, Said G. Symptomatic diabetic and non-diabetic neuropathies in a series of 100 diabetic patients. *J Neurol* 2002;249(5): 569–575.
53. McNeely MJ, Boyko EJ, Ahroni JH, et al. The independent contributions of diabetic neuropathy and vasculopathy in foot ulceration. How great are the risks? *Diabetes Care* 1995;18(2):216–219.

54. Lavery LA, Armstrong DG, Vela SA, Quebedeaux TL, Fleischli JG. Practical criteria for screening patients at high risk for diabetic foot ulceration. *Arch Intern Med* 1998;158(2):157–162.
55. Rith-Najarian SJ, Stolusky T, Gohdes DM. Identifying diabetic patients at high risk for lower-extremity amputation in a primary health care setting. A prospective evaluation of simple screening criteria. *Diabetes Care* 1992;15(10):1386–1389.
56. Young MJ, Breddy JL, Veves A, Boulton AJ. The prediction of diabetic neuropathic foot ulceration using vibration perception thresholds. A prospective study. *Diabetes Care* 1994;17(6):557–560.
57. Pham H, Armstrong DG, Harvey C, Harkless LB, Giurini JM, Veves A. Screening techniques to identify people at high risk for diabetic foot ulceration: a prospective multicenter trial. *Diabetes Care* 2000;23(5):606–611.
58. Boyko EJ, Ahroni JH, Stensel V, Forsberg RC, Davignon DR, Smith DG. A prospective study of risk factors for diabetic foot ulcer. The Seattle Diabetic Foot Study. *Diabetes Care* 1999;22(7):1036–1042.
59. Eriksson KF, Nilsson H, Lindgarde F, et al. Diabetes mellitus but not impaired glucose tolerance is associated with dysfunction in peripheral nerves. *Diabetes Med* 1994;11:279–285.

3
Genomics of Diabetic Neuropathy

Andrew G. Demaine and Bingmei Yang

SUMMARY

Diabetes is associated with considerable mortality and morbidity due to the long term complications of the disease. Diabetic neuropathy is a major complication of diabetes and there is increasing evidence to implicate genetic factors together with elevated blood glucose in the susceptibility to this condition. The majority of the studies on the genomics of diabetic neuropathy have focussed on the gene coding for aldose reductase *(AKR1B1)*. Polymorphisms of this gene have been associated with neuropathy. However, the Human Genome Project is likely to provide many more novel candidate genes that play a key role in the pathogenesis of this condition.

Key Words: Aldose reductase; diabetes; diabetic nephropathy; genetics; neuropathy; polyol pathway; retinopathy.

INTRODUCTION

Diabetes mellitus is characterized in the later stages of the disease by several chronic disorders often termed "diabetic complications." These diabetic complications arise from a combination of factors including genetic, metabolic, and vascular factors. Diabetic neuropathy is one of the most common diabetes complications, but remains the least understood *(1)*. The prevalence of diabetic neuropathy varies according to duration of diabetes ranging from 10% within 1 year of diagnosis to more than 50% after 25 years of the disease *(2–4)*. Diabetic neuropathy is a heterogeneous condition that includes acute reversible syndromes as well as a chronic disease state *(5–7)*. This heterogeneity strongly implicates multiple factors contributing to the disease process *(8)*.

The environmental factors that have been associated with the susceptibility, development, and progression of diabetic microvascular complications include gender, HLA type, age at onset of diabetes mellitus, duration of disease, degree of metabolic control, pubertal development, growth hormone secretion, and presence of proteinuria as well as C-peptide *(9–14)*. There are several metabolic and vascular pathways that have been identified as contributors to the pathogenesis of diabetic neuropathy. These include increased flux through the polyol pathway, nonenzymatic glycosylation, altered neurotrophism, insulin and C-peptide action, activation of protein kinase-C, apoptosis, and oxidative-nitrosative stress. Gene expression promoters such as transforming growth factors-α, vascular endothelial growth factors (VEGF) and the transcription factor nuclear factor-κB (NF-κB) have attracted a great deal of interest (Fig. 1).

From: *Contemporary Diabetes: Diabetic Neuropathy: Clinical Management, Second Edition*
Edited by: A. Veves and R. Malik © Humana Press Inc., Totowa, NJ

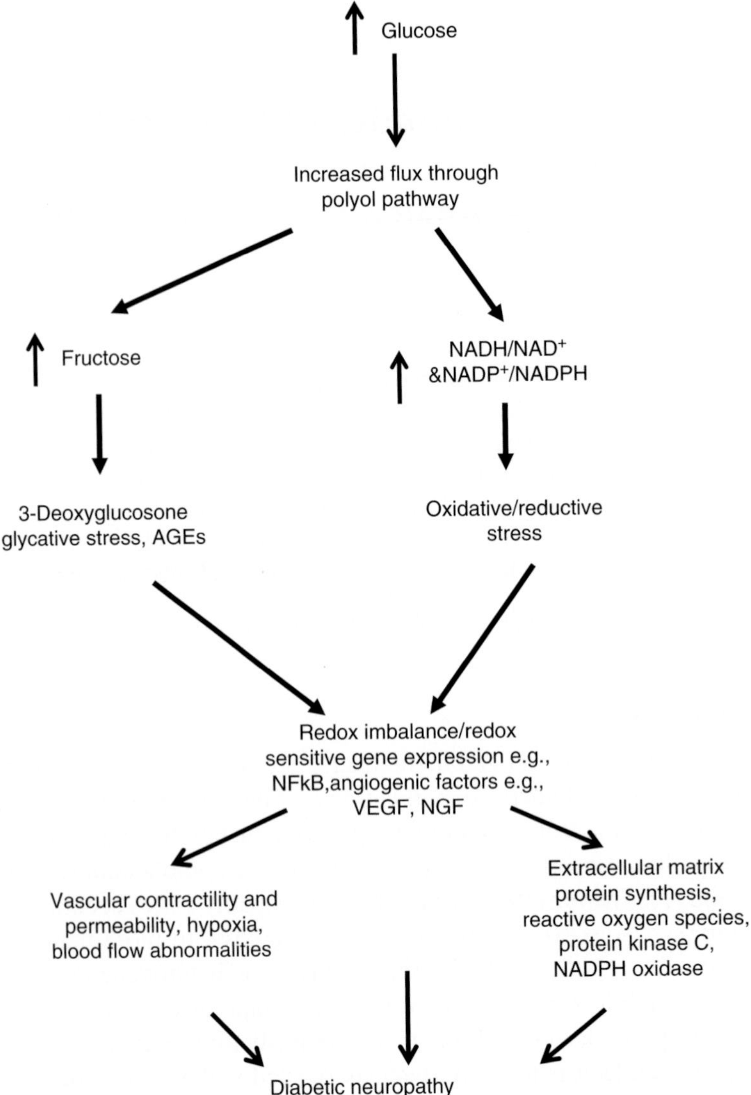

Fig. 1. Hyperglycemia-induced metabolic abnormalities because of increased flux through the polyol pathway.

GENETIC FACTORS AND DIABETIC NEUROPATHY

Over the past few years considerable data have emerged showing that genetic factors make an important contribution to the pathogenesis of diabetic microvascular complications *(15)*. This explains why certain patients with good glucose control still develop diabetic microvascular complications, whereas, there are those with poor control who appear to escape the long-term complications of diabetes. The United Kingdom Prospective Diabetes Study showed that strict glycemic control can modify the risk of microvascular disease in patients with type 2 diabetes mellitus (T2DM). Previously, the Diabetes Control of Complications Trial (DCCT) in patients with type 1 diabetes mellitus (T1DM) showed that strict glycemic control can both delay the onset of microvascular complications and slow the rate of progression of already established complications. The DCCT was able to demonstrate a nonlinear relationship between the life-time risk of complications and mean levels of HbA1c *(16,17)*.

CANDIDATE GENES

A number of genetic models have been proposed for the interaction of the diabetic milieu with genetic background of the individual. These include models in which the genetic factors modify the progression of the disease or possibly glycemic control *(18,19)*. Clearly, this would explain why some patients with well-controlled diabetes still develop complications, wheras others with poorly controlled diabetes "escape" any complications. There is a wide-spectrum in the incidence of microvascular disease between patients. For example, it is well-known that the majority of patients with nephropathy have retinopathy, but there are those who have retinopathy and normal renal function even after many years of diabetes. This heterogeneity in phenotype is a major problem in the design and interpretation of genetic studies. Until the genetic factors that contribute to each phenotype are known, it is unwise to assume that the same genes contribute to the same degree in all the tissues.

Previous family, transracial, and epidemiological studies strongly suggest that genetic factors are important in the susceptibility to diabetic nephropathy as well as retinopathy. These findings were supported by the DCCT showing familial clustering of diabetic microvascular complications *(20)*. The sequencing of the human genome now enables the positional cloning of multifactorial disease genes to be pursued. Several types of mutations exist including single nucleotide polymorphisms (SNPs), dinucleotide repeats, and microsatellites. These polymorphisms might be located in the promoter region of the gene and affect transcription or translation, and not infrequently determine the level of expression of the protein product *(21)*. High density SNP maps have been used to identify the potential genetic components of complex disease *(22)*. To date, there are only limited studies of whole genome screening for determinants of microvascular disease. Sib-pair linkage analysis was used to identify susceptibility loci for diabetic nephropathy in Pima Indians with T2DM *(23)*. The study suggested that chromosomes 3 and 9 might be important areas, but the strongest linkage was with the region harbouring *ALR2* on chromosome 7. Recently, chromosomes 10 has been identified as a possible region for determining the decline of renal function, whereas chromosome 18 has been postulated to be important in caucasoid T2DM patients *(24–26)*. Tanaka et al. *(27)* have reported association of solute-carrier family of 12 members, three with diabetic nephropathy, in a Japanese study by using the genome-wide analysis.

Genetic models can also be used to identify the susceptibility risk factor. Rogus et al. *(28)* have studied the genetic association between diabetic complications and diabetes duration by using a genetic model. Genetic models might be used to study a single major genetic effect whereby, carriage/noncarriage of a risk allele essentially indicates who will become affected, and a subtle minor genetic effect that simply shortens or lengthens the duration at which onset occurs. On a broader level, these results highlight the need to be cognizant of diabetes duration before onset of proteinuria or other late diabetic complications in family-based trio studies. To date, there have been no family studies looking at diabetic neuropathy.

The understanding of the mechanisms of brain and nervous system function has been greatly aided by the discovery of genes responsible for specific neurological disorders. These results will hopefully allow the genetic factors responsible for diabetic neuropathy to be identified and enable the following objectives to be realized:

1. Identification of the culprit gene(s) and the associated defect;
2. Understanding the mechanism by which the gene is regulated in the normal and diabetic state;
3. Developing molecular diagnostic approaches; and
4. Applications of this knowledge toward development of therapeutic regimens.

Any gene, that is involved in the aforementioned pathways could become a candidate gene. In the next sections the evidence for putative candidate genes will be reviewed (Tables 1–3).

Aldose Reductase (ALR2 or AKR1B1)

Under normal conditions glucose is metabolized by three key pathways, primarily by a hexokinase-dependent phosphorylating pathway to form glucose 6-phosphate, which then enters the glycolytic pathway to form lactate, or the hexose monophosphate shunt to form pentose-phosphate. Second, glucose might be oxidized to gluconic acid through an NAD^+-dependent glucose dehydrogenase. Finally, nonphosphorylated glucose might enter an accessory pathway of glucose metabolism known as the polyol pathway. Aldose reductase is the first and rate-limiting enzyme in the polyol pathway. It is widely distributed in human tissues including Schwann cells. Reduced glutathione synthesis, impaired nitric oxide synthesis, reduced Na^+, K^+-ATPase activity, increased protein kinase (PK)-C activity as well as a redox imbalance have all been identified as critical changes secondary to enhanced aldose reductase activity that precipitate the development of diabetic neuropathy *(29–34)*. Aldose reductase inhibitors can prevent excess polyol pathway flux, and hence these agents might prevent nerve conduction velocity deficits by preventing p38 MAP kinase activation *(35)*. The overexpression of human aldose reductase in mice with diabetes is associated with neuropathy and can be prevented by an aldose reductase inhibitor *(36)*. Transgenic mice overexpressing aldose reductase in Schwann cells show more severe nerve conduction velocity deficit and oxidative stress under hyperglycemic stress *(37)*. In those mice, the level of reduced glutathione (antioxidant) in the sciatic nerve was found to be correlated with the severity of motor nerve conduction velocity deficit. Growing evidence indicates that ALR2 has a key role in oxidative stress in the peripheral nerve and contributes to superoxide production by the vascular endothelium (review in ref. *38*).

ALR2 is a member of the NADPH-dependent monomeric aldo–keto oxidoreductases with a wide array of substrates. ALR2 can reduce the byproducts of glucose metabolism, such as methyglyoxal, 4-hydroxynonenal, and 3-deoxyglucosone *(39,40)*. Glucose is not the preferred substrate for ALR2. It is more efficient in reducing various aromatic and aliphatic aldehydes such as glyceraldehyde *(41)*.

ALR2 has been isolated from a number of tissues in man *(42–45)*. It is possible that the high levels of ALR2 enzyme activity and protein are genetically determined because of polymorphisms either in the coding or, promoter region of the gene. These genetic variations might in turn modulate the risk of diabetic microvascular complications in association with various other metabolic, genetic, and environmental factors.

Table 1
Summary of Studies Investigating Polymorphisms Within the Promoter Region of the Aldose Reductase Gene in T1DM and T2DM

Ethnic population	Microvascular complication	Polymorphisms studied	Association	References
T1DM				
Caucasian (Plymouth, UK) *N* = 159	Nephropathy	(CA)n	+	*57*
Caucasian (Plymouth, UK) *N* = 275	Neuropathy	(CA)n	+	*104*
Caucasian/Hispanic (USA) *N* = 108	Nephropathy	(CA)n	+	*70*
Caucasian (Milan, Italy) *N* = 70	Nephropathy	(CA)n	+	
Caucasian (Australian) *N* = 164	Retinopathy	(CA)n C(−106)T	+ +	*63,64*
Caucasian (Australian) *N* = 164	Retinopathy	(CA)n A(+11842)C	+ +	*63,64*
Caucasian (Birmingham, UK) *N* = 340	Nephropathy	(CA)n	−	*67*
Caucasian (Plymouth, UK) *N* = 229	Retinopathy	(CA)n C(−106)T	+ +	*58*
Caucasian (Boston, USA) *N* = 414	Nephropathy	(CA)n C(−106)T	+ +	*66*
Caucasian (Belfast, UK) *N* = 242	Nephropathy	(CA)n C(−106)T	− +	*67*
Caucasian (N of E, UK) *N* = 162	Nephropathy	(CA)n C(−106)T	− +	
Caucasian (Australian) *N* = 76	Nephropathy Neuropathy	(CA)n (CA)n	− −	*105*
T2DM				
Chinese (Hong Kong, China) *N* = 44	Retinopathy	(CA)n	+	*56*
Japanese (Osaka, Japan) *N* = 170	Retinopathy	(CA)n	+	*59*
Japanese (Kurume, Japan) *N* = 87	Retinopathy Nephropathy Neuropathy	(CA)n (CA)n (CA)n	+ − −	*106*
Japanese (Yamanashi, Japan) *N* = 61	Retinopathy	(CA)n	+	*60*

(Continued)

Table 1 ***(Continued)***

Ethnic population	Microvascular complication	Polymorphisms studied	Association	References
Caucasian (Boston, USA) $N = 576$	Nephropathy	(CA)n	–	*107*
Japanese (Shiga, Japan) $N = 304$	Nephropathy	(CA)n	–	*65*
Caucasian (Madrid, Spain) $N = 27$	Retinopathy	(CA)n	+	*108*
Caucasian (N of E, UK) $N = 223$	Nephropathy	(CA)n C(–106)T	– +	*67*
Pima Indian (Arizona, USA) $N = 327$	Nephropathy	(CA)n C(–106)T	– –	
Chinese (Hong Kong, China) $N = 384$	Retinopathy	(CA)n	–	*61*
Chinese (Changsha, China) $N = 145$	Retinopathy	C(–106)T C(–12)G	+	*55*
Chinese (Hong Kong, China) $N = 145$	Nephropathy	(CA)n	+	
Caucasoid (Finnish) $N = 85$	Neuropathy-progression	C–11G; C–106T (CA)n	+	*68*

The *ALR2* gene is localized on chromosome 7q35 *(AKR1B1, NM001628) (45)*. Pseudogenes have also been found on other chromosomes *(46)*. The gene extends more than 18 kb and contains 10 exons that code for a 1384 bp mRNA. The basal promoter activity is located between position –192 and +31. Several *cis*-regulatory elements have been isolated and point mutations in certain sequences such as the TATTTA reduced promoter activity to 35% of the wild-type DNA. The basal promoter region contains a consensus sequence for an androgen response element, three osmotic response element (ORE) sequences, ORE-A, ORE-B, and ORE-C, a sequence homologous to an Ap-1 site and also a microsatellite dinucleotide (AC) repeat sequence. In man, the ORE sequences are situated approximately 1200 bp upstream of the initiation site and maximum activity is obtained when all three ORE sequences are present *(47)*. The tonicity-binding protein (TonEBP), has recently been characterized and shown to bind to the ORE sequences and now known to be nuclear factor of activated T-cells-5 *(48,49)*. TonEBP is a homodimer that adopts a NF-κB-like structure to allow it to bind to DNA and completely encircle the helix to increase the kinetic stability of the TonEBP–DNA complex. High glucose increases nuclear factor of activated T-cells-5 binding to the OREs, which are located in the promoter region of the gene. This was significantly increased in patients with diabetic microvascular complications in comparison with those without.

AKR1B1 can be activated by a number of factors. For instance, tumor necrosis factor can initiate its expression possibly by the binding of the transcription factor NF-κB to the NF-κB regulatory element that shares extensive homology with the ORE *(49)*.

Table 2
Candidate Gene Studies in Diabetic Neuropathy

Gene	Variant	Result	Disease	References
SOD2 and *SOD3*	Mn-SOD Extracellular-SOD	+	DNu	*109*
PON	*Q192* allele	+	Complications	*110*
PON1	55 L/M	+	Complications	*110*
PON2	311 C/S	+	Complications	*110*
APOE	4/4	+	Severity of Nu	*111,112*
	2	Protective allele		
PON1	Gln192Arg	192Arg +	DR	*113*
Mn-SOD (*SOD2*)	Ala (–9)Val	+	Neu T1DM	*114*
EC-SOD (*SOD3*)	Arg213Gly	–	Neu T1DM	*114*
Neuro D	GCC45ACC Ala45Thr	+	Early-onset T2DM	*115*
CAT	T(–262)C	+	Neu T1DM	*116*
CAT	C1167T	–	Neu T1DM	*116*
GPX1	Pro/Leu	–	Neu T1DM	*116*
GSTT1	0/+	–	Neu T1DM	*116*
GSTM1	0/+	–	Neu T1DM	*116*
SOD2 (Mn-SOD)	Ala(–9)Val	+	Neu T1DM	*109*
SOD3 (EC-SOD)	Arg213Gly	+	Neu T1DM	*109*
NOS2	Microsatellite	+	Neu T1DM	*117*
SOD2	Ala(–9)Val	+	Neu T1DM	*118*
SOD3	Arg213Gly	+	Neu T1DM	*118*
APOE	Eplison4	–	DNu	*119*
Endothelial Nitric Oxidase Synthase	Glu 298ASP (G849T)	–	DN (n = 116) DR (n = 71) DNu (n = 103)	*120*
Na/K ATPase	A1 Bgl II	+	DNu	*91*
G protein β3 subunit	C825T		DN, DR, and DNu	*121*

The promoter region also has glucose (or carbohydrate) response elements (GRE) as it is stimulated by hyperglycemia *(50,51)*. Glucose-specific regulation of ALR2 has been demonstrated in human retinal pigment epithelial cells, although this effect was not apparent in Schwann cells of rats *(52,53)*.

5′ALR2

The first polymorphisms in the *AKR1B1* gene were identified in 1993 *(54)*. A number of additional polymorphisms have been identified in the *AKR1B1* gene. Of particular interest has been the (AC)*n* microsatellite dinucleotide repeat sequence polymorphism in the 5′ region of the gene. This dinucleotide repeat polymorphism designated *5′ALR2* is located approximately 2.1 kb upstream of the initiation site of *ALR2* close to the ORE sequences. A C–106T SNP situated in the basal promoter region of the *ALR2* gene has also been studied, as well as a A(+11842)C SNP within intron 8. Finally, a C(–12)G SNP has also been reported *(55)*.

Table 3
Functional Gene Studies in Diabetic Neuropathy

Gene	Result	Outcome	References
Glut5	Increase	Sciatic nerve in rats	*122*
Neurotrophin-3	Increase	Sensory nerve in rats	*123*
VEGF	Increase		*84*
AKR1B1 and *SDH*	Increase		*53*
AKR1B1	Increase		*124*
Insulin-like growth factor-1	Increase Delayed expression	Responsible for the delay in NGF response in diabetic rats	*125*
Nerve growth Factor	Decrease		*126*
Neuropeptides substance P			*126*
Calcitonin gene-related peptide			*126*
Adipocytokines (tumor necrosis factor-α, adiponectin, and leptin)	Affect nerve conduction velocity	T2DM with neuropathy	*127*
Activating transcription factor 3	Increased in neurons	STZ mice	*128*

More than 12 alleles of the 5′*ALR2* locus have been detected in different populations. The most common allele has been designated Z and consists of $(AC)_{24}$ repeats, whereas the *Z–2* allele contains $(AC)_{23}$ repeats and conversely, the *Z+2* allele $(AC)_{25}$ repeats. A similar nomenclature has been adopted for the remaining alleles. Interestingly, the Z 5′*ALR2* allele is the most common among all populations irrespective of the ethnic background.

The 5′*ALR2* locus has been associated with diabetic retinopathy, nephropathy, and also neuropathy in patients with T1DM as well as T2DM who are from different ethnic backgrounds (Table 1). In 1995, Ko et al. *(56)* showed that the frequency of the *Z–2* allele of the 5′*ALR2* locus is increased in early onset diabetic retinopathy in 44 unrelated Chinese (Hong Kong) patients with T2DM. The *Z–2* allele was found in 59% of patients with early onset diabetic retinopathy in comparison with only 9% with no microvascular complications. This was later confirmed in a British caucasoid population of patients with T1DM and nephropathy (and coexistent retinopathy). Whereas the frequency of the *Z–2* allele was increased in those subjects that had retinopathy alone, in comparison with uncomplicated subjects who had gone for at least 20 years without developing any retinopathy, proteinuria, or overt neuropathy this was not significant probably because of the small number of subjects *(57,58)*. There have now been numerous studies, the majority of which have shown a clear association between the *Z–2* allele and diabetic microvascular complications (Table 1).

An exception was the study by Fujisawa *(59)*, who investigated the 5′*ALR2* locus in T2DM subjects of Japanese origin. Eleven different alleles were found and a striking association was found with the length of the allele and diabetic retinopathy. The prevalence of short alleles (*Z–4* and *Z–2*) was higher in patients with retinopathy, whereas longer alleles were more common in those without retinopathy. Another study of the *5′ALR2* locus in Japanese patients with T2DM found an increased frequency of the *Z–4* "short" allele in those patients with proliferative retinopathy *(60)*. In contrast, the *Z+2* "long" allele was associated with the absence of retinopathy. A study of 384 late onset T2DM subjects of Hong Kong Chinese origin found no significant difference in the frequency of *Z+2/Z* and *Z–2* alleles between patients with or without diabetic retinopathy *(61)*. However, there was a significant increase in the frequency of the *Z–4* allele in those with retinopathy in comparison with those without. The high rate of progression of proliferative retinopathy might be associated with the *Z–2* allele in caucasoid patients with T2DM. The *Z* allele (long allele) was associated with a fivefold reduction in the appearance of retinopathy *(62)*. In a study of young Caucasoid adolescents with T1DM, Kao *(63,64)* showed that the *Z–2* allele was significantly higher in those with retinopathy in comparison with those without. The patients with retinopathy tended to be much younger and had more rapidly progressive form of the disease. These results have since been replicated and confirmed in a British Caucasoid population *(58)*.

It is intriguing why the length of the microsatellite should be associated with diabetic microvascular complications. It is possible that the microsatellite might alter the tertiary structure of the promoter and regulatory regions. This could modify the efficiency of binding of transcription factors such as TonEBP or, glucose (carbohydrate) response element binding protein. Alternatively, the allelic variation might be in linkage disequilibrium with another mutation that might affect the expression or function of the gene. There has been remarkable consistency between the published studies. There have been reports where no association has been found (Table 1). Maeda *(65)* studied Japanese patients with T2DM and found no association between any of the alleles and retinopathy.

C(–106)T

This is a C to T SNP located close to the basal promoter region at position –106. Kao *(63,64)* studied young adolescent Caucasiod T1DM subjects with or without diabetic retinopathy and found the *C(–106)* allele was associated with the *Z–2 5′ALR2* allele in patients with retinopathy, whereas the *C* as well as the *T* alleles were associated with the *Z+2* allele in the uncomplicated group. Similar results were found by Demaine *(58)*, who showed that the *C–106* and *Z–2 5′ALR2* alleles are strongly associated with retinopathy in a large cohort of British Caucasoid patients with T1DM. In patients with T1DM as well as T2DM with nephropathy associations have been found with the *T–106* allele rather than the *C–106 allele (66,67)*. The reason for this discrepancy is unclear, but probably is a reflection of the heterogeneity of patient populations and the disease.

Sivenius *(68)* recently showed in Finnish patients with T2DM that the *T–106* allele was associated with lower sensory response amplitudes in the peroneal, sural, and radial nerves. During follow-up for more than 10 years, the *T–106* allele was associated with a higher decrease in the conduction velocity of the motor peroneal nerve in comparison with those with the CC–106 genotype. No association was found with the *5′ALR2* alleles.

The study by Moczulski was the first to investigate the *5′ALR2* and –106 polymorphisms in a family based study using the transmission disequilibrium test. Families used in this study had T1DM with or without persistent proteinuria or diabetic nephropathy, and were of Caucasoid origin. There was a trend for preferential transmission of the *Z–2* allele in the case of comparison with the control trios (54% vs 46%, respectively). There was preferential transmission of the *T–106* allele in the case trios in comparison with the controls (54% vs 37%, respectively).

A(+11842)C

This SNP occurs at the 95th nucleotide of intron 8 and is the BamHI restriction endonuclease site that had previously been reported by Patel *(54,63,64)*. This polymorphism is strongly associated with diabetic retinopathy in adolescent T1DM subjects of Caucasoid (Australia) origin.

ALR2 *Haplotypes*

The presence of the three polymorphisms across the *ALR2* gene enables haplotypes to be defined. This might increase the specificity and sensitivity of the association. Using this approach it was found that the Z–2/C/A (5′*ALR2*/–106/+11842) haplotype accounted for more than 30% of all those found in patients with T1DM and nephropathy and in only 12.5% of the long-term uncomplicated subjects. More than 33% of the latter group had either *Z+2/C/C* or, *Z+2/T/C*, or *Z+2/T/A* haplotype. The odds ratio of having a "protective" haplotype and not developing microvascular complications of diabetes after 20 years duration was more than 9.

ALR2 Polymorphisms and Gene Expression

Marked differences in ALR2 enzyme activity and protein levels have been found between patients with or without diabetic microvascular complications. Recently, these studies have been extended to include expression of the *AKR1B1* gene. Patients with T1DM and nephropathy have been found to have threefold higher *ALR2* mRNA levels in comparison with those without nephropathy or nondiabetic renal disease and using highly sensitive ribonuclease protection assays, this increase was found to be closely linked with the *Z–2 5′ALR2* allele *(69,70)*. Patients with at least one copy of the *Z–2* allele had more than twofold higher levels of *ALR2* mRNA in comparison with those without the *Z–2* allele. Among the nondiabetic subjects there was no effect of the *Z–2* allele on mRNA levels. Hodgkinson used ribonuclease protection assays to investigate the expression of both *ALR2* as well as sorbitol dehydrogonase (SORD) in peripheral blood mononuclear cells of British caucasoid patients with T1DM that have been exposed to hyperglycemia (31 m*M* D-glucose) for 5 days in vitro *(51)*. Those patients with nephropathy and coexistent retinopathy had markedly increased levels of ALR2 mRNA in comparison with those with no microvascular disease after 20 years duration of T1DM or normal healthy controls. Those subjects with the *Z–2 5′ALR2* allele had the greatest abundance of mRNA confirming the linkage between this site and expression of the gene.

Attempts have also been made to ascertain the functional role of the *5′ALR2* alleles. Ikegishi *(60)* used luciferase reporter assays to show that promoter region containing the *Z–4* allele had significantly higher transcriptional activity than constructs containing a "long" allele. In preliminary studies, Yang *(71)* showed that the 2.1 kb promoter region that contains both *Z–2* and *C–106* alleles had significantly higher transcriptional activity than promoter regions containing any other combination of alleles. This increase was most apparent at normal tissue culture conditions, whereas the "protective" haplotype *Z+2/T–106* had a considerably reduced level of activity.

In a preliminary study, the *C–106* allele alone has been associated with enhanced transcriptional activity in cultured human retinal pigmented epithelial cells.

Protein Kinase-C

There is ample evidence supporting the hypothesis that abnormal activation of PKC in the diabetic state is important for the development of diabetic microvascular complications. There are at least 12 isoforms of PKC. High glucose-induced damage of mesangial cells is associated with the preferential activation of specific PKC isoforms: PKCB1 and PKCB2. Araki et al. *(72)* studied 9 SNP in *PKCB1* gene and identified the DNA sequence differences in the promoter of *PKCB1* that might contribute to diabetic nephropathy in T1DM. These results have not been confirmed in other studies.

Advanced Glycation End Product and Receptor of Advanced Glycation End Product

Nonenzymatic glycation is a process in which glucose can covalently attach itself to amino groups of proteins without the aid of enzymes to form advanced glycation end products (AGEs). Inhibition of AGE formation can ameliorate some of the features of diabetic neuropathy as well as nephropathy and retinopathy *(73,74)*. Misur et al. *(75)* observed that AGE localization was present in the endoneurium, perineurium, and microvessels in diabetic peripheral nerves.

Neuronal dysfunction is closely associated with activation of NF-κB *(76)*, and several studies have indicated that ligation of the receptor of advanced glycation end product (RAGE) results in sustained activation of NF-κB *(77,78)*. The ligand-RAGE-interaction results in an activation of NF-κB, increased expression of cytokines, chemokines, and adhesion molecules, and induces oxidative stress. Haslbeck et al. *(79)* study has shown that RAGE, NF-κB, and the RAGE ligand N(ε)-carboxymethyl lysine as well as interleukins are all present in sural nerve biopsies of patients with vasculitic neuropathy. N(ε)-carboxymethyl lysine, RAGE, NF-κB, and interleukin-6 were expressed by CD4(+), CD8(+), and CD68(+) cells, whereas control tissue showed only weak staining. These data suggest that the RAGE pathway might have a critical proinflammatory role in vasculitic neuropathy. Polymorphisms have been identified in the *RAGE* gene, but to date have not been associated with diabetic neuropathy.

Vascular Endothelial Growth Factor

VEGF is a cytokine that has been proposed to play a key role in the pathogenesis of diabetic microvascular complications *(80–82)*. The expression of the gene is regulated by changes in oxygen tension and redox imbalance in the cell *(83)*. VEGF induces vascular endothelial cell proliferation, migration, and vasopermeability in many types of tissues. Its expression is increased under hyperglycemic conditions in the peripheral nerves and dorsal root ganglia in rodent models of diabetic neuropathy *(84)*. This increase might play a role in complete nerve regeneration under diabetic conditions. *VEGF* gene transfer for neuropathy was performed in patients with diabetic neuropathy and experimental diabetic neuropathy in animals *(85,86)*. These studies supported the notion that diabetic neuropathy results from microvascular ischemia involving the vasa nervorum and raise the feasibility of a novel treatment strategy for patients with neuropathy. Polymorphisms in the promoter region of VEGF have been studied in diabetic nephropathy and retinopathy *(87)*.

Oxidative and Nitrosative Stress

Oxidative stress is a major risk factor in the development of diabetic complications. There are several enzymes involved in these processes. The related metabolic abnormalities that are implicated in diabetic neuropathy include an imbalance between nicotinamide adenine dinucleotide phosphate (NADP) and its reduced form, NADPH. The increased flux through the polyol pathway decreases NADPH:NADP$^+$ and NADH:NAD$^+$ ratios with accumulation of reactive oxygen species. During this process, NADPH oxidase generates reactive oxygen species (ROS), including superoxide and hydrogen peroxidase, highlighting the important role of NADPH oxidase as a source of ROS in the vascular system. NADPH oxidase is made up of a number of subunits and is distributed widely in various tissues. The gene coding for the p22 subunit of NADPH oxidase is polymorphic, including a C242T and A640G transitions. C242T results in the replacement of histidine by tyrosine at amino acid 72 of the putative heme-binding site and A649G is in the 3′ untranslated region. These two polymorphisms are associated with diabetic nephropathy in patients with T1DM although no association was found with neuropathy *(88)*. Hyperglycemia induced oxidative stress and apoptosis occurs in dorsal root neurons *(89)*. Table 2 summarizes a number of studies looking at genes involved in oxidative and nitrosative stress for instance superoxide dismutase (SOD), endothelial nitric oxide synthase, and catalase (CAT). A small number of studies have been carried out looking at genes involved in lipid metabolism such as ApoE and paraoxonase (PON). Table 3 summarizes functional studies of genes in diabetic neuropathy.

Poly(ADP-Ribose) Polymerase

Oxidative and nitrosative stress play a key role in the pathogenesis of diabetic neuropathy. Some studies have shown that the PARP (PARP-1; EC2.4.5.30) activation, a downstream effector of oxidant-induced DNA damage, is an obligatory step in the functional and metabolic changes in the diabetic nerve *(97)*. PARP-1 is a nuclear enzyme which is activated by oxidant-induced DNA single-strand breakage and transfers ADP-ribose residues from NAD$^+$ to nuclear proteins *(98–101)*. PARP-1 is present in both endothelial cells *(99,102)* and Schwann cells of the peripheral nerve *(103)*.

There is increasing interest in poly(ADP-ribose) polymerase (PARP) in the development of diabetic neuropathy. Reactive oxygen and nitrogen species trigger activation of mitogen-activated protein kinases and PARP as well as the inflammatory cascade and these downstream mechanisms are also involved in the pathogenesis of diabetes complications. The interactions among various hyperglycemia-initiated mechanisms are not completely understood and the relationship between increased aldose reductase activity and oxidative-nitrosative stress/PARP activation has recently become a focus of interest. Some studies have shown that increased aldose reductase activity leads to oxidative stress. However, others reported that increased aldose reductase activity is a consequence rather than a cause of oxidative stress (in particular, mitochondrial superoxide production) and PARP activation in the pathogenesis of diabetes complications. High blood glucose causes chemical changes in nerves and impairs the nerves ability to transmit signals. It also has the potential to damage blood vessels that carry oxygen and nutrients to the nerves. There is now evidence to suggest that insulin and C-peptide deficiencies are mainly responsible for perturbations of neurotrophic factors and contribute to oxidative stress in diabetic nerve (review ref. *90*).

Na/K ATPase

Diabetes mellitus induces a decrease in Na/K ATPase activity and this decrease plays a role in the development of diabetic neuropathy *(91)*. Na/K ATPase is encoded by various genes. Among them, the ATPase *A1* gene (α1-isoform) is expressed predominantly in peripheral nerves and in erythrocytes. The ATPase *A1* variant is associated with diabetic neuropathy in patients with T1DM *(92)*. A further study showed that the association between the ATPase *A1* variant and decreased enzyme activity in patients with a low C-peptide level *(93)*. This suggests that both genetic and environmental factors might regulate Na/K ATPase activity in patients with diabetes, although these studies need to be confirmed in larger cohorts.

Nerve Growth Factors and Other Neurotrophic Factors

The degenerative pathology including the loss or degeneration of neurons, Schwann cells, and neuronal fibers implicates nerve growth factors (Table 3). Endogenous growth factors might promote survival of neurons, whereas the expression of nerve growth factors (NGFs) are altered in diabetic neuropathy and peripheral neuron injury. NGFs induce neuronal regeneration in vitro and in vivo models of diabetic injury *(94)*. Therefore, a failure of neurotrophic factors to regulate neuronal phenotype might result in diabetic neuropathy *(95)*. Deficient neurotrophic support might contribute to the pathogenesis of diabetic neuropathy, and exogenous neurotrophins or other strategies might be useful tools to correct their deficiency *(96)*. Nothing is known about genetic variants of neurotrophic factors in susceptibility to diabetic neuropathy and is clearly an important area to be studied.

In conclusion, now at this stage it is possible to identify candidate genes that might be implicated in the pathogenesis of diabetic neuropathy and other microvascular complications of diabetes. To date, the most consistent finding has been the association with aldose reductase *(129–136)*. However, there will be other candidate genes that contribute to the polygenic background of diabetic neuropathy. The search for these genes is hampered by clinical heterogeneity of diabetic neuropathy and the interaction with other late complications of diabetes as well as the disease itself *(137–140)*. Hopefully, the next few years will bring major advances in this area. This should provide new vehicles for treating neuropathy, for instance, by specific targeting using "gene silencing technology;" and screening for "at risk" subjects to name just two.

REFERENCES

1. Greene DA, Sima AF, Pfeifer MA, Albers JW. Diabetic neuropathy. *Annu Rev Med* 41;303–317, 1990.
2. Pirart J. Diabetes mellitus and its degenerative complications: a prospective study of 4400 patients observed between 1947 and 1973. Part 2. *Diabetes Care* 1978;1:252–294.
3. Vinik AI, Liuzze FJ, Holland MT, Stansberry KB, LeBean JM, Coleb LB. Diabetic neuropathies. *Diabetes Care* 1992;15:1926–1975.
4. Sima AAF. Pathological definition and evaluation of diabetic neuropathy and clinical correlations. *Can J Neurol Sci* 1994;21(Suppl 4):513–517.

5. Sima AA, Cherian PV. Neuropathology of diabetic neuropathy and its correlations with neurophysiology. *Clin Neurosci* 1997;4:359–364.
6. Thomas PK. Classification, differential diagnosis, and staging of diabetic peripheral neuropathy. *Diabetes* 1997;46(Suppl 2):S54–S57.
7. Duby JJ, Campbell RK, Setter SM, White JR, Rasmussen KA. Diabetic neuropathy: an intensive review. *Am J Health Syst Pharm* 2004;61:160–173.
8. Greene DA, Sima AAF, Stevens MJ, Feldman EL, Lattimer SA. Complications: neuropathy, pathogenetic considerations. *Diabetes Care* 1992;15:1902–1925.
9. Annunzio d' G, Malvezzi F, Vitali L, et al. A 3-19 year follow up study on diabetic retinopathy in patients diagnosed in childhood and treated with conventional therapy. *Diabetic Med* 1997;14:951–955.
10. D'Angio CT, Ambati J, Phelps DL. Do urinary levels of vascular endothelial growth factors predict proliferative retinopathy? *Curr Eye Res* 2001;22:90.
11. Kalter-Leibovici O, Leibovici L, Loya N, et al. The development and progression of diabetic retinopathy in type 1 diabetic patients: a cohort study. *Diabetic Med* 1997;14:858–866.
12. Cohen RA, Hennekens CH, Christen WG, et al. Determinants of retinopathy progression in type 1 diabetes mellitus. *Am J Med* 1999;107:45–51.
13. DCCT Research Group. The absence of a glycaemic threshold for the development of long term complications: the perspective of the Diabetes Control and Complications Trial. *Diabetes* 1996;45:1289–1298.
14. Forst T, Kunt T, Pf utzner A, Beyeer J, Wahren J. New aspects on biological activity of C-peptide in IDDM patients. *Exp Clin Enocriol* 1998;106:270–276.
15. Rich SS, Freedman BI, Bowden DW. Genetic epidemiology of diabetic complications. *Diabetic Revs* 1997;5:165–173.
16. DCCT Research Group. The effect of intensive treatment of diabetes on the development and progression of long term complications in insulin dependent diabetes mellitus. *New Engl J Med* 1993;329;977–986.
17. DCCT Research Group. The relationship of glycaemic exposure (HbA1c) to the risk of development and progression of retinopathy in the diabetes controls and complications trial. *Diabetes* 1995;44:968–983.
18. Krolewski AS, Doria A, Magre J, Warram JH, Housman D. Molecular genetic approaches to the identification of genes involved in the development of nephropathy in insulin-dependent diabetes mellitus. *J Am Soc Nephrol* 1992;3(4 Suppl):S9–17.
19. Krolewski AS. Genetics of diabetic nephropathy: evidence for major and minor gene effects. *Kidney Int* 1999;55:1582–1596.
20. DCCT Research Group. Clustering of long term complications in families with diabetes in the diabetes control and complications trial. *Diabetes* 1997;46:1829–1839.
21. Connolly SB, Sadlier D, Kieran NE, Doran P, Brady HR. Transcriptome profiling and the pathogenesis of diabetic complications. *J Am Soc Nephrol* 2003;14(Suppl 3):S279–S283.
22. Antonellis A, Rogus JJ, Canani LH, et al. A method for developing high-density SNP maps and its application at the type 1 angiotensin II receptor (AGTR1) locus. *Genomics* 2002; 79:326–332.
23. Imperatore G, Hanson RL, Pettitt DJ, Kobes S, Bennett PH, Knowler WC. Sib-pair linkage analysis for susceptibility genes for microvascular complications among Pima Indians with type 2 diabetes. Pima Diabetes Genes Group. *Diabetes* 1998;47:821–830.
24. Freedman BI, Rich SS, Yu H, Roh BH, Bowden DW. Linkage heterogeneity of end-stage renal disease on human chromosome 10. *Kidney Int* 2002;62:770–774.
25. Hunt SC, Hasstedt SJ, Coon H, Camp NJ, Cawthon RM, Wu LL, Hopkins PN. Linkage of creatinine clearance to chromosome 10 in Utah pedigrees replicates a locus for end-stage renal disease in humans and renal failure in the fawn-hooded rat. *Kidney Int* 2002; 62:1143–1148.

26. Vardarli I, Baier LJ, Hanson RL, et al. Gene for susceptibility to diabetic nephropathy in type 2 diabetes maps to 18q22.3-23. *Kidney Int* 2002;62:2176–2183.
27. Tanaka N, Babazono T, Saito S, et al. Association of solute carrier family 12 (sodium/chloride) member 3 with diabetic nephropathy, identified by genome-wide analyses of single nucleotide polymorphisms. *Diabetes* 2003;52:2848–2853.
28. Rogus JJ, Warram JH, Krolewski AS. Genetic studies of late diabetic complications: the overlooked importance of diabetes duration before complication onset. *Diabetes* 2002;51(6):1655–1662.
29. Williamson JR, Chang K, Frangos M, et al. Hyperglycemic pseudohypoxia and diabetic complications. *Diabetes* 1993;42:801–813.
30. Stevens MJ, Dannanberg J, Feldman EL, et al. The linked roles of nitric oxide, aldose reductase, and (Na+, K+)-ATPase in the slowing bof nerve conduction in the streptozotocin diabetic rat. *J Clin Invest* 1994;94:853–859.
31. Cameron NE, Cotter MA, Hohman TC. Interactions between essential fatty acid, prostanoid, polyol pathway and nitric oxide mechanisms in the neurovascular deficit of diabetic rats. *Diabetologia* 1996;39:172–182.
32. Cameron NE, Cotter MA, Basso M, Hohman TC. Comparison of the effects of inhibitors of aldose reductase and sorbitol dehydrogenase on neurovascular function, nerve conduction and tissue polyol pathway metabolites in streptozotocin-diabetic rats. *Diabetologia* 1997;40:271–281.
33. Cameron NE, Cotter MA, Jack AM, Basso MD, Hohman TC. Protein kinase C effects on nerve fuction, perfusion, Na+, K+-ATPase activity and glutathione contents in diabetic rats. *Diabetologia* 1999;42:1120–1130.
34. Keogh RJ, Dunlop ME, Larkins RG. Effect of inhibition of aldose reductase on glucose of flux, diacylglycerol formation, protein kinase C, and phospholipase A2 activation. *Metabolism* 1997;46:41–47.
35. Price SA, Agthong S, Middlemas AB, Tomlinson DR. Mitogen-activated protein kinase p38 mediates reduced nerve conduction velocity in experimental diabetic neuropathy: interactions with aldose reductase. *Diabetes* 2004;53:1851–1856.
36. Yagihashi S, Yamagishi SI, Wada Ri R, et al. Neuropathy in diabetic mice overexpressing human aldose reductase and effects of aldose reductase inhibitor. *Brain* 2001; 124(Pt 12):2448–2458.
37. Song Z, Fu DT, Chan YS, Leung S, Chung SS, Chung SK. Transgenic mice overexpressing aldose reductase in Schwann cells show more severe nerve conduction velocity deficit and oxidative stress under hyperglycemic stress. *Mol Cell Neurosci* 2003;23(4):638–647.
38. Obrosova IG. How does glucose generate oxidative stress in peripheral nerve? *Int Rev Neurobiol* 2002;50:3–35.
39. Van der Jagt DL, Robinson B, Taylor KK, Hunsaker LA. Reduction of trioses by NADPH-dependent aldo-keto reductases. Aldose reductase, methylglyoxal and diabetic complications. *J Biol Chem* 1992;267:4364–4369.
40. Van der Jagt DL, Kolb NS, Van der Jagt TJ, et al. Substrate specificity of human aldose reductase: identification of 4-hydroxynonenal as an endogenous substrate. *Biochim Biophys Acta* 1995;1249:117–126.
41. Inazu N, Nagashima Y, Satoh T, Fugi T. Purification and properties of six aldo-keto reductases from rat adrenal gland. *J Biochem* 1994;115:991–999.
42. Bohren KM, Bullock B, Gabbays KH. The aldo-keto reductase superfamily. *J Bio Chem* 1989;264:9547–9551.
43. Chung S, La Mendola J. Cloning and sequence determination of human placental aldose reductase gene. *J Biol Chem* 1989;264:14,775–14,777.
44. Nishimura C, Matsuura Y, Kokai Y, et al. Cloning and expression of human aldose reductase. *J Biol Chem* 1990;265:9788–9792.

45. Graham A, Brown L, Hedge PJ, Gammack AJ, Markham AF. Structure of the human aldose reductase gene. *J Biol Chem* 1991;266:6872–6877.
46. Bateman JB, Kojis T, Heinzmann C, et al. Mapping of aldose reductase gene sequences to human chromosomes 1, 3, 7, 9, 11, and 13. *Genomics* 1993;17:560–565.
47. Ko BCB, Ruepp B, Bohren KM, Gabbay KH, Chung SSM. Identification and characterisation of multiple osmotic response sequences in the human aldose reductase gene. *J Biol Chem* 1997;272:16,431–16,437.
48. Lopez-Rodriguez C, Aramburu J, Rakeman AS, Rao R. NFAT, a constitutively expressed nuclear NFAT protein that does not co-operate with Fos and Jun. *Biochemistry* 1999;96:7214–7219.
49. Iwata T, Sato S, Jimenez J, et al. Osmotic response element is required for the induction of aldose reductase by tumour necrosis factor-alpha. *J Biol Chem* 1999;274:7993–8001.
50. Aida K, Tawata M, Ikegishi Y, Onaya T. Induction of rat aldose reductase gene transcription is mediated through cis-element, osmotic response element (ORE): increased synthesis and/or activation by phosphorylation of ORE-binding protein is a key step. *Endocrinology* 1999;140:609–617.
51. Hodgkinson AD, Sondergaard KL, Yang B, Cross DF, Millward BA, Demaine AG. Aldose reductase expression is induced by hyperglycaemia in diabetic nephropathy. *Kidney Int* 2001;60:211–218.
52. Henry DN, Frank RN, Hootman SR, Rood SE, Helig CW, Busik JV. Glucose-specific regulation of aldose reductase in human retinal pigment epithelial cells in vitro. *Invest Opthal Vis Sci* 2000;41:1554–1560.
53. Maekawa K, Tanimoto T, Okada S, Susuki T, Suzuki T, Yabe-Nichimura C. Expression of aldose reductase and sorbitol dehydrogenase genes in Schwann cells isolated from rats: effects of high glucose and osmotic stress. *Mol Brain Res* 2001;87:251–256.
54. Patel A, Hibberd ML, Millward BA, Demaine AG. Chromosome 7q35 and susceptibility to diabetic microvascular complications. *J Diabetic Compl* 1996;10:62–67.
55. Li Q, Xie P, Huang J, Gu Y, Zeng W, Song H. Polymorphisms and functions of the aldose reductase gene 5′regulatory region in Chinese patients with type 2 diabetes mellitus. *Chin Med J* 2002;115:209–213.
56. Ko BCB, Lam KSL, Wat NMS, Chung SSM. An (A-C)n dinucleotide repeat polymorphic marker at the 5′end of the aldose reductase gene is associated with early onset diabetic retinopathy in NIDDM patients. *Diabetes* 1995;44:727–732.
57. Heesom AE, Hibberd ML, Millward BA, Demaine AG. Polymorphisms in the 5′end of the aldose reductase gene is strongly associated with the development of diabetic nephropathy in type 1 diabetes. *Diabetes* 1997;46:287–291.
58. Demaine A, Cross D, Millward A. Polymorphisms of the aldose reductase gene and susceptibility to retinopathyin type 1 diabetes mellitus. *Invest Ophthalmol Vis Sci* 2000; 41:4064–4068.
59. Fujisawa T, Ikegami H, Kawaguchi Y, et al. Length rather than a specific allele of dinucleotide repeat in the 5′ upstream region of the aldose reductase gene is associated with diabetic retinopathy. *Diabet Med* 1999;16:1044–1047.
60. IkegishiY, Tawata M, Aida K, Onaya T. Z-4 allele upstream of the aldose reductase gene is associated with proliferative retinopathy in Japanese patients with NIDDM, and elevated luciferase gene transcription in vitro. *Life Sci* 1999;65:2061–2070.
61. Lee SC, Wang Y, Ko GT, et al. Association of retinopathy with a microsatellite at 5′end of the aldose reductase gene in Chinese patients with late-onset type 2 diabetes. *Opthal Genetic* 2001;22:63–67.
62. Olmos et al. 2000.
63. Kao YL, Donaghue K, Chan A, Knight J, Silink M. A novel polymorphism in the aldose reductase gene promoter region is strongly associated with diabetic retinopathyin adolescents with type 1 diabetes. *Diabetes* 1999;48:1338–1340.

64. Kao YL, Donaghue K, Chan A, Knight J, Silink M. An aldose reductase intragenic polymorphism associated with diabetic retinopathy. *Diabetes Res Clin Prac* 1999;46:155–160.
65. Maeda S, Haneda M, Yasuda H, et al. Diabetic nephropathy is not associated with the dinucleotide repeat polymorphism upstream of the aldose reductase (ALR2) gene but with erythrocyte aldose reductase content in Japanese subjects with type 2 diabetes. *Diabetes* 1999;48:420–422.
66. Moczulski DK, Burak W, Doria A, Zukowska-Szczechowska E, Warram JH, Grzeszczak W. The role of aldose reductase in the susceptibility to diabetic nephropathy in type II (non-insulin dependent) diabetes mellitus. *Diabetologia* 1999;42:94–97.
67. Neamat-Allah M, Feeney SA, Savage DA, et al. Analysis of the association between diabetic nephropathy and polymorphisms in the aldose reductase gene in type 1 and type 2 diabetes mellitus. *Diabet Med* 2001;18:906–914.
68. Sivenius K, Niskanen L, Pihlajamaki J, Laakso M, Partanen J, Uusitupa M. Aldose reductase gene polymorphisms and peripheral nerve function in patients with type 2 diabetes. *Diabetes care* 2004;27:2021–2026.
69. Shah VO, Dorin RI, Braun SM, Zager PG. Aldose reductase gene expression is increased in diabetic nephropathy. *J Clin Endo Metab* 1997;82:2294–2298.
70. Shah VO, Scavini M, Nikolic J, et al. Z-2 microsatellite allele is linked to increased expression of the aldose reductase gene in diabetic nephropathy. *J Clin Endo Metab* 1998;83: 2886–2891.
71. Yang BM, Millward A, Demaine A. Functional differences between the susceptibility Z-2/C-106 and protective Z+2/T-106 promoter region polymorphisms of the aldose reductase gene may account for the association with diabetic microvascular complications. *Biochm Biophys Acta* 2003;1639:1–7.
72. Araki SI, Daniel PK, Ng K. Identification of a common risk haplotype for diabetic nephropathy at the protein kinase C-β1 (PKCB1) gene locus. *J Am Soc Nephrol* 2003; 14:2015–2024.
73. Hammes HP, Martin S, Federlin K, Geisen K, Brownlee M. Aminoguanidine treatment inhibits the development of experimental diabetic retinopathy. *Proc Natl Acad Sci* 1991;88:11,555–11,558.
74. Soulis-Liparota T, Cooper M, Papazoglou D, Clarke B, Jerums G. Retardation by aminoguanidine of development of albuminuria, mesangial expansion, and tissue fluorescence in streptozocin-induced diabetic rat. *Diabetes* 1991;40:1328–1334.
75. Misur I, Zarkovic K, Barada A, Batelja L, Milicevic Z, Turk Z. Advanced glycation endproducts in peripheral nerve in type 2 diabetes with neuropathy. *Acta Diabetol* 2004;41:158–166.
76. Mattson MP, Camandola S. NF-kappaB in neuronal plasticity and neurodegenerative disorders. *J Clin Invest* 2001;107:247–254.
77. Bierhaus A, Schiekofer S, Schwaninger M, et al. Diabetes-associated sustained activation of the transcription factor nuclear factor-kappaB. *Diabetes* 2001;50:2792–2808.
78. Bierhaus A, Haslbeck KM, Humpert PM, et al. Loss of pain perception in diabetes is dependent on a receptor of the immunoglobulin superfamily. *J Clin Invest* 2004;114:1741–1751.
79. Haslbeck KM, Bierhaus A, Erwin S, et al. Receptor for advanced glycation endproduct (RAGE)-mediated nuclear factor-kappaB activation in vasculitic neuropathy. *Muscle Nerve* 2004;29:853–860.
80. Aiello LP, Avery RL, Arrigg PG, et al. Vascular endothelial growth factor in ocular fluid of patients with diabetic retinopathy and other retinal disorders. *N Engl J Med* 1994;331: 1480–1487.
81. Gröne HJ. Angiogenesis and vascular endothelial growth factor (VEGF): is it relevant in renal patients? Nephrology Dialysis *Transplantation* 1995;10:761–763.
82. Williams B. Factors regulating the expression of vascular permeability/vascular endothelial growth factor by human vascular tissue. *Diabetologia* 1997;40(Suppl 2):118–120.

83. Shweki D, Itin A, Soffer D, Keshet E. Vascular endothelial growth factor induced by hypoxia may mediate hypoxia-initiated angiogenesis. *Nature* 1992;359:843–845.
84. Samii A, Unger J, Lange W. Vascular endothelial growth factor expression in peripheral nerves and dorsal root ganglia in diabetic neuropathy in rats. *Neurosci Lett* 1999; 262:159–162.
85. Isner JM, Ropper A, Hirst K. VEGF gene transfer for diabetic neuropathy. *Hum Gene Ther* 2001;12:1593–1594.
86. Schratzberger P, Walter DH, Rittig K, et al. Reversal of experimental diabetic neuropathy by VEGF gene transfer. *J Clin Invest* 2001;107:1083–1092.
87. Yang BM, Cross DF, Ollerenshaw M, Millward BA, Demaine AG. Polymorphisms of vascular endothelial growth factor and susceptibility to diabetic microvascular complications in patients with type 1 diabetes mellitus. *J Diabetes Compl* 2003;17:1–6.
88. Hodgkinson AD, Millward BA, Demaine AG. Association of the p22phox component of NAD(P)H oxidase with susceptibility to diabetic nephropathy in patients with type 1 diabetes. *Diabetes Care* 2003;26:3111–3115.
89. Vincent AM, Olzmann JA, Brownlee M, Sivitz WI, Russell JW. Uncouping proteins prevent glucose-induced neuronal oxidative stress and programmed cell death. *Diabetes* 2004; 53:726–734.
90. Sima AA. New insights into the metabolic and molecular basis for diabetic neuropathy. *Cell Mol Life Sci* 2003;60(11):2445–2464.
91. Vague P, Coste TC, Jannot MF, Raccah D, Tsimaratos M. C-peptide, Na+/K(+)-ATPase, and diabetes. *Exp Diabesity Res* 2004;5:37–50.
92. Vague P, Dufayet D, Coste T, Moriscot C, Jannot MF, Raccah D. Association of diabetic neuropathy with Na/K ATPase gene polymorphism. *Diabetologia* 1997;40(5):506–511.
93. Jannot MF, Raccah D, De La Tour DD, Coste T, Vague P. Genetic nad environmental regulation of Na/K adenosine triphosphotase activity in diabetic patients. *Metabolism* 2002;51(3):284–291.
94. Leinninger GM, Vincent AM, Feldman EL. The role of growth factors in diabetic peripheral neuropathy. *J Peripher Nerv Syst* 2004;9:26–53.
95. Brewster WJ, Femyhough P, Diemel LT, Mohiuddin L, Tomlinson DR. Diabetic neuropathy, nerve growth factor and other neurotrophic factors. *Trends Neurosci* 1994;17:321–325.
96. Fernyhough P, Diemel LT, Hardy J, Brewster WJ, Mohiuddin L, Tomlinson DR. Human recombinant nerve growth factor replaces deficient neurotrophic support in the diabetic rat. *Eur J Neurosci* 1995;7:1107–1110.
97. Obrosova IG, Li F, Abatan OI, et al. Role of poly(ADP-ribose) polymerase activation in diabetic neuropathy. *Diabetes* 2004;53:711–720.
98. Garcia Soriano F, Virag L, Jagtap P, et al. Diabetic endothelial dysfunction: the role of poly (ADP-ribose) polymerase activation. *Nat Med* 2001;7:108–113.
99. Pacher P, Liaudet L, Soriano FG, Mabley JG, Szabo E, Szabo C. The role of poly(ADP-ribose) polymerase activation in the development of myocardial and endothelial dysfunction in diabetes. *Diabetes* 2002;51(2):514–521.
100. Virag L, Szabo C. The therapeutic potential of poly(ADP-ribose) polymerase inhibitors. *Pharmacol Rev* 2002;54:375–429.
101. Yu SW, Wang H, Poitras MF, et al. Mediation of poly(ADP-ribose) polymerase-1-dependent cell death by apoptosis-inducing factor. *Science* 2002;297:259–263.
102. Soriano FG, Virag L, Szabo C. Diabetic endothelial dysfunction: role of reactive oxygen and nitrogen species production and poly(ADP-ribose) polymerase activation. *J Mol Med* 2001;79:437–448.
103. Berciano MT, Fernandez R, Pena E, Calle E, Villagra NT, Lafarga M. Necrosis of Schwann cells during tellurium-induced primary demyelination: DNA fragmentation, reorganization

of splicing machinery, and formation of intranuclear rods of actin. *Neuropathol Exp Neurol* 1999;58:1234–1243.
104. Heesom AE, Millward A, Demaine AG. Susceptibility to diabetic neuropathy in patients with insulin dependent diabetes mellitus is associated with a polymorphism at the 5′ end of the aldose reductase gene. *J Neurol Neurosurg Psychiatry* 1998;64:213–216.
105. Ng DP, Conn J, Chung SS, Larkins RG. Aldose reductase (AC)n microsatellite polymorphism and diabetic microvascular complications in Caucasian type 1 diabetes mellitus. *Diabetes Res Clin Prac* 2001;52:21–27.
106. Ichikawa F, Yamada K, Ischiyama-Shigemotu S, Yuan X, Nonaka K. Association of an (A-C)n dinucleotide repeat polymorphic marker at the 5′-region of the aldose reductase gene with retinopathy but not with nephropathy or neuropathy in Japanese patients with Type 2 diabetes mellitus. *Diabet Med* 1999;16:744–748.
107. Moczulski DK, Burak W, Doria A, et al. The role of aldose reductase gene in the susceptibility to diabetic nephropathy in Type II (non-insulin-dependent) diabetes mellitus. *Diabetologia* 1999;42:94–97.
108. Olmos P, Futers S, Acosta AM, et al. (AC)23 [Z-2] polymorphism of the aldose reductase gene and fast progression of retinopathy in Chilcan type 2 diabetics. *Diabetes Res Clin Pract* 2000;47:169–176.
109. Strokov IA, Bursa TR, Drepa OI, Zotova EV, Nosikov VV, Ametov AS. Predisposing genetic factors for diabetic polyneuropathy in patients with type 1 diabetes: a population-based case-control study. *Acta Diabetol* 2003;40(Supp 2):S375–379.
110. Letellier C, Durou MR, Jouanolle AM, Le Gall JY, Poirier JY, Ruelland A. Serum paraoxonase activity and paraoxonase gene polymorphism in type 2 diabetic patients with or without vascular complications. *Diabetes Metab* 2002;28:297–304.
111. Bedlack RS, Strittmatter WJ, Morgenlander JC. Apolipoprotein E and neuromuscular disease: a critical review of the literature. *Arch Neurol* 2000;57:1561–1565.
112. Bedlack RS, Edelman D, Gibbs JW 3rd, et al. APOE genotype is a risk factor for neuropathy severity in diabetic patients. *Neurology* 2003;60:1022–1024.
113. Murata M, Maruyama T, Suzuki Y, Ikeda Y. Paraoxonase 1 192Gln/Arg polymorphism is associated with the risk of microangiopathy in type 2 diabetes mellitus. *Diabetic Med* 2004;21:837–844.
114. Chistyakov DA, Savost'anov KV, Zotova EV, Nosikov VV. Polymorphisms in the Mn-SOD and EC-SOD genes and their relationship to diabetic neuropathy in type 1 diabetes mellitus. *BMC Med Genet* 2001;2:4.
115. Ye L, Xu Y, Zhu Y, Fan Y, Deng H, Zhang J. Association of polymorphism in neurogenic differentiation factor 1 gene with type 2 diabetes. *Zhonghua Yi Xue Yi Chuan Xue Za Zhi* 2002;19:484–487.
116. Zotova EV, Savost'ianov KV, Chistiakov DA, et al. Search for the association of polymorphic markers for genes coding for antioxidant defence enzymes, with development of diabetic polyneuropathies in patients with type 1 diabetes mellitus. *Mol Biol (Mosk)* 2004;38:244–249.
117. Nosikov VV. Genomics of type 1 diabetes mellitus and its late complications. *Mol Biol (Mosk)* 2004;38:150–164.
118. Zotova EV, Chistiakov DA, Savost'ianov KV, et al. Association of the SOD2 Ala(-9)val and SOD3 Arg213Gly polymorphisms with diabetic polyneuropathy in patients with diabetes mellitus type 1. *Mol Biol (Mosk)* 2004;37:404–408.
119. Zhou Z, Hoke A, Cornblath DR, Griffin JW, Polydefkis M. APOE epsilon4 is not a susceptibility gene in idiopathic or diabetic sensory neuropathy. *Neurology* 2005;64(1):139–141.
120. Cai H, Wang X, Colagiuri S, Wilcken DEL. A common Glu298↔Asp (849G↔T) mutation at exon 7 of the endothelial nitric oxide synthase gene and vascular complications in type 2 diabetes. *Diabetes Care* 1998;21:2195–2196.

121. Shcherbak NS, Schwartz EI. The C825T polymorphism in the G-protein beta3 subunit gene and diabetic complications in IDDM patients. *J Hum Genet* 2001;46(1):188–191.
122. Asada T, Takakura S, Ogawa T, Iwai M, Kobayashi M. Overexpression of glucose transport protein 5 in sciatic nerve of streptozotocin-induced diabetic rats. *Neurosci Lett* 1998;14:111–114.
123. Cai F, Tomlinson DR, Fernyhough P. Elevated expression of neurotrophin-3 mRNA in sensory nerve of streptozotocin-diabetic rats. *Neurosci Lett* 1999;263:81–84.
124. Shimizu H, Ohtani KI, Tsuchiya T, et al. Aldose reductase mRNA expression is associated with rapid development of diabetic microangiopathy in Japanese Type 2 diabetic (T2DM) patients. *Diabetes Nutr Metab* 2000;13:75–79.
125. Xu G, Sima AA. Altered immediate early gene expression in injured diabetic nerve: implications in regeneration. *J Neuropathol Exp Neurol* 2001;60:972–983.
126. Pittenger G, Vinik A. Nerve growth factor and diabetic neuropathy. *Exp Diabesity Res* 2003;4:271–285.
127. Matsuda M, Kawasaki F, Inoue H, et al. Possible contribution of adipocytokines on diabetic neuropathy. *Diabet Res Clin Pract* 2004;66(Suppl 1):S121–S123.
128. Wright DE, Ryals JM, McCarson KE, Christianson JA. Diabetes-induced expression of activating transcription factor 3 in mouse primary sensory neurons. *J Perpher Nerv Syst* 2004;8:242–254.
129. Sozmen EY, Sozmen B, Delen Y, Onat T. Catalase/superoxide dismutase (SOD) and catalase/paraoxonase (PON) ratios may implicate poor glycemic control. *Arch Med Res* 2001;32:283–287.
130. Harjutsalo V, Katoh S, Sarti C, Tajima N, Tuomilehto J. Population-based assessment of familial clustering of diabetic nephropathy in type 1 diabetes. *Diabetes* 2004;53(9):2449–2454.
131. Kasajima H, Yamagishi S, Sugai S, Yagihashi N, Yagihashi S. Enhanced in situ expression of aldose reductase in peripheral nerve and renal glomeruli in diabetic patients. *Virchows Arch* 2001;439(1):46–54.
132. Murthy KG, Salzman AL, Southan GJ, Szabo C. Diabetic endothelial dysfunction: the role of poly(ADP-ribose) polymerase activation. *Nat Med* 2001;7:108–113.
133. Rossell JW, Golovov D, Vincent AM, et al. High glucose-induced oxidative trsess and mitochondrial dysfunction in neurons. *FASEB J* 2002;16:1738–1748.
134. Samaii A, Unger J, Lange W. Vascular endothelial growth factor expression in peripheral nerves and dorsal root ganglia in diabetic neuropathy in rats. *Neurosci Lett* 1999; 262:159–162.
135. Schimizu H, Ohtani KI, Tsuchiya T, et al. Aldose reductase mRNA expression is associated with rapid development of diabetic microangiopathy in Japanese type 2 diabetic (T2DM) patients. *Diabetes Nutr Metab* 2000;13:75–79.
136. Shangguan Y, Hall KE, Neubig RR, Wiley JW. Diabetic neuropathy: inhibitory G protein dysfunction involves PKC-dependent phosphorylation of Goalpha. *Neurochemistry* 2003; 86(4):1006–1014.
137. UK Prospective Diabetes Study (UKPDS) Group. Tight blood pressure control and risk of macrovascular and microvascular complications in type 2 diabetes. *Brit Med J* 1998; 317:703.
138. UK Prospective Diabetes Study (UKPDS) Group. Intensive blood-glucose control with sulphonylureas or insulin compared with conventional treatment and risk of complications in patients with type 2 diabetes (UKPDS 33). *Lancet* 1998;352:837–853.
139. Pirart J. Diabetes mellitus and its degenerative complications: a prospective study of 4,400 patients observed between 1947 and 1973. *Diabetes Metab* 1997;3:97–107.
140. Zochodne DW. Diabetic neuropathies: features and mechanisms. *Brain Pathol* 1999;9: 369–391.

4

Transgenic and Gene Knockout Analysis of Diabetic Neuropathy

Sookja K. Chung and Stephen S. M. Chung

SUMMARY

Neuropathy is one of the major complications of long-term diabetes. Despite many years of intense research by a number of laboratories, the pathogenetic mechanisms of this disease are still not completely understood. Likely contributing factors of this disease include the polyol pathway, nonenzymatic glycation, protein kinase-C activation, hexosamine pathway, and overproduction of superoxide by the mitochondrial respiratory chain. Their roles in the pathogenesis of diabetic neuropathy are mainly supported by pharmacological studies, which often have inherent problem of uncertain drug specificity and availability. This article reviews the recent studies using transgenic and gene knockout mice to examine the role of polyol pathway, nonenzymatic glycation, poly(adenosine 5′-diphosphate [ADP]-ribose) polymerase, and neurofilaments in diabetic neuropathy. The results of these studies confirm some of the findings from drug experiments and also settle some controversies. These genetic studies avoid some of the problems of using chemical inhibitors, but they also have inherent problems of their own. The prospect of using more sophisticated inducible transgene expression, and conditional gene ablation technologies to circumvent these problems are discussed. It is expected that the number of genetically engineered mutant mice will increase exponentially in the near future and some of them will undoubtedly contribute to our understanding of diabetic neuropathy.

Key Words: Diabetic neuropathy; gene knockout, glycation; polyol pathway; neurofilaments; PARP; transgenic.

INTRODUCTION

It is well-established that diabetic neuropathy as well as other complications of diabetes are consequences of chronic hyperglycemia. However, the mechanism is still unclear. Several models have been proposed to account for the deleterious effects of hyperglycemia on nerve tissue. They include the polyol pathway *(1,2)*, nonenzymatic glycation *(3,4)*, protein kinase-C (PKC) *(5,6)*, and overproduction of reactive oxygen species by the mitochondrial respiratory chain *(7)*. Pharmacological analyses has yielded much information on the pathogenesis of the disease. More recently, genetic analyses, particularly transgenic (TG) and gene knockout (KO) mouse models provided confirmatory as well as novel information.

From: *Contemporary Diabetes: Diabetic Neuropathy: Clinical Management, Second Edition*
Edited by: A. Veves and R. Malik © Humana Press Inc., Totowa, NJ

A major drawback of using chemical inhibitors to determine the function of an enzyme is that the drugs seldom inhibit the target enzyme alone without affecting other enzymes, and their availability and stability in target tissues are difficult to ascertain. Gene KO removes only the enzyme encoded by the gene, and the enzyme activity in all tissues is absent, avoiding the problem of drug specificity and availability. However, while the window of action of drugs can be selected as desired, the effect of gene KO might occur throughout the entire life span of the animal, sometimes affecting embryonic development. There is also the possibility that during development, there might be activation of genes to compensate for the lack of an enzyme activity. Thus, there is always a concern that the effects of gene KO on a disease might be the consequences of developmental abnormalities rather than the result of a lack of enzyme activity. Therefore, it is important that the gene KO mice do not exhibit any pathology before the induction of the disease.

Overexpression of genes in TG mice is another approach to determine the role of the genes in the pathogenesis of the disease. This is particularly useful when the mice express low level of the gene product, and consequently they do not develop the disease or develop only a mild form of the disease. A good example is that of mice with a low level of aldose reductase (AR) in their lens and they do not develop cataracts. TG mice that overexpress AR in their lens become susceptible to develop diabetic cataract, demonstrating the role of AR in this disease *(8)*. Another advantage of the TG approach is that human genes can be expressed in mice, producing authentic human enzymes for drug inhibition studies. However, there are also drawbacks in TG experiments. One is similar to gene ablation, wherein the transgenes might exert their effects during embryonic development. The other is that the transgenes are often expressed in other locations besides the target tissues because the expression of the transgene is heavily influenced by the neighboring sequences at the site of integration. It is difficult to determine if expression of the transgene in nontarget tissues would affect the development of the disease.

With these caveats in mind, the TG and KO studies that have been conducted in recent years to investigate the pathogenesis of diabetic neuropathy will be reviewed. Currently, only the studies on the polyol pathway, nonenzymatic glycation, poly(ADP-ribose) polymerase (PARP), and neurofilaments have been reported. Although PKC-βII has been implicated to be involved in this disease, and PKC-β gene KO mice are available *(9)*, the use of these KO mice to study the development of diabetic neuropathy has not yet been reported.

THE POLYOL PATHWAY

The polyol pathway is a glucose shunt that diverts excess glucose to form fructose. AR is the first and rate-limiting enzyme of the pathway. It reduces glucose to sorbitol, and in the process its cofactor NADPH is oxidized to NADP. Sorbitol dehydrogenase (SDH) then converts sorbitol to fructose, whereas its cofactor NAD^+ is converted to NADH. The polyol pathway was first recognized as a key factor in the development of diabetic cataracts, and soon afterwards, it was found to be involved in diabetic neuropathy, retinopathy, and nephropathy. AR also reduces galactose to form galactitol. Because a high galactose diet also produces tissue lesions similar to diabetic lesions, galactosemia has been used as an experimental surrogate for diabetes. It has also been suggested that conversion of sorbitol to fructose by SDH causes reduction of

NAD^+/NADH ratio, creating a "pseudohypoxic" state that might contribute to the deleterious effects of hyperglycemia *(10)*. As galactitol is not metabolized by SDH, galactosemia does not simulate some aspects of hyperglycemia. The key evidence for AR's involvement in diabetic neuropathy is that several structurally different AR inhibitors were shown to be effective in preventing the development of this disease in animal models *(11)*, suggesting that the beneficial effects of these drugs is because of the inhibition of AR and not other nonintended target enzymes. However, these drugs did not demonstrate a significant beneficial effect in clinical trials *(12,13)*, raising doubts on the validity of this model. In particular, it was pointed out that the amount of ARI required to normalize nerve blood flow and nerve conduction velocity (NCV) deficit in diabetic rats, exceeds that required to normalize the sorbitol level in the nerves, indicating the lack of correlation between polyol pathway activity and diabetic neuropathy *(14)*. However, this observation does not disprove AR's role in the disease because, as discussed later, sorbitol accumulation is not the cause of diabetic lesions in the nerve. Rather, it is the flux of glucose through the polyol pathway that produces the toxic effect of hyperglycemia. Kinetic calculations demonstrate that when there is a rapid conversion of sorbitol to fructose by SDH, even partial inhibition of AR activity would appear to completely normalize sorbitol levels in diabetic tissue *(2)*. Thus, normalizing nerve sorbitol level does not equate to complete blockage of the polyol pathway activity. However, this theory has not been proven in animal model. Genetic studies to determine AR's role in this disease become essential.

TG Mice Expressing AR in All Tissues

Because it is easier to develop TG mice than KO mice, TG approach was first used to investigate the role of AR in diabetic neuropathy. The first reported mouse model utilized the major histocompatibility complex (MHC) promoter, which is active in all tissues, to drive the expression of human AR (hAR) complementary DNA (cDNA) in TG mice. Indeed all tissues from the MHC-hAR TG mice tested were found to express the hAR mRNA, including liver, skeletal muscle, heart, kidney, brain, and lung. Under normal rearing condition, these mice developed thrombi of the renal vessels, but no abnormality was evident in the brain, lung, heart, thymus, spleen, intestine, liver, muscle, spinal cord, and sciatic nerve when examined under light microscopy *(15)*. Under nondiabetic condition, sorbitol and fructose contents in the sciatic nerve of the TG mice were similar to that of the wild-type (WT). When induced to become diabetic, sciatic nerve sorbitol and fructose levels in the TG mice were twice that of their WT littermates, suggesting that the *hAR* transgene increased the nerve AR activity by about twofold. Under normoglycemic condition, there was no difference in the motor NCV (MNCV) or the structure of the sciatic nerve, indicating that overexpression of AR did not affect the normal development and function of this tissue. When fed with a diet consisting of 30% galactose, they developed more severe neuropathy than the WT mice as indicated by higher reduction of MNCV and in the mean myelinated fiber size of the sciatic nerve *(16)*. When induced to become diabetic by streptozotocin, the MHC-hAR mice also exhibited a greater reduction of tibial MNCV and more severe myelinated fiber atrophy of the sciatic nerve *(17)*. Further, membrane-associated PKC and Na^+/K^+-adenosine triphosophatase (ATPase) activities were significantly reduced in the diabetic MHC-hAR mice sciatic nerves with the perineurial tissues removed.

Reduction of PKC activity in diabetic nerves is particularly intriguing. In other tissues of diabetic animals such as retina and kidney, PKC activity is thought to be activated *(18)*, and an inhibitor of PKC-βII isoform has been shown to prevent the development of diabetic lesions in these tissues *(19,20)*. PKC inhibitors have been shown to prevent the development of diabetic neuropathy in animal models *(5,21)*. To clarify these apparently contradictory observations, PKC activity and PKC isoforms were examined in the perineurial tissues of MHC-hAR and WT mice, and the results revealed a complex response of PKC isoforms to hyperglycemia *(22)*. In the membrane fraction of endoneurial tissues there was a significant reduction of PKC activity in the diabetic MHC-hAR mice but not in the non-TG mice. On the other hand, in the membrane fraction of the epineurial tissues diabetes led to similar increases in PKC activity in the both TG and WT mice, indicating that AR transgene contributed little to the activation of PKC in this tissue. Western blot analysis showed that in the epineurial tissues of WT mice diabetes caused a reduction in PKC-α protein level in the membrane fraction with a concomitant rise in the cytosol fraction, suggesting translocation induced by hyperglycemia. The hyperglycemia-induced redistribution of PKC-α is even more exaggerated in the MHC-hAR mice. On the other hand, hyperglycemia induced the translocation of PKC-βII protein from the cytosol to the membrane, opposite to that of PKC-α. There was slightly more PKC-βII translocated to the membrane in the TG mice than in the WT mice, but the difference was statistically insignificant. Hyperglycemia had no effect on the level or cellular distribution of PKC-βI in this tissue. In the endoneurial tissues PKC-α was not affected by hyperglycemia, whereas PKC-βI and -βII translocation from the cytosol to the membrane was increased. Again, the *AR* transgene only contributed a small and statistically insignificant increase in their membrane translocation. The hyperglycemia-induced membrane translocation of PKC-βI and -βII suggests activation of these PKC isoforms. As the perineurial tissues contain microvessels, these findings lend support to the notion that vascular lesions contribute to the pathology in diabetic nerves, and explain the beneficial effects of a PKC-βII inhibitor on diabetic neuropathy. These changes in PKC activity and translocation of different PKC isoforms in the endoneurial and epineurial tissues were all normalized by ARI, indicating that hyperglycemia-induced activation of PKC is mediated by AR activity. The fact that the AR transgene did not make a statistically significant difference in the translocation of some of the PKC isoforms is probably a reflection of the modest (more than twofold) increase in AR activity contributed by the transgene in these tissues.

TG Mice Expressing AR in Schwann Cells

Another controversial issue in diabetic neuropathy is whether it is because of metabolic dysfunction of the nerve or because of lesions in the vessels resulting in ischemia in the nerve tissues they supply. The fact that administration of different vasodilators prevented the development of diabetic neuropathy strongly supports the vascular theory *(23–25)*. To determine if the nerve tissue also contributes to diabetic neuropathy, TG mice containing the hAR cDNA fused to the rat myelin protein zero (P_0) promoter were developed *(26)*. These P_0-hAR mice express *hAR* specifically in the Schwann cells and not in other tissues. To better illustrate increased severity of diabetic neuropathy contributed by the increased level of AR, the *hAR* transgene was maintained in the F1 (hybrid of CBA mouse strain × C57BL) genetic background that is quite resistant to the development of this disease. Under normal rearing condition, the TG mice did not exhibit any structural or functional abnormality in their sciatic nerve. In both galactosemic and hyperglycemic conditions the WT (F1) control mice showed small and statistically insignificant reduction in MNCV in their sciatic nerve. On the other hand, the P_0-hAR mice exhibited a significant decrease in sciatic nerve MNCV, indicating that Schwann cell-specific overexpression of AR led to more severe functional deficits in this tissue. Diabetes did not lead to any drop in the reduced glutathione (GSH) level in the sciatic nerve of the WT mice, but caused a significant drop in the nerve GSH content in the TG mice, indicating that overexpression of AR increases oxidative stress. Interestingly, although there was a twofold increase in the sorbitol and fructose levels in the sciatic nerve of the diabetic TG mice compared with that of the diabetic WT mice, there was no significant difference in the galactitol levels in the sciatic nerve of the galactosemic WT and TG mice. This is probably because the galactitol level in the nerve of the galactosemic WT mice was already very high. The nerve galactitol level in the galactosemic WT or TG mice was about 30-fold higher than the sorbitol level in the nerve of diabetic TG mice, a reflection of the fact that galactitol is not metabolized by SDH or other enzymes. Such a high level of polyol might cause severe osmotic stress leading to leakage, reducing the increased accumulation of galactitol contributed by the *hAR* transgene.

AR Gene KO Mice

Although the MHC-hAR and P_0-hAR TG mice experiments clearly showed that increased AR activity exacerbates diabetic neuropathy, it might be argued that such a high level of AR activity is not found in normal animals and therefore, the transgene created an artificial disease mechanism irrelevant to the pathogenesis of the disease in WT animals. Therefore, *AR* gene KO mice provide an important animal model to complement ARI and TG studies. AR-deficient mice appear normal in every respect except that they drink and urinate twice as much the WT mice because of impairment in their urine concentrating mechanism *(27)*. This mild polyuric behavior does not affect their serum electrolyte levels. To detect the potential protective effect of AR deficiency on diabetic neuropathy in a better manner, the AR null mutation was maintained in C57BL mice, which developed more severe diabetic neuropathy than the F1 mice. Under normal rearing condition, MNCV and morphology of the sciatic nerve of the KO mice were normal. When induced to become diabetic the WT (C57BL) mice showed a significant decrease in the sciatic nerve MNCV, whereas there was no change in the KO mice. Further, diabetes caused a significant reduction in the sciatic nerve GSH level, but had no effect on the nerve GSH level in the AR null mice *(28)*. These results demonstrated that AR is a key enzyme in the pathogenesis of diabetic neuropathy and that hyperglycemia-induced oxidative stress is primarily the consequence of increased flux of glucose through the polyol pathway.

SDH-Deficient Mice

There were suggestions that the polyol pathway-mediated diabetic lesion is primarily the consequence of the activity of SDH rather than AR. Conversion of sorbitol to fructose by SDH leads to increase in the NADH/NAD$^+$ ratio similar to that experienced by hypoxic cells. This "pseudohypoxic state" is thought to induce PKC, increase prostaglandin synthesis, increase free radical production, and increase nitric oxide production *(10)*. However, attempts to use SDH inhibitors (SDI) to test this hypothesis gave contradictory results. A SDI called S-0773 has been shown to partially attenuate hyperglycemia-induced vascular dysfunction in the eye, sciatic nerve, and aorta in rats *(29)*. However, other SDIs were found to exacerbate diabetic peripheral and autonomic neuropathy *(30,31)*. A spontaneous SDH null mutation in mice had been characterized *(32)*. There is no apparent abnormality in the SDH-deficient mice and their sciatic nerve MNCV and morphology are normal. When these mice were induced to become diabetic there was a slightly higher reduction in their sciatic nerve MNCV than that of the WT mice. However, the difference was not statistically significant *(33)*. Nonetheless, the result indicates that blocking the SDH activity did not improve diabetic neuropathy, demonstrating that pseudohypoxia is unlikely to be the pathogenic mechanism of this disease. This set of experiments also revealed that nerve sorbitol level does not correlate to nerve dysfunction. The sorbitol level in the sciatic nerve of nondiabetic SDH null mice was about four times higher than that of diabetic WT mice. Yet the nondiabetic SDH null mice had normal MNCV, whereas the diabetic WT mice had significant slowing of MNCV. This, and the fact that the sorbitol level in the sciatic nerve of diabetic mice was only in the range of 0.2–0.6 nmol/mg dry weight, whereas myoinositol level was around 20 nmol/mg dry weight, indicate that polyol pathway-induced osmotic stress is unlikely to be a contributing factor in the pathogenesis of diabetic neuropathy in mice. Indeed, the increase in sorbitol in the diabetic nerve did not cause a compensatory decrease in myoinositol. Therefore, myoinositol depletion does not contribute to the development of diabetic neuropathy in mice.

Conclusions

The results of AR, TG, and KO mice experiments confirmed the findings from AR inhibitors studies. Although each of these studies might leave room for alternate interpretations, the complete agreement of these three experimental approaches unequivocally demonstrate that AR plays a key role in the pathogenesis of diabetic neuropathy. The experiments with Schwann cell-specific AR-overexpressing TG mice clearly showed that metabolic dysfunction in the nerve tissue also contribute to the pathogenesis of the disease. Further, the experiments with SDH null mice showed that blocking this point of the polyol pathway has no beneficial effect on diabetic neuropathy, putting to rest the controversies arising from contradictory findings of the SDI studies. These experiments also demonstrated that accumulation of sorbitol does not contribute to the development of diabetic neuropathy in mice. The pathogenesis of the disease most likely involves oxidative stress generated from the flux of glucose through the polyol pathway. This is in agreement with a number of studies, which showed that antioxidants were able to prevent the development of diabetic neuropathy *(34–36)*.

NONENZYMATIC GLYCATION

In diabetic animals and patients increased advanced glycation end products (AGE) covalently attach to intracellular, plasma and extracellular matrix proteins in the nerve, and other tissues *(37,38)*. It has been postulated that such modifications might affect neural metabolism, axonal transport, and tissue repair, thus enhancing neural degeneration and impairing neural regeneration. The strongest evidence in support of this model is that administration of aminoguanidine, an AGE inhibitor, attenuated MNCV, and sensory NCV (SNCV) deficits in diabetic rats *(39,40)*. However, besides inhibition of AGE formation, aminoguanidine is known to inhibit the activity of other enzymes including the inducible-, neuronal-, and endothelial-nitric oxide synthases, and the semicarbazide-sensitive amine oxidase *(41)*. It is likely that there might be still other enzymes that are affected by this drug. Therefore, it is not clear if the beneficial effect of this drug on diabetic neuropathy is the consequence of inhibition of AGE formation.

One of the mechanisms by which AGE exerts its toxic effects is its interaction with its receptor for advanced glycation end products (RAGE) *(42,43)*. This leads to the activation of a cascade of cytotoxic pathways, including the activation of the transcription factor, which is nuclear factor (NF)-κB, thought to contribute to diabetic neuropathy *(44)*. Infusion into diabetic rats containing the soluble fragment of RAGE (sRAGE), which consists of the AGE-binding domain that attenuated vascular dysfunction, indicated that the AGE–RAGE interaction plays an important role in diabetic microvascular complications *(45)*. Administration of sRAGE also appeared to be beneficial to diabetic neuropathy *(44)*. When 3-months WT mice with diabetes were placed on 55°C hot-plate, the latency or the time it takes for them to respond was significantly longer than that for the mice without diabetes, indicating impairment of pain perception as a result of diabetes. Treatment with sRAGE for 3 weeks completely normalized the delayed latency in mice with diabetes, indicating that RAGE is involved in the hyperglycemia-induced loss of pain perception. When the RAGE null mutant mice were induced to become diabetic, the nociceptive threshold was lower than that of the WT mice with diabetes but significantly higher than that of the WT or RAGE-null mice without diabetes, indicating that RAGE deficiency provides partial protection against diabetic sensory neuropathy *(44)*. Examination of the footpad skin of these mice revealed that diabetes led to a significant decrease in the PGP9.5-positive small nerve fibers in this tissue in the WT mice. However, a similar decrease in nerve fibers also occurred in the footpad of the diabetic RAGE null mice, indicating that RAGE deficiency did not protect against diabetes-induced small fiber loss, although it partially restored the function of the remaining nerve fibers.

The RAGE null mice and the WT control mice in these experiments were offspring of SVEV129 × C57BL. Perhaps, because of their hybrid genetic background, diabetes did not cause a significant reduction in their MNCV or SNCV. Interestingly, diabetes led to a dramatic induction of NF-κB activity in the sciatic nerve of the WT mice as judged by electrophorectic mobility shift assay. Activation of NF-κB is thought to be the key contributor to hyperglycemia-induced tissue lesions. Yet the large increase in NF-κB in the sciatic nerve did not lead to any significant change in the MNCV or SNCV, indicating that this transcription factor might not play an important role in the pathogenesis of diabetic neuropathy. It would be interesting to cross the RAGE null mutation into pure C57BL genetic background where the WT mice exhibit significant reduction in MNCV and SNCV when induced to become diabetic. Then one can determine if RAGE deficiency has any protective effect on diabetes-induced MNCV and SNCV reduction.

It is interesting that while sRAGE completely restored the nociceptive threshold of the diabetic mice, RAGE deficiency only partially restored it. One explanation is that there are other AGE receptors such as the macrophage scavenger receptor and the galectin-3 that might have similar deleterious effect as RAGE when they interact with AGE *(46)*. With the removal of RAGE, AGEs would bind to other receptors to exert their toxic effects. On the other hand, infusion of sRAGE might engage all the AGEs, making them unavailable to interact with their receptors. However, treatment with antibodies against RAGE that should only block RAGE, also has a strong protective effect similar to sRAGE, suggesting that there are other contributing factors to the diabetes-induced neural dysfunction. Further, intracellular AGE and AGE attached to extracellular matrix are also thought to contribute to diabetic lesions *(47,48)*. However, these AGEs are not able to interact with cell surface RAGE or other AGE receptors. Removing RAGE is unlikely to block their deleterious effects.

PARP ACTIVATION

Increased oxidative stress, presumably from polyol pathway activity, AGE and its interaction with RAGE, PKC activation, and hyperactivity of mitochondrial respiratory chain, damages lipids, proteins, and DNA *(49)*. DNA strand breaks activate PARP, which is an enzyme that transfers ADP-ribose from NAD^+ to nuclear proteins as part of the DNA repair process *(50)*. However, overactivation of PARP has deleterious consequences, including the activation of the proinflammatory transcription factors NF-κB and activating protein-1 (AP-1), and the induction of the apoptosis-inducing factor, which might lead to cell death *(51–53)*. PARP has been shown to be involved in the diabetes-induced endothelial dysfunction of the aorta *(54,55)*.

The *PARP-1* gene KO mice were used to determine if PARP contributes to diabetic neuropathy. These mice showed no obvious abnormality. Under normal rearing condition, the MNCV of their sciatic nerve, the SNCV of their digital nerve, and the morphology of their sciatic nerve all appeared normal *(56)*. When the WT mice were induced to become diabetic by streptozotocin, their MNCV and SNCV decreased significantly. In the sciatic nerve of the diabetic WT mice there was significant increase in immunostaining of PAR, the product of PARP activity, indicating that hyperglycemia activates PARP. The PARP-1 null mice on the other hand, showed no reduction in MNCV and SNCV when induced to become diabetic. The blood glucose level in the diabetic PARP null mice was not different from that of the diabetic WT mice, indicating that PARP did not affect diabetes, but plays an important role in the diabetes-induced functional impairment in the peripheral nerves. When fed a high galactose diet, which simulates and exaggerates the AR-mediated glucose toxicity, the WT mice showed even higher reduction in sciatic nerve MNCV and digital nerve SNCV than that of diabetic WT mice. PARP deficiency partially protected these mice against galactosemia-induced MNCV reduction, and completely protected them against galactosemia-induced SNCV reduction, suggesting that hyperglycemia-induced activation of PARP is mediated by AR activity. This was confirmed by experiments that showed that ARI blocked the hyperglycemia-induced oxidative stress and activation of PARP in the sciatic nerve *(57)*. The deleterious effect of overactivation of PARP is because of the depletion of its cofactor NAD^+, which leads to the depletion of ATP. In the sciatic nerve of the diabetic and galactosemic WT mice, the ratio of phosphocreatine (PCr)/Cr, an indicator of cytosolic ATP/ADP ratio, was significantly decreased. There was no change in PCr/Cr ratio in the sciatic nerve of the diabetic or galactosemic PARP-deficient mice. These results indicate that hyperglycemia activation of PARP depletes cellular PCr level, and by inference, energy stores.

Two structurally unrelated inhibitors of PARP were administered to diabetic rats. Both drugs were able to normalize diabetes-induced reduction in MNCV, SNCV, nerve blood flow, blood pressure, and vascular conductance in rats, confirming the findings in PARP-1 null mice *(56)*. These PARP inhibitors are potential drugs for the prevention and treatment of diabetic neuropathy and other complications. However, studies are needed to determine if inhibition of PARP activity would leave unrepaired the hyperglycemia-induced DNA breaks that might lead to mutations and cancers.

NEUROFILAMENT

NF, consisting of heavy, medium, and light subunits, form the major structural lattice of axon. The function of the neurofilaments (NF) is not clear, but abnormal phosphorylation of these proteins is associated with neurodegenerative diseases such as amyotrophic lateral sclerosis, Parkinson disease, Alzheimer disease, and diabetes *(58,59)*. In diabetes, stress-activated protein kinases are thought to be involved in their aberrant phosphorylation *(60,61)*. Further, abnormal NF accumulation was found in the proximal axon segments of diabetic dorsal root ganglia sensory neurons in human *(62)*, whereas loss of NF in distal nerve terminals of sensory neurons was observed in long-term diabetic rats *(63)*. Impairment in the transport of NF proteins was suspected *(64)*. However, it is not clear whether these changes are the cause or consequences of diabetic lesion.

A line of TG mice that express a fusion protein, where the carboxyl terminus of heavy NF was replaced by β-galactosidase, was found to be completely devoid of peripheral axonal NF, as the fusion protein causes aggregates of NF to precipitate in the perikarya *(65)*. Interestingly, there was no obvious abnormality in the NF-deficient mice except that the caliber of their axons was smaller. In the tibial nerve of these mice the number of fibers and fiber density were higher than that of the WT mice, whereas the axon diameter and axon area were smaller *(66)*. Under normal condition there was no obvious degeneration of their neurons, but the NCV was slower and the amplitude of the nerve action potential was dramatically lower than that of the WT mice, presumably because of the smaller caliber axons. The reduction in SNCV was much more pronounced than the reduction in MNCV. These mice were of Swiss genetic background. When induced to become diabetic, the WT mice exhibited no significant reduction in MNCV and SNCV in their sciatic nerve. The diabetic NF-deficient mice on the other hand, showed significant slowing of MNCV and SNCV. The reduction of the NCV was attenuated by the administration of insulin. Although there was no significant change in the structure of the tibial and sural nerves in the diabetic WT mice, diabetes caused significant decreases in the number of fibers, fiber density, fiber size, axon diameter, and axon area in the tibial nerve of the NF-deficient mice. Similar structural changes were also observed in their sural nerve, except that there was no significant change in the fiber number.

The fact that the NF-deficient mice were more susceptible to diabetes-induced lesions indicates that NF has protective effect on diabetic neuropathy. However, it is not clear whether this finding is relevant to the pathogenesis of the disease in WT animals where slowing of NCV is associated with aberrant phosphorylation of NF rather than the lack of it *(60)*. The decrease in NCV is one of the earliest sign of hyperglycemia-induced lesion, whereas loss of NF occurs only after prolonged hyperglycemia *(63)*. It is possible that loss of NF is the consequence of neuropathy rather than a contributing factor of the disease. The significant NCV slowing and structural abnormalities in the peripheral nerve of the NF-deficient mice before induction of diabetes make interpretation of the results difficult. At this point, it is not clear how the aberrant phosphorylation of NF might contribute to the pathogenesis of diabetic neuropathy.

PERSPECTIVE

In this brief review, the applications of TG and gene KO technologies to investigate the pathogenesis of diabetic neuropathy have been discussed. The results of the genetic analyses on the polyol pathway are in complete agreement with findings from ARI studies, thus unambiguously confirming the role of the polyol pathway in the pathogenesis of this disease. These studies also demonstrated that the polyol pathway-induced oxidative stress rather than osmotic stress is the cause of the diabetes-induced toxicity, and that the mechanism involves the activation of PARP. The experiments with RAGE null mice demonstrated that interaction between plasma AGE and RAGE is the main source of toxicity induced by nonenzymatic glycation. The contribution by intracellular AGE and AGE attached to extracellular matrix to diabetic neuropathy remains unclear. The finding that the development of diabetic neuropathy is accelerated in NF-deficient mice is difficult to interpret because these mice already showed functional and structural abnormalities in the nerve before the induction of diabetes. Perhaps a more appropriate model would be mice lacking the kinase that phosphorylates NF under hyperglycemia.

Genetic analysis of the pathogenic mechanism of a disease has its advantages and disadvantages. The main advantage is that it avoids the uncertainty of drug specificity and availability. Further, with the advent of genome sequence information and DNA array and proteomic analysis of diseases, there will be exponential increase in the number of genes implicated in various diseases that need to be verified. Currently, it is faster to inactivate gene functions by gene KO, antisense RNA, or siRNA technology than by developing specific chemical inhibitors of the gene products. However, gene manipulation by conventional TG and gene KO technologies might affect tissue development, making them unsuitable for adult disease studies. The NF-deficient mice described earlier illustrate this point. More sophisticated TG and gene KO technologies developed in recent years circumvent some of these problems *(67)*. Several inducible transgene expression systems have been developed. In these systems the expression of the transgenes is under the control of a promoter that is regulated by a ligand-activated transcriptional enhancer. Usually, the ligands are cell-permeable small molecules not found in mammalian cells such as tetracycline, ecdysone, or isopropyl-β-thiogalactosidase. Although expression systems based on hormone receptor-activated promoters have also been developed. Thus, tissue specificity (determined by the specificity of the promoter that express the ligand-activated transcriptional enhancer) and time of induction (determined by the administration of the ligand) of the transgene can be selected as desired. However, development of these inducible transgene expression systems is quite

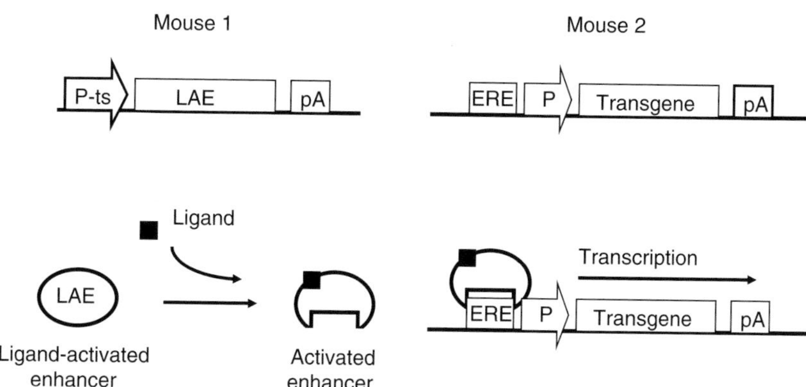

Fig. 1. Inducible transgene expression. Mouse line 1 carries the *LAE* gene that is under the control of a tissue-specific promoter. The transcription termination signal is indicated by (pA). Mouse 2 carries the transgene of interest that is under the control of the minimal promoter (P) together with the enhancer responsive element to which the activated LAE binds. Mating of mouse 1 and 2 brings the two transgenes together. Administration of the ligand to the mice activates the LAE, which then binds to enhancer responsive element to initiate the transcription of the transgene in tissues where LAE is expressed.

cumbersome because two separate TG lines have to be developed (Fig. 1) one carrying the ligand-activated enhancer (LAE) (Fig. 1, Mouse 1), and the other the transgene under the control of the ligand/enhancer inducible promoter (Fig. 1, Mouse 2). Mating between these two TG lines brings the two transgenes into the same host. Conditional gene KO methods have also been developed (Fig. 2). Again this involves the development of two separate mouse lines. First, by conventional gene-targeting technique, the site-specific recombination sequence loxP is introduced into both sides of the gene to be removed (Fig. 2, Mouse 1). Second, by mating of the loxP mice with a TG mouse line that carries the recombinase (Cre) (Fig. 2, mouse 2) will activate recombination between two loxP sequences resulting in the removal of the gene in between. Ablation of the gene in a specific tissue can be obtained by engineering the expression of the *Cre* transgene in the target tissue using an appropriate promoter. Temporal specificity of gene ablation can be obtained by engineering the *Cre* transgene expression under the control of an inducible promoter.

There are other genetically engineered mice that are useful for analyzing the pathogenic mechanisms of diabetic neuropathy. An example is the mice carrying a reporter gene under the control of the NF-κB promoter *(68)*. Abnormal NF-κB activity is thought to be an important part of the mechanisms leading to diabetic neuropathy *(69–71)*. In this case the reporter gene β-globin, is not normally found in nerve tissues, and its transcript is readily detectable by reverse transcriptase-polymerase chain reaction. Generally, this type of reporter transgene is applicable to study the transcriptional regulation of transcription factors, structural proteins, or enzymes that do not have a convenient assay to determine their activity or abundance. Other reporter genes such as β-galactosidase *(72)*, luciferase *(73)*, or fluorescence proteins *(74)* provide even more convenient in vitro and *in situ* assessment of gene induction or suppression. However, some of these reporter genes do have toxic effect in some cells. Another useful tool is

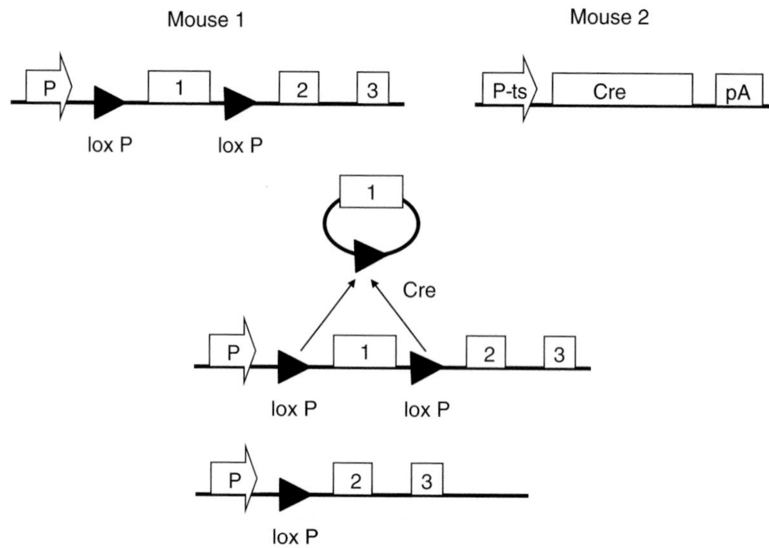

Fig. 2. Conditional gene knockout. For mouse line 1, by conventional homologous gene replacement technique, two site-specific recombination sequences (lox P) are introduced into each side of the sequence to be deleted. Open boxes with numbers indicate the introns. Conventional transgenic technology generates mouse line 2, where the site-specific *Cre* gene is under the control of a tissue-specific promoter. The transcription termination signal for the transgene is indicated by (pA). Mating between mouse 1 and 2 brings the Cre and lox P together. Expression of Cre in the target tissue activates the removal of the intron 1 as indicated.

the line of TG mice that express the yellow fluorescence protein (YFP) specifically in the neurons *(75)*. The transgene in these mice is the YFP cDNA under the control of the thymas cell antigen (thy1.2) promoter. All sensory and motor neurons in these thy1.2-YFP mice emit yellow fluorescence when viewed under the fluorescence microscope. When the hairs of these mice are shaved to expose their skin, the dermal nerve fibers are visible under fluorescence microscope without sectioning of tissue. When induced to become diabetic, the loss of fluorescence nerve fibers was evident *(76)*. Thus, these mice provide a noninvasive method of monitoring small fiber degeneration and regeneration during the progression of diabetes, and they will be useful for testing the efficacy of drugs in the treatment and prevention of diabetic neuropathy (Fig. 3).

The advantage of having a variety of techniques to manipulate their genome made mice a favorite animal model to study various biomedical problems. Consequently, a large number of TG and KO mice have been developed, and many more will be developed in the future. The RAGE, PARP, and NF null mice were not originally developed to study diabetic neuropathy. Undoubtedly, many other mutant mice will also be useful for investigating the pathogenesis of this disease. Although, mice do not exhibit the full spectrum of the pathology of diabetic neuropathy as in human, using them to determine the mechanisms leading to common pathology, and find out the reasons for the differences, will surely help us better understand the pathogenesis of this debilitating disease in human.

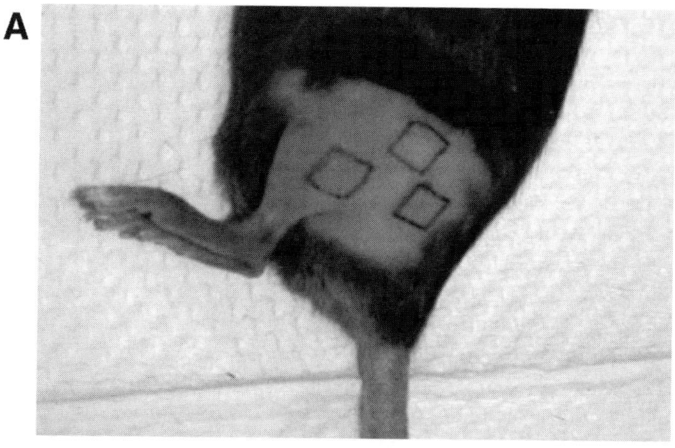

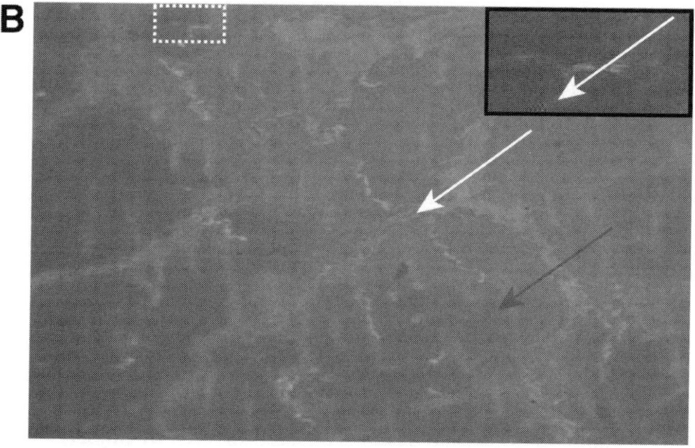

Fig. 3. YFP-positive fibers in the skin from live animal. **(A)** The hair was removed from the leg of Thy1-YFP mice. **(B)** YFP-positive fibers in the skin showing the primary small fibers (red arrow) and the secondary small fibers (white arrows). Original magnification: ×100.

ACKNOWLEDGMENTS

The authors wish to thank Ms. Marcella Ma for her technical assistance with the DNA and ES cell microinjection for generating HAR TG and AR KO mice. The genetic analyses of polyol pathway enzymes in diabetic complications have been possible because of support from the Research Grant Council of Hong Kong.

REFERENCES

1. Gabbay KH, Merola LO, Field RA. Sorbitol pathway: presence in nerve and cord with substrate accumulation in diabetes. *Science* 1966;151:209–210.
2. Oates PJ. Polyol pathway and diabetic peripheral neuropathy. *Int Rev Neurobiol* 2002;50: 325–392.
3. King RH. The role of glycation in the pathogenesis of diabetic polyneuropathy. *Mol Pathol* 2001;54:400–408.

4. Thornalley PJ. Glycation in diabetic neuropathy: characteristics, consequences, causes, and therapeutic options. *Int Rev Neurobiol* 2002;50:37–57.
5. Cameron NE, Cotter MA. Effects of protein kinase Cbeta inhibition on neurovascular dysfunction in diabetic rats: interaction with oxidative stress and essential fatty acid dysmetabolism. *Diabetes Metab Res Rev* 2002;18:315–323.
6. Eichberg J. Protein kinase C changes in diabetes: is the concept relevant to neuropathy? *Int Rev Neurobiol* 2002;50:61–82.
7. Nishikawa T, Edelstein D, Du XL, et al. Normalizing mitochondrial superoxide production blocks three pathways of hyperglycaemic damage. *Nature* 2000;404:787–790.
8. Lee AY, Chung SK, Chung SS. Demonstration that polyol accumulation is responsible for diabetic cataract by the use of transgenic mice expressing the aldose reductase gene in the lens. *Proc Natl Acad Sci USA* 1995;92:2780–2784.
9. Leitges M, Schmedt C, Guinamard R, et al. Immunodeficiency in protein kinase cbeta-deficient mice. *Science* 1996;273:788–791.
10. Williamson JR, Chang K, Frangos M, et al. Hyperglycemic pseudohypoxia and diabetic complications. *Diabetes* 1993;42:801–813.
11. Sarges R, Oates PJ. Aldose reductase inhibitors: recent developments. *Prog Drug Res* 1993;40:99–161.
12. Pfeifer MA, Schumer MP, Gelber DA. Aldose reductase inhibitors: the end of an era or the need for different trial designs? *Diabetes* 1997;46(Suppl 2):S82–S89.
13. Tsai SC, Burnakis TG. Aldose reductase inhibitors: an update. *Ann Pharmacother* 1993;27:751–754.
14. Cameron NE, Cotter MA. Dissociation between biochemical and functional effects of the aldose reductase inhibitor, ponalrestat, on peripheral nerve in diabetic rats. *Br J Pharmacol* 1992;107:939–944.
15. Yamaoka T, Nishimura C, Yamashita K, et al. Acute onset of diabetic pathological changes in transgenic mice with human aldose reductase cDNA. *Diabetologia* 1995;38:255–261.
16. Yagihashi S, Yamagishi S, Wada R, et al. Galactosemic neuropathy in transgenic mice for human aldose reductase. *Diabetes* 1996;45:56–59.
17. Yagihashi S, Yamagishi SI, Wada RR, et al. Neuropathy in diabetic mice overexpressing human aldose reductase and effects of aldose reductase inhibitor. *Brain* 2001;124: 2448–2458.
18. Koya D, King GL. Protein kinase C activation and the development of diabetic complications. *Diabetes* 1998;47:859–866.
19. Frank RN. Potential new medical therapies for diabetic retinopathy: protein kinase C inhibitors. *Am J Ophthalmol* 2002;133:693–698.
20. Koya D, Haneda M, Nakagawa H, et al. Amelioration of accelerated diabetic mesangial expansion by treatment with a PKC beta inhibitor in diabetic db/db mice, a rodent model for type 2 diabetes. *FASEB J* 2000;14:439–447.
21. Kim H, Sasaki T, Maeda K, Koya D, Kashiwagi A, Yasuda H. Protein kinase Cbeta selective inhibitor LY333531 attenuates diabetic hyperalgesia through ameliorating cGMP level of dorsal root ganglion neurons. *Diabetes* 2003;52:2102–2109.
22. Yamagishi S, Uehara K, Otsuki S, Yagihashi S. Differential influence of increased polyol pathway on protein kinase C expressions between endoneurial and epineurial tissues in diabetic mice. *J Neurochem* 2003;87:497–507.
23. Cameron NE, Cotter MA. Metabolic and vascular factors in the pathogenesis of diabetic neuropathy. *Diabetes* 1997;46(Suppl 2):S31–S37.
24. Low PA, Lagerlund TD, McManis PG. Nerve blood flow and oxygen delivery in normal, diabetic, and ischemic neuropathy. *Int Rev Neurobiol* 1989;31:355–438.
25. Malik RA, Williamson S, Abbott C, et al. Effect of angiotensin-converting-enzyme (ACE) inhibitor trandolapril on human diabetic neuropathy: randomised double-blind controlled trial [see comments]. *Lancet* 1998;352:1978–1981.

26. Song Z, Fu DT, Chan YS, Leung S, Chung SS, Chung SK. Transgenic mice overexpressing aldose reductase in Schwann cells show more severe nerve conduction velocity deficit and oxidative stress under hyperglycemic stress. *Mol Cell Neurosci* 2003;23: 638–647.
27. Ho HT, Chung SK, Law JW, et al. Aldose reductase-deficient mice develop nephrogenic diabetes insipidus. *Mol Cell Biol* 2000;20:5840–5846.
28. Chung SS, Ho EC, Lam KS, Chung SK. Contribution of polyol pathway to diabetes-induced oxidative stress. *J Am Soc Nephrol* 2003;14:S233–S236.
29. Tilton RG, Chang K, Nyengaard JR, van den EM, Ido Y, Williamson JR. Inhibition of sorbitol dehydrogenase. Effects on vascular and neural dysfunction in streptozocin-induced diabetic rats. *Diabetes* 1995;44:234–242.
30. Obrosova IG, Fathallah L, Lang HJ, Greene DA. Evaluation of a sorbitol dehydrogenase inhibitor on diabetic peripheral nerve metabolism: a prevention study. *Diabetologia* 1999;42:1187–1194.
31. Schmidt RE, Dorsey DA, Beaudet LN, Plurad SB, Williamson JR, Ido Y. Effect of sorbitol dehydrogenase inhibition on experimental diabetic autonomic neuropathy. *J Neuropathol Exp Neurol* 1998;57:1175–1189.
32. Lee FK, Chung SK, Chung SS. Aberrant mRNA splicing causes sorbitol dehydrogenase deficiency in C57BL/LiA mice. *Genomics* 1997;46:86–92.
33. Ng TF, Lee FK, Song ZT, et al. Effects of sorbitol dehydrogenase deficiency on nerve conduction in experimental diabetic mice [published erratum appears in Diabetes 1998 Aug;47(8):1374]. *Diabetes* 1998;47:961–966.
34. Cameron NE, Tuck Z, McCabe L, Cotter MA. Effect of the hydroxyl radical scavenger, dimethylthiourea, on peripheral nerve tissue perfusion, conduction velocity and nociception in experimental diabetes. *Diabetologia* 2001;44:1161–1169.
35. Kishi Y, Schmelzer JD, Yao JK, et al. Alpha-lipoic acid: effect on glucose uptake, sorbitol pathway, and energy metabolism in experimental diabetic neuropathy. *Diabetes* 1999;48: 2045–2051.
36. Stevens MJ, Obrosova I, Cao X, Van Huysen C, Greene DA. Effects of DL-alpha-lipoic acid on peripheral nerve conduction, blood flow, energy metabolism, and oxidative stress in experimental diabetic neuropathy. *Diabetes* 2000;49:1006–1015.
37. Cerami A, Vlassara H, Brownlee M. Role of advanced glycosylation products in complications of diabetes. *Diabetes Care* 1988;11(Suppl 1):73–79.
38. Ryle C, Donaghy M. Non-enzymatic glycation of peripheral nerve proteins in human diabetics. *J Neurol Sci* 1995;129:62–68.
39. Cameron NE, Cotter MA, Dines K, Love A. Effects of aminoguanidine on peripheral nerve function and polyol pathway metabolites in streptozotocin-diabetic rats. *Diabetologia* 1992;35:946–950.
40. Yagihashi S, Kamijo M, Baba M, Yagihashi N, Nagai K. Effect of aminoguanidine on functional and structural abnormalities in peripheral nerve of STZ-induced diabetic rats. *Diabetes* 1992;41:47–52.
41. Thornalley PJ. Use of aminoguanidine (Pimagedine) to prevent the formation of advanced glycation endproducts. *Arch Biochem Biophys* 2003;419:31–40.
42. Schmidt AM, Hasu M, Popov D, et al. Receptor for advanced glycation end products (AGEs) has a central role in vessel wall interactions and gene activation in response to circulating AGE proteins. *Proc Natl Acad Sci USA* 1994;91:8807–8811.
43. Stern DM, Yan SD, Yan SF, Schmidt AM. Receptor for advanced glycation endproducts (RAGE) and the complications of diabetes. *Ageing Res Rev* 2002;1:1–15.
44. Bierhaus A, Schiekofer S, Schwaninger M, et al. Diabetes-associated sustained activation of the transcription factor nuclear factor-kappaB. *Diabetes* 2001;50:2792–2808.

45. Wautier JL, Zoukourian C, Chappey O, et al. Receptor-mediated endothelial cell dysfunction in diabetic vasculopathy. Soluble receptor for advanced glycation end products blocks hyperpermeability in diabetic rats. *J Clin Invest* 1996;97:238–243.
46. Vlassara H. The AGE-receptor in the pathogenesis of diabetic complications. *Diabetes Metab Res Rev* 2001;17:436–443.
47. Brownlee M. Advanced protein glycosylation in diabetes and aging. *Annu Rev Med* 1995;46:223–234.
48. Vlassara H, Palace MR. Diabetes and advanced glycation endproducts. *J Intern Med* 2002;251:87–101.
49. Rosen P, Nawroth PP, King G, Moller W, Tritschler HJ, Packer L. The role of oxidative stress in the onset and progression of diabetes and its complications: a summary of a Congress Series sponsored by UNESCO-MCBN, the American Diabetes Association and the German Diabetes Society. *Diabetes Metab Res Rev* 2001;17:189–212.
50. Herceg Z, Wang ZQ. Functions of poly(ADP-ribose) polymerase (PARP) in DNA repair, genomic integrity and cell death. *Mutat Res* 2001;477:97–110.
51. Ha HC, Snyder SH. Poly(ADP-ribose) polymerase is a mediator of necrotic cell death by ATP depletion. *Proc Natl Acad Sci USA* 1999;96:13,978–13,982.
52. Liaudet L. Poly(adenosine 5′-diphosphate) ribose polymerase activation as a cause of metabolic dysfunction in critical illness. *Curr Opin Clin Nutr Metab Care* 2002;5: 175–184.
53. Yu SW, Wang H, Poitras MF, et al. Mediation of Poly(ADP-Ribose) Polymerase-1-Dependent Cell Death by Apoptosis-Inducing Factor. *Science* 2002;297:259–263.
54. Garcia SF, Virag L, Jagtap P, et al. Diabetic endothelial dysfunction: the role of poly(ADP-ribose) polymerase activation. *Nat Med* 2001;7:108–113.
55. Soriano FG, Pacher P, Mabley J, Liaudet L, Szabo C. Rapid Reversal of the Diabetic Endothelial Dysfunction by Pharmacological Inhibition of Poly(ADP-Ribose) Polymerase. *Circ Res* 2001;89:684–691.
56. Obrosova IG, Li F, Abatan OI, et al. Role of poly(ADP-ribose) polymerase activation in diabetic neuropathy. *Diabetes* 2004;53:711–720.
57. Obrosova IG, Pacher P, Szabo C, et al. Aldose Reductase Inhibition Counteracts Oxidative-Nitrosative Stress and Poly(ADP-Ribose) Polymerase Activation in Tissue Sites for Diabetes Complications. *Diabetes* 2005;54:234–242.
58. Al Chalabi A, Miller CC. Neurofilaments and neurological disease. *Bioessays* 2003;25:346–355.
59. Liu Q, Xie F, Siedlak SL, et al. Neurofilament proteins in neurodegenerative diseases. *Cell Mol Life Sci* 2004;61:3057–3075.
60. Fernyhough P, Gallagher A, Averill SA, et al. Aberrant neurofilament phosphorylation in sensory neurons of rats with diabetic neuropathy. *Diabetes* 1999;48:881–889.
61. Fernyhough P, Schmidt RE. Neurofilaments in diabetic neuropathy. *Int Rev Neurobiol* 2002;50:115–144.
62. Schmidt RE, Dorsey D, Parvin CA, Beaudet LN, Plurad SB, Roth KA. Dystrophic axonal swellings develop as a function of age and diabetes in human dorsal root ganglia. *J Neuropathol Exp Neurol* 1997;56:1028–1043.
63. Scott JN, Clark AW, Zochodne DW. Neurofilament and tubulin gene expression in progressive experimental diabetes: failure of synthesis and export by sensory neurons. *Brain* 1999;122(Pt 11):2109–2118.
64. Medori R, Autilio-Gambetti L, Monaco S, Gambetti P. Experimental diabetic neuropathy: impairment of slow transport with changes in axon cross-sectional area. *Proc Natl Acad Sci USA* 1985;82:7716–7720.
65. Tu PH, Robinson KA, de Snoo F, et al. Selective degeneration fo Purkinje cells with Lewy body-like inclusions in aged NFHLACZ transgenic mice. *J Neurosci* 1997;17:1064–1074.

66. Zochodne DW, Sun HS, Cheng C, Eyer J. Accelerated diabetic neuropathy in axons without neurofilaments. *Brain* 2004;127:2193–2200.
67. Bockamp E, Maringer M, Spangenberg C, et al. Of mice and models: improved animal models for biomedical research. *Physiol Genomics* 2002;11:115–132.
68. Lernbecher T, Muller U, Wirth T. Distinct NF-kappa B/Rel transcription factors are responsible for tissue-specific and inducible gene activation. *Nature* 1993;365:767–770.
69. Mezzano S, Aros C, Droguett A, et al. NF-kappaB activation and overexpression of regulated genes in human diabetic nephropathy. *Nephrol Dial Transplant* 2004;19:2505–2512.
70. Purves TD, Tomlinson DR. Diminished transcription factor survival signals in dorsal root ganglia in rats with streptozotocin-induced diabetes. *Ann NY Acad Sci* 2002;973:472–476.
71. Ramana KV, Friedrich B, Srivastava S, Bhatnagar A, Srivastava SK. Activation of nuclear factor-kappaB by hyperglycemia in vascular smooth muscle cells is regulated by aldose reductase. *Diabetes* 2004;53:2910–2920.
72. Cui C, Wani MA, Wight D, Kopchick J, Stambrook PJ. Reporter genes in transgenic mice. *Transgenic Res* 1994;3:182–194.
73. Contag CH, Bachmann MH. Advances in in vivo bioluminescence imaging of gene expression. *Annu Rev Biomed Eng* 2002;4:235–260.
74. Hadjantonakis AK, Nagy A. The color of mice: in the light of GFP-variant reporters. *Histochem Cell Biol* 2001;115:49–58.
75. Brendza RP, O'Brien C, Simmons K, et al. PDAPP; YFP double transgenic mice: a tool to study amyloid-beta associated changes in axonal, dendritic, and synaptic structures. *J Comp Neurol* 2003;456:375–383.
76. Chen YS, Chung SSM, Chung SK. Noninvasive Monitoring of Diabetes-Induced Cutaneous Nerve Fiber Loss and Hypoalgesia in thy1-YFP Transgenic Mice. *Diabetes* 2005;54(11):3112–3118.

5
Hyperglycemia-Initiated Mechanisms in Diabetic Neuropathy

Irina G. Obrosova, PhD

SUMMARY

Peripheral diabetic neuropathy (PDN) is one of the most devastating complications of diabetes mellitus. The pathogenesis of PDN involves hyperglycemia-initiated mechanisms as well as other factors, i.e., impaired insulin signaling, hypertension, disturbances of fatty acid and lipid metabolism. This review describes new findings in animal and cell culture models:

1. Supporting the importance of previously established hyperglycemia-initiated mechanisms, such as increased aldose reductase activity, nonenzymatic glycation/glycoxidation, activation of protein kinase-C, and enhanced oxidative stress;
2. Addressing the role of nitrosative stress and downstream effectors of oxidative-nitrosative injury, such as poly(ADP-ribose) polymerase activation, mitogen-activated protein kinase activation, cyclooxygenase-2 activation, activation of nuclear factor-κB, and impaired Ca^{2+} homeostasis and signaling; and
3. Suggesting the contribution of two newly discovered mechanisms, such as 12/15-lipoxygenase activation and Na^+/H^+-exchanger-1 activation, in PDN.

Key Words: Aldose reductase; calcium signaling; cyclooxygenase-2; diabetic neuropathy; 12/15-lipoxygenase; mitogen-activated protein kinases; nuclear factor-κB; nonenzymatic glycation; oxidative-nitrosative stress; protein kinase-C; poly(ADP-ribose) polymerase.

INTRODUCTION

Diabetic distal symmetric sensorimotor polyneuropathy affects at least 50% of patients with diabetes, and is the leading cause of foot amputation *(1)*. The pathogenesis of peripheral diabetic neuropathy (PDN) is studied better than the pathogenesis of autonomic neuropathy. However, two largest clinical trials in subjects with type 1 and type 2 diabetes, i.e., diabetes control and complication trial (DCCT) and United Kingdom Prospective Diabetes Study (UKPDS), indicate that intensive therapy and improved blood glucose control reduce incidence and slow progression of both complications, thus implicating hyperglycemia as a leading causative factor *(1,2)*. In particular, the DCCT has shown that the incidence of neuropathy in type 1 diabetes can be reduced by more than 50% with intensive therapy and optimal glycemic control *(3)*. Intensive therapy in the DCCT caused a significant risk reduction of developing autonomic nerve abnormalities at 5 years only

From: *Contemporary Diabetes: Diabetic Neuropathy: Clinical Management, Second Edition*
Edited by: A. Veves and R. Malik © Humana Press Inc., Totowa, NJ

in the primary prevention group (4 vs 9%) *(4)*. A number of mechanisms have been proposed to link chronic hyperglycemia to diabetes-induced deficits in motor and sensory nerve conduction velocities (MNCV and SNCV) and other manifestations of PDN. The vascular concept of PDN implies that diabetes-induced endothelial dysfunction with resulting decrease in nerve blood flow (NBF) and endoneurial hypoxia has a key role in functional and morphological changes in the diabetic nerve *(5)*. Endothelial changes in *vasa nervorum* have been attributed to multiple mechanisms including increased aldose reductase (AR) activity, nonenzymatic glycation and glycoxidation, activation of protein kinase C (PKC), oxidative-nitrosative stress, changes in arachidonic acid, and prostaglandin metabolism *(5)*. Recently, they have also been attributed to decreased expression of the vanilloid receptor 1 in *vasa nervorum (6)*, increased production of angiotensin (AT) II, and activation of the AT1-receptor *(7)*, activation of poly(ADP-ribose) polymerase (PARP)-1 *(8)*, nuclear factor (NF)-κB *(9)*, and cyclooxygenase-2 (COX-2) *(10)*, and others. The neurochemical concept of PDN suggests the importance of similar mechanisms in the *neural* elements of peripheral nervous system (PNS), i.e., Schwann cells and neurons. Other pathobiochemical mechanisms in PNS have also been invoked.

Those include:

1. Metabolic abnormalities, such as downregulation of Na^+/K^+ ATP-ase activity *(11)*, "pseudohypoxia," i.e., increase in free cytosolic $NADH/NAD^+$ ratio attributed to increased conversion of sorbitol to fructose by sorbitol dehydrogenase (SDH) *(12)*, changes in fatty acid and phospholipid metabolism *(13)*, and recently, 12/15-lipoxygenase (12/15-LO) activation *(14)*;
2. Impaired neurotrophic support *(15,16)*;
3. Changes in signal transduction *(17)*; and
4. Dorsal root ganglion (DRG) and Schwann cell mitochondrial dysfunction and premature apoptosis *(18,19)*.

The present review of the findings obtained in the last 5 years has two major objectives, i.e., (1) to evaluate new experimental evidence that supports or disproves previously formulated concepts of the pathogenesis of PDN and (2) to characterize newly discovered mechanisms.

ROLE FOR VASCULAR VS NONVASCULAR MECHANISMS

Over past several years, the importance of vascular vs nonvascular mechanisms in the pathogenesis of PDN remained a subject of debate. The key role of reduced NBF and resulting endoneurial hypoxia in diabetes-associated nerve conduction deficit appears to be supported by the findings with a variety of vasodilators; for example, the α_1-adrenoceptor antagonist prazosin *(20)*, the K(ATP) channel openers, celikalim and WAY135201 *(21)*, the AT-converting enzyme (ACE) inhibitor enalapril, and the AT II receptor antagonist L158809 *(7)*. In author's study *(20)*, prazosin prevented diabetes-induced neurovascular dysfunction and MNCV deficit, without counteracting accumulation of sorbitol pathway intermediates, depletion of myo-inositol and taurine, downregulation of Na, K-ATPase activity, and enhanced lipid peroxidation in the peripheral nerve. Therefore, none of these neurochemical changes appears to be of critical importance for the development of nerve conduction slowing in, at least, short-term diabetes. However, it is unclear whether the aforementioned and other vasodilators can affect peripheral nerve metabolism and conduction independent from their vasodilator properties (*see* the information on lisinopril and salbutamol provided on page 70).

The vascular concept of PDN is seemingly supported by the recent findings with the high molecular weight metal chelator, hydroxyethyl starch-deferoxamine (HESD), known to be confined to vascular space when administered intravenously and therefore, not to penetrate into neural elements of the peripheral nerve. Alleviation of both NBF and nerve conduction deficits *(22,23)*, combined with reduced superoxide and peroxynitrite formation in *vasa nervorum (23)*, in HESD-treated streptozotocin (STZ)-diabetic rats in comparison with the corresponding untreated group could be interpreted as a proof for the key role of vascular mechanism in MNCV and SNCV deficit in early diabetes. However, it is not excluded that in vascular space, HESD is metabolized with formation of deferoxamine, with its subsequent delivery to a neural compartment of the peripheral nerve. In addition, such reactive oxygen species (ROS) as hydrogen peroxide, lipid peroxide (free form), and peroxynitrite can move from vascular to nonvascular space, and alleviation of oxidative stress in one nerve compartment will automatically diminish ROS abundance in others. The role of NBF in early PDN is also seemingly supported by the studies with the endothelial nitric oxide synthase inhibitor N^G-nitro-L-arginine (L-NNA). Cotreatment with L-NNA abolished the effects of pharmacological agents, i.e., vasodilators, antioxidants, AR inhibitors (ARIs), and so on, on both NBF and nerve conduction velocity *(5)*. However, the spectrum of pharmacological effects of L-NNA is not studied to the extent that would allow to exclude adverse effects on MNCV and SNCV through some unidentified mechanism.

The neurochemical consequences of nerve ischemia in the peripheral nerve have not been studied in detail. *Retinal* response to ischemia involves a compensatory upregulation of several neurotrophic factors partially protecting retinal neurons from the lack of oxygen and nutrients *(24)*. Correspondingly, administration of neurotrophic factors to rats with experimental PDN prevents nerve conduction slowing, without counteracting a decrease in NBF. This phenomenon has been observed with neurotrophin-3, brain-derived neurotrophic factor as well as prosaposin *(16)*. Furthermore, the most recent study by Calcutt et al. *(25)* demonstrated that treatment of diabetic rats with a sonic hedgehog-IgG fusion protein (1) ameliorated retrograde transport of nerve growth factor (NGF) increased sciatic nerve concentrations of calcitonin-gene related product and neuropeptide Y, (2) restored normal MNCV and SNCV, and (3) maintained the axonal caliber of large myelinated fibers.

These beneficial effects have been observed in the absence of any improvement in NBF. The importance of neurochemical mechanisms in diabetes-associated nerve conduction deficits, energy failure, and abnormal sensation and pain is also supported by several other reports *(26–29)*. In the study *(26)*, the PARP inhibitor PJ34 caused only a modest 17% increase of NBF, but essentially normalized nerve energy state and completely reversed diabetes-induced MNCV and SNCV deficits. Therefore, a complete normalization of NBF is not required for correction of MNCV or SNCV in diabetic rats. Furthermore, in the recent low-dose PARP inhibitor-containing combination therapy study *(27)*, two combination therapies, i.e., the PARP inhibitor 1,5-isoquinolinediol (ISO) plus the ACE inhibitor lisinopril and ISO plus the β_2-adrenoceptor agonist salbutamol equally efficiently counteracted diabetes-associated neurovascular dysfunction, but only ISO plus salbutamol corrected MNCV deficit, whereas the effect of ISO plus lisinopril was statistically nonsignificant. Thus, correction of NBF is insufficient for correction of MNCV deficit. Note that both lisinopril and salbutamol have signal transduction and metabolic effects that could be completely independent of vasodilator properties of these agents. Lisinopril acts as a weak antioxidant *(30)* and nitric oxide scavenger *(31)*. The spectrum of pharmacological effects of salbutamol is even more impressive: the agent inhibits expression of intercellular adhesion molecule-1, CD-40, and CD-14 *(32)* as well as eicosanoid biosynthesis *(33)*, increases intracellular cyclic adenosine monophosphate concentration, cyclic adenosine monophosphate-dependent PKA, adenylyl cyclase, phosphatase PP2A and L-type Ca^{2+} channel activities, modulates G protein signaling *(34)*, and stimulates pentose phosphate pathway *(35)*. At least, several of these effects might account for better MNCV response to ISO plus salbutamol in comparison with ISO plus lisinopril treatment.

The most impressive evidence for dissociation of NBF and nerve conduction changes has recently been generated in two studies in animal models of type 2 diabetes *(28,29)*. In type 2 BBZDR/Wor rats, neurovascular defects were not accompanied by sensory nerve conduction slowing or hyperalgesia *(28)*. Furthermore, in type 2 Zucker diabetic fatty rats development of motor nerve conduction deficit at 12–14 weeks of age markedly preceded decrease in sciatic endoneurial nutritive blood flow (at 24–28 weeks of age *[29]*). In contrast, in Zucker rats with impaired glucose tolerance, but absent fasting hyperglycemia (a model of the initial stage of type 2 diabetes) neurovascular dysfunction developed earlier than motor nerve conduction deficit (at 24–28 weeks of age and 32 weeks of age, respectively *[29]*).

ROLE FOR AR

The sorbitol pathway of glucose metabolism consists of two reactions. First, glucose is reduced to its sugar alcohol sorbitol by NADPH-dependent AR. Then, sorbitol is oxidized to fructose by NAD-dependent SDH. Negative consequences of the sorbitol pathway hyperactivity under diabetic or hyperglycemic conditions include intracellular sorbitol accumulation and resulting osmotic stress, and generation of fructose, which is 10-times more potent glycation agent than glucose. One group reported that increased flux through SDH leads to so called "pseudohypoxia," i.e., an increased free cytosolic $NADH/NAD^+$ *(12)* ratio, whereas others *(36)* did not find a relation between cytosolic or mitochondrial $NAD^+/NADH$ redox state and SDH activity in the peripheral nerve. Two groups obtained the results indicating that increased AR, but not SDH, activity contributes to PDN *(37,38)*. Furthermore, SDH inhibition appeared detrimental rather than beneficial, for autonomic neuropathy *(39)*.

The role for AR in PDN has been reviewed in detail *(40)*. New evidence for the key role of AR in the pathogenesis of PDN has been generated in both experimental studies in animal and cell culture models of diabetes and clinical trials of ARIs. The results implicating increased AR activity in high glucose- and diabetes-induced oxidative-nitrosative stress *(41–45)* and downstream events such as mitogen-activated PK (MAPK) activation *(46,47)*, PARP activation *(45)*, COX-2 activation (Calcutt et al., unpublished), and activation of NF-κB *(46,47)* are of particular interest. In particular, it has been demonstrated that AR inhibition counteracts high glucose- and diabetes-induced superoxide formation in aorta *(42)*, epineurial vessels *(45)*, and endothelial cells *(43–45)*; nitrotyrosine formation in peripheral nerve *(45)*, *vasa nervorum (46)*, kidney glomeruli and tubuli *(48)*, endothelial cells *(43)* and mesangial cells *(48)*, lipid peroxidation in peripheral nerve *(41),* and retina *(44)*; loss of two major nonenzymatic antioxidants, reduced glutathione (GSH), and ascorbate in peripheral nerve *(45)*, and downregulation of several major antioxidative defense enzymes in the retina *(44)*.

The author's group has also demonstrated the key role for AR in diabetes-associated PARP activation in peripheral nerve, retina, kidney, human Schwann cells, and mesangial cells *(45,48)*. Two groups have demonstrated the key role for AR in diabetes-induced MAPK activation in rat lens and DRG neurons *(46,47)*. Both PARP activation and MAPK activation are involved in transcriptional regulation of gene expression, through the transcription factors NF-κB, activator protein-1, p53, and others *(49,50)*. Activation of these transcription factors leads to upregulation of inducible nitric oxide synthase, COX-2, endothelin-1, cell-adhesion molecules, and inflammatory genes *(49,51)*. Thus, the demonstration of a major contribution of AR to oxidative-nitrosative stress and PARP and MAPK activation in tissue-sites for diabetic complications allows to predict that in the near future the link between increased AR activity and altered transcriptional regulation and gene expression will be established. Any product of genes controlled through PARP- and MAPK-dependent transcription factors, regardless of how unrelated to the sorbitol pathway this product looks from a biochemical point of view, will be affected by a diabetes-associated increase in AR activity and amenable to control by AR inhibition. In accordance with this prediction, the most recent findings have shown that increased AR activity is responsible for diabetes-induced COX-2 upregulation in the spinal cord (Calcutt et al., unpublished), and NF-κB activation in high-glucose exposed vascular smooth muscle cells *(52)*.

The role for AR in the pathogenesis of PDN is supported by findings obtained in AR-overexpressing and AR-knockout mice. Yagihashi et al. *(53)* demonstrated that induction of STZ-diabetes in the mice transgenic for human AR resulted in more severe peripheral nerve sorbitol and fructose accumulation, MNCV deficit, and nerve fibre atrophy than in their nontransgenic littermates. Treatment of diabetic transgenic mice with the ARI WAY121-509 significantly prevented the accumulation of sorbitol, the decrease in MNCV, and the increased myelinated fibre atrophy in diabetic transgenic mice. Similar findings had been obtained in another transgenic mouse model that overexpressed AR specifically in the Schwann cells of peripheral nerve under the control of the rat myelin protein zero promoter *(54)*. The transgenic mice exhibited a significantly higher reduction in MNCV under both diabetic and galactosemic conditions than the nontransgenic mice with normal AR content. In contrast, AR-deficient mice appeared protected from motor nerve conduction slowing after 4 and 8 weeks of STZ-diabetes *(55)*. These data lend further support to the important role of AR in functional, metabolic, and morphological abnormalities characteristic of PDN.

The findings in transgenic and knockout mouse models are in line with new studies with structurally diverse ARIs. Coppey et al. *(56)* implicated AR in diabetes-induced impairment of vascular reactivity of epineurial vessels, an early manifestation of PND, which precedes motor nerve conduction slowing. The author's group has demonstrated that established functional and metabolic abnormalities of, at least, early PDN, can be reversed with an adequate dose of ARI, i.e., the dose that completely suppressed diabetes-associated sorbitol pathway hyperactivity *(41)*. Calcutt et al. *(57)* have shown that the ARI statil prevented thermal hypoalgesia in STZ-diabetic rats; furthermore, another ARI IDD 676, given from the onset of diabetes, prevented the development of thermal hyperalgesia and also, stopped progression to thermal hypoalgesia when delivered in the last 4 weeks of an 8-week period of diabetes. In a recent study *(58)*, the ARI fidarestat partially prevented thermal hypoalgesia in type 2 diabetic ob/ob mice. Tactile allodynia was not prevented by an ARI treatment in either Calcutt et al. *(57)* study in STZ-diabetic rats or the study in ob/ob mice *(58)*, although paw withdrawal thresholds in response to light touch with flexible von Frey filaments tended to increase in ob/ob mice treated with fidarestat in comparison with the corresponding untreated group.

New evidence supports the role of AR in the pathogenesis of advanced PDN. A 15-month AR inhibition with fidarestat dose-dependent corrected slowed F-wave, MNCV, and SNCV in STZ-diabetic rats *(55)*. In the same study, diabetes-induced paranodal demyelination, and axonal degeneration were reduced to the normal with such low dose of fidarestat as 2 mg/kg. Other manifestations of advanced PDN, such as axonal atrophy, distorted axon circularity, and reduction of myelin sheath thickness were also inhibited. The results of two double-blind placebo-controlled clinical trials of fidarestat in patients with type 1 and type 2 diabetes are also encouraging (*60*, and Arezzo et al., unpublished). Fidarestat improved electrophysiological measures of median and tibial MNCV, F-wave minimum latency, F-wave conduction velocity, and median SNCV (forearm and distal) as well as subjective symptoms of PDN, such as numbness, spontaneous pain, sensation of rigidity, paresthesia in the sole upon walking, heaviness in the foot, and hypesthesia. These results support the applicability of the AR concept to the pathogenesis of human PDN, and are consistent with the findings of another clinical trial with the ARI zenarestat, indicating that robust inhibition of AR in diabetic human nerve improves nerve physiology and fiber density *(51)*. Recently, improvement of sensory nerve conduction velocity in patients with diabetic sensorimotor polyneuropathy was also found with the new ARI AS-3201 *(62)*. The role for AR in human diabetic neuropathy is also supported by the genetic polymorphism data *(40)*.

ROLE FOR NONENZYMATIC GLYCATION

Glycation is the nonenzymatic reaction of glucose, α-oxoaldehydes, and other saccharide derivatives with proteins, nucleotides, and lipids, with formation of early glycation adducts (fructosamines) and advanced glycation end products (AGE). Formation of some AGE, i.e., pentosidine and N^{ε}-[carboxymethyl]-lysine, combines both glycation and oxidative steps in a process termed "glycooxidation." In the last several years, the role for glycation/glycoxidation in diabetic complications including diabetic neuropathy has been extensively reviewed *(63–65)*. A number of new studies in animal models of diabetes and human subjects support the role of this mechanism.

Using the state-of-the art technique, i.e., liquid chromatography with tandem mass spectrometry (MS) detection, Karachalias et al. *(66)* produced evidence of accumulation of fructosyl-lysine and AGE in peripheral nerve of STZ-diabetic rats. In particular, sciatic nerve concentrations of N^{ε}-[carboxymethyl]-lysine and N^{ε}-[carboxyethyl]-lysine were markedly increased in diabetic rats in comparison with controls. Hydroimidazolone AGEs derived from glyoxal, nethylglyoxal, and deoxyglucosone were major AGEs quantitatively. The receptor for AGE (RAGE) was localized both in endothelial and Schwann cells of the peripheral nerve *(67)*. Recently generated RAGE–/– mice appeared partially protected from diabetes-associated pain perception loss, an indicator of long-standing diabetic neuropathy *(68)*. Furthermore, in the same study, loss of pain perception was reversed in the diabetic wild-type mice treated with soluble RAGE. The new inhibitor of AGE and advanced lipoxidation end product (ALE) formation, pyridoxamine, previously reported to be effective against diabetic nephropathy and retinopathy was found to reverse established sciatic endoneurial NBF, MNCV, and SNCV deficits in STZ-diabetic rats with 8-week duration of diabetes *(69)*. Of interest, this correction was achieved in the absence of any significant effect of the agent on the levels of AGE/ALEs, *N*-(carboxymethyl)lysine, and *N*-(carboxyethyl)lysine in total sciatic nerve protein, which suggests that short-term diabetes and pyridoxamine treatment target AGE/ALE in *vasa nervorum* rather than neural components of the peripheral nerve. Another new antiglycation agent OPB-9195 reduced sciatic nerve immunoreactive AGE expression, and prevented the slowing of tibial motor nerve conduction, downregulation of Na^+, K^+-ATPase activity, and accumulation of 8-hydroxy-2′-deoxyguanosine (a marker of DNA oxidative damage) in STZ-diabetic rats with 24-week duration of diabetes *(70)*.

High-dose therapy of thiamine and benfotiamine, suppressed AGE accumulation in the peripheral nerve *(66)* and reversed diabetic neuropathy *(71)*, potentially by reducing the levels of triose phosphates through activation of transketolase. Several in vitro studies describe adverse effects of AGE precursors and AGE *per se* in Schwann cells *(72,73)*. In particular, methylglyoxal was found to induce rat Schwann cell apoptosis through oxidative stress-mediated activation of p38 MAPK *(72)*. AGE derived from glyceraldehyde and glycolaldehyde, but not from glucose induced rat Schwann cell apoptosis, decreased cell viability and replication, decreased mitochondrial membrane potential, activated NF-κB, and enhanced production of inflammatory cytokines, i.e., tumor necrosis factor (TNF-α) and interleukin-β *(73)*.

Several new studies support the presence of AGE accumulation in patients with diabetes mellitus. The AGE pyrraline immunoreactivity was more intense in the optic nerve head of diabetic subjects in comparison with nondiabetic controls *(74)*. Pronounced AGE immunoreactivity was detected in axons and myelin sheaths in 90% of patients with type 2 diabetes, but not in control subjects, and the intensity of axonal AGE positivity significantly correlated with the severity of morphological alterations characteristic for PDN *(75)*. In the same study, AGE positivity was clearly present in endoneurium, perineurium, and microvessels of patients with diabetes. Bierhaus et al. *(68)* have demonstrated that ligands of RAGE, the receptor itself, activated NF-κB, p65, and interleukin-6 colocalized in the microvasculature of sural nerve biopsies obtained from human subjects with diabetic neuropathy. Furthermore, N^{ε}-[carboxymethyl]-lysine, RAGE, and NF-κB were found in the sural nerve perineurium, epineurial vessels, and endoneurial vessels of subjects with impaired glucose tolerance-related polyneuropathy *(76)*. Several clinical studies support the role of glycation in the pathogenesis of PDN and other diabetes complications *(77–79)*. In particular, it has been reported that increased accumulation of skin AGE precedes and correlates with clinical manifestations of diabetic neuropathy *(77)*. In another study, AGE accumulation in skin, serum, and saliva increased with progression of neuropathy, nephropathy, and retinopathy *(78)*.

Furthermore, serum N^{ε}-[carboxymethyl]-lysine concentrations were found significantly higher in children and adolescents with type 1 diabetes and diabetes complications (background retinopathy, microalbuminuria, and neuropathy) in comparison with the uncomplicated group *(79)*.

ROLE FOR PKC ACTIVATION

PKC includes a superfamily of isoenzymes, many of which are activated by 1,2-diacylglycerol in the presence of phosphatidylserine. PKC isoforms phosphorylate a wide variety of intracellular target proteins and have multiple functions in signal transduction-mediated cellular regulation. The role for PKC in the pathogenesis of PDN has been reviewed in detail *(80)*. PKC is activated in *vasa nervorum* of diabetic rats *(81)*, and vessel-rich epineurial vessels of diabetic mice *(82)*. PKC has been reported decreased *(83)*, unchanged *(81)*, or increased *(84)* in the diabetic rat nerve, and decreased in endoneurial tissue of diabetic mouse nerve *(82)*. PKC activity was markedly reduced in DRG neurons of the wild-type STZ-diabetic mice and furthermore, in the diabetic mice overexpressing human AR *(85)*. These changes were associated with reduced expression and activity of the membrane PKC-α isoform that translocated to cytosol. The membrane PKC-IIβ isoform expression was increased in AR-overexpressing diabetic transgenic mice, but not in the wild-type mice *(85)*.

The experimental evidence obtained with various PKC inhibitors as well as the diacylglycerol complexing agent cremophor by several groups *(81,86–88)* suggests the detrimental role of PKC activation in *vasa nervorum*. The PKC inhibitors, WAY151003, chelerythrine, and LY333531 as well as cremophor prevented or reversed NBF and conduction deficits *(81,86,87)*, and the PKC inhibitor *bis*-indolylmaleimide-1HCl corrected acetylcholine-mediated vascular relaxation in epineurial arterioles in the STZ-diabetic rat model *(88)*. The role for neural PKC in the pathogenesis of PDN remains unclear. However, recent findings suggest that neuronal PKC might be related to diabetes-associated changes in expression, phosphorylation, and function of the vanilloid receptor 1, known to play an important role in diabetic neuropathic pain *(89)*. The novel PKC-β isoform selective inhibitor JTT-010 was found to ameliorate nerve conduction deficits, hyperalgesia (formalin test in its first phase), and hypoalgesia (formalin test in its second phase, tail flick test) in STZ-diabetic rats *(90)*.

ROLE FOR OXIDATIVE-NITROSATIVE STRESS

Enhanced oxidative stress, resulting from imbalance between production and neutralization of ROS is a well-recognized mechanism in the pathogenesis of PDN. Recently, considerable progress has been made in the detection of diabetes-associated oxidative injury in PNS. New studies *(20,21,36,41,45,81)* have confirmed previously established lipid peroxidation product accumulation, GSH depletion and increase in GSSG/GSH ratio, and downregulation of superoxide dismutase (SOD) activity in the diabetic peripheral nerve. In addition, new markers of ROS-induced injury have been identified in peripheral nerve, *vasa nervorum*, and DRG in experimental PDN. Those include decreased catalase and total quinone reductase activities, depletion of ascorbate and taurine, and increase in dehydroascorbate/ascorbate ratio in peripheral nerve *(91,92)*, increased production of superoxide in *vasa nervorum (23)*, and accumulation of

8-hydroxy-2′-deoxyguanosine in DRG of STZ-diabetic rats *(19)*. Diabetes-induced changes of the aforementioned indices were corrected by antioxidant treatment. Accumulation of nitrotyrosine (a footprint of peroxynitrite-induced protein nitration) has been documented in peripheral nerve *(45)*, *vasa nervorum (23,45)*, and DRG *(93)* in diabetic rats, and peripheral nerve of diabetic mice *(92)* indicating that diabetes creates not just oxidative, but oxidative-nitrosative stress in PNS. Enhanced nitrosative stress has been documented in human subjects with PDN *(95)*.

Numerous new studies reveal the important role of oxidative stress in nerve functional, metabolic, neurotrophic, and morphological abnormalities characteristic of PDN. The role for ROS in diabetes-associated nerve conduction and blood flow deficits has been demonstrated in studies with the "universal" antioxidant DL-α-lipoic acid *(5,23,91)*, which is known to combine free radical and metal chelating properties with an ability (after conversion to dehydrolipoic acid) to regenerate levels of other antioxidants, i.e., GSH, ascorbate, α-tocopherol, catalase, and glutathione peroxidase. It has also been confirmed with other antioxidants including the potent hydroxyl radical scavenger dimethylthiourea *(96)*, HESD *(22,23)*, and the SOD mimetic M40403 *(97)*. Furthermore, diabetes-induced MNCV and SNCV deficits were reversed by the peroxynitrite decomposition catalyst FP15 treatment *(94)*. Two groups produced experimental evidence of an important role for oxidative stress in diabetes-associated impairment of neurotrophic support to the peripheral nerve by demonstrating that (1) diabetes and pro-oxidant treatment caused NGF and NGF-regulated neuropeptide, i.e., substance P and neuropeptide Y deficits in the sciatic nerve that were, at least partially, counteracted by α-lipoic acid *(98)*, (2) taurine alleviated oxidative stress and prevented diabetes-induced NGF deficit in the sciatic nerve of STZ-diabetic rats *(92)*.

Several reports suggest involvement of oxidative-nitrosative stress in the mechanisms underlying diabetic neuropathic pain and abnormal sensory responses. In the author's study *(94)*, the tail-flick response latency was increased in diabetic NOD mice in comparison with nondiabetic mice, and this variable was normalized by short-term treatment with the peroxynitrite decomposition catalyst FP15. Studies in the "mature" short-term rat model of STZ-diabetes revealed thermal and mechanical hyperalgesia (exaggerated pain state), which was corrected by lipoic acid *(99)*, and alleviated by the hydroxyl radical scavenger dimethylthiourea *(96)*. The mechanisms underlying diabetes-associated tactile allodynia have not been studied in detail; however, a beneficial effect of nitecapone, an inhibitor of catechol-*O*-methyltransferase and antioxidant, suggests the involvement of oxidative-nitrosative stress *(100)*.

Over past several years, the continuing debate about a "primary mechanism" of diabetic complications has centered on the origin of oxidative stress in tissue-sites for diabetic complications and its relation to other factors. According to the "unifying concept" of Brownlee derived from the studies in bovine aortic endothelial cell culture model *(101,102)*, mitochondrial superoxide production is the primary source of oxidative stress in tissue-sites for diabetes complications, and this mechanism is responsible for sorbitol pathway hyperactivity, formation of AGE, and activation of PKC. Whereas the important role of mitochondria as a ROS-producing factory in diabetes is beyond doubt, this hypothesis has several major problems. First, it is unclear whether similar relations exist in other cell types, i.e., Schwann cells, and DRG neurons, and whether the mitochondrial mechanism of ROS generation is so important in high glucose-exposed human cells. Second, several extramitochondrial mechanisms have been demonstrated to be of similar, if not greater importance in endothelial cells of *vasa nervorum* as well as other cells. Those include xanthine oxidase, a multifunctional enzyme of an iron-sulfur molybdenum flavoprotein composition, present in high concentrations in capillary endothelial cells and producing oxygen free radicals, uric acid, and superoxide. Xanthine oxidase is increased in ischemia-reperfusion injuries, anoxia, inflammation, and diabetes mellitus *(103)*. The importance of xanthine oxidase in PDN has been recently demonstrated by Cameron et al. (unpublished) who found a complete correction of diabetes-associated NBF and conduction deficits by the xanthine oxidase inhibitor allopurinol. The same group produced evidence suggesting that two other extramitochondrial mechanisms of ROS generation, i.e., NAD(P)H oxidase and semicarbazide sensitive amine oxidase are also involved in the pathogenesis of PDN *(104,105)*. A recent study *(106)* demonstrated the important role for NAD(P)H oxidase as well as the lipid ceramide in palmitate-induced oxidative stress in bovine retinal pericytes, and several reports suggest the key role for NAD(P)H oxidase in the diabetic kidney *(107,108)*. Evidence for the important contribution of other factors, i.e., 12/15-LO *(109)*, COX-2 *(110)*, and endothelin-1 *(111)*, is emerging. Moreover, inhibition of Na^+/H^+-exchanger (NHE)-1 was found to counteract diabetes-associated superoxide generation in aorta (M.A.Yorek., unpublished). Third, the "unifying concept" is in disagreement with numerous findings supporting the role for AR in oxidative-nitrosative stress in tissue sites for diabetic complications *(41,42,44,45,48)* as well as in high glucose-exposed endothelial cells *(43–45)*. Note that the role for AR in high glucose-induced superoxide production in endothelial cells has been demonstrated by several groups that used different techniques and structurally diverse ARIs *(42–45)*. The author's group has shown that AR inhibition normalized indices of oxidative stress including lipid peroxidation product, GSH, and ascorbate concentrations as well as SOD activity and nitrotyrosine and poly(ADP-ribose) immunoreactivities in the diabetic peripheral nerve *(41,45,112)*.

ROLE FOR DOWNSTREAM EFFECTORS OF ROS INJURY AND OTHER NEWLY DISCOVERED MECHANISMS

PARP Activation

One of the important effectors of oxidative-nitrosative injury and associated DNA single-strand breakage is activation of the nuclear enzyme PARP *(113)*. Once activated, PARP cleaves nicotinamide adenine dinucleotide (NAD^+) with formation of nicotinamide and ADP-ribose residues, which are attached to nuclear proteins and to PARP itself, with formation of poly(ADP-ribosyl)ated protein polymers. The process leads to:

1. NAD^+ depletion and energy failure *(26,27,113,114)*;
2. Changes of transcriptional regulation and gene expression *(49,51)*; and
3. Poly(ADP-ribosyl)ation and inhibition of the glycolytic enzyme glyceraldehyde 3-phosphate dehydrogenase, resulting in diversion of the glycolytic flux toward several pathways implicated in diabetes complications *(115)*.

Recent studies of the author's group *(8,26,27)* revealed that PARP activation is an early and fundamental mechanism of PDN. It is clearly manifest in peripheral nerve, *vasa nervorum*, and DRG neurons of STZ-diabetic rats *(8,26,27,93)* as well as peripheral nerves of STZ-diabetic *(94)* and ob/ob mice *(58)*. Using endothelial and Schwann cell markers and double immunostaining *(8)*, the author's group localized PARP activation in endothelial and Schwann cells of diabetic rat nerve. The group was first to develop the Western blot analysis of poly(ADP)-ribosylated proteins in rat sciatic nerve *(27)*; using this approach, it was found that poly(ADP)-ribosylated protein abundance increased by 74% in rats with 4-weeks duration of STZ-diabetes in comparison with nondiabetic controls. Furthermore, accumulation of poly(ADP)-ribosylated proteins was found to develop very early, i.e., within about 12–24 hours of exposure of cultured human endothelial and Schwann cells to high glucose *(27)*. PARP-1 protein abundance was not affected by high glucose or PARP inhibitor treatment in either cell type consistent with the current knowledge on PARP-1 as abundantly expressed enzyme with very minor, if any, transcriptional regulation *(113)*.

Studies with several structurally unrelated PARP inhibitors and PARP-deficient (*PARP–/–*) mice revealed the important role for PARP activation in diabetes-associated MNCV and SNCV deficits, neurovascular dysfunction and peripheral nerve energy failure *(8,26)*. *PARP–/–* mice were protected from both diabetic and galactose-induced MNCV and SNCV deficits and nerve energy failure that were clearly manifest in the wild-type (*PARP+/+*) diabetic or galactose-fed mice *(8)*. Two structurally unrelated PARP inhibitors, 3-aminobenzamide and 1,5-ISO, reversed established NBF and conduction deficits as well as energy deficiency in STZ-diabetic rats *(8)*. The third inhibitor, PJ34, essentially corrected nerve conduction deficits and energy deficiency despite relatively modest (17%) reversal of NBF deficit *(26)*. From these observations, it was concluded that PARP inhibition counteracts diabetes-induced changes in nerve energy state (the variable that correlates best with nerve conduction) primarily through recently discovered effect on the glycolytic enzyme glyceraldehyde 3-phosphate dehydrogenase *(115)* and resulting improvement of glucose utilization in Schwann cells. The latter is consistent with normalization of free NAD^+/NADH ratio, an index of tricarboxylic cycle activity and glucose utilization, in the peripheral nerve mitochondrial matrix of PJ34-treated diabetic rats *(26)*. In the same study, PJ34 treatment counteracted accumulation of lactate and glutamate, as well as depletion of α-glutarate in diabetic peripheral nerve. Nerve glucose and sorbitol pathway intermediate concentrations were similarly elevated in PJ34-treated and untreated rats *(26)*, which is consistent with the downstream localization of PARP activation, consequent to increased AR activity and resulting oxidative-nitrosative stress, in the pathogenesis of diabetic complications. In other two studies of the author's group, diabetes-induced peripheral nerve protein poly(ADP)-ribosylation was blunted by the ARI fidarestat and the peroxynitrite decomposition catalyst FP15 *(45,94)*, thus, indicating the importance of increased AR activity and nitrosative stress among the upstream mechanisms underlying PARP activation.

The low-dose PARP inhibitor-containing combination therapies (with two vasodilators, the ACE-inhibitor lisinopril and β–adrenoceptor agonist salbutamol), reversed neurovascular dysfunction, SNCV deficit (MNCV deficit was reversed by salbutamol-, but not lisinopril-containing drug combination) as well as thermal and mechanical hyperalgesia in rats with short-term STZ-diabetes *(27)*. Theoretically, PARP activation can contribute to diabetic neuropathic pain and abnormal sensory responses through several mechanisms including, but not limited to:

1. Upregulation of TNF-α and other inflammatory genes;
2. Activation of p38 MAP kinase in the spinal cord and Schwann cells; and
3. Ca^{2+}-regulated excitotoxic insults, all of which have been implicated in the pathogenesis of painful neuropathy *(116–118)*.

PARP-dependence of TNF-α overexpression, p38 MAP kinase activation, and Ca^{2+}-regulated excitotoxic insults in pathological conditions associated with oxidative stress have been experimentally documented *(113,119–121)*. Furthermore, recent studies from the author's group revealed that PARP activation not only results from, but also exacerbates oxidative-nitrosative stress in peripheral nerve, *vasa nervorum*, and human Schwann cells *(122)*. Detailed studies of the role for PARP activation in diabetic neuropathic pain are in progress in the laboratory.

Activation of MAPKs

Numerous findings indicate that ROS and reactive nitrogen species cause MAPK activation *(17,123)*, and increasing evidence supports the importance of MAPKs in the pathogenesis of PDN. ERK, p38 MAPK, and JNK are activated in DRG neurons of STZ-diabetic rats *(17)*. Enhanced p38 MAPK activation in response to endothelin-1 or platelet-derived growth factor has been observed in immortalized Schwann cells cultured in 25 m*M* glucose in comparison with those in 5 m*M* glucose *(124)*. Sural nerve JNK activation and increases in total levels of p38 and JNK have been observed in patients with both type 1 and type 2 diabetes *(17)*. MAPKs are implicated in aberrant neurofilament phosphorylation, a phenomenon involved in the etiology of the diabetic sensory polyneuropathy *(125)*. Fernyhough et al. *(125)* have reported a two- to threefold elevation of neurofilament phosphorylation in lumbar DRG of STZ-diabetic and spontaneously diabetic BB rats as well as 2.5-fold elevation in neurofilament M phosphorylation in sural nerve of BB rats. Diabetes-induced three- to fourfold increase in phosphorylation of a 54-kDa isoform of JNK in DRG and sural nerve correlated with elevated *c*-Jun and neurofilament phosphorylation. p38 activation in DRG neurons of STZ-diabetic rats is prevented by the ARIs sorbinil and fidarestat, which suggests the important role of AR in diabetes-related alterations in MAPK signaling *(126)*. The p38 MAPK inhibitor SB239063 corrected MNCV and SNCV deficits in STZ-diabetic rats, thus implicating p38 MAPK in motor and sensory nerve dysfunction *(47,126)*. In the same animal model, the p38-α MAPK inhibitor SD-282 counteracted mechanical allodynia, C-, but not a delta-fiber-mediated thermal hyperalgesia, and attenuated flinching behavior during the quiescent period and the second phase of the formalin response *(127)*. Spinal p38 MAPK has also been implicated in the neuropathic pain induced by inflammation *(128)*.

Activation of NF-kB

Both PARP-1 and MAPKs are involved in transcriptional regulation of gene expression, through the transcription factors NF-κB, activator protein-1, p53, and others *(113,114,129)*. Activated NF-κB has been identified in perineurium, epineurial vessels, and endoneurium in sural nerve biopsies of subjects with impaired glucose tolerance *(76)* and overt diabetes *(68)*. NF-κB activation was also found in isolated Schwann cells cultured in high glucose medium in comparison with those in low glucose *(130)* and such activation was prevented by the ARI fidarestat. Similar effect of AR inhibition on NF-κB activation was observed in high glucose-exposed vascular smooth muscle cells *(52)*. Activation of NF-κB and other transcription factors by high glucose *(52,130)* and oxidative stress *(131)* leads to upregulation of inducible nitric oxide synthase, COX-2, endothelin-1, cell adhesion molecules, and inflammatory genes *(49,51)*. Growing evidence indicates that the aforementioned transcription factors and their target genes are involved in the pathogenesis of diabetic complications, and, in particular, PDN *(9,10, 68,132)*. Thus, it is not surprising that inhibition of NF-κB by pyrrolidine dithiocarbamate and the serine protease inhibitor *N*-α-tosyl-L-lysine chloro-methylketone, i.e., IκB protease activity-blocking agent, corrected nerve conduction and blood flow deficits in STZ-diabetic rats *(9)*. In the same animal model, *N*-α-tosyl-L-lysine chloro-methylketone also partially reversed gastric autonomic neuropathy *(9)*.

Activation of COX-2 and 12/15-LO

Evidence for the important role of arachidonic acid metabolic pathways, i.e., COX-1 and COX-2, cytochrome P450 epoxygenase, and LOs in diabetes complications is emerging. The lipid products of these pathways include thromboxane, prostaglandins, leukotrienes, lipoxins, epoxyetraenoic acid, 12-hydroperoxy-eicosatetraenoic acid, 12-(HETE) hydroxy-eicosatetraenoic acid, 15-HETE, and a whole variety of their derivatives. COX-1 protein expression was reported unchanged in the diabetic peripheral nerve *(10)* and reduced in the spinal cord *(133)*, whereas COX-2 protein abundance was increased in both tissues *(10,133)*. Selective COX-2 inhibition with meloxicam prevented motor nerve conduction and endoneurial nutritive blood flow deficits in the diabetic rats *(10)*. The same group *(134)* found diabetic COX-2 deficient mice protected from MNCV and SNCV slowing that was clearly manifest in the diabetic wild-type mice. Several studies implicate COX-2 overexpression in increased production of hydroxyl radicals and hydrogen peroxide as well as lipid peroxidation *(110,135)*, and STZ-diabetic COX-2–/– mice have been reported to develop less severe peripheral nerve oxidative stress than the diabetic wild-type mice *(134)*.

One of the most interesting members of the LO family is 12/15-LO, a nonheme iron-containing dioxygenase that forms 12-hydroperoxy-eicosatetraenoic acid and 12- and 15-HETEs and oxidizes esterified arachidonic acid in lipoproteins (cholesteryl esters) and phospholipids *(109,136)*. 12/15-LO is abundantly expressed in endothelial cells (i.e., aortic and retinal endothelial cells), smooth muscle cells, monocyte/macrophages as well as renal mesangial cells, tubular epithelial cells, and podocytes, and the enzyme expression is increased under diabetic and hyperglycemic conditions *(109,136)*.

Recent in vivo and cell culture studies *(109,136,137)* revealed that high glucose-induced 12/15-LO activation affects multiple metabolic and signal transduction pathways, transcriptional regulation, and gene expression. The major consequences include increased free radical production and lipid peroxidation, MAPK and NF-κB activation, inflammatory response, excessive growth as well as adhesive and chemoattractant effects *(109,136,137)*. Recent findings from the author's group suggest an important role for 12/15-LO activation in peripheral DN *(14)*. In particular, it was found that:

1. 12/15-LO is abundantly expressed in mouse peripheral nerve and its expression increases in diabetic conditions;

2. 12/15-LO−/− mice with both type 1 (streptozotocin-induced) and type 2 (high fat diet-induced) diabetes develop less severe peripheral DN than wild-type mice;
3. Some manifestations of peripheral DN in STZ-diabetic mice are reversed by a short-term 12/15-LO inhibitor treatment;
4. 12/15-LO is abundantly expressed in human Schwann cells (HSC), one of the major cell targets in human DN, and its overexpression is clearly manifest after a short-term (24 h) exposure to high glucose; and
5. 12/15-LO overexpression in high glucose-exposed HSC contributes to activation (phosphorylation) of all three subtypes of MAPKs including p38 MAPK, ERK ½, and JNK-1, recently implicated in the pathogenesis of both experimental and human DN *(17,47,125–127)*.

These results provide the rationale for detailed studies of the role for 12/15-LO pathway in diabetic neuropathic changes.

Altered Ca^{2+} Homeostasis and Signaling

Growing evidence suggests that diabetic sensory neuropathy is associated with abnormal Ca^{2+} homeostasis and signaling in DRG neurons *(138,139)*. Enhanced Ca^{2+} influx through multiple high-threshold calcium currents is present in sensory neurons of several rat models of diabetes mellitus, including the spontaneously diabetic BioBred/Worchester (BB/W) rats and STZ-diabetic rats *(139)*. Sensory neurons of STZ-diabetic rats have increased mRNA expression of voltage-gated calcium channels *(140)*. Enhanced calcium entry in diabetes is also linked to the impairment of G protein-coupled modulation of calcium channel function *(138)*. Increased AR activity and taurine deficiency contribute to diabetes-related enhancement of voltage-dependent calcium currents in DRG neurons *(138,139)*. These two mechanisms probably converge at the level of oxidative stress and result in PARP activation known to promote $[Ca^{2+}]_i$ accumulation and impair calcium signaling. Resting $[Ca^{2+}]_i$ increased in rat lumbar nociceptive neurons with the duration of STZ diabetes, whereas calcium mobilization from the endoplasmic reticulum reduced *(140)*. $[Ca^{2+}]_i$ is essentially required for 12/15-LO catalytic activity *(141)* predominantly confined to cytoplasm *(142)*.

Evidence for important role of $[Ca^{2+}]_i$ in neuropathic pain of different origin and in particular, diabetic neuropathic pain is emerging. Luo et al. *(143)* found that injury to type-specific calcium channel alpha 2delta-1 subunit upregulation in rat neuropathic pain models (mechanical nerve injuries, diabetic neuropathy, chemical neuropathy) correlated with antiallodynic effect of the anticonvulsant gabapentin. Furthermore, a recent 6-week, randomized, double-blind, multicenter clinical trial in 246 patients with painful diabetic neuropathy revealed that pregabalin, a new drug that interacts with the alpha 2delta-1 protein subunit of the voltage-gated calcium channel, is a efficacious and safe treatment for diabetic neuropathic pain *(144)*. Similar findings have been obtained in another 12-week, randomized, double-blind, multicenter, placebo-controlled trial of pregabalin that revealed a significant pain relief in patients with chronic postherpetic neuralgia or painful diabetic neuropathy *(145)*.

Activation of NHE-1

Recent studies from the author's group suggest an important role for NHE-1 in PDN *(146)*. The NHE-1 specific inhibitor cariporide, at least, partially prevented MNCV and SNCV deficits, thermal hypoalgesia, mechanical hyperalgesia, and tactile allodynia in

STZ-diabetic rats. STZ-diabetic NHE-1+/– mice developed less severe early PDN than the wild-type mice. Increased NHE-1 protein expression was found early (about 24 hours) after exposure of human endothelial and Schwann cells to high glucose, thus suggesting that this mechanism can be of importance in human PDN *(147)*.

CONCLUSION

Multiple mechanisms are involved in the pathogenesis of PDN. New findings support the role for previously discovered mechanisms, such as increased AR activity, nonenzymatic glycation, PKC activation, and oxidative stress in functional and morphological abnormalities in the diabetic nerve. Evidence for the important role for nitrosative stress, MAPK activation, PARP activation, COX-2 activation, and Ca^{2+} signaling is emerging. Several newly discovered mechanisms include activations of NF-κB, the 12/15-LO pathway, and NHE-1. Studies of the role for these mechanisms in PDN and their interactions with other pathogenetic factors are in progress.

REFERENCES

1. Writing Team for the Diabetes Control and Complications Trial/Epidemiology of Diabetes Interventions and Complications Research Group. Effect of intensive therapy on the microvascular complications of type 1 diabetes mellitus. *JAMA* 2002;287:2563–2569.
2. Stratton I, Adler AI, Neil H, et al. Association of glycaemia with macrovascular and microvascular complications of type 2 diabetes (UKPDS 35): prospective observational study. *BMJ* 2000;321:405–412.
3. Boulton A. Lowering the risk of neuropathy, foot ulcers and amputations. *Diab Medicine* 1998;15(Suppl 4):S57–S59.
4. Donaghue K. Autonomic neuropathy: diagnosis and impact on health in adolescents with diabetes. *Horm Res* 1998;50(Suppl 1):33–37.
5. Cameron NE, Eaton SE, Cotter MA, Tesfaye S. Vascular factors and metabolic interactions in the pathogenesis of diabetic neuropathy. *Diabetologia* 2001;44:1973–1988.
6. Davidson EP, Coppey LJ, Yorek MA. Activity and expression of the vanilloid receptor 1 (TRPV1) is altered by long-term diabetes in epineurial arterioles of the rat sciatic nerve. *Diabetes Metab Res Rev* 2006;22:211–219.
7. Coppey LJ, Davidson EP, Rinehart TW, et al. ACE inhibitor or angiotensin II receptor antagonist attenuates diabetic neuropathy in streptozotocin-induced diabetic rats. *Diabetes* 2006;55:341–348.
8. Obrosova I, Li F, Abatan O, et al. Role of poly(ADP-ribose) polymerase activation in diabetic neuropathy. *Diabetes* 2004;53:711–720.
9. Cotter MA, Gibson TM, Cameron NE. Nuclear factor kappa B inhibition improves nerve function in diabetic rats. *Diabetologia* 2003;46:A70.
10. Pop-Busui R, Marinescu V, Van Huysen C, et al. Dissection of metabolic, vascular, and nerve conduction interrelationships in experimental diabetic neuropathy by cyclooxygenase inhibition and acetyl-L-carnitine administration. *Diabetes* 2002;51:2619–2628.
11. Sima AA, Sugimoto K. Experimental diabetic neuropathy: an update. *Diabetologia* 1999; 42:773–788.
12. Williamson JR, Chang K, Fringes M, et al. Hyperglycemia pseudohypoxia and diabetic complications. *Diabetes* 1993;42:801–813.
13. Kuruvilla R, Eichberg J. Depletion of phospholipid arachidonoyl-containing molecular species in a human Schwann cell line grown in elevated glucose and their restoration by an aldose reductase inhibitor. *J Neurochem* 1998;71:775–783.

14. Obrosova IG, Lyzogubov V, Marchand J, Bai F, Nadler JL, Drel VR. Role for 12/15-lipoxygenase in diabetic neuropathy. *Diabetes* 2006;55(Suppl 1):A189 [Abstract].
15. Tomlinson DR, Fernyhough P, Diemel LT. Role of neurotrophins in diabetic neuropathy and treatment with nerve growth factors. *Diabetes* 1997;46(Suppl 2):S43–S49.
16. Calcutt NA, Campana WM, Eskeland NL, et al. Prosaposin gene expression and the efficacy of a prosaposin-derived peptide in preventing structural and functional disorders of peripheral nerve in diabetic rats. *J Neuropathol Exp Neurol* 1999;58:628–636.
17. Purves T, Middlemas A, Agthong S, et al. A role for mitogen-activated protein kinases in the etiology of diabetic neuropathy. *FASEB J* 2001;15:2508–2514.
18. Russell JW, Sullivan KA, Windebank AJ, Herrmann DN, Feldman EL. Neurons undergo apoptosis in animal and cell culture models of diabetes *Neurobiol* 1999;6:347–363.
19. Schmeichel AM, Schmelzer JD, Low PA. Oxidative injury and apoptosis of dorsal root ganglion neurons in chronic experimental diabetic neuropathy. *Diabetes* 2003;52:165–171.
20. Obrosova IG, Van Huysen C, Fathallah L, Cao X, Stevens MJ, Greene DA. Evaluation of alpha(1)-adrenoceptor antagonist on diabetes-induced changes in peripheral nerve function, metabolism, and antioxidative defense. *FASEB J* 2000;14:1548–1558.
21. Hohman TC, Cotter MA, Cameron NE. ATP-sensitive $K(^{+})$ channel effects on nerve function, Na(+), K(+) ATPase, and glutathione in diabetic rats. *Eur J Pharmacol* 2000; 397:335–341.
22. Cameron NE, Cotter MA. Effects of an extracellular metal chelator on neurovascular function in diabetic rats. *Diabetologia* 2001;44:621–628.
23. Coppey LJ, Gellett JS, Davidson EP, Dunlap JA, Lund DD, Yorek MA. Effect of antioxidant treatment of streptozotocin-induced diabetic rats on endoneurial blood flow, motor nerve conduction velocity, and vascular reactivity of epineurial arterioles of the sciatic nerve. *Diabetes* 2001;50:1927–1937.
24. Chidlow G, Schmidt KG, Wood JP, Melena J, Osborne NN. Alpha-lipoic acid protects the retina against ischemia-reperfusion. *Neuropharmacology* 2002;43:1015–1025.
25. Calcutt NA, Allendoerfer K, Mizisin AP, et al. Therapeutic efficacy of sonic hedgehog protein in experimental diabetic neuropathy. *J Clin Invest* 2003;111:507–514.
26. Li F, Szabo C, Pacher P, et al. Evaluation of orally active poly(ADP-ribose) polymerase inhibitor in streptozotocin-diabetic rat model of early peripheral neuropathy. *Diabetologia* 2004;47:710–717.
27. Li F, Drel VR, Szabo C, Stevens MJ, Obrosova IG. Low-dose poly(ADP-ribose) polymerase inhibitor-containing combination therapies reverse early peripheral diabetic neuropathy. *Diabetes* 2005;54:1514–1522.
28. Stevens MJ, Zhang W, Li F, Sima AA. C-peptide corrects endoneurial blood flow but not oxidative stress in type 1 BB/Wor rats. *Am J Physiol Endocrinol Metab* 2004;287: E497–E505.
29. Oltman CL, Coppey LJ, Gellett JS, Davidson EP, Lund DD, Yorek MA. Progression of vascular and neural dysfunction in sciatic nerves of Zucker diabetic fatty and Zucker rats. *Am J Physiol Endocrinol Metab* 2005;289:E113–E122.
30. Mantle D, Patel VB, Why HJ, et al. Effects of lisinopril and amlodipine on antioxidant status in experimental hypertension. *Clin Chim Acta* 2000;299:1–10.
31. Noda Y, Mori A, Packer L. Free radical scavenging properties of alacepril metabolites and lisinopril. *Res Commun Mol Pathol Pharmacol* 1997;96:125–136.
32. Kuroki K, Takahashi HK, Iwagaki H, et al. Beta2-adrenergic receptor Stimulation-induced immunosuppressive effects possibly through down-regulation of co-stimulatory molecules, ICAM-1, CD40 and CD14 on monocytes. *J Int Med Res* 2004;32:465–483.
33. Meliton AY, Munoz NM, Liu J, et al. Blockade of LTC4 synthesis caused by additive inhibition of gIV-PLA2 phosphorylation: effect of salmeterol and PDE4 inhibition in human eosinophils. *J Allergy Clin Immunol* 2003;112:404–410.

34. Davare MA, Avdonin V, Hall DD, et al. A beta2 adrenergic receptor signaling complex assembled with the Ca^{2+} channel Cav1.2. *Science* 2001;293:98–101.
35. Zimmer HG, Ibel H, Suchner U. Beta-adrenergic agonists stimulate the oxidative pentose phosphate pathway in the rat heart. *Circ Res* 1990;67:1525–1534.
36. Obrosova IG, Fathallah L, Lang HJ, Greene DA. Evaluation of a sorbitol dehydrogenase inhibitor on diabetic peripheral nerve metabolism: a prevention study. *Diabetologia* 1999; 42:1187–1194.
37. Cameron NE, Cotter MA, Basso M, Hohman TC. Comparison of the effects of inhibitors of aldose reductase and sorbitol dehydrogenase on neurovascular function, nerve conduction and tissue polyol pathway metabolites in streptozotocin-diabetic rats. *Diabetologia* 1997;40:271–281.
38. Ng TF, Lee FK, Song ZT, et al. Effects of sorbitol dehydrogenase deficiency on nerve conduction in experimental diabetic mice. *Diabetes* 1998;47:961–966.
39. Schmidt RE, Dorsey DA, Beaudet LN, et al. A potent sorbitol dehydrogenase inhibitor exacerbates sympathetic autonomic neuropathy in rats with streptozotocin-induced diabetes. *Exp Neurol* 2005;192:407–419.
40. Oates PJ. Polyol pathway and diabetic peripheral neuropathy. *Int Rev Neurobiol* 2002; 50:325–392.
41. Obrosova IG, Van Huysen C, Fathallah L, Cao XC, Greene DA, Stevens MJ. An aldose reductase inhibitor reverses early diabetes-induced changes in peripheral nerve function, metabolism, and antioxidative defense. *FASEB J* 2002;16:123–125.
42. Gupta S, Chough E, Daley J, et al. Hyperglycemia increases endothelial superoxide that impairs smooth muscle cell Na^+-K^+-ATPase activity. *Am J Physiol* 2002;282:C560–C566.
43. Remessy AB, Abou-Mohamed G, Caldwell RW, Caldwell RB. High glucose-induced tyrosine nitration in endothelial cells: role of eNOS uncoupling and aldose reductase activation. *Invest Ophthalmol Vis Sci* 2003;44:3135–3143.
44. Obrosova IG, Minchenko AG, Vasupuram R, et al. Aldose reductase inhibitor fidarestat prevents retinal oxidative stress and vascular endothelial growth factor overexpression in streptozotocin-diabetic rats. *Diabetes* 2003;52:864–871.
45. Obrosova IG, Pacher P, Szabo C, et al. Aldose reductase inhibition counteracts oxidative-nitrosative stress and poly(ADP-ribose) polymerase activation in tissue sites for diabetes complications. *Diabetes* 2005;54:234–242.
46. Zatechka DS, Jr, Kador PF, Garcia-Castineiras S, Lou MF. Diabetes can alter the signal transduction pathways in the lens of rats. *Diabetes* 2003;52:1014–1022.
47. Price SA, Agthong S, Middlemas AB, Tomlinson DR. Mitogen-activated protein kinase p38 mediates reduced nerve conduction velocity in experimental diabetic neuropathy: interactions with aldose reductase. *Diabetes* 2004;53:1851–1856.
48. Drel VR, Pacher P, Stevens MJ, Obrosova IG. Aldose reductase inhibition counteracts nitrosative stress and poly(ADP-ribose) polymerase activation in diabetic rat kidney and high-glucose-exposed human mesangial cells. *Free Radic Biol Med* 2006;40:1454–1465.
49. Ha HC, Hester LD, Snyder SH. Poly(ADP-ribose) polymerase-1 dependence of stress-induced transcription factors and associated gene expression in glia. *Proc Natl Acad Sci USA* 2002;99:3270–3275.
50. Yang SH, Sharrocks AD, Whitmarsh AJ. Transcriptional regulation by the MAP kinase signaling cascades. *Gene* 2003;320:3–21.
51. Minchenko AG, Stevens MJ, White L, et al. Diabetes-induced overexpression of endothelin-1 and endothelin receptors in the rat renal cortex is mediated via poly(ADP-ribose) polymerase activation. *FASEB J* 2003;17:1514–1516.
52. Ramana KV, Friedrich B, Srivastava S, Bhatnagar A, Srivastava SK. Activation of nuclear factor-kappaB by hyperglycemia in vascular smooth muscle cells is regulated by aldose reductase. *Diabetes* 2004;53:2910–2920.

53. Yagihashi S, Yamagishi SI, Wada R, et al. Neuropathy in diabetic mice overexpressing human aldose reductase and effects of aldose reductase inhibitors. *Brain* 2001;124:2448–2458.
54. Song Z, Fu DT, Chan YS, Leung S, Chung SS, Chung SK. Transgenic mice overexpressing aldose reductase in Schwann cells show more severe nerve conduction velocity deficit and oxidative stress under hyperglycemic stress. *Mol Cell Neurosci* 2003;23:638–647.
55. Ho EC, Lam KS, Chen YS, et al. Aldose reductase-deficient mice are protected from delayed motor nerve conduction velocity, increased c-Jun NH2-terminal kinase activation, depletion of reduced glutathione, increased superoxide accumulation, and DNA damage. *Diabetes* 2006;55:1946–1953.
56. Coppey LJ, Gellett JS, Davidson EP, Dunlap JA, Yorek MA. Effect of treating streptozotocin-induced diabetic rats with sorbinil, myo-inositol or aminoguanidine on endoneurial blood flow, motor nerve conduction velocity and vascular function of epineurial arterioles of the sciatic nerve. *Int J Exp Diabetes Res* 2002;3:21–36.
57. Calcutt NA, Freshwater JD, Mizisin AP. Prevention of sensory disorders in diabetic Sprague-Dawley rats by aldose reductase inhibition or treatment with ciliary neurotrophic factor. *Diabetologia* 2004;47:718–724.
58. Drel VR, Mashtalir N, Ilnystska O, et al. The leptin-deficient (ob/ob) mouse: a new animal model of peripheral neuropathy of type 2 diabetes and obesity. *Diabetes* 2006;55:3335–3343.
59. Kato N, Mizuno K, Makino M, Suzuki T, Yagihashi S. Effects of 15-month aldose reductase inhibition with fidarestat on the experimental diabetic neuropathy in rats. *Diab Res Clin Pract* 2000;50:77–85.
60. Hotta N, Toyota T, Matsuoka K, et al. The SNK-860 Diabetic Neuropathy Study Group: Clinical efficacy of fidarestat, a novel aldose reductase inhibitor, for diabetic peripheral neuropathy. *Diabetes Care* 2001;24:1776–1782.
61. Greene DA, Arezzo JC, Brown MB. Effect of aldose reductase inhibition on nerve conduction and morphometry in diabetic neuropathy. Zenarestat Study Group. *Neurology* 1999;53:580–591.
62. Bril V, Buchanan RA. Aldose reductase inhibition by AS-3201 in sural nerve from patients with diabetic sensorimotor polyneuropathy. *Diabetes Care* 2004;27:2369–2375.
63. Thornalley PJ. Glycation in diabetic neuropathy: characteristics, consequences, causes, and therapeutic options. *Int Rev Neurobiol* 2002;50:37–57.
64. Dickinson PJ, Carrington AL, Frost GS, Boulton AJ. Neurovascular disease, antioxidants and glycation in diabetes. *Diab Metab Res Rev* 2002;18:260–272.
65. Ahmed N. Advanced glycation endproducts—role in pathology of diabetic complications. *Diab Res Clin Pract* 2005;67:3–21.
66. Karachalias N, Babaei-Jadidi R, Ahmed N, Thornalley PJ. Accumulation of fructosyllysine and advanced glycation end products in the kidney, retina and peripheral nerve of streptozotocin-induced diabetic rats. *Biochem Soc Trans* 2003;31(Pt 6):1423–1425.
67. Wada R, Yagihashi S. Role of advanced glycation end products and their receptors in development of diabetic neuropathy. *Ann NY Acad Sci* 2005;1043:598–604.
68. Bierhaus A, Haslbeck KM, Humpert PM, et al. Loss of pain perception in diabetes is dependent on a receptor of the immunoglobulin superfamily. *J Clin Invest* 2004;114:1741–1751.
69. Cameron NE, Gibson TM, Nangle MR, Cotter MA. Inhibitors of advanced glycation end product formation and neurovascular dysfunction in experimental diabetes. *Ann NY Acad Sci* 2005;1043:784–792.
70. Wada R, Nishizawa Y, Yagihashi N, et al. Effects of OPB-9195, anti-glycation agent, on experimental diabetic neuropathy. *Eur J Clin Invest* 2001;31:513–520.
71. Cameron NE, Nangle MR, Gibson TM, Cotter MA. Benfotiamine treatment improves vascular endothelium and nerve function in diabetic rats. *Diabetes* 2004;53:A35 [Abstract].

72. Fukunaga M, Miyata S, Liu BF, et al. Methylglyoxal induces apoptosis through activation of p38 MAPK in rat Schwann cells. *Biochem Biophys Res Commun* 2004;320:689–695.
73. Sekido H, Suzuki T, Jomori T, Takeuchi M, Yabe-Nishimura C, Yagihashi S. Reduced cell replication and induction of apoptosis by advanced glycation end products in rat Schwann cells. *Biochem Biophys Res Commun* 2004;320:241–248.
74. Amano S, Kaji Y, Oshika T, et al. Advanced glycation end products in human optic nerve head. *Br J Ophthalmol* 2001;85:52–55.
75. Misur I, Zarkovic K, Barada A, Batelja L, Milicevic Z, Turk Z. Advanced glycation end-products in peripheral nerve in type 2 diabetes with neuropathy. *Acta Diabetol* 2004; 41:158–166.
76. Haslbeck KM, Schleicher E, Bierhaus A, et al. The AGE/RAGE/NF-(kappa)B pathway may contribute to the pathogenesis of polyneuropathy in impaired glucose tolerance (IGT). *Exp Clin Endocrinol Diab* 2005;113:288–291.
77. Meerwaldt R, Links TP, Graaff R, et al. Increased accumulation of skin advanced glycation end-products precedes and correlates with clinical manifestation of diabetic neuropathy. *Diabetologia* 2005;48;1637–1644.
78. Garay-Sevilla ME, Regalado JC, Malacara JM, et al. Advanced glycosylation end products in skin, serum, saliva and urine and its association with complications of patients with type 2 diabetes mellitus. *J Endocrinol Invest* 2005;28:223–230.
79. Hwang JS, Shin CH, Yang SW. Clinical implications of N epsilon-(carboxymethyl)lysine, advanced glycation end product, in children and adolescents with type 1 diabetes. *Diab Obes Metab* 2005;7:263–267.
80. Eichberg J. Protein kinase C changes in diabetes: is the concept relevant to neuropathy. *Int Rev Neurobiol* 2002;50:61–82.
81. Cameron NE, Cotter MA, Jack AM, Basso MD, Hohman TC. Protein kinase C effects on nerve function, perfusion, Na(+), K(+)-ATPase activity and glutathione content in diabetic rats. *Diabetologia* 1999;42:1120–1130.
82. Yamagishi S, Uehara K, Otsuki S, Yagihashi S. Differential influence of increased polyol pathway on protein kinase C expressions between endoneurial and epineurial tissues in diabetic mice. *J Neurochem* 2003;87:497–507.
83. Kim J, Rushovich EH, Thomas TP, Ueda T, Agranoff BW, Greene DA. Diminished specific activity of cytosolic protein kinase C in sciatic nerve of streptozocin-induced diabetic rats and its correction by dietary myo-inositol. *Diabetes* 1991;40:1545–1554.
84. Kishi Y, Schmelzer JD, Yao JK, et al. Alpha-lipoic acid: effect on glucose uptake, sorbitol pathway, and energy metabolism in experimental diabetic neuropathy. *Diabetes* 1999;48:2045–2051.
85. Uehara K, Yamagishi S, Otsuki S, Chin S, Yagihashi S. Effects of polyol pathway hyperactivity on protein kinase C activity, nociceptive peptide expression, and neuronal structure in dorsal root ganglia in diabetic mice. *Diabetes* 2004;53:3239–3247.
86. Jack AM, Cameron NE, Cotter MA. Effects of the diacylglycerol complexing agent, cremophor, on nerve-conduction velocity and perfusion in diabetic rats. *J Diab Compl* 1999;13:2–9.
87. Nakamura J, Kato K, Hamada Y, et al. A protein kinase C-beta-selective inhibitor ameliorates neural dysfunction in streptozotocin-induced diabetic rats. *Diabetes* 1999;48: 2090–2095.
88. Coppey LJ, Gellett JS, Davidson EP, Yorek MA. Preventing superoxide formation in epineurial arterioles of the sciatic nerve from diabetic rats restores endothelium-dependent vasodilation. *Free Radic Res* 2003;37:33–40.
89. Hong S, Wiley JW. Early painful diabetic neuropathy is associated with differential changes in the expression and function of vanilloid receptor 1. *J Biol Chem* 2005;7(280):618–627.

90. Sasase T, Yamada H, Sakoda K, et al. Novel protein kinase C-beta isoform selective inhibitor JTT-010 ameliorates both hyper- and hypoalgesia in streptozotocin- induced diabetic rats. *Diab Obes Metab* 2005;7:586–594.
91. Stevens MJ, Obrosova I, Cao X, Van Huysen C, Greene DA. Effects of DL-alpha-lipoic acid on peripheral nerve conduction, blood flow, energy metabolism, and oxidative stress in experimental diabetic neuropathy. *Diabetes* 2000;49:1006–1105.
92. Obrosova IG, Fathallah L, Stevens MJ. Taurine counteracts oxidative stress and nerve growth factor deficit in early experimental diabetic neuropathy. *Exp Neurol* 2001;172:211–219.
93. Cheng C, Zochodne DW. Sensory neurons with activated caspase-3 survive long-term experimental diabetes. *Diabetes* 2003;52:2363–2371.
94. Obrosova IG, Mabley JG, Zsengeller Z, et al. Role for nitrosative stress in diabetic neuropathy: evidence from studies with a peroxynitrite decomposition catalyst. *FASEB J* 2005;19: 401–403.
95. Hoeldtke RD, Bryner KD, McNeill DR, et al. Nitrosative stress, uric Acid, and peripheral nerve function in early type 1 diabetes. *Diabetes* 2002;51:2817–2825.
96. Cameron NE, Tuck Z, McCabe L, Cotter MA. Effect of the hydroxyl radical scavenger, dimethylthiourea, on peripheral nerve tissue perfusion, conduction velocity and nociception in experimental diabetes. *Diabetologia* 2001;44:1161–1169.
97. Coppey LJ, Gellett JS, Davidson EP, et al. Effect of M40403 treatment of diabetic rats on endoneurial blood flow, motor nerve conduction velocity and vascular function of epineurial arterioles of the sciatic nerve. *Br J Pharmacol* 2001;134:21–29.
98. Hounsom L, Corder R, Patel J, Tomlinson DR. Oxidative stress participates in the breakdown of neuronal phenotype in experimental diabetic neuropathy. *Diabetologia* 2001;44:424–428.
99. Cameron NE, Jack AM, Cotter MA. Effect of alpha-lipoic acid on vascular responses and nociception in diabetic rats. *Free Radic Biol Med* 2001;31:125–135.
100. Pertovaara A, Wei H, Kalmari J, Ruotsalainen M. Pain behavior and response properties of spinal dorsal horn neurons following experimental diabetic neuropathy in the rat: modulation by nitecapone, a COMT inhibitor with antioxidant properties. *Exp Neurol* 2001;167:425–434.
101. Nishikawa T, Edelstein D, Du XL, et al. Normalizing mitochondrial superoxide production blocks three pathways of hyperglycaemic damage. *Nature* 2000;404:787–790.
102. Brownlee M. The pathobiology of diabetic complications: a unifying mechanism. *Diabetes* 2005;54:1615–1625.
103. Meneshian A, Bulkley GB. The physiology of endothelial xanthine oxidase: from urate catabolism to reperfusion injury to inflammatory signal transduction. *Microcirculation* 2002;9:161–175.
104. Cotter MA, Cameron NE. Effect of the NAD(P)H oxidase inhibitor,apocynin, on peripheral nerve perfusion and function in diabetic rats. *Life Sci* 2003;73:1813–1824.
105. Cameron NE, Cotter MA. Effects of inhibition of semicarbazide-sensitive amine oxidase (SSAO) on neurovascular function in diabetic rats. *Diabetes* 2002;51:A194 [Abstract].
106. Cacicedo JM, Benjachareowong S, Chou E, Ruderman NB, Ido Y. Palmitate-induced apoptosis in cultured bovine retinal pericytes: roles of NAD(P)H oxidase, oxidant stress, and ceramide. *Diabetes* 2005;54:1838–1845.
107. Gorin Y, Kim NH, Feliers D, Bhandari B, Choudhury GG, Abboud HE. Angiotensin II activates Akt/protein kinase B by an arachidonic acid/redox-dependent pathway and independent of phosphoinositide 3-kinase. *FASEB J* 2001;15:1909–1920.
108. Gorin Y, Ricono JM, Wagner B, et al. Angiotensin II-induced ERK1/ERK2 activation and protein synthesis are redox-dependent in glomerular mesangial cells. *Biochem J* 2004; 381(Pt 1):231–239.
109. Natarajan R, Nadler JL. Lipid inflammatory mediators in diabetic vascular disease. *Arterioscler Thromb Vasc Biol* 2004;24:1542–1548.
110. Agha AM, El-Khatib AS, Al-Zuhair H. Modulation of oxidant status by meloxicam in experimentally induced arthritis. *Pharmacol Res* 1999;40:385–392.

111. Ergul A, Johansen JS, Stromhaug C, et al. Vascular dysfunction of venous bypass conduits is mediated by reactive oxygen species in diabetes: role of endothelin-1. *J Pharmacol Exp Ther* 2005;313:70–77.
112. Obrosova IG, Greene DA, Lang HJ. Antioxidative Defense in Diabetic Peripheral Nerve Effect of DL-α-lipoic acid, Aldose Reductase Inhibitor and Sorbitol Dehydrogenase Inhibitor, in *Antioxidants in Diabetes Management* (Packer L, Roesen P, Tritschler H, King G, Azzi A, eds.), Marcel Dekker, New York, NY, 2000, pp. 93–110.
113. Jagtap P, Szabo C. Poly(ADP-ribose) polymerase and the therapeutic effects of its inhibitors. *Nat Rev Drug Discov* 2005;4:421–440.
114. Garcia Soriano F, Virag, L, Jagtap P, et al. Diabetic endothelial dysfunction: the role of poly(ADP-ribose) polymerase activation. *Nature Med* 2001;7:108–113.
115. Du X, Matsumura T, Edelstein D, et al. Inhibition of GAPDH activity by poly(ADP-ribose) polymerase activates three major pathways of hyperglycemic damage in endothelial cells. *J Clin Invest* 2003;112:1049–1057.
116. Empl M, Renaud S, Erne B, et al. TNF-alpha expression in painful and nonpainful neuropathies. *Neurology* 2001;56:1371–1377.
117. Svensson C, Marsala M, Westerlund A, et al. Activation of p38 mitogen-activated protein kinase in spinal microglia is a critical link in inflammation-induced spinal pain processing. *J Neurochem* 2003;86:1534–1544.
118. Wallace M. Calcium and sodium channel antagonists for the treatment of pain. *Clin J Pain* 2000;16(Suppl 2):S80–S85.
119. Scott G, Kean R, Mikheeva T, et al. The therapeutic effects of PJ34 [N-(6-oxo-5, 6-dihydrophenanthridin-2-yl)-N,N-dimethylacetamide.HCl], a selective inhibitor of poly(ADP-ribose) polymerase, in experimental allergic encephalomyelitis are associated with immunomodulation. *J Pharmacol Exp Ther* 2004;310:1053–1061.
120. Veres B, Radnai B, Gallyas F, et al. Regulation of kinase cascades and transcription factors by a poly(ADP-ribose) inflammation in mice. *J Pharmacol Exp Ther* 2004;310: 247–255.
121. Aarts M, Tymianski M. Molecular mechanisms underlying specificity of excitotoxic signaling in neurons. *Cur Mol Med* 2004;4:137–147.
122. Obrosova IG, Drel VR, Pacher P, et al. Oxidative-nitrosative stress and poly(ADP-ribose) polymerase (PARP) activation in experimental diabetic neuropathy: the relation is revisited. *Diabetes* 2005;54:3435–3441.
123. Torres M, Forman HJ. Redox signaling and the MAP kinase pathways. *Biofactors* 2003; 17:287–296.
124. Almhanna K, Wilkins PL, Bavis JR, Harwalkar S, Berti-Mattera LN. Hyperglycemia triggers abnormal signaling and proliferative responses in Schwann cells. *Neurochem Res* 2002;27:1341–1347.
125. Fernyhough P, Gallagher A, Averill SA, et al. Aberrant neurofilament phosphorylation in sensory neurons of rats with diabetic neuropathy. *Diabetes* 1999;48:881–889.
126. Agthong S, Tomlinson DR. Inhibition of p38 MAP kinase corrects biochemical and neurological deficits in experimental diabetic neuropathy. *Ann NY Acad Sci* 2002;973:359–362.
127. Sweitzer SM, Medicherla S, Almirez R, et al. Antinociceptive action of a p38alpha MAPK inhibitor, SD-282, in a diabetic neuropathy model. *Pain* 2004;109:409–419.
128. Svensson CI, Marsala M, Westerlund A, et al. Activation of p38 mitogen-activated protein kinase in spinal microglia is a critical link in inflammation-induced spinal pain processing. *J Neurochem* 2003;86:1534–1544.
129. Yang SH, Sharrocks AD, Whitmarsh AJ. Transcriptional regulation by the MAP kinase signaling cascades. *Gene* 2003;320:3–21.
130. Suzuki T, Sekido H, Kato N, Nakayama Y, Yabe-Nishimura C. Neurotrophin-3-induced production of nerve growth factor is suppressed in Schwann cells exposed to high glucose: involvement of the polyol pathway. *J Neurochem* 2004;91:1430–1438.

131. Kabe Y, Ando K, Hirao S, Yoshida M, Handa H. Redox regulation of NF-kappaB activation: distinct redox regulation between the cytoplasm and the nucleus. *Antioxid Redox Signal* 2005;7:395–403.
132. Dyck PJ, Windebank AJ. Diabetic and nondiabetic lumbosacral radiculoplexus neuropathies: new insights into pathophysiology and treatment. *Muscle Nerve* 2002;25:477–491.
133. Freshwater JD, Svensson CI, Malmberg AB, Calcutt NA. Elevated spinal cyclooxygenase and prostaglandin release during hyperalgesia in diabetic rats. *Diabetes* 2002;51: 2249–2255.
134. Pop-Busui R, Kellogg A, Li F, Larkin D, Stevens MJ. Effects of COX-2 gene inactivation on nerve conduction velocity and oxidative stress in experimental diabetes. *Diabetes* 2004; 53:A33 [Abstract].
135. Tardieu D, Jaeg JP, Deloly A, Corpet DE, Cadet J, Petit CR. The COX-2 inhibitor nimesulide suppresses superoxide and 8-hydroxy-deoxyguanosine formation, and stimulates apoptosis in mucosa during early colonic inflammation in rats. *Carcinogenesis* 2000;21:973–976.
136. Natarajan R, Nadler JL. Lipoxygenases and lipid signaling in vascular cells in diabetes. *Front Biosci* 2003;8:783–795.
137. Reilly KB, Srinivasan S, Hatley ME, et al. 12/15-Lipoxygenase activity mediates inflammatory monocyte/endothelial interactions and atherosclerosis in vivo. *J Biol Chem* 2004; 279:9440–9450.
138. Hall KE, Liu J, Sima AA, Wiley JW. Impaired inhibitory G-protein function contributes to increased calcium currents in rats with diabetic neuropathy. *J Neurophysiol* 2001; 86:760–770.
139. Li F, Obrosova IG, Abatan O, et al. Taurine replacement attenuates hyperalgesia and abnormal calcium signaling in sensory neurons of STZ-D rats. *Am J Physiol Endocrinol Metab* 2005;288:E29–E36.
140. Hall KE, Sima AA, Wiley JW. Voltage-dependent calcium currents are enhanced in dorsal root ganglion neurones from the Bio Bred/Worchester diabetic rat. *J Physiol* 1995; 486(Pt 2):313–322.
141. Yusaf SP, Goodman J, Gonzalez IM, et al. Streptozocin-induced neuropathy is associated with altered expression of voltage-gated calcium channel subunit mRNAs in rat dorsal root ganglion neurones. *Biochem Biophys Res Commun* 2001;289:402–406.
142. Natarajan R, Bai W, Rangarajan V, et al. Platelet-derived growth factor BB mediated regulation of 12-lipoxygenase in porcine aortic smooth muscle cells. *J Cell Physiol* 1996; 169:391–400.
143. Zhu H, Takahashi Y, Xu W, et al. Low density lipoprotein receptor-related protein-mediated membrane translocation of 12/15-lipoxygenase is required for oxidation of low density lipoprotein by macrophages. *J Biol Chem* 2003;278:13,350–13,355.
144. Luo ZD, Calcutt NA, Higuera ES, et al. Injury type-specific calcium channel alpha 2 delta-1 subunit up-regulation in rat neuropathic pain models correlates with antiallodynic effects of gabapentin. *J Pharmacol Exp Ther* 2002;303:1199–1205.
145. Richter RW, Portenoy R, Sharma U, Lamoreaux L, Bockbrader H, Knapp LE. Relief of painful diabetic peripheral neuropathy with pregabalin: a randomized, placebo-controlled trial. *J Pain* 2005;6:253–260.
146. Freynhagen R, Strojek K, Griesing T, Whalen E, Balkenohl M. Efficacy of pregabalin in neuropathic pain evaluated in a 12-week, randomised, double-blind, multicentre, placebo-controlled trial of flexible- and fixed-dose regimens. *Pain* 2005;115:254–263.
147. Drel VR, Li F, Obrosova IG. Na^+/H^+ exchanger-1 inhibition counteracts multiple manifestations of early diabetic neuropathy. *Diabetes* 2005;54:A214 [Abstract].

6
Effectors—Sonic Hedgehog and p38 Mitogen-Activated Protein Kinase

Sally A. Price, Rebecca C. Burnand, and David R. Tomlinson

SUMMARY

This chapter covers the identification of mitogen-activated protein kinases as early stage transducers of the damaging effects of glucose on peripheral nerves. They are activated by several metabolic consequences of hyperglycemia, in particular oxidative stress, osmotic stress, and advanced glycation end products. Inhibition of one group of mitogen-activated protein kinases—the p38 group—prevents the development of reduced nerve conduction velocity in experimental diabetes; such inhibition can also be achieved by an aldose reductase inhibitor, giving an explanation for the mechanism underlying the damaging effect of the polyol pathway. The effect of treatment is also described with sonic hedgehog in preventing reduced nerve conduction velocity and normalising expression of genes coding for endoskeletal proteins, which may be instrumental in preserving the integrity of the distal axon.

Key Words: Sonic hedgehog; p38 MAP kinase; nerve conduction; gene expression; axonal endoskeleton.

INTRODUCTION

The development of potential new therapies for diabetic neuropathy has been sporadic over the last 20 years. In general, the process has been boosted by a prospective aetiological mechanism reaching consensus among scientists together with the development of drugs to counteract it. The polyol pathway and aldose reductase inhibitors provide a classical example. As is shown in Fig. 1, interest in the polyol pathway rose dramatically in the 1980s, peaking at around 1990; thereafter there has been a steady decline as clinical findings indicated that the hypothesis was inapplicable to complications, at least as a sole explanation of pathogenesis. Subsequently, no hypothesis has reached such a consensus and the development of potential novel therapeutics has virtually stalled.

This chapter attempts to revitalize the process by proposing two new hypotheses to explain the development of diabetic neuropathy. These are not mutually exclusive; indeed it is instrumental that more than one set of pathogenetic mechanisms coexist and act in concert. If these hypotheses are cogent, then new avenues for development of therapeutics open up.

It has been obvious for many years that, if glucose itself is the damaging agent in the initial aetiology of neuropathy, then there must be some processes that are sensitive to

From: *Contemporary Diabetes: Diabetic Neuropathy: Clinical Management, Second Edition*
Edited by: A. Veves and R. Malik © Humana Press Inc., Totowa, NJ

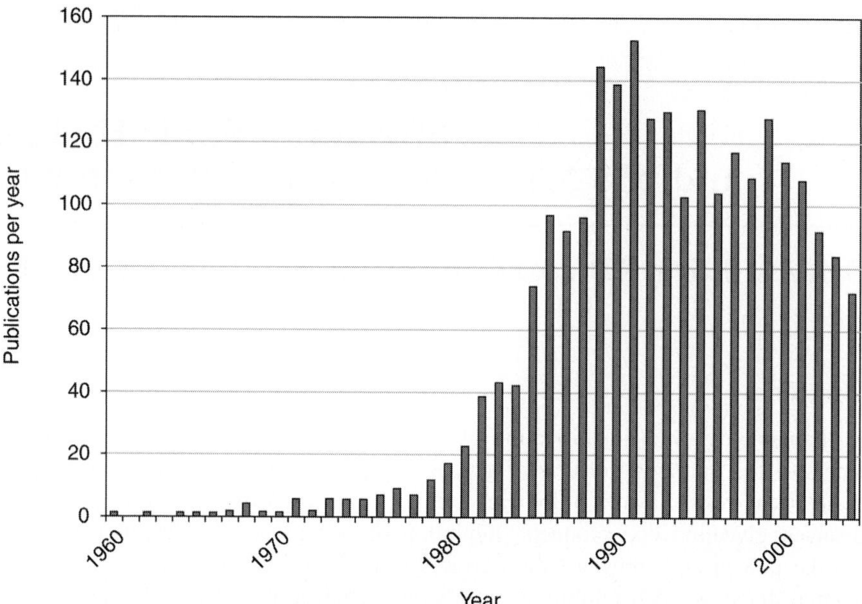

Fig. 1. Publications per year on the sorbitol/polyol pathway as indexed by PubMed (http://www.ncbi.nlm.nih.gov/PubMed/).

glucose and are interpolated between hyperglycemia and the onset of neurodegeneration. We have made an extensive study of the way in which the mitogen-activated protein kinases (MAPKs), and especially p38 MAPK, are activated directly by glucose and indirectly by the osmotic and oxidative stresses that it induces in diabetes *(1,2)*. In this chapter is presented and discussed evidence for involvement of p38 MAPK in functional changes and its inhibition as a therapeutic strategy considered.

The influence of long-term trophic support and its defects in diabetes on the development of neuropathy have been examined *(3)*. It is clear from this that more than one neurotrophic factor is defective in diabetes and reversal of this possibly requires a pleiotypic response characteristic of several factors. It is possible that agents that govern multiple developmental changes may exert just such a broad–based influence. Such a factor is sonic hedgehog (Shh) and this chapter begins with consideration of its potential influence and the novel therapeutic opportunities that it might present *(4)*.

SONIC HEDGEHOG AND DIABETIC NEUROPATHY

The hedgehog proteins are a highly homologous family of proteins that are widely expressed during development. There are three known mammalian homologues sonic (Shh), desert (Dhh), and indian (Ihh). Treatment of the streptozotocin (STZ) rat model of diabetes with a fusion protein containing human recombinant Shh and rat immunoglobin G (Shh–IgG) ameliorates a range of diabetes-induced functional and structural disorders of the peripheral nerve. For example, motor and sensory nerve conduction velocities in the lower limbs are both increased to values comparable to that of nondiabetic animals *(4)*. In addition, deficits in nerve growth factor and the related peptide substance P, shown in diabetic rats *(5)*, are not present in rats treated with Shh–IgG *(4)*.

There is a clear disruption in the gene expression of hedgehog genes in the peripheral nervous system of diabetic animals. The mRNA encoding Dhh is reduced in the sciatic nerve of the diabetic rat *(4)*. In addition, *shh* was downregulated in the dorsal root ganglion (DRG) neurons of diabetic animals at 8 weeks duration of diabetes (Burnand et al., unpublished observations). The mechanism by which treatment with Shh–IgG restores functional deficits in the nerve is unknown.

The Hedgehog Family of Proteins

The name hedgehog comes from the spiky processes that cover the larval cuticle in *hh* homozygotes. The hedgehog proteins (Hh) are a family of morphogens that act in a dose dependent manner after being secreted from their tissue source; they exert their effect by altering gene expression. The hedgehog gene (*Hh*) was first identified in *Drosophila* embryos, as a gene encoding for a protein implicated in segment polarity *(6)*. Since then, most studies in *Drosophila* have focused on the role of hedgehog in regulating the growth and patterning of the wing and other appendages *(7)*.

Three mammalian hedgehog homologues have been found and are named Shh, Dhh, and Ihh *(8)*. Two homologues have been found in fish and are named echidna and tiggywinkle hedgehog *(9,10)*.

The multiple *hh* genes of vertebrates have presumably arisen by duplication and subsequent divergence of a single ancestral *hh* gene. Although *shh*, *ihh*, and *dhh* are highly homologous, *shh* is closer to *ihh* than *dhh* in sequence identity. Pathi et al. *(11)* have shown that the three proteins have the ability to function similarly, but with different potencies, hence the proteins can substitute for each other. They showed that the rank order of potencies in each of the contexts they tested was Shh > Ihh > Dhh.

Shh is expressed in numerous tissues including the central nervous system, the peripheral nervous system, limbs, somites, the skeleton, and skin. It has numerous roles during mammalian development, directing pattern formation, and inducing cell proliferation.

Humans or mice lacking Shh develop holoprosencephaly and cyclopia because of a failure of separation of the lobes of the forebrain *(12)*. Shh organises the developing neural tube by establishing distinct regions of homeodomain transcription factor production along the dorsoventral axis *(13)*. These transcription factors, including Nkx, Pax, and Dbx family members, specify neuronal identity. Shh acts directly on target cells and not through other secreted mediating factors, to specify neuronal cell fate *(14)*. It also has important known patterning roles in the formation of other tissues including the brain *(15)* and the eye *(9)*. In addition to the many functions of Shh in determining cell fate, it also has roles in controlling cell proliferation and differentiation in neuronal and nonneuronal cell types.

The numerous responses to Shh are achieved by controlling the production, amount, and biochemical nature of the signal itself, including covalent modification of Shh.

During development, the expression of *Dhh* mRNA is highly restricted. Its expression has been shown in the Sertoli cells of the developing testes *(16,17)* and in the Schwann cells of the peripheral nerve *(18)*. Male *Dhh*-null mice are sterile and fail to produce mature spermatozoa *(16)*. The peripheral nerves of Dhh-null mice are also highly abnormal. The perineurial sheaths surrounding the nerve fascicles are abnormally thin and extensive microfasicles consisting of perineurial like cells are formed within the endoneurium. The nerve tissue barrier is permeable, and the tight junctional arrays between, adjacent perineurial cells are abnormal and incomplete *(18)*.

Ihh has two known roles in vertebrate development. The first is in the formation of the endoderm where Ihh is critical for the differentiation of the visceral endoderm *(19)*. The second is in postnatal bone growth *(20)* where Ihh appears to coordinate growth and morphogenesis, a suggestion has also been made proposing a role for Ihh in healing long bone fractures *(21)*.

Until recently, it was thought that hedgehog proteins directly bind to a single receptor named Patched (Ptc). Ptc, located on the surface of responding cells, is a 1500 amino acid glycoprotein that constitutes 12 membrane-spanning domains *(22,23)*. Two human homologues of Ptc have been identified named Ptc1 and Ptc2 *(24)*. Ptc1 is the main receptor for Shh, Ihh, and Dhh, the function of Ptc2 is unknown. It has been shown that a number of isoforms of Ptc2 exist it is proposed that the expression of the different isoforms is associated with the "fine-tuning" of the Hh response *(25)*.

Ptc is required for the repression of target genes in the absence of Hh. The Hh signal induces target gene expression by binding to and inactivating Ptc. Inactivation of Ptc allows smoothened to become active; Smo is a 115 kDa transmembrane protein that is essential for transducing the Shh signal, only one human homolog is known. It is not yet clear whether the inhibition of Smo by Ptc is the result of direct or indirect interaction. Either way, the binding of Hh to Ptc results in a change that allows smoothened to transduce the signal. In humans and mice, the loss of *ptc* function causes medulloblastomas, tumors of the cerebullum, and other developmental abnormalities resulting from the inappropriate expression of Shh target genes *(26,27)*.

In addition to repressing target gene transcription, Ptc also regulates the movement of Hh through tissues; the binding of Hh to Ptc limits the spread of Hh from its source. In *Drosophila* producing mutant Ptc, Hh can be detected at distances greater than those producing the wide-type protein *(28)*. The binding of Shh to Ptc induces rapid internalization of Shh into endosomes, the fate of Shh after internalization is not yet known *(29)*.

In 2002 it was shown that Shh also directly binds to another protein called megalin *(30)*. This single chain protein is approx 600 KDa and consists of a C-terminal cytoplasmic domain, a single transmembrane domain and an extremely large ectodomain *(31)*. Megalin functions as an endocytic receptor which mediates the endocytosis of ligands including insulin *(32)*, the presence of functional motifs at the C-terminal cytoplasmic domain suggest that this protein may also have a role in signal transduction *(33)*. The phenotypes of megalin deficient mice are consistent with phenotypes of mice deficient in Shh and Smo *(34,35)*.

The signal transduction pathway downstream to Ptc and Smo is not well understood. Ultimately, it results in the nuclear translocation of the Gli proteins. The Gli genes encode transcription factors that share five highly conserved tandem C_2–H_2 zinc fingers and a consensus histidine–cysteine linker sequence between the zinc fingers *(36)*. The *Drosophila* homolog is called cubitus interruptus (Ci). Ci is regulated post-transcriptionally; the full length Ci protein consists of 155 amino acid residues (Ci-155) *(37,38)*.

In the absence of a Hh signal, Ci forms a tetrameric complex with proteins named: Costal-2, Fused, and Suppressor of fused at the microtubules *(39,40)*. In this complex form Ci is cleaved to form a 75 amino acid residue ($Ci_{[rep]}$) *(41)* that retains the zinc finger domain and translocates to the nucleus to repress downstream target genes *(42)*. In some cells, proteolysis of Ci seems to be dependent on protein kinase-A mediated phosphorylation *(43)*. Transduction of the Hh signal inhibits proteolysis of Ci, resulting in an accumulation of the full-length protein. On translocation to the nucleus this activator form stimulates transcription of target genes. In the absence of Hh signal not all full length Ci is cleaved, a residual amount escapes but is prevented from activating target genes by its retention in the cytoplasm and active nuclear export *(41,44)* thus, it seems likely that there are many levels of control over Ci activity that remain to be fully elucidated.

There are three known Gli homologues in mammals: Gli1 (also referred to as Gli), Gli 2, and Gli 3. All three Gli homologues have been tested for separate functional domains. C-terminally truncated forms of both Gli2 and Gli3 that resemble the truncated form of Ci have been shown to repress reporter gene expression in cell lines or Shh targets in vivo *(45,46)*. Gli1 does not seem to contain a represser domain, instead only functioning as a transcription activator *(46)*.

Effects on Indices of Diabetic Neuropathy

As previously mentioned, treatment of the diabetic rat with Shh–IgG reverses a number of indices of diabetic neuropathy including, deficits in nerve conduction velocity. Figure 2 shows sensory and motor nerve conduction velocity values at 8 and 12 weeks duration of diabetes in the STZ model of diabetes. There are clear deficits in the diabetic animals that are reversed by treatment with Shh–IgG. Shh–IgG treatment had no effect on body weight or glycemia in diabetic rats, implying that the severity of diabetes was unaffected by Shh–IgG. Shh–IgG administration had no effect on the concentration of polyol pathway components in peripheral nerve (Burnand et al., unpublished).

Shh protein signaling ultimately leads to the translocation of the Gli proteins to the nucleus where they act as transcription factors. Therefore, the mechanism by which Shh–IgG exerts its effects is likely to be transcription based. In both human and experimental models of diabetes there are a wide range of structural changes in the peripheral nerve. These changes include a loss in the number of myelinated fibres and paranodal demyelination *(47,48)*. There is also a reduction in the capacity of peripheral nerves to regenerate following injury *(49,50)*. Actin, tubulin, and the neurofilament proteins are the main cytoskeletal proteins essential for structural integrity of the axon. Other accessory proteins including numerous actin binding proteins are present in the peripheral nerve and produce a structure of extreme complexity and versatility. Abnormalities in the production and processing of structural proteins have been widely reported in diabetic neuropathy *(5,51,52)*. Evidence gathered in our laboratory shows that treatment of the diabetic rat with Shh–IgG reverses abnormalities in the gene expression of a range of structural proteins as shown in Fig. 3. This restoration in gene expression may form part of the mechanism by which treatment with Shh–IgG corrects deficits in nerve conduction velocity in diabetic rats.

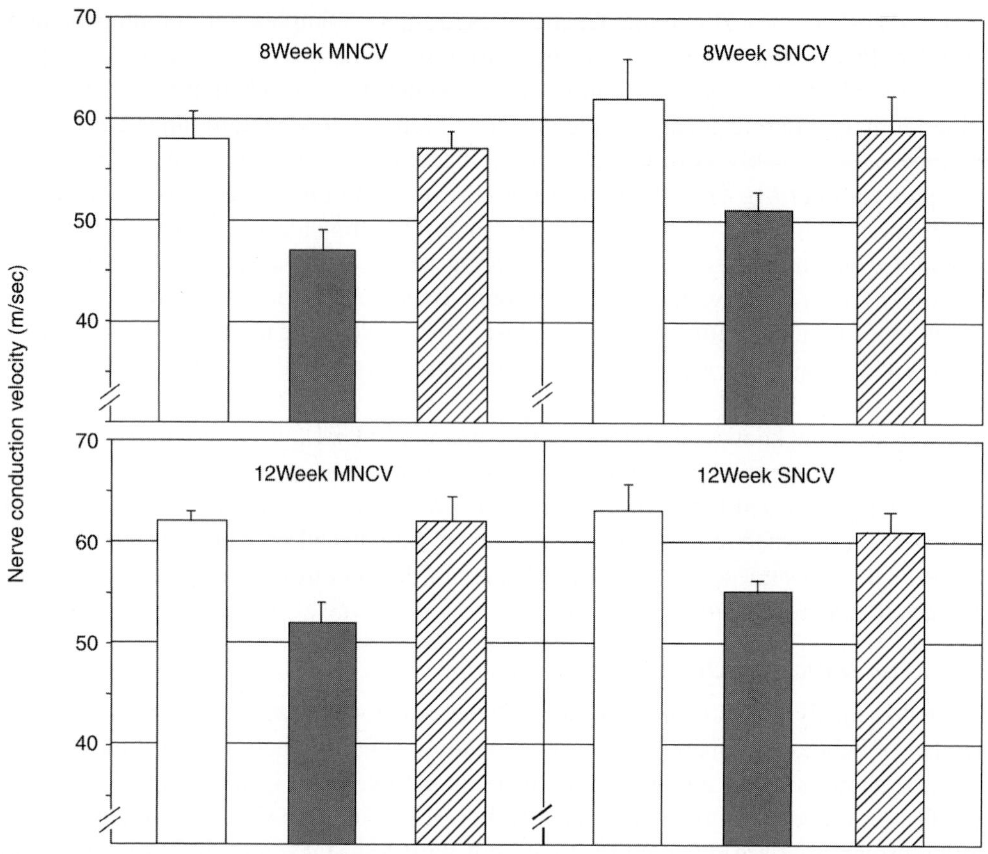

Fig. 2. Motor and sensory nerve conduction velocities in control (open columns), diabetic (gray columns) and sonic hedgehog (diagonal hatching)-treated diabetic rats. Diabetes caused significant ($p < 0.01$) slowing of both at 8 and 12 weeks, which was normalised by sonic hedgehog at both durations.

To date, the work conducted on the use of Shh–IgG as a potential therapeutic agent in the treatment of diabetic neuropathy has resulted in positive outcomes. No adverse side effects have been observed at 12 weeks duration of diabetes. A longer term study is now necessary to determine the longer term potential of this promising new therapy.

MITOGEN-ACTIVATED PROTEIN KINASES

MAPKs are a family of enzymes involved in transducing signals derived from the extracellular environment. There are three main subtypes of MAPKs: extracellular regulated kinases (ERKs), *c-Jun* N-terminal kinases (JNKs), and p38 MAPKs. All family members are activated by dual phosphorylation of a consensus sequence, Thr-Xxx-Tyr by MAPK kinases. Upstream of these are the MAPK kinase kinases, thereby forming a three kinase cascade. There are fewer different kinases at each subsequent level of the cascade, resulting in refinement of the signal. Specificity may be achieved by stimulus-selective pathways, distinct cellular pools of kinases, or the presence of scaffold proteins required for the interaction of certain kinases. Activated MAPKs can phosphorylate targets within the cytoplasm, such as cytoskeletal proteins and other

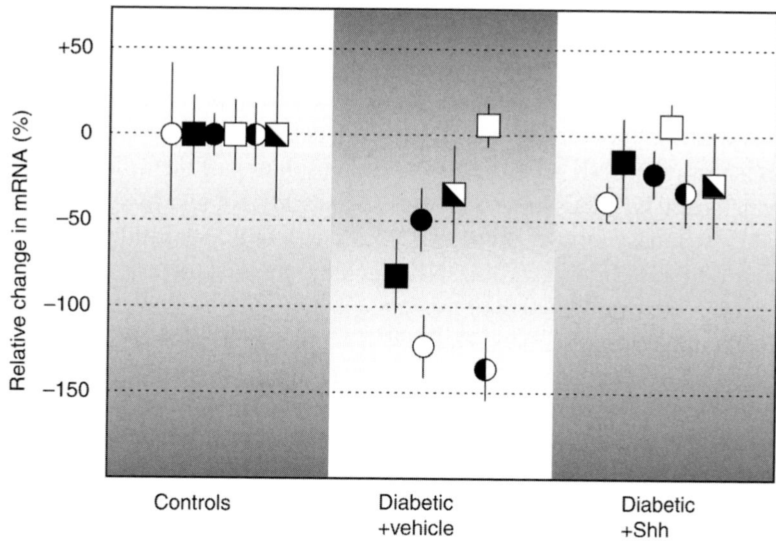

Fig. 3. In dorsal root ganglia of rats with 12 weeks streptozotocin diabetes there was a general reduction in gene expression (mRNA levels) for endoskeletal proteins; some of these reductions were normalised by treatment with sonic hedgehog. Coding: open circles—β-actin; filled squares—γ-actin; filled circles—NFL, neurofilament light subunit; open squares—NFM, neurofilament medium subunit; half-filled circles—NFH, neurofilament heavy subunit; half-filled squares—α-tubulin.

kinases, or they may be translocated to the nucleus where they activate transcription factors and mediate gene expression.

Extracellular Signal-Regulated Kinases

ERK1 was identified as a kinase activated by insulin, having a pivotal role in transducing mitogenic signals by converting tyrosine phosphorylation into the serine/threonine phosphorylations that regulate downstream events *(53)*. ERK2 and ERK3 were subsequently identified *(54)*. ERK1 and ERK2 have 83% amino acid homology, are expressed in most tissues to varying degrees, and are activated by growth factors, phorbol esters and serum. ERK1/2 activation is typically triggered by receptor tyrosine kinases and G protein-coupled receptors at the cell surface. These activate the small GTP-binding protein Ras, allowing signaling through the Raf/MEK/ERK cascade. Downstream, ERK1/2 activates other kinases (e.g., RSKs, MSKs, and MNKs), membrane components (e.g., CD120a, Syk, and calnexin), cytoskeletal proteins (e.g., neurofilament) or nuclear targets (e.g., SRC1, Pax6, NF-AT, Elk1, MEF2). ERK3 displays ubiquitous expression and responds to various growth factors *(54)*. It is only 42% identical to ERK1 and differs from ERK1/2 in that it is a constitutively active nuclear kinase and does not phosphorylate typical MAPK substrates *(54,55)*. The fifth mammalian ERK kinase is designated ERK5 or big MAPK1 (BMK1) because it is twice the size of the other ERK family members and has a distinct C-terminal *(56,57)*. Erk5 contributes to Ras/Raf signaling *(56,58)* and is activated in response to growth factors and stress *(56,59)*. ERK6 is a protein kinase involved in myoblast differentiation *(60)* but is usually referred to as p38γ. ERK7 and ERK8 have also been cloned recently *(61,62)*.

C-Jun N-Terminal Kinases

JNK was identified as the kinase that phosphorylated *c-Jun* after exposure of cells to transforming oncogenes and ultraviolet light *(63)*. It was thus recognized as an important signaling cascade for modulating the activity of distinct nuclear targets. There are 10 mammalian isoforms of JNK arising from alternate splicing of the 3 JNK genes. The JNK proteins are activated by MAP kinase kinases such as MKK4 and MKK7 and upstream of these MAP kinase kinase kinases including MLKs and ASK. Scaffold proteins such as JIP and β-arrestin 2 are also integral to the JNK signaling module, determining proximity and specificity. JNK proteins differ in their associations with scaffold proteins and also in their interaction with downstream targets. Defined substrates of JNK total at about 50–60 protein and include cytoskeletal proteins (e.g., neurofilament, tau, and microtubule associated proteins), mitochondria (e.g., bim), and nuclear proteins (c-Jun, ATF-2, and Elk-1) *(64)*. Roles for the different isoforms of JNK are gradually becoming elucidated. It is known that basal activity of JNK1 is far greater than that of JNK2 and JNK3. Coupled with the fact that JNK1 knockout mice are defective/embryonically lethal, this suggests a greater role for JNK1 under physiological conditions. JNK3 knockout mice are healthy and are resistant to excitotoxic brain insults *(65)*, suggesting a greater pathological role for this isoform. In addition tissue specific effects of the role have been described. In most situations, inhibition of JNK is detrimental, however in cells such as cardiac myocytes and sensory neurones inhibition of JNK may confer protection.

Mitogen-Activated Protein Kinase p38

The p38 MAPK signal transduction pathway is activated by proinflammatory cytokines and environmental stresses such as osmotic shock, ultraviolet radiation, heat, and chemicals (*see* refs. *66–68* for reviews). There are four members of the p38 MAPK family: p38α *(69,70)*, p38β *(71)*, p38γ *(72)*, and p38δ *(73)*, each encoded by a different gene. The p38 MAPKs are phosphorylated and activated by MKK3 and MKK6 at threonine and tyrosine residues and can mediate signaling to the nucleus *(74)*. A large number of substrates have been described for p38, these include the transcription factors ATF-2, Elk-1, cAMP response element binding proteins (CREB), and cytoplasmic targets such as tau, MAPKAPK-2. p38 MAPKs are widely expressed, with at least 3 of the genes being expressed in the peripheral nervous system (S Price, personal observation). The effect of p38 activation in response to cellular stress is diverse, although the majority of reports favour a role in cell death rather than cell survival for neuronal cells. p38 signaling has been proposed to mediate apoptotic signaling in response to a variety of stimuli in neurons including oxidative stress in primary forebrain cultures *(75)*, mesencephalic cells *(76)*, and cortical neurons *(77)*, and NGF withdrawal in PC12 cells *(78)*. Conversely, p38 activation was not observed following NGF withdrawal in primary cultures of sympathetic neurons *(79)* and NGF has been shown to increase p38 activation in DRG in vivo *(80)*. This suggests that activation of p38 alone does not predict a detrimental outcome. High basal activity of p38 has been described in the adult rat brain *(81)*, although the physiological roles of p38 activation have been sparsely investigated.

Stress Kinases—Mechanism of Damage

In 1993, the Diabetes Control and Complications Trial Research Group concluded that the incidence and severity of diabetic complications are increased by poor glycaemic control, indicating that hyperglycemia is likely to be the major causative factor. Several consequences are known to result from excess glucose these include hyperosmolarity, increased polyol pathway flux, oxidative stress, formation of advanced glycation end products (AGE), and activation of protein kinase C. These pathways are integrally linked with each other and with a variety of other cellular pathways. MAPK activation is implicated in all these pathways, suggesting a pivotal role in transducing the effects of high glucose in diabetic neuropathy.

Uptake of extracellular glucose without the dependency for insulin is a common feature of tissues affected by diabetic macrovascular complications. One major consequence is an increased flux through the polyol pathway (Fig. 4). In this pathway, aldose reductase converts glucose to sorbitol, and this is subsequently converted to fructose by sorbitol dehydrogenase. Excessive flux through the polyol pathway leads to accumulation of the poorly membrane permeable metabolites sorbitol and fructose in diabetic rats *(82)*. One consequence is that cells may be subjected to osmotic stress. This mechanism is thought to account for the formation of sugar-induced cataractogenesis in diabetic rat lens *(83)*. The contribution of osmotic stress resulting from increased polyol pathway flux in peripheral nerve is less well defined *(84)*.

Extracellular osmotic stress may also occur in diabetic nerves as these are subject to serum hyperosmolarity. Demonstrated a reduction in axonal size in myelinated fibres and suggested this was, at least in part, because of shrinkage as a result of increased tissue osmolarity *(85)*.

Hyperosmolarity activates MAPKs in a variety of cell types *(69,86,87)*, and therefore it is plausible that hyperosmotic stress can activate MAPKs in diabetic neuropathy. In aortic smooth muscle cells from normal rats, glucose activates p38 by a PKC-δ isoform-dependent mechanism *(88)*. However, at higher levels of glucose, p38 is activated by hyperosmolarity through a PKC independent pathway. This suggests that different pathways may be activated simultaneously by high glucose. Furthermore, p38 has been shown to mediate the effects of hyperglycemia-induced osmotic stress in vivo in the rat mesenteric circulation *(89)*.

In recent years, oxidative stress has come to the forefront of hypotheses proposed to be causative of diabetic neuropathy. Numerous studies have shown that antioxidants such as vitamin E *(90–92)*, DL-α-lipoic acid *(93–95)*, and taurine *(96,97)* can prevent abnormalities in diabetic nerve. Oxidative stress results from an imbalance in the production of reactive oxygen species and cellular antioxidant defence mechanisms. The increased free radical production may then result in oxidization of various cellular components including lipids, proteins, and nucleic acids. Components that are modified by ROS may have decreased activity leading to widespread dysfunction including disturbances in metabolism and defective signaling pathways.

Oxidative stress in diabetic nerve may result from a variety of mechanisms including increased flux through the polyol pathway (Fig. 4), endoneurial hypoxia, hyperlipidaemia, increases in free fatty acids, activation of PKC, activation of receptors for AGE, and glucose itself. The major source of oxidative stress in cells is the production of reactive oxygen species (ROS) and reactive nitrogen species (RNS). Naturally occurring ROS and RNS usually have oxygen or nitrogen based unpaired electrons resulting from enzymatic or nonenzymatic reactions. Examples include superoxide anion, hydroxyl radical, nitrogen oxide, and peroxynitrite. High glucose inhibits ATP synthase resulting

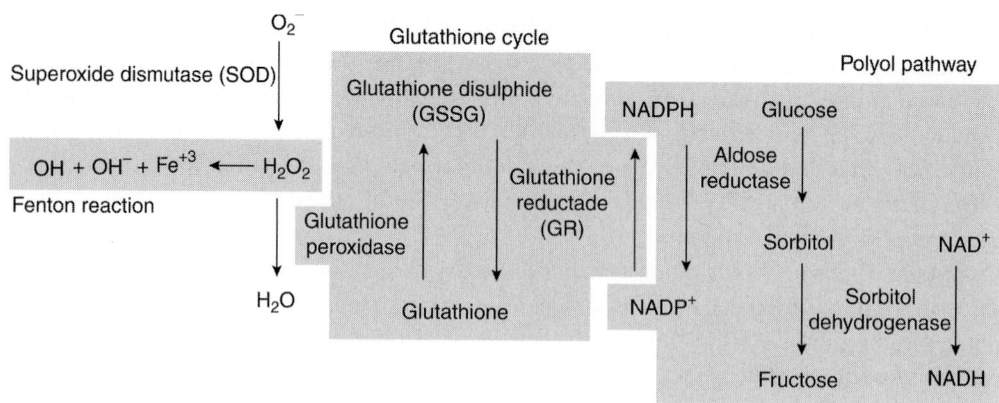

Fig. 4. Interconnecting pathways for oxidative stress. The polyol pathway consumes NADPH, compromising the glutathione cycle, reducing levels of oxidized glutathione and impairing conversion of hydrogen peroxide to water by glutathione peroxidase. This favours the Fenton reaction generating super-hydroxyl radicals.

in slowing of electron transfer in the mitochondria and increased production of superoxide ions *(98)*. Superoxide ions are normally converted to hydrogen peroxide and water by the enzyme superoxide dismutase. Hydrogen peroxide is also produced by enzymatic transfer of two electrons to molecular oxygen by enzymes such as monoamine oxidase and urate oxidase. Hydrogen peroxide is reduced by glutathione peroxidase, myeloperoxidase, and catalase or nonenzymatic decomposition occurs through the fenton reaction, producing the highly reactive hydroxyl radical (OH). The activity of both superoxide dismutase and catalase was found to be decreased (but not reaching statistical significance) in peripheral nerve after 6 weeks of diabetes *(99,100)*. Longer durations of diabetes (3 or 12 months) failed to show a decrease in either gene expression or activity of either enzyme, an increase in catalase expression was reported at 12 months. These results suggest that changes in SOD and catalase may be dynamic in diabetic nerve. Superoxides can also react with NO, forming peroxynitrite (ONOO-), which rapidly causes protein nitration or nitrosylation, lipid peroxidation, DNA damage, and cell death. In sciatic nerve of rats given a peroxynitrite decomposition catalyst, immunoreactivity for nitrotyrosine and poly ADP-ribose (PARP) was present only in diabetic animals *(101)*, indicating that nitrosative stress is indeed present in animal models of diabetic neuropathy.

Glutathione is another important cellular antioxidant that acts as a non-enzymatic reducing agent, helping to keep cysteine thiol side chains in a reduced state on the surface of proteins. The reduction of oxidized glutathione to reduced glutathione (GSH), catalysed by glutathione reductase is dependent on NADPH as a cofactor (Fig. 4). Increased flux through the polyol pathway can cause depletion of GSH *(102,103)*, possibly as a result of competition between aldose reductase and glutathione reductase for NADPH resulting in NADPH deficiency *(104,105)* but more likely because of a decrease in total glutathione *(106,107)*. Increased polyol pathway flux can also create oxidative stress because of the reaction of NADH with NADH oxidase and mitochondrial overloading with NADH. The significance of polyol-induced oxidative stress is highlighted by the fact that an aldose reductase inhibitor can prevent diabetes induced lipid peroxidation in peripheral nerve *(107)*.

ROS and RNS such as hydrogen peroxide, superoxide, and peroxynitrite activate ERK, JNK, and p38 in a variety of in vitro models *(108–112)*, whereas MAPK activation is now well documented in these in vitro models, there is a lack of evidence for MAPK activation by ROS and RNS in vivo. Recently, however *(113)*, showed that ConA induced liver failure in mice resulted in TNF-α induced ROS production leading to sustained activation of JNK, which could be prevented by an antioxidant. Depleted GSH was also a consequence whereas there was less depletion in JNK1–/– mice, thus establishing a link between ROS activation and MAPK activation in vivo. β-adrenoreceptor stimulation in cardiac tissues was also found to increase superoxide production and lipid peroxidation with concomitant activation of p38, JNK, and ERK. These changes could be prevented with the antioxidant Tempol *(114)*. The relationship between high glucose, oxidative stress, and MAPK activation may only be apparent with more chronic hyperglycemia because acute (3h) glucose infusion in rats resulted in oxidative stress as measured by MDA and total glutathione but not in activation of ERK1/2 or p38 in liver *(115)*. It will be of great significance to establish the existence of oxidative stress-induced MAPK activation in diabetic neuropathy.

AGE exert their cellular effects by interacting with cell surface receptors, the best characterized of these is the receptor for advanced glycation end products (RAGE). In rat pulmonary smooth muscle cells it was demonstrated that RAGE activation can induce ERK1/2 activated p21 (ras) and nuclear factor kB (NFkB) signaling *(116)*. Subsequently a role for p38 in RAGE-induced NF-κB-dependent secretion of proinflammatory cytokines was established *(117)*. RAGE-induced activation of JNK is not well documented but has been shown in RAGE-amphoterin induced tumour growth *(118)* and high-mobility group protein-1 (HMGB1—a novel inflammatory molecule) induced RAGE activation in human microvascular endothelial cells *(119)*.

MAPK Activation in Sensory Neurones

In vitro models cannot replicate the chronic conditions of diabetes because primary cells slowly, but progressively die in culture. Furthermore, the interaction between neuronal and non-neuronal cells and the supply of nutrients cannot be mimicked directly. However cell culture models do provide a means of isolating components known to be important in diabetes and reduce the use of in vivo models. In primary cultures of dorsal root ganglia neurons, high glucose activated p38, and JNK but not ERK in a concentration-dependent manner (10–200 m*M*) following 16 hours treatment *(1)*. Oxidative stress in the form of hydrogen peroxide or diethyl maleate resulted in activation of p38 and ERK but not JNK. Treatment with high glucose and oxidative stress had an additive effect on activation of p38, suggesting different mechanisms of activation.

Exposure of DRG neurones to high glucose and oxidative stress also resulted in a decrease in cell viability as indicated by lactate dehydrogenase and MTT assays, measurements of intact plasma membranes and mitochondrial function, respectively. Concomitant treatment with a specific ERK pathway inhibitor (U0126) or a specific p38 pathway inhibitor (SB20210) prevented activation of ERK or p38, respectively and prevented the decrease in cell viability. This suggests that activation of p38 and ERK by glucose or oxidative stress is detrimental in sensory neurones.

Commercially available specific inhibitors of the JNK pathway that are easily soluble have been lacking and therefore less is known about the role of the JNK pathway in sensory neurons. Treatment with the peptide inhibitor JNK inhibitor 1 *(120)* resulted in death of primary cultures of DRG neurons *(121)*. This inhibitor appeared to be selective for JNK because c-Jun phosphorylation was prevented, whereas there was no effect on other MAPKs. The recent development of new and more soluble JNK inhibitors may help elucidate the effects of JNK signaling in sensory neurones in diabetic neuropathy.

MAPK Activation and Neuropathy in Diabetes

To investigate the effect of diabetes on MAPK activation, antibodies were used that either recognize an epitope found on all forms of a particular MAPK (total, -T) or an epitope specific to the phosphorylated (activate) form (phosphorylated, -P). Immunohistochemical studies on normal rats showed that ERK was expressed in both neurones and satellite cells of the DRG, whereas ERK-P was found exclusively in satellite cells. In the sciatic nerve ERK-T and ERK-P immunoreactivity was seen in both axons and Schwann cells. Western blotting indicated that DRG from diabetic animals showed an increase in ERK-P relative to ERK-T for both the p42 (ERK2) and p44 (ERK1) isoforms after 8, 10, or 12 weeks diabetes *(1,122)*. The increase in ERK-P was because of activation in the satellite cells in the DRG. Activated p44 ERK was also found to be significantly increased in the sural nerve of 12 week STZ rats *(123)*. However, no changes were found in ERK-P in the sural nerve in a separate study with the same duration of diabetes *(122)*.

In control DRG, JNK-T staining was found predominantly in neurones. JNK-P showed a similar distribution; staining was observed in the cytoplasm of neurones, but was absent from the nuclei. In sciatic nerve, JNK immunohistochemistry was restricted to axons. JNK staining has also been documented in the ventral horn and motoneuron perikarya *(122)*. In diabetic animals, Western blotting revealed increased JNK activation (p46 and p54/56) in the DRG *(1,121,122)*. Increased levels of JNK-P in sciatic and sural nerve from 12 weeks STZ-rats were also observed *(123)*. p54 JNK has also been shown to be elevated in the DRG and sural nerve in an alternative model of type 1 diabetes, the BB rat *(122)*. Immunohistochemistry of diabetic DRG showed that JNK-P is translocated from the cytoplasm to the nucleus of neurones. In axons of the sciatic nerve, staining is increased in large myelinated fibers. In other studies carried out in STZ-rats in the same laboratory, only certain isoforms of JNK were shown to be activated (S. A. Price and D. R. Tomlinson, personal observations) or were shown to be increased but not reaching statistical significance. Activation of JNK was related to the duration of diabetes (increased activation with longer durations) and to the blood glucose levels (increased with higher blood glucose levels). Activated *c-Jun*, a transcription factor known to be downstream of JNK, displays a similar pattern of activation to that of JNK in diabetic rats *(122)*.

Immunohistochemistry demonstrated that p38-T was also located in neuronal cells in the DRG of control rats (Fig. 5). Similar to JNK-T, immunoreactivity was largely restricted to the cytoplasm and appeared to be absent from the nuclei and satellite cells.

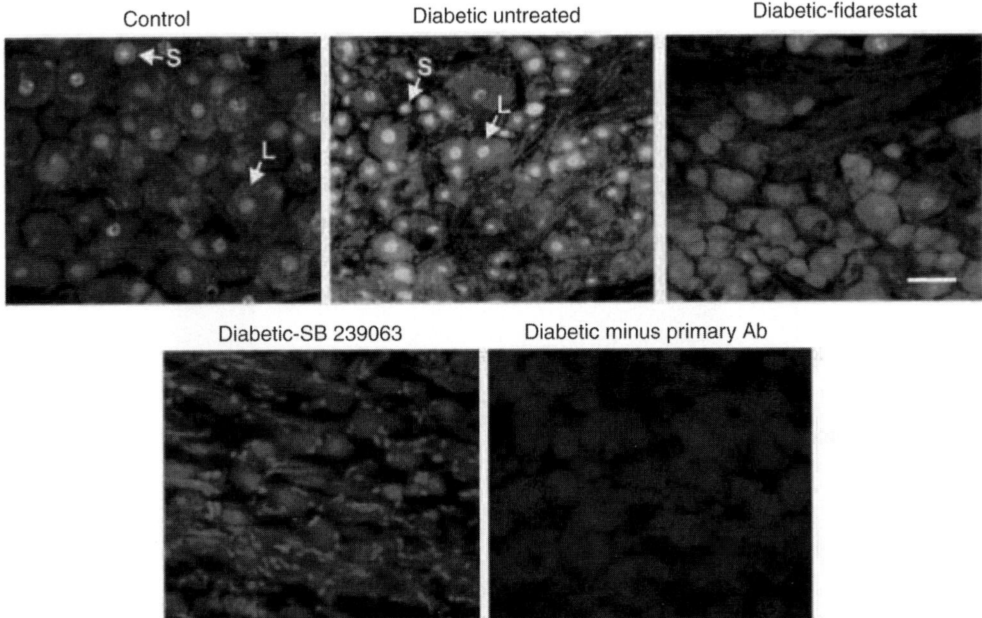

Fig. 5. Bar charts and Western blots showing the effects of Insulin, fidarestat and the p38 mitogen-activated protein kinases inhibitor, SB239063 on activation of mitogen-activated protein kinases p38 in dorsal root ganglia. The Western blot shows the effect of diabetes (UD), compared with controls (C), and fidarestat-treated diabetes (DF) on total (p38-T) and phosphorylated p38 (p38-P).

p38-P was present in the cytoplasm of neurones but more intense staining was also observed in the nuclei of some cells. In sciatic nerve p38-T was expressed in axons and Schwann cells and p-38-P was expressed in axons. Western blotting showed an increase in p38-P in the DRG of diabetic animals *(1)*, accompanied by predominantly nuclear staining observed with immunohistochemistry. p38-P staining was also increased in the sciatic nerve of diabetic animals *(124)* and staining became visible in Schwann cells as well as axons. In the L1 spinal cord, diabetes also promoted p38 activation in motoneuron cell bodies, as identified by colocalization of choline acetyltransferase. There was also intense p38 activation in microglia and diffuse labeling in neuronal and non-neuronal cells of the gray matter. Interestingly, in sural nerve biopsies from diabetic patients there is an increase in both p38-T and p38-P *(1)*.

All changes that have been observed in diabetic animals could be reversed with insulin and also the aldose reductase inhibitor, fidarestat, indicating that activation is a consequence of hyperglycemia (Figs. 5 and 6). Treatment of STZ-diabetic rats with the second-generation p38 inhibitor SB 239063 (20 mg/kg per day) prevents activation of p38 in DRG and sciatic nerve and also deficits in nerve conduction velocity observed in untreated diabetic rats *(124)*. The inhibitor used specifically inhibits the α- and β-isoforms of p38 that are the isoforms predominantly expressed in neuronal tissue *(125)* and has no effect on other MAP, tyrosine, or lipid kinases *(126)*. Treatment of diabetic rats with the aldose reductase inhibitor fidarestat or insulin also prevented activation of p38 (Figs. 5 and 6)

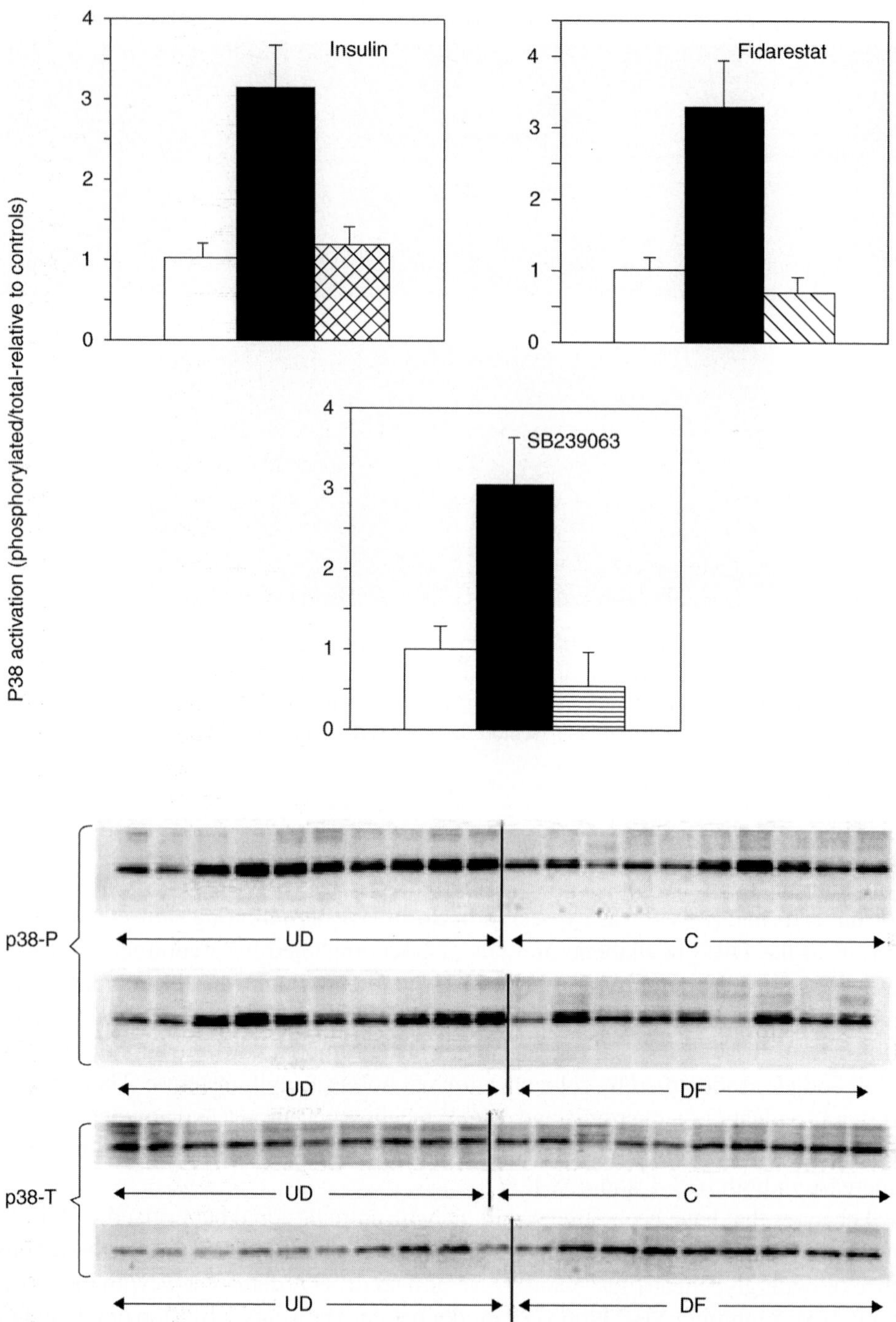

Fig. 6. Immunocytochemistry showing activated (phosphorylated) p38 in cytoplasm and, especially, nuclei of both small and large neurone cell bodies in dorsal root ganglia. There was marked activation in diabetes, which was specific, as is shown by the sections exposed to secondary, but no primary antibody. Both fidarestat and the p38 inhibitor, SB239063 prevented the activation of p39 mitogen-activated protein kinase.

suggesting that p38 activation is a consequence of hyperglycemia and lies downstream of the polyol pathway *(124)*. This evidence supports the in vitro work by *(1)* and indicates that MAPK activation is detrimental in diabetic neuropathy. Elucidation of the down stream targets of p38 in sensory neurons may suggest therapeutic targets for diabetic neuropathy in the future.

CONCLUSION

This account makes it clear that one group of glucose transducers—the MAPKs—has been identified. There can be little doubt of their involvement in early stages of the registration of damaging effects of glucose to neurones and Schwann cells. This probably extends to other cell types and may contribute to vasculopathy, retinopathy, and nephropathy. In so far as p38 MAPK might be pivotal, it is clear that aldose reductase inhibitors that are as effective as fidarestat can remove that source of cellular damage. This might be seen to negate the relevance of p38 because of the lack of clinical efficacy of the aldose reductase inhibitors tested to date. However, it is clear that early intervention is paramount and it is also likely that the level of inhibition may need to be greater than has yet been achieved clinically.

It will be interesting to see the development of Shh analogues and to determine whether these affect activation of MAPKs. If the two approaches to the consequences of glucose intoxication are complimentary then we will have a clear gateway to what some of us consider to be inevitable—multiple therapeutic approaches. This will add interest as well as difficulty to clinical trials.

REFERENCES

1. Purves TD, Middlemas A, Agthong S, et al. A role for mitogen-activated protein kinases in the aetiology of diabetic neuropathy. *FASEB J* 2001;15:2508–2514.
2. Tomlinson DR. Mitogen-activated protein kinases as glucose transducers for diabetic complications. *Diabetologia* 1999;42:1271–1281.
3. Fernyhough P, Tomlinson DR. The therapeutic potential of neurotrophins for the treatment of diabetic neuropathy. *Diabetes Reviews* 1999;7:300–311.
4. Calcutt NA, Allendoerfer KL, Mizisin AP, et al. Therapeutic efficacy of sonic hedgehog protein in experimental diabetic neuropathy. *J Clin Invest* 2003;111:507–514.
5. Fernyhough P, Diemel LT, Hardy J, Brewster WJ, Mohiuddin L, Tomlinson DR. Human recombinant nerve growth factor replaces deficient neurotrophic support in the diabetic rat. *Eur J Neurosci* 1995;7:1107–1110.
6. Nusslein-Volhard C, Wieschaus E. Mutations affecting segment number and polarity in Drosophila. *Nature* 1980;287:795–801.
7. Diaz-Benjumea FJ, Cohen SM. Wingless acts through the shaggy/zeste-white 3 kinase to direct dorsal-ventral axis formation in the Drosophila leg. *Development* 1994;120:1661–1670.
8. Echelard Y, Epstein DJ, St-Jacques B, et al. Sonic hedgehog, a member of a family of putative signaling molecules, is implicated in the regulation of CNS polarity. *Cell* 1993;75:1417–1430.
9. Ekker SC, Ungar AR, Greenstein P, et al. Patterning activities of vertebrate hedgehog proteins in the developing eye and brain. *Curr Biol* 1995;5:944–955.
10. Currie PD, Ingham PW. Induction of a specific muscle cell type by a hedgehog-like protein in zebrafish. *Nature* 1996;382:452–455.
11. Pathi S, Pagan-Westphal S, Baker DP, et al. Comparative biological responses to human Sonic, Indian, and Desert hedgehog. *Mech Dev* 2001;106:107–117.

12. Chiang C, Litingtung Y, Lee E, et al. Cyclopia and defective axial patterning in mice lacking Sonic hedgehog gene function. *Nature* 1996;383:407–413.
13. Briscoe J, Pierani A, Jessell TM, Ericson J. A homeodomain protein code specifies progenitor cell identify and neuronal fate in the ventral neural tube. *Cell* 2000;101:435–445.
14. Briscoe J, Chen Y, Jessell TM, Struhl G. A hedgehog-insensitive form of patched provides evidence for direct long-range morphogen activity of sonic hedgehog in the neural tube. *Mol Cell* 2001;7:1279–1291.
15. Kohtz JD, Baker DP, Corte G, Fishell G. Regionalizaton within the mammalian telencephalon is mediated by changes in responsiveness to Sonic Hedgehog. *Development* 1998;125:5079–5089.
16. Bitgood MJ, Shen L, McMahon AP. Sertoli cell signaling by Desert hedgehog regulates the male germline. *Curr Biol* 1996;6:298–304.
17. Bitgood MJ, McMahon AP. Hedgehog and Bmp genes are coexpressed at many diverse sites of cell-cell interaction in the mouse embryo. *Dev Biol* 1995;172:126–138.
18. Parmantier E, Lynn B, Lawson D, et al. Schwann cell-derived Desert hedgehog controls the development of peripheral nerve sheaths. *Neuron* 1999;23:713–724.
19. Becker S, Wang ZJ, Massey H, et al. A role for Indian hedgehog in extraembryonic endoderm differentiation in F9 cells and the early mouse embryo. *Dev Biol* 1997;187:298–310.
20. Vortkamp A, Pathi S, Peretti GM, Caruso EM, Zaleske DJ, Tabin CJ. Recapitulation of signals regulating embryonic bone formation during postnatal growth and in fracture repair. *Mech Dev* 1998;71:65–76.
21. Ito M, Yoshioka K, Akechi M, et al. JSAP1, a novel Jun N-terminal protein kinase (JNK)-binding protein that functions as a scaffold factor in the JNK signaling pathway. *Mol Cell Biol* 1999;19:7539–7548.
22. Hooper JE, Scott MP. The Drosophila patched gene encodes a putative membrane protein required for segmental patterning. *Cell* 1989;59:751–765.
23. Nakano Y, Guerrero I, Hidalgo A, Taylor A, Whittle JR, Ingham PW. A protein with several possible membrane-spanning domains encoded by the Drosophila segment polarity gene patched. *Nature* 1989;341:508–513.
24. Motoyama J, Takabatake T, Takeshima K, Hui C. Ptch2, a second mouse Patched gene is co-expressed with Sonic hedgehog. *Nat Genet* 1998;18:104–106.
25. Rahnama F, Toftgard R, Zaphiropoulos PG. Distinct roles of PTCH2 splice variants in Hedgehog signalling. *Biochem J* 2004;378:325–334.
26. Goodrich LV, Milenkovic L, Higgins KM, Scott MP. Altered neural cell fates and medulloblastoma in mouse patched mutants. *Science* 1997;277:1109–1113.
27. Milenkovic L, Goodrich LV, Higgins KM, Scott MP. Mouse patched1 controls body size determination and limb patterning. *Development* 1999;126:4431–4440.
28. Chen Y, Struhl G. Dual roles for patched sequestering and transducing Hedgehog. *Cell* 1996;87:553–563.
29. Incardona JP, Lee JH, Robertson CP, Enga K, Kapur RP, Roelink H. Receptor-mediated endocytosis of soluble and membrane-tethered Sonic hedgehog by Patched-1. *Proc Natl Acad Sci USA* 2000;97:12,044–12,049.
30. McCarthy RA, Barth JL, Chintalapudi MR, Knaak C, Argraves WS. Megalin functions as an endocytic sonic hedgehog receptor. *J Biol Chem* 2002;277:25,660–25,667.
31. Oleinikov AV, Zhao J, Makker SP. Cytosolic adaptor protein Dab2 is an intracellular ligand of endocytic receptor gp600/megalin. *Biochem J* 2000;347Pt 3:613–621.
32. Orlando RA, Rader K, Authier F, et al. Megalin is an endocytic receptor for insulin. *J Am Soc Nephrol* 1998;9:1759–1766.
33. Hjalm G, Murray E, Crumley G, et al. Cloning and sequencing of human gp330, a Ca(2+)-binding receptor with potential intracellular signaling properties. *Eur J Biochem* 1996;239:132–137.

34. Chen W, Burgess S, Hopkins N. Analysis of the zebrafish smoothened mutant reveals conserved and divergent functions of hedgehog activity. *Development* 2001:128:2385–2396.
35. Litingtung Y, Chiang C. Specification of ventral neuron types is mediated by an antagonistic interaction between Shh and Gli3. *Nat Neurosci* 2000;3:979–985.
36. Ruppert JM, Kinzler KW, Wong AJ, et al. The GLI-Kruppel family of human genes. *Mol Cell Biol* 1988;8:3104–3113.
37. Orenic TV, Slusarski DC, Kroll KL, Holmgren RA. Cloning and characterization of the segment polarity gene cubitus interruptus Dominant of Drosophila. *Genes Dev* 1990;4:1053–1067.
38. Motzny CK, Holmgren R. The Drosophila cubitus interruptus protein and its role in the wingless and hedgehog signal transduction pathways. *Mech Dev* 1995;52:137–150.
39. Sisson JC, Ho KS, Suyama K, Scott MP. Costal2, a novel kinesin-related protein in the Hedgehog signaling pathway. *Cell* 1997;90:235–245.
40. Robbins E, Dobrzansky P, Haun K, et al. Efficacy of orally-administered CB-1093, an NGF-inducing vitamin D receptor ligand, in the fimbria fornix lesion model (Abstract). *Society for Neuroscience Abstracts* 1997;23:881.
41. Aza-Blanc P, Ramirez-Weber FA, Laget MP, Schwartz C, Kornberg TB. Proteolysis that is inhibited by hedgehog targets Cubitus interruptus protein to the nucleus and converts it to a repressor. *Cell* 1997;89:1043–1053.
42. Ohlmeyer JT, Kalderon D. Dual pathways for induction of wingless expression by protein kinase A and Hedgehog in Drosophila embryos. *Genes Dev* 1997;11:2250–2258.
43. Jiang J, Struhl G. Protein kinase A and hedgehog signaling in Drosophila limb development. *Cell* 1995;80:563–572.
44. Chen CH, von Kessler DP, Park W, Wang B, Ma Y, Beachy PA. Nuclear trafficking of Cubitus interruptus in the transcriptional regualation of Hedgehog target gene expression. *Cell* 1999;98:305–316.
45. Dai P, Akimaru H, Tanaka Y, Maekawa T, Nakafuku M, Ishii S. Sonic Hedgehog-induced activation of the Gli1 promoter is mediated by GLI3. *J Biol Chem* 1999;274:8143–8152.
46. Shin SH, Kogerman P, Lindstrom E, Toftgard R, Biesecker LG. GLI3 mutations in human disorders mimic Drosophila cubitus interruptus protein functions and localizaton. *Proc Natl Acad Sci USA* 1999;96:2880–2884.
47. Thomas PK, Tomlinson DR. Diabetic and hypoglycaemic neuropathy. In Peripheral Neuropathy 3 ed. Dyck PJ, Thomas PK, Griffin JW, Low PA, Poduslo JF, eds. W. B. Saunders Co., Philadelphia, 1992, pp.1219–1250.
48. Yagihashi S. Nerve structural defects in diabetic neuropathy: Do animals exhibit similar changes? *Neurosci Res Commun* 1997;21:25–32.
49. Longo FM, Powell HC, Lebeau J, Gerrero MR, Heckman H, Myers RR. Delayed nerve regeneration in streptozotocin diabetic rats. *Muscle Nerve* 1986;9:385–393.
50. Ekstrom AR, Tomlinson DR. Impaired nerve regeneraton in streptozotocin-diabetic rats. Effects of treatment with an aldose reductase inhibitor. *J Neurol Sci* 1989;93:231–237.
51. Mohiuddin L, Fernyhough P, Tomlinson DR. Reduced levels of mRNA encoding endoskeletal and growth-associated proteins in sensory ganglia in experimental diabetes mellitus. *Diabetes* 1995;44:25–30.
52. Scott JN, Clark AW, Zochodne DW. Neurofilament and tubulin gene expression in progressive experimental diabetes—failure of synthesis and export by sensory neurons. *Brain* 1999;122:2109–2117.
53. Boulton TG, Yancopoulos GD, Gregory JS, et al. An insulin-stimulated protein kinase similar to yeast kinases involved in cell cycle control. *Science* 1990;249:64–67.
54. Boulton TG, Nye SH, Robbins DJ, et al. ERKs: a family of protein-serine/threonine kinases that are activated and tyrosine phosphorylated in response to insulin and NGF. *Cell* 1991;65:663–675.

55. Boulton TG, Cobb MH. Identification of multiple extracellular signal-regulated kinases (ERKs) with antipeptide antibodies. *Cell Regul* 1991;2:357–371.
56. Zhou G, Bao ZQ, Dixon JE. Components of a new human protein kinase signal transduction pathway. *J Biol Chem* 1995;270:12,665–12,669.
57. Lee JD, Ulevitch RJ, Han J. Primary structure of BMK1: a new mammalian map kinase. *Biochem Biophys Res Commun* 1995;213:715–724.
58. English JM, Pearson G, Hockenberry T, Shivakumar L, White MA, Cobb MH. Contribution of the ERK5/MEK5 pathway to Ras/ Raf signaling and growth control. *J Biol Chem* 1999;274:31,588–31,592.
59. Hayashi M, Lee JD. Role of the BMK1/ERK5 signaling pathway: lessons from knockout mice. *J Mol Med* 2004;82:800–808.
60. Lechner C, Zahalka MA, Giot JF, Moller NP, Ullrich A: ERK6, a mitogen-activated protein kinase involved in C2C12 myoblast differentiation. *Proc Natl Acad Sci U S A* 1996;93:4355–4359.
61. Abe MK, Kuo WL, Hershenson MB, Rosner MR. Extracellular signal-regulated kinase 7 (ERK7), a novel ERK with a C-terminal domain that regulates its activity, its cellular localization, and cell growth. *Mol Cell Biol* 1999;19:1301–1312.
62. Abe MK, Saelzler MP, Espinosa R III, et al. ERK8, a new member of the mitogen-activated protein kinase family. *J Biol Chem* 2002;277:16,733–16,743.
63. Hibi M, Lin A, Smeal T, Minden A, Karin M. Identification of an oncoprotein-and UV-responsive protein kinase that binds and potentiates the c-Jun activation domain. *Genes Dev* 1993;7:2135–2148.
64. Waetzig V, Herdegen T. Neurodegenerative and physiological actions of c-Jun N-terminal kinases in the mammalian brain. *Neurosci Lett* 2004;361:64–67.
65. Yang DD, Kuan CY, Whitmarsh AJ, et al. Absence of excitotoxicity-induced apoptosis in the hippocampus of mice lacking the Jnk3 gene. *Nature* 1997;389:865–870.
66. Davis RJ. Transcriptional regulation by MAP kinases. *Mol Reprod Dev* 1995;42:459–467.
67. Cohen DM. Mitogen-activated prot ein kinase cascades and the signaling of hyperosmotic stress to immediate early genes. *Comp Biochem Physiol A Physiol* 1997;117:291–299.
68. Whitmarsh AJ, Davis RJ. Signal transduction by MAP kinases: regulation by phosphorylation-dependent switches. *Sci STKE* 1999;E1.
69. Han J, Lee JD, Bibbs L, Ulevitch RJ. A MAP kinase targeted by endotoxin and hyperosmolarity in mammalian cells. *Science* 1994;265:808–811.
70. Lee JC, Laydon JT, McDonnell PC, et al. A protein kinase involved in the regulation of inflammatory cytokine biosynthesis. *Nature* 1994;372:739–746.
71. Jiang Y, Chen C, Li Z, et al. Characterization of the structure and function of a new mitogen-activated protein kinase (p38β). *J Biol Chem* 1996;271:17,920–17,926.
72. Li Z, Jiang Y, Ulevitch RJ, Han J. The primary structure of p38 gamma: a new member of p38 group of MAP kinases. *Biochem Biophys Res Commun* 1996;228:334–340.
73. Goedert M, Cuenda A, Craxton M, Jakes R, Cohen P. Activation of the novel stress-activated protein kinase SAPK4 by cytokines and cellular stresses is mediated by SKK3 (MKK6); comparison of its substrate specificity with that of other SAP kinases. *EMBO J* 1997;16:3563–3571.
74. Raingeaud J, Whitmarsh AJ, Barrett T, Derijard B, Davis RJ. MKK3- and MKK6-regulated gene expression is mediated by the p38 mitogen-activated protein kinase signal transduction pathway. *Mol Cell Biol* 1996;16:1247–1255.
75. McLaughlin B, Pal S, Tran MP, et al. p38 activation is required upstream of potassium current enhancement and caspase cleavage in thiol oxidant-induced neuronal apoptosis. *J Neurosci* 2001;21:3303–3311.
76. Choi WS, Eom DS, Han BS, et al. Phosphorylation of p38 MAPK induced by oxidative stress is linked to activation of both caspase-8- and -9-mediated apoptotic pathways in dopaminergic neurons. *J Biol Chem* 2004;279:20,451–20,460.

77. Wang JY, Shum AY, Ho YJ, Wang JY. Oxidative neurotoxicity in rat cerebral cortex neurons: synergistic effects of H2O2 and NO on apoptosis involving activation of p38 mitogen-activated protein kinase and caspase-3. *J Neurosci Res* 2003;72:508–519.
78. Xia Z, Dickens M, Raingeaud J. Davis RJ, Greenberg ME. Opposing effects of ERK and JNK-p38 MAP kinases on apoptosis. *Science* 1995;270:1326–1331.
79. Eilers A, Whitfield J, Babij C, Rubin LL, Ham J. Role of the Jun kinase pathway in the regulation of c-Jun expression and apoptosis in sympathetic neurons. *J Neurosci* 1998;18:1713–1724.
80. Delcroix JD, Valletta JS, Wu C, Hunt SJ, Kowal AS, Mobley WC. NGF signaling in sensory neurons: evidence that early endosomes carry NGF retrograde signals. *Neuron* 2003;39:69–84.
81. Mielke K, Brecht S, Dorst A, Herdegen T. Activity and expression of JNK1, p38 and ERK kinases, c-Jun N-terminal phosphorylation, and *c-jun* promoter binding in the adult rat brain following kainate-induced seizures. *Neurosci* 1999;91:471–483.
82. Gabbay KH, Merola LO, Field RA. Sorbitol pathway: presence in nerve and cord with substrate accumulation in diabetes. *Science* 1966;151:209–210.
83. Kinoshita JH. A thirty year journey in the polyol pathway. *Exp Eye Res* 1990;50:567–573.
84. Oates PJ. Polyol pathway and diabetic peripheral neuropathy. *Int Rev Neurobiol* 2002;50:325–392.
85. Sugimura K, Windebank AJ, Natarajan V, Lambert EH, Schmid HHO, Dyck PJ. Interstitial hyperosmolarity may cause axis cylinder shrinkage in streptozotocin diabetic nerve. *J Neuropathol Exp Neurol* 1980;39:710–721.
86. Galcheva-Gargova Z, Derijard B, Wu IH, Davis RJ. An osmosensing signal transduction pathway in mammalian cells. *Science* 1994;265:806–808.
87. Duzgun SA, Rasque H, Kito H, et al. Mitogen-activated protein phosphorylation in endothelial cells exposed to hyperosmolar conditions. *J Cell Biochem* 2000;76:567–571.
88. Igarashi M, Wakasaki H, Takahara N, et al. Glucose or diabetes activates p38 mitogen-activated protein kinase via different pathways. *J Clin Invest* 1999;103:185–195.
89. Schaffler A, Arndt H, Scholmerich J, Palitzsch KD. Amelioration of hyperglycemic and hyperosmotic induced vascular dysfunction by in vivo inhibition of protein kinase C and p38 MAP kinase pathway in the rat mesenteric microcirculation. *Eur J Clin Invest* 2000;30:586–593.
90. Nickander KK, Schmelzer JD, Rohwer DA, Low PA. Effect of α-tocopherol deficiency on indices of oxidative stress in normal and diabetic peripheral nerve. *J Neurol Sci* 1994;126:6–14.
91. Karasu Ç, Dewhurst M, Stevens EJ, Tomlinson DR. Effects of anti-oxidant treatment on sciatic nerve dysfunction in streptozotocin-diabetic rats; comparison with essential fatty acids. *Diabetologia* 1995;38:129–134.
92. Tutuncu NB, Bayraktar M, Varli K. Reversal of defective nerve conduction with vitamin E supplementation in type 2 diabetes: a preliminary study. *Diabetes Care* 1998;21:1915–1918.
93. Nagamatsu M, Nickander KK, Schmelzer JD, et al. Lipoic acid improves nerve blood flow, reduces oxidative stress, and improves distal nerve conduction in experimental diabetic neuropathy. *Diabetes Care* 1995;18:1160–1167.
94. Ziegler D, Hanefeld M, Ruhnau KJ, et al. Treatment of symptomatic diabetic peripheral neuropathy with the anti-oxidant α-lipoic acid—a 3-week multicentre randomized controlled trial (ALADIN study). *Diabetologia* 1995;38:1425–1433.
95. Garrett NE, Malcangio M, Dewhurst M, Tomlinson DR. α-Lipoic acid corrects neuropeptide deficits in diabetic rats via induction of trophic support. *Neurosci Lett* 1997;222:191–194.
96. Pop-Busui R, Sullivan KA, Van Huysen C, et al. Depletion of taurine in experimental diabetic neuropathy: implications for nerve metabolic, vascular, and functional deficits. *Exp Neurol* 2001;168:259–272.

97. Obrosova IG, Fathallah L, Stevens MJ. Taurine counteracts oxidative stress and nerve growth factor deficit in early experimental diabetic neuropathy. *Exp Neurol* 2001;172:211–219.
98. Brownlee M. Biochemistry and molecular cell biology of diabetic complications. *Nature* 2001;414:813–820.
99. Obrosova IG, Fathallah L, Greene DA. Early changes in lipid peroxidation and antioxidative defense in diabetic rat retina: effect of DL-alpha-lipoic acid. *Eur J Pharmacol* 2000;398:139–146.
100. Stevens MJ, Obrosova I, Cao XH, Van Huysen C, Greene DA. Effects of DL-α-lipoic acid on peripheral nerve conduction, blood flow, energy metabolism, and oxidative stress in experimental diabetic neuropathy. *Diabetes* 2000;49:1006–1015.
101. Obrosova IG, Mabley JG, Zsengeller Z, et al. Role for nitrosative stress in diabetic neuropathy: evidence from studies with a peroxynitrite decomposition catalyst. *FASEB J* 2005;19:401–403.
102. Gonzalez A-M, Sochor M, McLean P. The effect of an aldose reductase inhibitor (sorbinil) on the level of metabolites in lenses of diabetic rats. *Diabetes* 1983;32:482–485.
103. Bravi MC, Pietrangeli P, Laurenti O, et al. Polyol pathway activation and glutathione redox status in non-insulin-dependent diabetic patients. *Metabolism* 1997;46:1194–1198.
104. Cameron NE, Cotter MA, Basso M, Hohman TC. Comparison of the effects of inhibitors of aldose reductase and sorbitol dehydrogenase on neurovascular function, nerve conduction and tissue polyol pathway metabolites in streptozotocin-diabetic rats. *Diabetologia* 1997;40:271–281.
105. Lee AY, Chung SS. Contributions of polyol pathway to oxidative stress in diabetic cataract. *FASEB J* 1999;13:23–30.
106. Cameron NE, Cotter MA, Jack AM, Basso MD, Hohman TC. Protein kinase C effects on nerve function, perfusion, Na^+,K^+-ATPase activity and glutathione content in diabetic rats. *Diabetologia* 1999;42:1120–1130.
107. Obrosova IG, Van Huysen C, Fathallah L, Cao XC, Greene DA, Stevens MJ. An aldose reductase inhibitor reverses early diabetes-induced changes in peripheral nerve function, metabolism, and antioxidative defense. *FASEB J* 2002;16:123–125.
108. Guyton KZ, Liu Y, Gorospe M, Xu Q, Holbrook NJ. Activation of mitogen-activated protein kinase by H_2O_2. Role in cell survival following oxidant injury. *J Biol Chem* 1996;271:4138–4142.
109. Clerk A, Fuller SJ, Michael A, Sugden PH. Stimulation of "stress-regulated" mitogen-activated protein kinases (stress-activated protein kinases/c-Jun N-terminal kinases and p38-mitogen-activated protein kinases) in perfused rat hearts by oxidative and other stresses. *J Biol Chem* 1998;273:7228–7234.
110. Kanterewicz BI, Knapp LT, Klann E. Stimulation of p42 and p44 mitogen-activated protein kinases by reactive oxygen species and nitric oxide in hippocampus. *J Neurochem* 1998;70:1009–1016.
111. Oh-hashi K, Maruyama W, Yi H, Takahashi T, Naoi M, Isobe K. Mitogen-activated protein kinase pathway mediates peroxynitrite-induced apoptosis in human dopaminergic neuroblastoma SH-SY5Y cells. *Biochem Biophys Res Commun* 1999;263:504–509.
112. Go YM, Patel RP, Maland MC, et al. Evidence for peroxynitrite as a signaling molecule in flow-dependent activation of c-Jun NH(2)-terminal kinase. *Am J Physiol* 1999;277:H1647–H1653.
113. Kamata H, Honda S, Maeda S, Chang L, Hirata H, Karin M. Reactive oxygen species promote TNFalpha-induced death and sustained JNK activation by inhibiting MAP kinase phosphatases. *Cell* 2005;120:649–661.
114. Zhang GX, Kimura S, Nishiyama A, et al. Cardiac oxidative stress in acute and chronic isoproterenol-infused rats. *Cardiovasc Res* 2005;65:230–238.
115. Ling PR, Mueller C, Smith RJ, Bistrian BR. Hyperglycemia induced by glucose infusion causes hepatic oxidative stress and systemic inflammation, but not STAT3 or MAP kinase activation in liver in rats. *Metabolism* 2003;52:868–874.

116. Lander HM, Tauras JM, Ogiste JS, Hori O, Moss RA, Schmidt AM. Activation of the receptor for advanced glycation end products triggers a p21(ras)-dependent mitogen-activated protein kinase pathway regulated by oxidant stress. *J Biol Chem* 1997;272:17,810–17,814.
117. Yeh CH, Sturgis L, Haidacher J, et al. Requirement for p38 and p44/p42 mitogen-activated protein kinases in RAGE-mediated nuclear factor-kappaB transcriptional activation and cytokine secretion. *Diabetes* 2001;50:1495–1504.
118. Taguchi A, Blood DC, del Toro G, et al. Blockade of RAGE-amphoterin signalling suppresses tumour growth and metastases. *Nature* 2000;405:354–360.
119. Fiuza C, Bustin M, Talwar S, et al. Inflammation-promoting activity of HMGB1 on human microvascular endothelial cells. *Blood* 2003;101:2652–2660.
120. Barr RK, Kendrick TS, Bogoyevitch MA. Identification of the critical features of a small peptide inhibitor of JNK activity. *J Biol Chem* 2002;277:10,987–10,997.
121. Price SA, Hounsom L, Purves-Tyson TD, Fernyhough P, Tomlinson DR. Activation of JNK in sensory neurons protects against sensory neuron cell death in diabetes and on exposure to glucose/oxidative stress in vitro. *Ann N Y Acad Sci* 2003;1010:95–99.
122. Fernyhough P, Gallagher A, Averill SA, Priestley JV, Hounsom L, Patel J, Tomlinson DR. Aberrant neurofilament phosphorylation in sensory neurons of rats with diabetic neuropathy. *Diabetes* 1999;48:881–889.
123. Purves TD, Tomlinson DR. Are mitogen-activated protein kinases glucose transducers for diabetic neuropathies? *Int Rev Neurobiol* 2002;50:83–114.
124. Price SA, Agthong S, Middlemas AB, Tomlinson DR. Mitogen-activated protein kinase p38 mediates reduced nerve conduction velocity in experimental diabetic neuropathy: interactions with aldose reductase. *Diabetes* 2004;53:1851–1856.
125. Jiang Y, Gram H, Zhao M, et al. Characterization of the structure and function of the fourth member of p38 group mitogen-activated protein kinases, p38delta. *J Biol Chem* 1997;272:30,122–30,128.
126. Underwood DC, Osborn RR, Kotzer CJ, et al. SB 239063, a potent p38 MAP kinase inhibitor, reduces inflammatory cytokine production, airways eosinophil infiltration, and persistence. *J Pharmacol Exp Ther* 2000;293:281–288.

7
Neuronal and Schwann Cell Death in Diabetic Neuropathy

James W. Russell, MD, MS, Rita M. Cowell, PhD, and Eva L. Feldman, MD, PhD

SUMMARY

The balance of evidence supports the concept that programmed cell death (PCD) occurs in cells of the peripheral nervous system (PNS) in the presence of diabetes, elevated glucose levels, or insulin deprivation. The morphological appearance of apoptosis, the severity of cell death, and the mechanism of cell death might vary between different cell types in the PNS and between different mammalian models of diabetes. However, most cells show evidence of mitochondrial (Mt) damage and some, if not all, the features of the original morphological descriptions of apoptosis. PCD has mainly been described in cell culture and animal models of diabetes, although there is also morphological evidence of apoptosis in Schwann cells from human sural nerve. Evidence of PCD or organellar damage often exceeds the observed dorsal root ganglion neuronal loss. Apoptosis represents only the final pathological observation in this state of organellar failure or suboptimal organelle function. It is likely that even nonapoptotic neurons exhibit impaired metabolic function and protein synthesis and this dysregulation will in part induce neuropathy. One potential mechanism for induction of apoptosis in the PNS is diabetes-induced generation of reactive oxygen species and dysregulation of Mt function. During Mt dysfunction, several essential players of apoptosis, including procaspases and cytochrome-*c* are released into the cytosol and result in the formation of multimeric complexes that induce apoptotic cell death. Antioxidants and certain regulators of the inner Mt membrane potential, for example B-cell lymphoma (BCL) proteins, uncoupling proteins, and growth factors might prevent apoptosis in the PNS. The primary precipitating events leading to apoptosis in the PNS need to be clearly delineated if it is to be understood how to intervene or prevent the most common complication of diabetes, namely neuropathy.

Key Words: Apoptosis; programmed cell death; diabetes; neuropathy; oxidative stress; mitochondria; growth factors; uncoupling proteins; BCL.

INTRODUCTION

Apoptosis or programmed cell death (PCD) is essential for the normal functioning and survival of most cells including those in the peripheral nervous system (PNS). The morphological appearance of apoptosis, the severity of cell death, and the mechanism of cell death might vary between different cell types in the PNS and between different mammalian models of diabetes. However, most cells show evidence of mitochondrial (Mt)

From: *Contemporary Diabetes: Diabetic Neuropathy: Clinical Management, Second Edition*
Edited by: A. Veves and R. Malik © Humana Press Inc., Totowa, NJ

damage and some, if not all, the features of the original morphological descriptions of apoptosis *(1–3)*. PCD has mainly been described in cell culture and animal models of diabetes, although there is also morphological evidence of apoptosis in Schwann cells (SC) from human sural nerve. Reactive oxygen species and the resulting oxidative stress play a pivotal role in apoptosis and are likely to primarily mediate their effect by causing dysregulation of Mt function. During Mt dysfunction, several essential players of apoptosis, including procaspases and cytochrome-*c* are released into the cytosol and result in the formation of multimeric complexes that induce apoptotic cell death. Antioxidants and certain regulators of the inner Mt membrane potential, for example, BCL proteins, uncoupling proteins (UCPs), and growth factors might prevent apoptosis in the PNS. Despite disagreements over the nature of apoptosis in some cells in the PNS, the actual importance of apoptosis in the PNS rests mainly in the pathways leading to apoptosis, and how intervention in these pathways might result in a reduction in the severity of peripheral neuropathy. This review will describe the pathological changes that distinguish apoptosis from other forms of cell death, describe known mechanisms of PCD, and finally discuss both evidence of PCD and mechanisms of PCD in the PNS.

DISTINGUISHING APOPTOSIS FROM NECROSIS

Cell death takes two distinct forms, necrosis and apoptosis. Necrosis is a degenerative process that follows irreversible injury to the cell. Apoptosis, a Greek word that refers to the dropping of leaves from the tree, is an active process requiring protein synthesis for its execution and might perform either a homeostatic or a pathological role. As a simple distinction, apoptosis requires activation of cell signaling whereas necrosis does not. Apoptosis produces characteristic morphological changes including shrinkage of the cell, cytoplasmic blebbing, rounding of the cell (loss of adhesion or anoikis), condensation of the nuclear chromatin and cytoplasm, fragmentation of the nucleus, and budding of the whole cell to produce membrane-bounded bodies in which organelles are initially intact *(1–3)*. These bodies are phagocytosed and digested by adjacent cells without evidence of inflammation. An important and overlooked characteristic is the presence of cell shrinkage, hence the original term of shrinking necrosis *(1,2)*. Other distinguishing features between apoptosis and necrosis include rupture of lysosomes and the internucleosome cleavage of DNA observed in apoptosis that does not resemble the random DNA degradation observed in necrosis *(4)*.

Despite the morphological and biochemical distinctions, it is important to realize that under pathological conditions both apoptosis and necrosis might result from the same process and that the difference in pathology might represent the degree of response to the same stimulus. For example, intracellular adenosine triphosphate (ATP) concentration might be critical in selection of the cell death pathway. A high ATP concentration favors apoptosis, whereas a low concentration promotes necrosis *(5–8)*. The activity of poly(ADP-ribose) polymerase (PARP)-1 might be the pivotal point in this cell death decision, and as in other pathological conditions is important in the pathogenesis of diabetic complications *(9–11)*. Although, poly ADP-ribosylation contributes to DNA repair and helps to maintain the genome, under conditions of oxidative stress there is overactivation of PARP that in turn consumes NAD(+), depletes ATP, and culminates in cell necrosis. If the ATP remains relatively high then PCD will occur by activation of caspases.

CASPASES AND PCD

The name caspase is derived from the specificity of these cysteine proteases to cleave their substrates after an aspartic acid. All caspases are synthesized as inactive zymogens called procaspases. At the onset of apoptosis, caspases undergo intramolecular cleavage and often this is followed by a second cleavage to remove the prodomain from the protease domain. The caspases form two primary groups, initiator caspases that include caspase-2, -8, -9, and -10, and effector caspases. Initiator caspases are the proximal death-inducing caspases that are activated in response to apoptotic stimuli; their primary function is to activate downstream effector caspases by catalyzing a single proteolytic cleavage. Activation of an effector caspase zymogen involves a specific intrachain cleavage, which is mediated by a specific initiator caspase. As a consequence of the intrachain cleavage, the catalytic activity of the effector caspase is enhanced by several orders of magnitude, thus magnifying the cell death inducing effect. Classically, PCD is induced by either extrinsic or intrinsic pathways.

EXTRINSIC PCD PATHWAY

The receptor-linked pathway is known as the extrinsic pathway and this pathway requires binding of a ligand to a death receptor on the cell surface *(4)*. In this system, tumor necrosis factor (TNF) and Fas ligand (FasL) bind to their cell surface death receptors, TNF receptor type 1 and Fas receptor, respectively. Once activated, these receptors recruit the signal-producing moieties TNF receptor type 1-associated death domain, Fas-associated death domain *(4)*, and caspase-8 forming an oligomeric complex called the death-inducing signaling complex. Formation of the death-inducing signaling complex activates the initiator caspase, caspase-8, which then cleaves and activates the effector caspase-3, resulting in PCD *(12–14)*. Although the extrinsic pathway is less well-characterized in diabetic complications, there is evidence of FasL activation in association with diabetic neuropathy. Circulating soluble Fas and soluble FasL, two transmembrane glycoproteins involved in apoptosis are significantly increased in diabetic patients with neuropathy compared with patients without complications or nondiabetic subjects. However, it is unclear if Fas has a neuronal origin *(15)*.

INTRINSIC PCD PATHWAY

In contrast to the extrinsic pathway, the intrinsic pathway (Fig. 1) is mediated primarily by Mt and Mt stress *(3,16–21)*. One of the pivotal events in the process is Mt outer membrane permeabilization. This leads to release of several Mt inducers, for example, cytochrome-*c*, which are normally found in the space between the inner and outer Mt membrane. Under high glucose conditions and in the diabetic state, Mt outer membrane permeabilization is often preceded by hyperpolarization of the inner Mt membrane potential ($\Delta\Psi_M$), followed by a depolarization step, an event associated with induction of PCD *(16,20,22,23)*. In dorsal root ganglion (DRG) neurons, the hyperpolarization wave is observed early after an added glucose load and this corresponds to early cleavage of caspase-3 at the same point of time. One of the key events preceding apoptosis is a change in the Mt permeability transition. Mt permeability transition is associated with opening of the adenine nucleotide transporter (ANT)/voltage-dependent anion channel (VDAC) spanning the inner and outer Mt membranes. This change results in osmotic

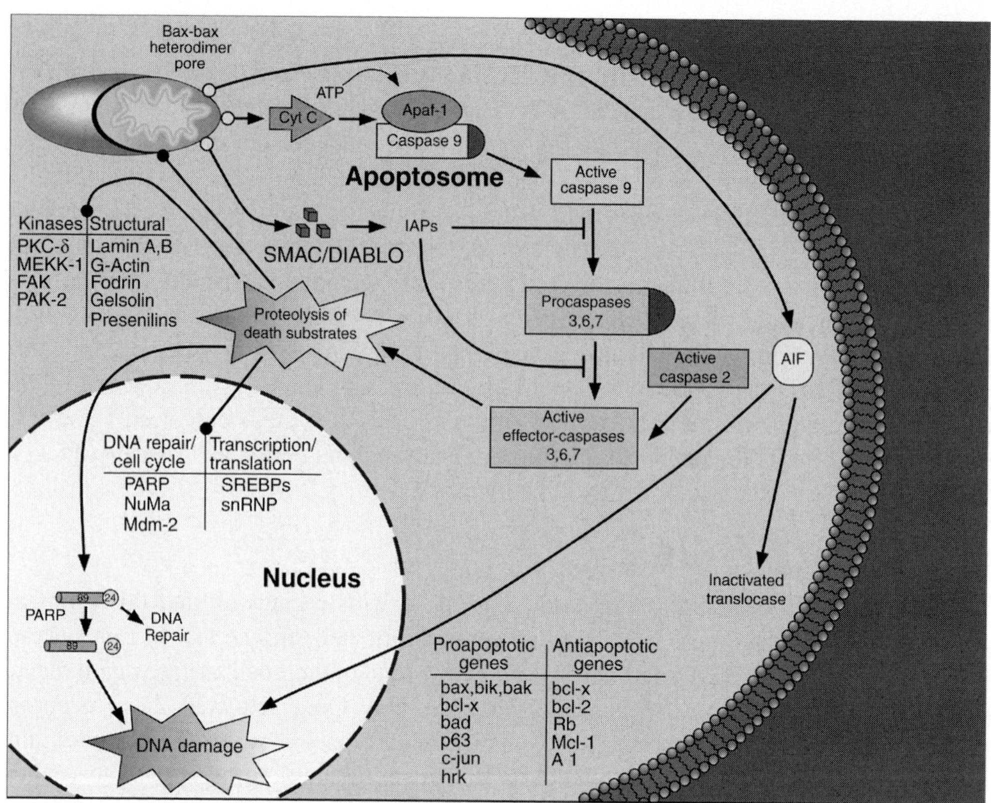

Fig. 1. Model for PCD pathways in neurons. Following inner Mt membrane depolarization, cytochrome-*c* (Cyt C) is released and combines with cell death pathway components to form the apoptosome complex, consisting of caspase-9 and apoptosis protease-activating factor 1 (Apaf-1). The formation of this complex leads to cleavage of caspase-9 and downstream activation of effector caspases-3, -6 and -7. The activation of the effector caspases is blocked by inhibitor of apoptosis proteins (IAPs). The IAPs in turn might be inhibited by second Mt activator of caspase (SMAC/DIABLO) that is released by apoptotic stimulation of the Mt. The effector caspases damage structural proteins, inhibit the DNA repair cycle, DNA transcription and translation, and cleave poly-ADP-ribose-polymerase (PARP). Cleavage of PARP facilitates the degradation of DNA. Apoptosis inducing factor (AIF) is released from the Mt with induction of apoptosis through a caspase independent pathway. AIF translocates to the nucleus causing DNA fragmentation. Genes that regulate apoptosis (both activators and inhibitors) are listed. (Reprinted from ref. *115*.)

swelling that in turn disrupts the integrity of the outer Mt membrane *(24)*, and is associated with release of proapoptotic factors into the cytoplasm that activate the caspase cascade *(17)*. In contrast, inhibition of the ANT/VDAC channel by bongkrekic acid or with cyclosporine stabilizes the $\Delta\Psi_m$ *(20,25,26)*, and inhibits downstream cleavage of caspase-3 indicating that stabilization of the $\Delta\Psi_M$ is important in preventing PCD. Moreover, kinetic data show that Mt undergo major changes in membrane permeability, polarity, and volume before other well-recognized signs of apoptosis such as caspase activation and chromatin condensation *(18)*. All these changes have been described in models of diabetic neuropathy *(16,20,27–31)*.

The BCL-2 family of apoptosis-regulating proteins might also prevent Mt outer membrane permeabilization. Certain Bcl proteins inhibit PCD. For example, BCL-2, BCL-xL, and BCL-2-associated athanogene (Bag-1) are part of the basic machinery that controls PCD by inhibiting a variety of stimuli including reactive oxygen species (ROS) generation and loss of trophic support *(32–34)*. BCL-2 and related proteins act directly on the outer Mt membrane to prevent permeabilization *(3,17,35,36)*, and suppress PCD *(37,38)* by regulating calcium fluxes through the Mt and endoplasmic reticulum *(39)*. BCL-xL appears to function in a similar manner to BCL-2. Bag-1 shares no significant homology with BCL-2, but interacts functionally and additively with BCL-2 to prevent PCD *(33)*.

In contrast, proapoptotic BCL proteins, such as BAX and BAK can bind to VDAC and might result in permeabilization of the outer Mt membrane *(40,41)*. In the presence of an apoptosis-inducing signal, BCL-2-associated protein (BAX) and BCL-2-homologous antagonist killer (BAK) oligomerize and insert into the outer Mt membrane *(42)*. In support of this concept, mice lacking BAX and BAK fail to undergo outer membrane permeabilization and apoptosis following numerous apoptotic signals *(43,44)*. When there is loss of outer Mt membrane permeability, this leads to release of proteins from the intermembrane space, although rather than being released simultaneously, release is likely dependent on secondary events for example remodeling of the matrix or change in polarity of the inner Mt membrane *(45)*.

Despite the intrinsic and extrinsic apoptosis pathways exhibiting well-characterized hierarchies, a potential interaction between the pathways exists. The extrinsic pathway interacts with the intrinsic pathway through caspase-8-mediated cleavage of BCL-2 interacting protein (BID), which triggers the release of proapoptotic proteins from the intermembrane space of Mt into the cytoplasm *(46)*.

CYTOSOLIC PCD PATHWAY

Induction of PCD might also occur independently of Mt depolarization *(47)* by primarily cytosolic mechanisms. One key component of the cell death machinery, Apaf-1, in the presence of dATP forms a complex with cytochrome-*c* and caspase-9 (the apoptosome) *(13,48,49)*. Selective binding of caspase-9 to Apaf-1 results in caspase-9-dependent hierarchical activation of caspases-2, -3, -6, -7, -8, and -10, resulting ultimately in DNA fragmentation seen in apoptosis *(50–53)*. In turn, caspase-3 activates caspase-2, -6, -8, and -10 and amplifies caspase-9 cleavage *(50)*. In contrast, BCL-2 and BCL-xL complex with Apaf-1 and caspase-9 through different binding sites to form a ternary complex *(48)* that inhibits cleavage of downstream caspases *(48)* and serve to inhibit PCD.

OXIDATIVE AND NITROSATIVE INDUCED CELL DEATH IN DIABETIC NEUROPATHY

Hyperglycemia promotes production of superoxides (O_2^-), increases flux through the Mt electron transport chain, and might be responsible for most of the key features of oxidative stress *(20,23,54,55)*. In cell culture models of hyperglycemia, inhibition of formation prevents glucose-induced formation of advanced glycation end products (AGEs) and activation of protein kinase-C *(56)*. O_2^- can also react with nitric oxide (NO) to form peroxynitrite ($ONOO^-$), which can damage intracellular lipids and proteins, resulting in lipid peroxidation, DNA fragmentation, and cell death. Accumulation of

NADH coupled with failure of the Mt creatine phosphate pump to regenerate ATP from ADP also results in disruption of the Mt electron transfer chain, and depletion of ATP *(56)*. Depletion of ATP is associated with apoptosis in vitro *(20)*, and similar changes are seen in chronic neuropathy in diabetic animals *(57)*. Oxidative stress can be prevented by inhibitors of the Mt electron transport chain, for example, Mt complex II or III inhibitors, for example, TTFA or myxothiazole *(20,58)*. Failure to prevent oxidative stress results in Mt DNA damage. DNA damage might be repaired by base excision repair, however, if not repaired there is furthermore disruption of the electron transport chain and production of further ROS. This vicious cycle of ROS production and Mt DNA damage ultimately leads to energy depletion in the cell and apoptosis *(29,59)*.

One potential stimulus for O_2^- generation is NO *(60)*. NO by interaction with the electron transport chain functions not only acts as a physiological regulator of cell respiration, but also augments the generation of ROS by Mt, and can trigger PCD *(61)*. Evidence of increased production of reactive nitrogen species (NO and $ONOO^-$) coupled with evidence of PCD implicate nitrosative injury in models of diabetic neuropathy *(62,63)*. NO is formed by activation of NO synthase (NOS), which analyzes the oxidation of L-arginine to NO and citrulline (for review *see* ref. *64*). Neuronal NOS is the primary constitutively active isoform in neurons. NO is relatively unstable in vivo, however, it can bind thiol-containing proteins, thereby substantially increasing its half-life. This process, called S-nitrosylation results in directed and rapid activation or deactivation of proteins and affects the signaling of specific proteins *(64–67)*.

NO might have both neuroprotective and neurotoxic roles depending on other modifying pathways. NO induced toxicity depends in general on the degree of local generation of NO and/or O_2^- *(68,69)*. $ONOO^-$ can inactivate electron transfer complexes I, II, and ATPase *(70)*, reversibly nitroslylate or irreversibly nitrate critical proteins and enzymes, including manganese superoxide dismutase, cytochrome-*c*, aconitase, and VDAC (reviewed in refs. *64,71*). In combination, these effects of NO increase oxidative stress and nitrosative stress through the overproduction of S-nitrosylated proteins *(72)*. Manganese superoxide dismutase, a superoxide scavenger, might protect from $ONOO^-$-induced cell death *(69)*.

Activation of neuronal NOS, endothelial NOS, or the inducible form of NOS might produce paradoxical responses in the peripheral nerve. Inducible NOS is increased in the arteries of diabetic rats *(73)*, but unchanged in DRG neurons from chronically diabetic rats *(74)*. Deficits in endothelial NO and other endothelial vasodilators can result in reduced nerve perfusion and function *(64,75,76)*. With ischemia, there is failure of the endothelial NOS:NO axis that will result in reduced perfusion of the peripheral nerve and further aggravate ischemic oxidative injury to the peripheral nerve.

APOPTOSIS IN DRG

Pathological changes consistent with apoptosis have been described in the PNS in models of diabetic neuropathy. Several pathological changes are observed in the diabetic DRG and dorsal roots (Fig. 2). Condensation of chromatin, shrinkage of the nucleus and cell cytoplasm, with preservation of the cytoplasmic membrane are seen in both DRG neurons as well as in satellite cells or SC from diabetic but not from control animals *(27)*. These apoptotic changes occur side-by-side with healthy cells, consistent with single cell deletion. The changes are evenly distributed throughout the DRG neurons and in addition are observed in dorsal root SC. Frequent large vacuoles are observed, evenly distributed throughout the cytoplasm and many correspond to enlarged ballooned Mt with disruption of the inner cristae structure. The abnormal vacuoles are most prominent in cells showing early apoptotic changes such as mild chromatin aggregation with neuronal and cytoplasmic shrinkage. Although occasional vacuolation is observed in DRG cells from control animals, the Mt structure appears normal. After acute induction of hyperglycemia in animals, there is evidence of chromatin compaction, shrinkage of the nucleus and cytoplasm with preservation of the cell membrane in the presence of intact lysosomes. These changes are more severe than in the chronically hyperglycemic rodent *(27)*. Similar to the changes observed in vivo, high glucose induces apoptosis in vitro: the degree of cell injury is dependent on the concentration of glucose present and occurs rapidly. In vitro, DRG cultured in extra glucose show compaction of chromatin into uniformly dense masses, deletion of single cells, cell shrinkage into apoptotic bodies, retention of membrane integrity with some membrane blebbing, and presence of intact lysosomes. This effect cannot be explained merely by glucose-induced hyperosmolarity, as similar changes are not observed when equiosmolar concentrations of mannitol or sodium chloride are used *(27)*.

One of the areas of controversy has been whether there is classical apoptosis in the PNS and if loss of DRG neurons by apoptosis is responsible for the observed neuropathic deficits observed in both animals and humans. Most studies to date indicate there is activation of caspases in DRG neurons both in vitro and in vivo *(16,20,27–31)*. There is also evidence of neuronal nuclear DNA fragmentation using in vivo studies with rigorously applied controls showing convincing positive TdT-mediated dUTP-biotin nick end labeling (TUNEL) staining with DNAse *(27–29)*. Most studies indicate some loss of DRG neurons *(27,31,77)*, and in particular there is a statistically significant loss of large DRG neurons *(31)*. In one study, using rigorous counting techniques of DRG nuclei in 6–12 pairs of sections from the whole DRG, it was concluded that there was no loss of neurons in the DRG from diabetic animals *(77)*. In fact, this study showed a 14.5% decrease in the mean number of neurons (determined by nuclei) per ganglia in 12-month diabetic compared with control animals. However, there was a large variance between animal groups and this likely resulted in inadequate power to detect a statistical difference. In fact, there is clear evidence that not all neurons are affected equally and that there is variability in the degree of neuronal loss in experimental animals similar to the observed variability in the severity of neuropathy in humans. Thus, the concept that a similar diabetic insult will always result in neuronal injury in all DRG neurons equally, and will produce the same degree of loss of sensory neurons is simplistic. Eventhough, there is evidence of DRG neuronal loss, the number of DRG neurons showing evidence of caspase-3 cleavage or TUNEL staining appears to be higher than the measured loss of neurons. This might occur because activation of caspases does not invariably result in neuronal death, or that there is an intrinsic capacity for repair within the neuron resulting either from DNA repair or by activation of neurotrophic protective signaling pathways *(78)*.

As indicated in the initial description of mechanisms of apoptosis, PCD is a balance between caspase activation and blocking by inhibitors of apoptosis. One possible repair

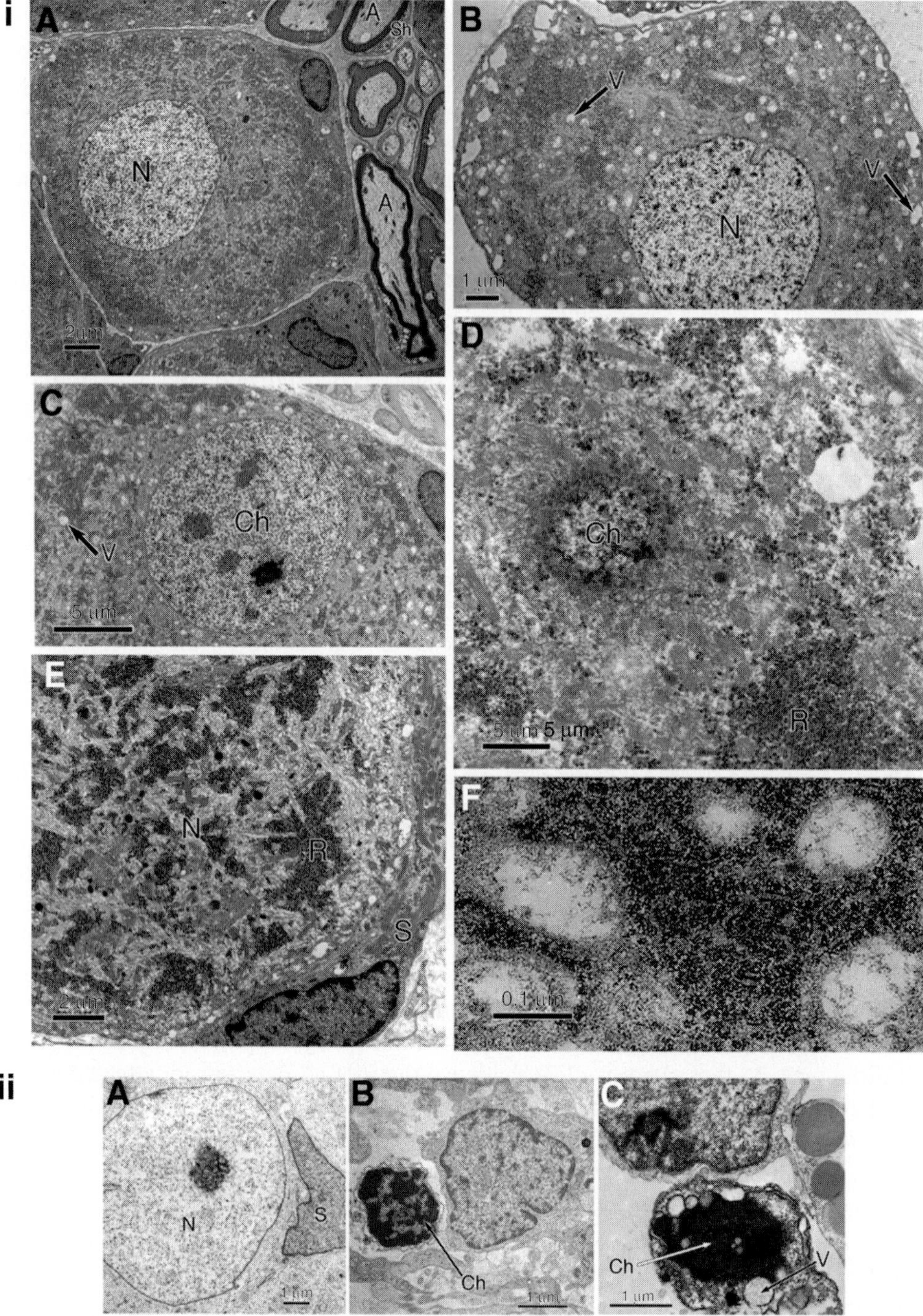

Fig. 2. Electron micrographs showing representative early apoptotic changes and vacuolation in DRG neurons, and SC in: **(I)** diabetic (1 month) and control animals. **(A)** Control DRG neurons and axons, showing normal diffuse chromatin staining in the nucleus (N), Schwann cell (Sh), and normal axons (A) with intact myelin lamellae showing little or no myelin splitting. **(B)** DRG neuron from a diabetic animal showing coarse chromatin staining, with early aggregation

mechanism would be by elevated expression of the DNA repair enzyme PARP *(30)*. DNA repair by PARP-1 is itself a double-edged regulator of cellular survival. When the DNA damage is moderate, PARP-1 participates in the DNA repair process. Conversely, in the case of massive DNA injury, elevated PARP-1 activation leads to rapid and massive NAD(+)/ATP consumption and cell death by necrosis *(10)*.

Studies in cell culture and diabetic animals indicate that there is dysfunction of the normal electron transfer chain function and that this is associated with induction of oxidative stress *(20)*. In a DRG cell culture model, the first 2 hour of hyperglycemia are sufficient to induce oxidative stress and PCD *(79)*. On exposure to elevated glucose concentrations, superoxide formation, inhibition of aconitase, and lipid peroxidation occurs within 1 hour of the hyperglycemic stress, and is followed rapidly by caspase-3 activation and DNA fragmentation *(20,79)*. Injury to the neurons can be prevented by the antioxidant α-lipoic acid *(79,80)*, consistent with a model in DRG neurons where oxidative stress induced apoptosis can be ameliorated or prevented by antioxidants. This finding is supported by in vivo data that antioxidants can prevent neuronal and axonal injury in the PNS *(11,23,57,64,81,82)*. In 1–12-month diabetic rats, 8-Hydroxy-2′-deoxyguanosine labeling is significantly increased at all time-points in DRG neurons consistent with oxidative DNA injury *(29)*. The changes in oxidative injury are coupled with an increase in caspase-3 labeling in acutely and chronically diabetic animals. These apoptotic changes are coupled with loss of DRG neurons that were higher in chronic in comparison with acutely diabetic animals and a progressive sensory neuropathy *(29)*.

Corresponding to this evidence of apoptosis, are changes in the intrinsic pathway of PCD. In the diabetic state, there is evidence of MMD *(20,28,83,84)*. In affected DRG neurons, there is a decrease in BCL-2 levels and translocation of cytochrome-*c*

Fig. 2. *(Continued)* in the nucleus (N) and vacuolation (V) in the cytoplasm. Remains of Mt cristae can be seen in many of the vacuoles, a change that is even more apparent at higher magnifications. **(C)** More severe chromatin aggregation (Ch), vacuolation (V) throughout the cytoplasm, and condensed rough endoplasmic reticulum associated with apparent loss of perikaryeal volume. **(D)** Further DRG neuronal chromatin clumping (Ch) and early dissolution of the nucleus. There is further ribosomal aggregation (R). Although blebbing of the cytoplasmic membrane is observed, the membrane remains intact with no evidence of inflammation or phagocytosis. **(E)** End stage changes in the DRG neuron. The nucleus is severely fragmented and the nuclear outline is no longer apparent. There is marked condensation of rough endoplasmic reticulum and ribosomes (R). Despite severe blebbing, the neuronal cytoplasmic membrane is still present. An adjacent satellite cell (S) has maintained its integrity consistent with single cell deletion of the DRG neuron during the process of apoptosis. **(F)** Enlarged Mt from DRG neuron in B showing disruption of cristae. **(II)** DRG cell culture. Whole DRG were cultured for 48 hours in the conditions described below: **(A)** Control DRG. Normal nucleus (N) and nucleolus, with evenly distributed chromatin. The satellite cell (S) shows darker staining, but non-aggregated chromatin, and a "cap shaped" nucleus, which is normal for this cell. **(B)** Twenty millimolar added glucose. There is well-developed chromatin compaction (Ch) in one neuron, and early compaction in another neuron. Both neurons show shrinkage of the perikaryon, but the outer cell membrane is intact. **(C)** High glucose (150 m*M*). There is early chromatin compaction (Ch) and shrinking of the cell nucleus and perikaryon similar to the changes seen in **B**. (Reprinted from ref. *27*, with permission from Elsevier.)

from the Mt to the cytoplasm *(85)*. One of the key events preceding apoptosis is a change in the permeability transit pore (PTP) associated with opening of the ANT/VDAC channel spanning the inner and outer Mt membranes *(19,20)*. In hyperglycemic conditions there is early serine phosporylation of BCL-2 followed by a reduction in BCL-2 expression and loss of $\Delta\Psi_M$ *(19)*.

UCPs also have sequence homology to Mt transporters including the BCL proteins suggesting that they might be Mt carriers *(70,86,87)*. When UCP levels are reduced, the $\Delta\Psi_M$ is abnormally high, and increases backpressure on the inner Mt membrane proton pumps. These events might further promote induction of PCD. *UCP3* expression is rapidly downregulated by hyperglycemia in diabetic rats and by high-glucose in cultured neurons *(16)*, and maintained by the presence of bongkrekic acid consistent with regulation of UCPs by the $\Delta\Psi_M$ *(16,19,22)*. Overexpression of UCP1, -2, or -3 prevents glucose-induced transient Mt membrane hyperpolarization, ROS formation, and induction of PCD *(16,22)*.

Interestingly, insulin-like growth factor (IGF)-I is neuroprotective by blocking Mt swelling, inner mitochondrial membrane depolarization (MMD), and caspase-3 activation. Two important IGF-I signaling pathways, phosphatidylinositol 3-kinase (PI3K) and mitogen-activated protein (MAP) kinase/MAP-extracellular signal regulated kinase (MEK) are implicated in regulation of apoptosis *(88,89)*. In neurons treated with high glucose, the PI3K pathway is the primary pathway regulating BCL-2 and BCL-xL, MMD, and apoptosis *(19,90)*. Although inhibition of MAPK/MEK signaling independently and partially blocks IGF-I inhibition of MMD, these signaling intermediates do not significantly affect IGF-I inhibition of Mt swelling, indicating that IGF-I regulates different components of Mt function through discrete signaling pathways *(19)*. IGF-I stimulation of the PI3K/Akt pathway phosphorylates three known Akt effectors: the survival transcription factor CREB and the proapoptotic effector proteins glycogen synthase kinase-3β and forkhead. IGF-I regulates DRG survival at the nuclear level by increasing accumulation of phospho-Akt in DRG neuronal nuclei, increased CREB-mediated transcription, and nuclear exclusion of forkhead *(90)*. A further mechanism by which IGF-I can reduce apoptosis in DRG neurons is by activating UCPs and in particular UCP3 through a PI3K regulated signaling pathway *(91–93)*. Similar changes have been observed with insulin treatment. Insulin increases the $\Delta\Psi_M$ and prevents MMD by activation of the PI3K signaling pathway and phosphorylation of Akt and cAMP response element binding (CREB) *(83,84)*. This in turn is associated with increased ATP levels.

Other signaling pathways might also be involved with regulation of PCD in DRG neurons: diabetes activates all three groups of MAP kinases in sensory ganglia *(94)*. Inhibition of ERK and p38, stress responsive members of the MAPK family, prevents nerve damage. Antioxidants and aldose reductase inhibitors that improve neuronal function in diabetic rats are also able to inhibit activation of ERK and p38 in DRG and increase activation of JNK *(94)*. In DRG from chronically diabetic rats, the p54/56 isoforms of JNK are activated and furthermore activated when these animals are treated with antioxidants. In contrast, cultured DRG neurons die when treated with JNK inhibitors. It is thus likely that activation of C-Jun N-terminal kinases (JNK) because of a combination of raised glucose and oxidative stress serves to protect DRG neurons from glycemic damage *(94)*. Alternative apoptosis pathways such as p53 activation have been shown to occur in an oxygen glucose deprivation model of ischemia observed in diabetic neuropathy *(80,95)*.

Specifically, there is an increase in phospho-p53 levels under hypoxic-glucose deprivation that is associated with DNA damage and cell-cycle disruption. These changes suggest a possible role for p53-mediated apoptosis in diabetic neuropathy *(95)*. DRG neuronal apoptosis in this system was prevented by increasing the concentration of NGF in the culture medium consistent with observations in both animal model of diabetes and human neuropathy that nerve growth factor (NGF) might protect against apoptosis *(96,97)*.

Metabotropic glutamate receptors (mGluRs) might also regulate CREB signaling intermediates and prevent neuronal cellular injury *(98–101)*. The mGluRs are a subfamily of glutamate receptors that are G protein-coupled and linked to second messenger systems *(101,102)*. In addition to strong mechanism-driven evidence that glutamate carboxypeptidase (GCP)II inhibitors and mGluR3 agonists are neuroprotective, there are preclinical data that GCPII inhibitors ameliorate diabetic neuropathy in animal models *(103)*. The GCPII inhibitor 2-(phosphonomethyl)pentanedioic acid (2-PMPA) is protective against glucose-induced PCD and neurite degeneration in DRG neurons in a cell culture model of diabetic neuropathy *(98)*. In this model, inhibition of neuronal PCD is mediated by the Group II mGluR, mGluR3. 2-PMPA neuroprotection is completely reversed by the mGluR3 antagonist, (S)-α-ethylglutamic acid, but not by Group I and III mGluR inhibitors. Other mGluR3 agonists, for example, (2R, 4R)-4-aminopyrrolidine-2,4-dicarboxylate (APDC) and *N*-acetyl-aspartyl-glutamate provide protection to neurons exposed to high glucose conditions, consistent with the concept that 2-PMPA neuroprotection is mediated by increased *N*-acetyl-aspartyl-glutamate activity. Furthermore, the direct mGluR3 agonist, APDC prevents induction of ROS *(104)*. Together these findings are consistent with an emerging concept that mGluRs might protect against cellular injury by regulating oxidative stress in the neuron, and might represent a novel mechanism to prevent ROS induced PCD in diabetic neuropathy.

APOPTOSIS IN AUTONOMIC NEURONS

Apoptosis in the diabetic autonomic nervous system has been less completely studied than in the somatic nervous system. Nevertheless, important information on the regulation of apoptosis in the autonomic nervous system has become available in the last 5 years. In rat superior cervical ganglion (SCG) cultures, there is evidence of glucose-induced apoptosis in SCG neurons, although they are considerably less sensitive to glucose toxicity than DRG neurons treated with the same high glucose conditions *(105)*. Apoptosis in SCG neurons is coupled with inhibition of neurite growth, reduction in neurite caliber, beading of neurites, and retraction of the neurite growth cone consistent with degeneration of autonomic fibers *(105)*. In agreement with these findings, acute streptozotocin diabetes is associated with evidence of PCD in a small number of autonomic neurons and activation of the apoptotic cascade occurs relatively early in diabetic autonomic neuropathy *(106)*. However, there is no significant neuron loss in chronic diabetes in either the rat superior mesenteric or superior cervical sympathetic ganglia, indicating that apoptotic neuronal cell death alone is unlikely to account for the severity of autonomic neuropathy observed in type 1 diabetes *(107)*.

As with DRG neurons, insulin and IGF-I inhibit both the induction of apoptosis and loss of autonomic neurons *(105,108)*. Furthermore, loss of autonomic neurons is more severe in animal models of type 1 in comparison with type 2 diabetes, suggesting a protective role for insulin and IGF-I and that failure of these protective systems may account for the severity of autonomic dysfunction in type 1 diabetes *(106,109)*. In support of this concept, differences in neuroaxonal dystrophy have been observed in different animal models of autonomic neuropathy: two models of type 1 diabetes, the streptozotocin diabetic and BB/W rat develop marked hyperglycemia and concomitant deficiency in both circulating insulin and IGF-I. These type 1 animals develop neuroaxonal dystrophy in nerve terminals in the prevertebral sympathetic ganglia and the distal portions of noradrenergic ileal mesenteric nerves. In contrast, the Zucker diabetic fatty rat, an animal model of type 2 diabetes, despite developing severe hyperglycemia comparable with that in the STZ- and BB/W-diabetic rat models does not develop neuroaxonal dystrophy. Unlike the type 1 models of diabetes, the Zucker diabetic fatty rats have significant hyperinsulinemia and normal levels of plasma IGF-I *(109)*.

APOPTOSIS IN THE SC

Despite the abundance of SC in the peripheral nerve, less is known about SC than DRG apoptosis in the diabetic PNS. Several lines of evidence support morphological changes of apoptosis in SC in vitro, in models of diabetic neuropathy, and in human diabetic neuropathy *(22,110)*. SC obtained from the dorsal root of diabetic animals exhibit chromatin clumping and disruption of the myelin surrounding atrophic axons (Fig. 3) *(110)*. Schwann-like satellite cells from corresponding diabetic DRG show severe chromatin clumping, and perikaryeal vacuolation consistent with Mt ballooning and disruption of the internal Mt cristae structure. Similar observations have been made in vitro using the chromatin stain bisbenzamide. Under high glucose conditions, SC nuclei break apart into brightly staining apoptotic clusters indicative of chromatin condensation and nuclear fragmentation, changes that are confirmed with TUNEL and propidium iodide staining. Furthermore, high glucose conditions promote cleavage of caspase-3 and -7. The antiapoptotic BCL family protein, BCL-xL is expressed in normal SC, but is not significantly increased or decreased under high glucose conditions. However, overexpression of BCL-xL protects SC from apoptosis in vitro *(110)*.

Changes in animal models of diabetes are reproduced in human SC. In human sural nerve SCs from patients with moderately severe diabetic neuropathy, several key changes consistent with SC apoptosis are observed in some, but not all SC. These include: nuclear chromatin condensation, shrinkage of the SC cytosol, swelling and disruption of the Mt and of the rough endoplasmic reticulum, disruption of the normal Mt cristae structure, and formation of cytoplasmic vacuoles *(21,22)*. Eventually, there is loss of the SC nucleus and cytosol with preservation of the plasma membrane and supporting collagen, forming ghost cells. These changes are consistent with single cell deletion observed in apoptosis, but rarely in necrosis. No inflammatory infiltrates are observed in the affected nerves, such as might be seen with necrosis of the peripheral nerve. One potential cause for glucose-induced apoptosis is by generation of AGEs. In SC treated with different isoforms of AGE, a change in the $\Delta\Psi_M$ leading to depolarization and SC apoptosis was induced by AGE-2 and -3, but not AGE-1. Apoptosis was ameliorated by the antioxidant α-lipoic acid and by inhibition of p38 signaling. In addition, AGE-2 and -3 significantly

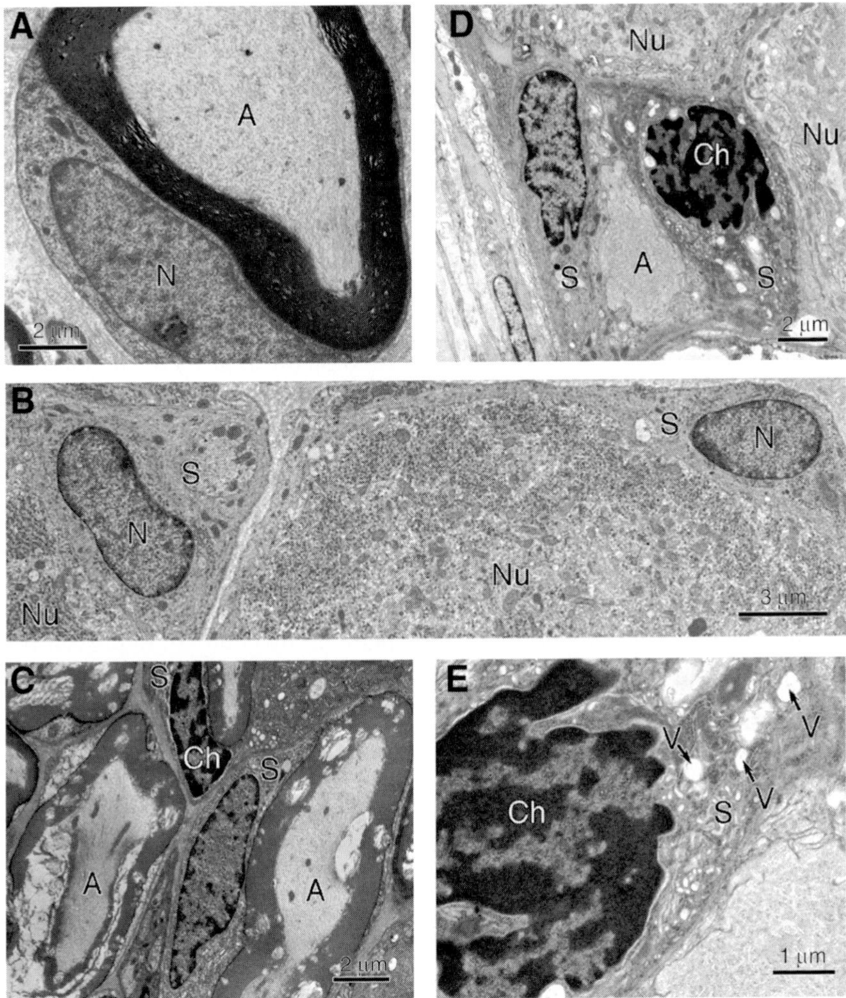

Fig. 3. Electron micrograph of SC from control and STZ-treated diabetic rats. Control animals **(A,B)** and STZ-treated rats made diabetic for 1 month **(C–E)**. Control SC, showing normal diffuse chromatin staining in the nucleus (N), and normal axon (A) with intact myelin lamellae showing little or no myelin splitting. **(A)** Satellite cells (S), which are Schwann-like cells, from a control animal showing normal diffuse chromatin staining in the nucleus (N), and cytoplasm. The satellite cells lie adjacent to DRG neurons (Nu) that show normal cytoplasmic components. **(B)** In the dorsal root, from diabetic animals, there is clumping of the chromatin (Ch) in the SC (S), atrophy of axons (A), and disruption of myelin surrounding the axons. **(C)** In Satellite cells (S) from a diabetic dorsal root ganglion, there is severe chromatin clumping (Ch), shrinkage of the perikaryeon, and prominent vacuolation. An atrophic axon (A) is seen, nestled between two Schwann-like satellite cells, adjacent to DRG neurons (Nu), which also show evidence of perikaryeal vacuolation. **(E)** End stage changes in a diabetic Schwann cell (S). There is nuclear chromatin clumping and fragmentation (Ch) coupled with prominent vacuolation (V) resulting from ballooning of mitochondria and disruption of their cristae. Bars in each panel indicate magnification. (Published with permission from ref. *110.*)

suppressed the SC replication rate, enhanced the release of TNF-α and IL-1β, and activated nuclear factor-κB *(111)*.

In contrast, certain growth factors can reduce SC apoptosis. Growth factors such as NGF might also serve as antioxidants and this function might contribute to their role as possible therapeutic entities in diabetic neuropathy *(112–114)*. NGF in physiological concentrations is able to reduce SC MMD *(22)*. In contrast, pretreatment with 50 μg/mL p75 neurotrophin receptor (p75 NTR) functional blocking antibody blocks the effect of NGF on the $\Delta\Psi_M$. High glucose induces dose-dependent cleavage of caspases in SC. NGF also reduces apoptosis in SC measured using caspase-3 or TUNEL. This reduction in apoptosis is reversed by pretreatment with p75 NTR function blocking antibody *(22)*. These results indicate that NGF mediates some of its Mt stabilizing effects and antiapoptotic effects through the p75 NTR. IGF-I is also protective to SC in culture at higher concentrations (10 n*M*) that active the IGF-I receptor but not the insulin receptor *(110)*. In contrast, PI3K, but not MAP/MEK kinase inhibitors block the protective effect of IGF-I. These findings are consistent with those in DRG neurons where IGF-I protects SC from apoptosis through PI3K signaling intermediates. Interestingly, the addition of IGF-I, in either normal glucose or high glucose, has no effect on BCL-xL expression in native SC or BCL-xL transfected SC suggesting a possible non-BCL-dependent mechanism in preventing apoptosis with glucose stress.

CONCLUSION

Because of the first observation of apoptosis in the PNS less than a decade ago, the balance of evidence supports the concept that PCD occurs in cells of the PNS in the presence of diabetes, elevated glucose levels, or insulin deprivation. In general, measured apoptosis is more severe in DRG neurons than in autonomic neurons, or SC. Ultimately, DRG neuronal death is a balance between finely regulated but often opposing pathways. Evidence of PCD or organellar damage often exceeds the observed DRG neuronal loss. This raises the question, is DRG neuronal loss of significance in the pathogenesis of diabetic neuropathy? Apoptosis represents only the final pathological observation in this state of organellar failure or suboptimal organelle function. It is likely that even nonapoptotic neurons exhibit impaired metabolic function and protein synthesis and this dysregulation will in part induce neuropathy. More importantly, the primary precipitating events leading to apoptosis in the PNS need to be clearly delineated if it is to be understood how to intervene or prevent the most common complication of diabetes, namely neuropathy.

ACKNOWLEDGMENTS

The authors would like to thank Ms. Denice Janus for secretarial support. This work was supported in part by NIH NS42056, The Juvenile Diabetes Research Foundation Center for the Study of Complications in Diabetes (JDRF), Office of Research Development (Medical Research Service), Department of Veterans Affairs (JWR); NS49863 (RMC); NIH NS36778, NIH NS38849, and grants from the JDRF and Program for Understanding Neurological Diseases (ELF) and the Michigan Imaging Laboratory.

REFERENCES

1. Kerr JF. Shrinkage necrosis: a distinct mode of cellular death. *J Pathol* 1971;105:13–20.
2. Kerr JF. History of the events leading to the formulation of the apoptosis concept. *Toxicology* 2002;181–182:471–474.
3. Green DR, Kroemer G. The pathophysiology of mitochondrial cell death. *Science* 2004; 305:626–629.
4. Kiechle FL, Zhang X. Apoptosis: biochemical aspects and clinical implications. *Clin Chim Acta* 2002;326:27–45.
5. Lemasters JJ, Qian T, He L, et al. Role of mitochondrial inner membrane permeabilization in necrotic cell death, apoptosis, and autophagy. *Antioxid Redox Signal* 2002;4:769–781.
6. Leist M, Single B, Naumann H, et al. Inhibition of mitochondrial ATP generation by nitric oxide switches apoptosis to necrosis. *Exp Cell Res* 1999;249:396–403.
7. Nicholls DG, Budd SL. Mitochondria and neuronal survival. *Physiol Rev* 2000;80:315–360.
8. van Loo G, Saelens X, van Gurp M, MacFarlane M, Martin SJ, Vandenabeele P. The role of mitochondrial factors in apoptosis: a Russian roulette with more than one bullet. *Cell Death Differ* 2002;9:1031–1042.
9. Zheng L, Szabo C, Kern TS. Poly(ADP-ribose) polymerase is involved in the development of diabetic retinopathy via regulation of nuclear factor-kappaB. *Diabetes* 2004;53: 2960–2967.
10. Virag L, Szabo C. The therapeutic potential of poly(ADP-ribose) polymerase inhibitors. *Pharmacol Rev* 2002;54:375–429.
11. Obrosova IG, Pacher P, Szabo C, et al. Aldose reductase inhibition counteracts oxidative-nitrosative stress and poly(ADP-ribose) polymerase activation in tissue sites for diabetes complications. *Diabetes* 2005;54:234–242.
12. Nagata S, Golstein P. The Fas death factor. *Science* 1995;267:1449–1456.
13. Shiozaki EN, Shi Y. Caspases, IAPs and Smac/DIABLO: mechanisms from structural biology. *Trends Biochem Sci* 2004;29:486–494.
14. Degli Esposti M. Mitochondria in apoptosis: past, present and future. *Biochem Soc Trans* 2004;32:493–495.
15. Guillot R, Bringuier AF, Porokhov B, Guillausseau PJ, Feldmann G. Increased levels of soluble Fas in serum from diabetic patients with neuropathy. *Diabetes Metab* 2001;27:315–321.
16. Vincent AM, Olzmann JA, Brownlee M, Sivitz WI, Russell JW. Uncoupling proteins prevent glucose-induced neuronal oxidative stress and programmed cell death. *Diabetes* 2004;53:726–734.
17. Green DR, Reed JC. Mitochondria and apoptosis. *Science* 1998;281:1309–1312.
18. Kroemer G, Zamzami N, Susin SA. Mitochondrial control of apoptosis. *Immunol Today* 1997;18:44–51.
19. Leinninger GM, Russell JW, van Golen CM, Berent A, Feldman EL. Insulin-like growth factor-I regulates glucose-induced mitochondrial depolarization and apoptosis in human neuroblastoma. *Cell Death Differ* 2004;11:885–896.
20. Russell JW, Golovoy D, Vincent AM, et al. High glucose-induced oxidative stress and mitochondrial dysfunction in neurons. *FASEB J* 2002;16:1738–1748.
21. Cowell RM, Russell JW. Peripheral Neuropathy and the Schwann Cell, in *Neuroglia* (Kettenmann H, Ransom BR, eds.), Oxford University Press, 2004, pp. 573–585.
22. Vincent AM, Brownlee M, Russell JW. Oxidative stress and programmed cell death in diabetic neuropathy. *Ann NY Acad Sci* 2002;959:368–383.
23. Vincent AM, Russell JW, Low P, Feldman EL. Oxidative stress in the pathogenesis of diabetic neuropathy. *Endocr Rev* 2004;25:612–628.

24. Kroemer G, Dallaporta B, Resche-Rigon M. The mitochondrial death/life regulator in apoptosis and necrosis. *Annu Rev Physiol* 1998;60:619–642.
25. Eskes R, Antonsson B, Osen-Sand A, et al. Bax-induced cytochrome C release from mitochondria is independent of the permeability transition pore but highly dependent on Mg^{2+} ions. *J Cell Biol* 1998;143:217–224.
26. Jurgensmeier JM, Xie Z, Deveraux Q, Ellerby L, Bredesen D, Reed JC. Bax directly induces release of cytochrome c from isolated mitochondria. *Proc Natl Acad Sci USA* 1998;95:4997–5002.
27. Russell JW, Sullivan KA, Windebank AJ, Herrmann DN, Feldman EL. Neurons undergo apoptosis in animal and cell culture models of diabetes. *Neurobiol Dis* 1999;6:347–363.
28. Srinivasan S, Stevens MJ, Wiley JW. Diabetic peripheral neuropathy: Evidence for apoptosis and associated mitochondrial dysfunction. *Diabetes* 2000;49:1932–1938.
29. Schmeichel AM, Schmelzer JD, Low PA. Oxidative injury and apoptosis of dorsal root ganglion neurons in chronic experimental diabetic neuropathy. *Diabetes* 2003;52:165–171.
30. Cheng C, Zochodne DW. Sensory neurons with activated caspase-3 survive long-term experimental diabetes. *Diabetes* 2003;52:2363–2371.
31. Kishi M, Tanabe J, Schmelzer JD, Low PA. Morphometry of dorsal root ganglion in chronic experimental diabetic neuropathy. *Diabetes* 2002;51:819–824.
32. Reed JC. Double identity for proteins of the Bcl-2 family. *Nature* 1997;387:773–776.
33. Schulz JB, Bremen D, Reed JC, et al. Cooperative interception of neuronal apoptosis by bcl-2 and bag-1 expression: prevention of caspase activaton and reduced production of reactive oxygen species. *J Neurochem* 1997;69:2075–2086.
34. Satoh T, Sakai N, Enokido Y, Uchiyama Y, Hatanaka H. Free radical-independent protection by nerve growth factor and Bcl-2 of PC12 cells from hydrogen peroxide-triggered apoptosis. *J Biochem* 1996;120:540–546.
35. Adams JM, Cory S. The Bcl-2 protein family: arbiters of cell survival. *Science* 1998;281:1322–1326.
36. Bouillet P, Metcalf D, Huang DC, et al. Proapoptotic Bcl-2 relative Bim required for certain apoptotic responses, leukocyte homeostasis, and to preclude autoimmunity. *Science* 1999;286:1735–1738.
37. Bissonette RP, Echeverri F, Mahboubi A, Green DR. Apoptotic cell death induced by c-myc is inhibited by bcl-2. *Nature* 1992;359:552–554.
38. Raff MC, Barres BA, Burne JF, Coles HS, Ishizaki Y, Jacobson MD. Programmed cell death and the control of cell survival: Lessons from the nervous system. *Science* 1994;262:695–700.
39. Lam M, Dubyak G, Chen L, Nunez G, Miesfeld RL, Distelhorst CW. Evidence that BCL-2 represses apoptosis by regulating endoplasmic reticulum-associated Ca^{2+} fluxes. *Proc Natl Acad Sci USA* 1994;91:6569–6573.
40. Cheng EH, Sheiko TV, Fisher JK, Craigen WJ, Korsmeyer SJ. VDAC2 inhibits BAK activation and mitochondrial apoptosis. *Science* 2003;301:513–517.
41. Zamzami N, El Hamel C, Maisse C, et al. Bid acts on the permeability transition pore complex to induce apoptosis. *Oncogene* 2000;19:6342–6350.
42. Ruffolo SC, Breckenridge DG, Nguyen M, et al. BID-dependent and BID-independent pathways for BAX insertion into mitochondria. *Cell Death Differ* 2000;7:1101–1108.
43. Korsmeyer SJ, Wei MC, Saito M, Weiler S, Oh KJ, Schlesinger PH. Pro-apoptotic cascade activates BID, which oligomerizes BAK or BAX into pores that result in the release of cytochrome c. *Cell Death Differ* 2000;7:1166–1173.
44. Wei MC, Zong WX, Cheng EH, et al. Proapoptotic BAX and BAK: a requisite gateway to mitochondrial dysfunction and death. *Science* 2001;292:727–730.
45. Karbowski M, Youle RJ. Dynamics of mitochondrial morphology in healthy cells and during apoptosis. *Cell Death Differ* 2003;10:870–880.

46. Li H, Zhu H, Xu CJ, Yuan J. Cleavage of BID by caspase 8 mediates the mitochondrial damage in the Fas pathway of apoptosis. *Cell* 1998;94:491–501.
47. Krohn AJ, Wahlbrink T, Prehn JH. Mitochondrial depolarization is not required for neuronal apoptosis. *J Neurosci* 1999;19:7394–7404.
48. Pan G, O'Rourke K, Dixit VM. Caspase-9, Bcl-XL, and Apaf-1 form a ternary complex. *J Biol Chem* 1998;273:5841–5845.
49. Song Q, Kuang Y, Dixit VM, Vincenz C. Boo, a novel negative regulator of cell death, interacts with Apaf-1. *EMBO J* 1999;18:167–178.
50. Slee EA, Harte MT, Kluck RM, et al. Ordering the cytochrome c-initiated caspase cascade: hierarchical activation of caspases-2,3,6,7,8, and 10 in a caspase-9 dependent manner. *J Cell Biol* 1999;144:281–292.
51. Ellis HM, Horvitz HR. Genetic control of programmed cell death in the nematode *C. elegans*. *Cell* 1986;44:817–829.
52. Jacobson MD, Evan GI. Breaking the ice. Structural and functional similarities have been discovered between two mammalian proteins, Bcl-2 and interleukin 1b-converting enzyme, and proteins encoded by nematode cell-death genes. *Curr Biol* 1994;4:337–340.
53. Corkins MR, Vanderhoof JA, Slentz DH, MacDonald RG, Park JHY. Growth stimulation by transfection of intestinal epithelial cells with an antisense insulin-like growth factor binding protein-2 construct. *Biochem Biophys Res Commun* 1995;211:707–713.
54. Du XL, Edelstein D, Rossetti L, et al. Hyperglycemia-induced mitochondrial superoxide overproduction activates the hexosamine pathway and induces plasminogen activator inhibitor-1 expression by increasing Sp1 glycosylation. *Proc Natl Acad Sci USA* 2000;97:12,222–12,226.
55. Brownlee M. Biochemistry and molecular cell biology of diabetic complications. *Nature* 2001;414:813–820.
56. Nishikawa T, Edelstein D, Du XL, et al. Normalizing mitochondrial superoxide production blocks three pathways of hyperglycaemic damage. *Nature* 2000;404:787–790.
57. Stevens MJ, Obrosova I, Cao X, Van Huysen C, Greene DA. Effects of DL-alpha-lipoic acid on peripheral nerve conduction, blood flow, energy metabolism, and oxidative stress in experimental diabetic neuropathy. *Diabetes* 2000;49:1006–1015.
58. Russell JW, Golovoy D, Vincent A, et al. High glucose induced-oxidative stress and mitochondrial dysfunction in neurons. *FASEB J* 2002;16:1738–1748.
59. Mandavilli BS, Santos JH, Van Houten B. Mitochondrial DNA repair and aging. *Mutat Res* 2002;509:127–151.
60. Poderoso JJ, Carreras MC, Lisdero C, Riobo N, Schopfer F, Boveris A. Nitric oxide inhibits electron transfer and increases superoxide radical production in rat heart mitochondria and submitochondrial particles. *Arch Biochem Biophys* 1996;328:85–92.
61. Moncada S, Erusalimsky JD. Does nitric oxide modulate mitochondrial energy generation and apoptosis? *Nat Rev Mol Cell Biol* 2002;3:214–220.
62. Cowell R, Cherian K, Russell JW. Regulation of neuronal nitric oxide synthase (nNOS) in models of diabetic neuropathy. *J Peripheral Nerv System* 2003;8:1–78.
63. Garcia SF, Virag L, Jagtap P, et al. Diabetic endothelial dysfunction: the role of poly(ADP-ribose) polymerase activation. *Nat Med* 2001;7:108–113.
64. Cowell RM, Russell JW. Nitrosative injury and antioxidant therapy in the management of diabetic neuropathy. *J Investig Med* 2004;52:33–44.
65. Jaffrey SR, Erdjument-Bromage H, Ferris CD, Tempst P, Snyder SH. Protein S-nitrosylation: a physiological signal for neuronal nitric oxide. *Nat Cell Biol* 2001;3:193–197.
66. Foster MW, McMahon TJ, Stamler JS. S-nitrosylation in health and disease. *Trends Mol Med* 2003;9:160–168.
67. Marshall HE, Merchant K, Stamler JS. Nitrosation and oxidation in the regulation of gene expression. *FASEB J* 2000;14:1889–1900.

68. Raoul C, Estevez AG, Nishimune H, et al. Motoneuron death triggered by a specific pathway downstream of Fas. potentiation by ALS-linked SOD1 mutations. *Neuron* 2002;35:1067–1083.
69. Gonzalez-Zulueta M, Ensz LM, Mukhina G, et al. Manganese superoxide dismutase protects nNOS neurons from NMDA and nitric oxide-mediated neurotoxicity. *J Neurosci* 1998;18:2040–2055.
70. Murphy MP. Nitric oxide and cell death. *Biochim Biophys Acta* 1999;1411:401–414.
71. Radi R, Cassina A, Hodara R, Quijano C, Castro L. Peroxynitrite reactions and formation in mitochondria. *Free Radic Biol Med* 2002;33:1451–1464.
72. Eu JP, Liu L, Zeng M, Stamler JS. An apoptotic model for nitrosative stress. *Biochemistry* 2000;39:1040–1047.
73. Reiss P, Casula M, de Ronde A, Weverling GJ, Goudsmit J, Lange JM. Greater and more rapid depletion of mitochondrial DNA in blood of patients treated with dual (zidovudine+didanosine or zidovudine+zalcitabine) vs. single (zidovudine) nucleoside reverse transcriptase inhibitors. *HIV Med* 2004;5:11–14.
74. Zochodne DW, Verge VM, Cheng C, et al. Nitric oxide synthase activity and expression in experimental diabetic neuropathy. *J Neuropathol Exp Neurol* 2000;59:798–807.
75. Cameron NE, Eaton SE, Cotter MA, Tesfaye S. Vascular factors and metabolic interactions in the pathogenesis of diabetic neuropathy. *Diabetologia* 2001;44:1973–1988.
76. Thomas SR, Chen K, Keaney JF, Jr. Oxidative stress and endothelial nitric oxide bioactivity. *Antioxid Redox Signal* 2003;5:181–194.
77. Zochodne DW, Verge VM, Cheng C, Sun H, Johnston J. Does diabetes target ganglion neurones? Progressive sensory neurone involvement in long-term experimental diabetes. *Brain* 2001;124:2319–2334.
78. Sayers NM, Beswick LJ, Middlemas A, et al. Neurotrophin-3 prevents the proximal accumulation of neurofilament proteins in sensory neurons of streptozocin-induced diabetic rats. *Diabetes* 2003;52:2372–2380.
79. Vincent AM, McLean LL, Backus C, Feldman EL. Short-term hyperglycemia produces oxidative damage and apoptosis in neurons. *FASEB J* 2005;19:638–640.
80. Honma H, Podratz JL, Windebank AJ. Acute glucose deprivation leads to apoptosis in a cell model of acute diabetic neuropathy. *J Peripher Nerv Syst* 2003;8:65–74.
81. Coppey LJ, Gellett JS, Davidson EP, Dunlap JA, Lund DD, Yorek MA. Effect of antioxidant treatment of streptozotocin-induced diabetic rats on endoneurial blood flow, motor nerve conduction velocity, and vascular reactivity of epineurial arterioles of the sciatic nerve. *Diabetes* 2001;50:1927–1937.
82. Obrosova IG. How does glucose generate oxidative stress in peripheral nerve? *Int Rev Neurobiol* 2002;50:3–35.
83. Huang TJ, Price SA, Chilton L, et al. Insulin prevents depolarization of the mitochondrial inner membrane in sensory neurons of type 1 diabetic rats in the presence of sustained hyperglycemia. *Diabetes* 2003;52:2129–2136.
84. Huang TJ, Verkhratsky A, Fernyhough P. Insulin enhances mitochondrial inner membrane potential and increases ATP levels through phosphoinositide 3-kinase in adult sensory neurons. *Mol Cell Neurosci* 2005;28:42–54.
85. Srinivasan S, Stevens M, Wiley JW. Diabetic peripheral neuropathy: evidence for apoptosis and associated mitochondrial dysfunction. *Diabetes* 2000;49:1932–1938.
86. Jezek P, Costa AD, Vercesi AE. Evidence for anion-translocating plant uncoupling mitochondrial protein in potato mitochondria. *J Biol Chem* 1996;271:32,743–32,748.
87. Bairoch A. The PROSITE dictionary of sites and patterns in proteins, its current status. *Nucleic Acids Res* 1993;21:3097–3103.
88. Russell JW, Windebank AJ, Schenone A, Feldman EL. Insulin-like growth factor-I prevents apoptosis in neurons after nerve growth factor withdrawal. *J Neurobiol* 1998;36:455–467.

89. Ghatan S, Larner S, Kinoshita Y, et al. p38 MAP kinase mediates bax translocation in nitric oxide-induced apoptosis in neurons. *J Cell Biol* 2000;150:335–347.
90. Leinninger GM, Backus C, Uhler MD, Lentz SI, Feldman EL. Phosphatidylinositol 3-kinase and Akt effectors mediate insulin-like growth factor-I neuroprotection in dorsal root ganglia neurons. *FASEB J* 2004;18:1544–1546.
91. Gustafsson H, Adamson L, Hedander J, Walum E, Forsby A. Insulin-like growth factor type 1 upregulates uncoupling protein 3. *Biochem Biophys Res Commun* 2001;287:1105–1111.
92. Guerra C, Benito M, Fernandez M. IGF-I induces the uncoupling protein gene expression in fetal rat brown adipocyte primary cultures: role of C/EBP transcription factors. *Biochem Biophys Res Commun* 1994;201:813–819.
93. Valverde AM, Lorenzo M, Navarro P, Benito M. Phosphatidylinositol 3-kinase is a requirement for insulin-like growth factor I-induced differentiation, but not for mitogenesis, in fetal brown adipocytes. *Mol Endocrinol* 1997;11:595–607.
94. Price SA, Hounsom L, Purves-Tyson TD, Fernyhough P, Tomlinson DR. Activation of JNK in sensory neurons protects against sensory neuron cell death in diabetes and on exposure to glucose/oxidative stress in vitro. *Ann NY Acad Sci* 2003;1010:95–99.
95. Honma H, Gross L, Windebank AJ. Hypoxia-induced apoptosis of dorsal root ganglion neurons is associated with DNA damage recognition and cell cycle disruption in rats. *Neurosci Lett* 2004;354:95–98.
96. Anand P, Terenghi G, Warner G, Kopelman P, Williams-Chestnut RE, Sinicropi DV. The role of endogenous nerve growth factor in human diabetic neuropathy. *Nat Med* 1996;2:703–707.
97. Unger JW, Klitzsch T, Pera S, Reiter R. Nerve growth factor (NGF) and diabetic neuropathy in the rat: morphological investigations of the sural nerve, dorsal root ganglion, and spinal cord. *Exp Neurol* 1998;153:23–34.
98. Berent-Spillson A, Robinson A, Golovoy D, Slusher B, Rojas C, Russell JW. Protection against glucose-induced neuronal death by NAAG and GCP II inhibition is regulated by mGluR3. *J Neurochem* 2004;89:90–99.
99. Flor PJ, Battaglia G, Nicoletti F, Gasparini F, Bruno V. Neuroprotective activity of metabotropic glutamate receptor ligands. *Adv Exp Med Biol* 2002;513:197–223.
100. Vincent AM, Maiese K. The metabotropic glutamate system promotes neuronal survival through distinct pathways of programmed cell death. *Exp Neurol* 2000;166:65–82.
101. De Blasi A, Conn PJ, Pin J, Nicoletti F. Molecular determinants of metabotropic glutamate receptor signaling. *Trends Pharmacol Sci* 2001;22:114–120.
102. Cartmell J, Schoepp DD. Regulation of neurotransmitter release by metabotropic glutamate receptors. *J Neurochem* 2000;75:889–907.
103. Zhang W, Slusher B, Murakawa Y, et al. GCPII (NAALADase) inhibition prevents long-term diabetic neuropathy in type 1 diabetic BB/Wor rats. *J Neurol Sci* 2002;194:21–28.
104. Berent Spillson A, Russell JW. Metabotropic glutamate receptor regulation of neuronal injury. *Exp Neurol* 2003;184:S97–S105.
105. Russell JW, Feldman EL. Insulin-like growth factor-I prevents apoptosis in sympathetic neurons exposed to high glucose. *Horm Metab Res* 1999;31:90–96.
106. Guo C, Quobatari A, Shangguan Y, Hong S, Wiley JW. Diabetic autonomic neuropathy: evidence for apoptosis in situ in the rat. *Neurogastroenterol Motil* 2004;16:335–345.
107. Schmidt RE. Neuronal preservation in the sympathetic ganglia of rats with chronic streptozotocin-induced diabetes. *Brain Res* 2001;921:256–259.
108. Schmidt RE, Dorsey DA, Beaudet LN, Plurad SB, Parvin CA, Miller MS. Insulin-like growth factor I reverses experimental diabetic autonomic neuropathy. *Am J Pathol* 1999;155:1651–1660.
109. Schmidt RE, Dorsey DA, Beaudet LN, Peterson RG. Analysis of the Zucker Diabetic Fatty (ZDF) type 2 diabetic rat model suggests a neurotrophic role for insulin/IGF-I in diabetic autonomic neuropathy. *Am J Pathol* 2003;163:21–28.

110. Delaney CL, Russell JW, Cheng H-L, Feldman EL. Insulin-like growth factor-I and over-expression of Bcl-xL prevent glucose-mediated apoptosis in Schwann cells. *J Neuropathol Exp Neurol* 2001;60:147–160.
111. Sekido H, Suzuki T, Jomori T, Takeuchi M, Yabe-Nishimura C, Yagihashi S. Reduced cell replication and induction of apoptosis by advanced glycation end products in rat Schwann cells. *Biochem Biophys Res Commun* 2004;320:241–248.
112. Pan Z, Sampath D, Jackson G, Werrbach-Perez K, Perez-Polo R. Nerve growth factor and oxidative stress in the nervous system. *Adv Exp Med Biol* 1997;429:173–193.
113. Park DS, Morris EJ, Stefanis L, et al. Multiple pathways of neuronal death induced by DNA-damaging agents, NGF deprivation, and oxidative stress. *J Neurosci* 1998;18:830–840.
114. Lieberthal W, Triaca V, Koh JS, Pagano PJ, Levine JS. Role of superoxide in apoptosis induced by growth factor withdrawal. *Am J Physiol* 1998;275(5 Pt 2):F691–F702.
115. Russell JW, Kaminsky A. Oxidative injury in diabetic neuropathy, in *Nutrition and Diabetes: Pathophysiology and Management* (Opara E, ed.), by courtesy of Taylor & Francis Group, LLC, Boca Raton, FL, 2006;381–397.

8

Metabolic–Functional–Structural Correlations in Somatic Neuropathies in the Spontaneously Type 1 and Type 2 Diabetic BB-Rats

Anders A. F. Sima, Weixian Zhang, and Hideki Kamiya

SUMMARY

Diabetic neuropathy (DPN) is a dynamic condition affecting both type 1 and type 2 diabetic subjects. It can be divided into an early and reversible metabolic phase of nerve dysfunction. This is caused by hyperglycemia-induced activation of the polyol-pathway, redox imbalances as well as by insulin/C-peptide deficiencies resulting in impaired neural Na^+/K^+-ATPase activity and impairment of endoneurial blood flow. Superimposed on these metabolic abnormalities, progressive structural changes evolve which become increasingly resistant to therapeutic interventions. These affect both unmyelinated and myelinated fiber populations and consist of axonal atrophy, degeneration, and loss occurring in a dying-back fashion. The underlying mechanisms include impaired neurotrophic support including perturbed insulin/C-peptide signaling, resulting in suppressed expression of neuroskeletal protein genes, and aberrant phosphorylation of these axonal building blocks. Both the early metabolic and later occurring molecular abnormalities underlying the structural abnormalities are more severely affected in type 1 DPN relating to insulin and C-peptide deficiencies, which are not present in type 2 diabetes. This distinction between the two forms of DPN also underlies nodal and paranodal degeneration unique to both human and experimental type 1 DPN. Impaired insulin action affects the expression of nodal and paranodal adhesive molecules and their post-translational modifications. Such aberrations result in disruption of the paranodal barrier function with decreased nodal Na^+-channels densities and worsening of the nerve conduction defect in type 1 DPN. In conclusion, major differences exist between type 1 and type 2 DPN, which can be directly related to the absence and presence of insulin action.

Key Words: Axonal degeneration; diabetic neuropathy; insulin action; neurotrophism; nodal degeneration; type 1 and type 2 diabetes.

INTRODUCTION

Diabetic polyneuropathies (DPN) are a heterogeneous group of dynamic conditions affecting somatic and autonomic peripheral nerves. It is the most common late complication of diabetes mellitus *(1–4)* and occurs in both type 1 and type 2 diabetes with a prevalence varying from 10% within 1 year of diagnosis to 50% in patients with diabetes for more than 25 years *(5–7)*. DPN complicating type 1 diabetes occurs

From: *Contemporary Diabetes: Diabetic Neuropathy: Clinical Management, Second Edition*
Edited by: A. Veves and R. Malik © Humana Press Inc., Totowa, NJ

more predictably and tend to progress more rapidly in comparison with DPN in type 2 diabetes *(3,8,9)*.

Despite decades of intense clinical and experimental research into DPN, their underlying pathogenetic factors, their dynamics, and how they correlate with emerging functional and structural abnormalities is still not fully understood *(10,11)*. The current understanding of early metabolic and molecular changes in DPN has heavily relied on acute experiments in the streptozotocin (STZ)-diabetic rat. Such data have then been extrapolated to established DPN in humans and have served as a basis for the development of various therapeutic drugs and the design and execution of clinical trials, thereby ignoring the dynamic of underlying mechanisms and changing spectrum of structural changes. No doubt, the STZ-rat model has served as a good and inexpensive model of hyperglycemia and its effects on peripheral nerve. However, it has several shortcomings and reflects poorly on human DPN in which for instance nerve fiber loss is the cardinal pathology, which is lacking in STZ-rats. STZ-induced diabetes causes a partial β-cell destruction and hyperglycemia. Hence, it is neither a good model of human type 1 insulin- and C-peptide-deficient diabetes nor is it a model of human type 2 hyperinsulinemic and insulin-resistant diabetes *(12)*. Furthermore, it lacks the comorbidities characteristic of human type 2 diabetes such as obesity, hypercholesterolemia, and hyperlipidemia.

Our laboratory has taken a different approach in an attempt to mimic the human disorders by using two models with spontaneous onset of diabetes: The type 1 Bio-Breeding Worcester (BB/Wor)-rat develops acute onset of diabetes at the age of 70–75 days, secondary to an immune-mediated selective destruction of pancreatic β-cell. This results in total insulin and C-peptide deficiencies and requires daily titration of insulin doses for maintenance of an even hyperglycemic level at 20–25 m*M* glucose *(13,14)*. In the type 2 Bio-Breeding Zucker derived Worcester (BBZDR/Wor)-rat, outbred on the same background as the type 1 model, diabetes occurs at 70–80 days of age and is preceded by obesity. It develops peripheral insulin resistance with hyperinsulinemia, hypercholesterolemia and triglyceridememia *(15)* and maintains spontaneously hyperglycemic levels equal to those of the type 1 BB/Wor-rat. Hence, these two models mimic more accurately the two major types of human diabetes which develop DPN, and can therefore be used advantageously to explore the pathological and pathogenetic differences *(1,16)* between type 1 and type 2 DPN.

This review will point out the basic underlying metabolic differences in peripheral nerve between the two models, the progression of functional deficits, structural abnormalities, and their correlations.

UNDERLYING METABOLIC ABNORMALITIES IN TYPE 1 AND TYPE 2 DPN

Several hyperglycemia-induced pathways have been invoked as the pathogenetic basis for DPN, such as

1. Activation of the polyol-pathway resulting in redox imbalances and perturbation of myoinositol and organic osmolyte imbalances *(17–19)*.
2. Nonenzymatic glycation yielding advanced glycation end products *(20)*.
3. Perturbations of neurotrophic homeostasis affecting particularly the nerve growth factor (NGF) and insulin-like growth factor (IGF) systems (Fig. 1) *(21–24)*.

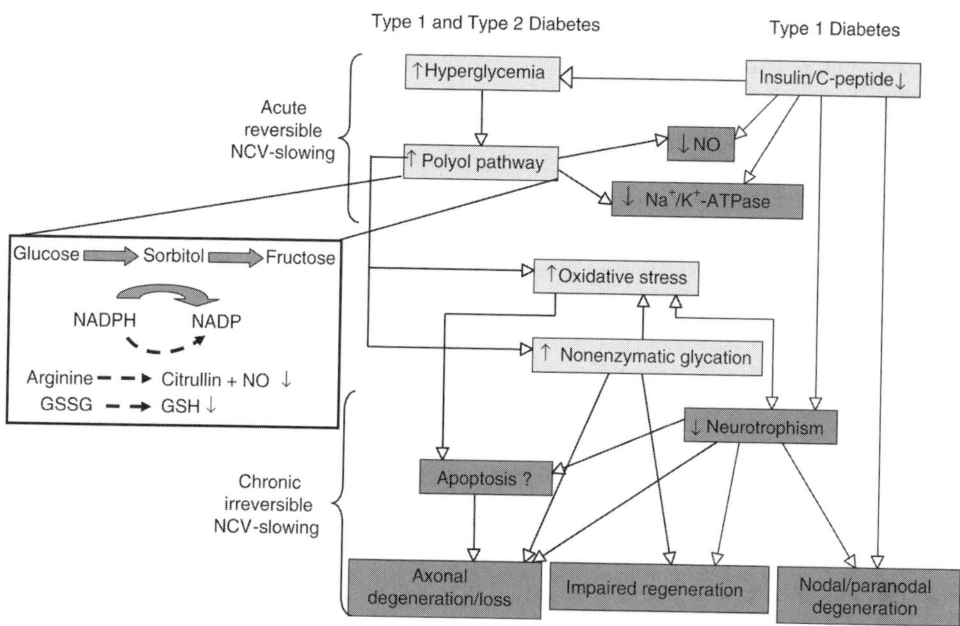

Fig. 1. Scheme of pathogenetic pathways involved in type 1 and type 2 DPN. Note that some of the early key metabolic abnormalities such as Na^+/K^+-ATPase and NO activities as well as oxidative stress are influenced both by hyperglycemia and insulin/C-peptide deficiencies. This is also true for some of the mechanisms involved in the "structural phase" with the exception of nodal/paranodal degeneration, which appears to be a direct consequence of impaired insulin action.

Several investigators have suggested that these factors eventually come together, causing mitochondrial dysfunction, superoxide overproduction, and oxidative and nitrosative stress, leading to NO depletion, impaired nerve perfusion, which would provide a common mechanism underlying the genesis of DPN *(25–27)*.

Recently, it was shown that endoneurial blood flow is decreased and oxidative stress increased in type 1 BB/Wor-rats. Insulinomimetic C-peptide replacement did not effect oxidative stress, but prevented nerve conduction velocity (NCV) and neurovascular deficits by NO-sensitive and -insensitive mechanisms, respectively. On the other hand, in type 2 BBZDR/Wor-rats, neurovascular deficits and increased oxidative stress were unaccompanied by sensory NCV slowing. These data suggest that sensory nerve deficits are not inevitably the consequence of oxidative stress and decreased endoneurial perfusion *(28)*. The vascular hypothesis of DPN therefore remains controversial.

Impaired neural Na^+/K^+-ATPase activity consequent to perturbed redox imbalances from an activated polyol-pathway has been implied as a major contributing factor to the acute nerve conduction defect (Fig. 1) *(17,29,30)*. Interestingly, despite exposure to the same levels of cumulative hyperglycemia, type 1 BB/Wor-rats exhibit a greater flux through the polyol-pathway in comparison with type 2 BBZDR/Wor-rats, and more severe defects in Na^+/K^+-ATPase activity and myoinositol depletion *(31)*, suggesting that additional factors must contribute to the Na^+/K^+-ATPase defect. Recent studies have demonstrated significant dose-dependent protective effects by proinsulin C-peptide on Na^+/K^+-ATPase activity in neural and other tissues, in the absence of an effect on hyperglycemia and polyol-pathway activity *(32–35)*. Therefore, it appears that both perturbed redox balances through the polyol-pathway *(36)* and direct effects of insulin/C-peptide deficiencies mediated through a putative G protein-linked receptor or through the insulin receptor itself *(37–39)* to contribute to the more severe Na^+/K^+-ATPase defect in type 1 diabetes (Fig. 1).

Neurotrophic factors are essential for the maintenance of neurons and their regenerative capacity and for the protection against apoptosis *(23,24,40)*. The major groups of neurotrophic factors are NGF and its receptors, other neurotrophins as well as the IGF family of neurotrophic factors. The latter consist of IGF-I, IGF-II, insulin, and their respective receptors, as well as the IGF binding proteins *(22)*. Various neurotrophic factors are responsible for the gene regulation of neuroskeletal proteins such as neurofilaments and neurotubules, and for the integrity of neuropeptide specific neuronal populations such as substance P (SP) and calcitonin-gene-related peptide (CGRP) dorsal root ganglion cells. Several lines of investigations have in the last number of years demonstrated that insulin and synergistically acting proinsulin C-peptide have direct gene-regulatory effects on both IGF-I and NGF family members of neurotrophic factors (Fig. 1), besides their own neurotrophic actions they also act as facilitators of ligand binding to TrkA, the high affinity NGF receptor *(41–44)*.

These regulatory functions by insulin/C-peptide are reflected in a more severe suppression of IGF's IGF-IR, insulin receptor and NGF and TrkA receptor expression in dorsal root ganglia and peripheral nerve in the type 1 BB/Wor-rat as in comparison with the type 2 counterpart *(45,46)*. Such differences therefore will have consequences such as regenerative capacities, survival of neuropeptide specific neuronal populations, and maintenance of axonal integrity *(41,45,46)*.

It is therefore clear that the metabolic and molecular insults in type 1 and type 2 DPN differ in magnitude and the predominant inciting defects (Fig. 1). Hyperglycemia common to both types of diabetes is a major contributing factor as demonstrated by large-scale clinical studies as well as experimentally. However, in recent years insulin and C-peptide deficiencies have emerged as perhaps equally important in the development of type 1 late complications including DPN *(32,47–51)*.

PROGRESSION AND MECHANISMS OF SOMATIC NERVE DYSFUNCTION

Myelinated Fiber Function

Dysfunction of myelinated fiber populations is reflected in decreased NCV, reflecting particularly large myelinated fibers. Motor nerve conduction velocity (MNCV) shows after 1 week's duration of diabetes significant deficits in the type 1 BB/Wor-rat, whereas the type 2 counterpart shows a milder but significant decrease only after 1 month's duration of diabetes (Fig. 2) *(31–32)*. These early deficits correlate with a milder degree of nodal axonal hydropic swelling in the type 2 model consistent with a milder Na^+/K^+-ATPase defect *(31)*. On the other hand, the endoneurial nutritive nerve blood flow is equally diminished in type 1 and type 2 BB-rats *(28)*, suggesting that diminished Na^+/K^+-ATPase activity is a stronger determinant for the acute metabolic nerve conduction defect than is endoneurial blood flow.

Earlier nodal clamp studies in the BB/Wor-rat has demonstrated decreased axolemmal Na^+ equilibrium potentials, and decreased nodal Na^+ permeability and currents,

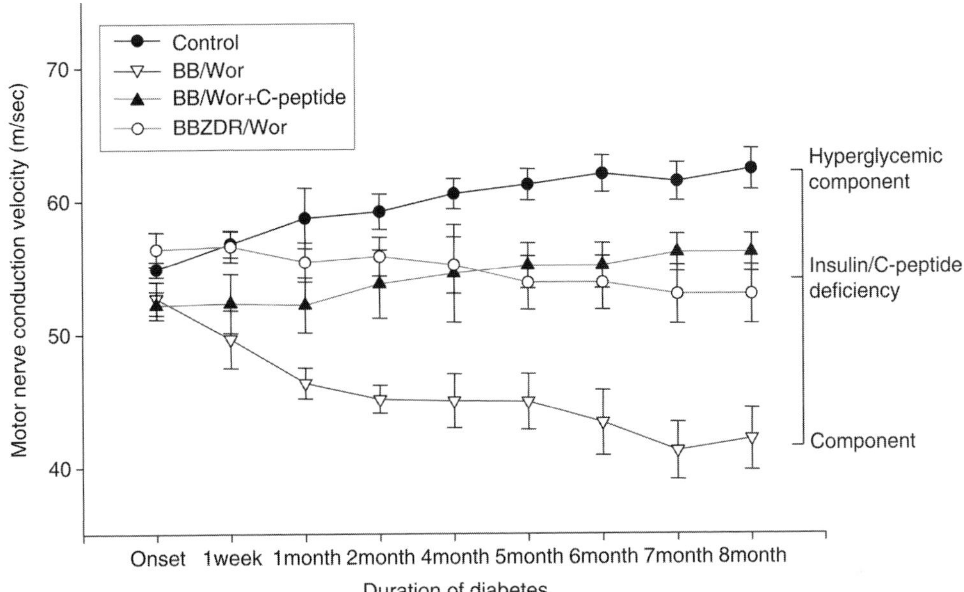

Fig. 2. Longitudinal data on motor nerve conduction velocities (MNCV) in control-, BB/Wor-, BBZDR/Wor-, and C-peptide replaced BB/Wor-rats. Note a severe acute immediate decline in MNCV in BB/Wor-rats which is probably associated with the more severe Na^+/K^+-ATPase defect in comparison with BBZDR/Wor-rats. In the BB/Wor-rat the MNCV then levels off to 5 months duration followed by a further progressive decline. This coincides with the emergence of nodal and paranodal degenerative changes. The type 2 BBZDR/Wor-rat, which shows milder early metabolic abnormalities and nodal and paranodal degenerative changes, shows a significantly milder progression of the MNCV deficit. Replenishment of C-peptide in BB/Wor-rats significantly prevents the MNCV defect, although not completely as these animals are still hyperglycemic. The MNCV profile of these animals is similar to that of type 2 BBZDR/Wor-rats. These comparisons therefore allow us to separate out a hyperglycemic NCV defect and in type 1 animals an additional insulin/ C-peptide deficiency component. Each data point represents means ± SD's from at least eight animals.

resulting in a blunted initial inward Na^+ current *(52–54)*. These findings correlate with increased intra-axonal $[Na^+]^i$ at the node. Hence the bioelectrical changes are in full agreement with impaired Na^+/K^+-ATPase activity at the nodal membrane and intra-axonal nodal swelling. This series of interrelated changes is correctable with insulin treatment *(53,55)*, aldose reductase inhibition *(56)*, acetyl-L-carnitine treatment *(57)*, or C-peptide replenishment *(32)*, all of which simultaneously correct the neural Na^+/K^+-ATPase defect. Recently Kitano et al. *(58)* using the threshold tracking technique, demonstrated reduced transaxolemmal Na^+ gradients in patients with mild DPN, changes which improved along with NCV after 4 weeks of intensive insulin treatment.

After this initial, so called *metabolic and reversible NCV-defect*, the MNCV starts to show a further progressive decline at 4–5 months duration of diabetes in the BB/Wor-rat (Fig. 2) and becomes increasingly uncorrectable by metabolic means. This is the initiation of the socalled *structural and irreversible NCV defect*. At this time, there are early axonal atrophy and the emergence of nodal and paranodal molecular and structural changes in the BB/Wor-rat.

Table 1
Progression of Axonal Atrophy and Fiber Loss in Sensory Myelinated Fibers in Sural Nerve

	Months of diabetes					
	4	6	8	10	11	14
Axonal size (% of normal)	91.3[a]	88.5[b]	82.9[b]	80.5[b]	79.3[b]	77.5[b]
Fiber member (% of normal)	89.6[c]	80.6[b]	76.8[b]	70.7[b]	67.1[b]	–

Values are percentages of control values.
[a] $p < 0.005$.
[b] $p < 0.001$ vs controls.
[c] $p < 0.05$.

Abnormalities of the nodal apparatus consist of a breach of the paranodal ion-channel barrier (axoglial dysjunction), allowing for the lateralization of nodal Na-channels, hence diminishing their concentration at the nodal axolemma *(1,55,59,60)*. Axoglial dysjunction leads to further perturbations of nodal Na^+ permeability and diminished excitability of the nodal membrane *(49,59)*, potentially resulting in conduction block. As large myelinated fibers are more susceptible to axoglial dysjunction, it will greatly impact on the nerve conduction velocity *(55)*, and contribute to the progressive increase in the chronic nerve conduction defect in type 1 DPN. Additional contributing factors are progressive axonal atrophy and eventually myelinated fiber loss (Table 1). These changes occur only late and to a significantly milder extent in the type 2 BBZDR/Wor-rat, explaining the milder progression of the nerve conduction defects in this model (Fig. 2).

Recently the molecular abnormalities underlying axoglial dysjunction were described and demonstrated that they are mainly caused by impaired gene regulatory mechanisms secondary to perturbed insulin signaling *(61)*. Therefore, these findings are in keeping with insulin/C-peptide deficiencies in type 1 diabetes mellitus, which are not present in type 2 diabetes. To provide further evidence for this notion, it was demonstrated that C-peptide replacement, which does not effect hyperglycemia, prevented underlying molecular abnormalities and restored significantly MNCV to values similar to those exhibited by the type 2 BBZDR/Wor-rat. From these data it was concluded that the NCV defect in type 1 DPN consists of a hyperglycemia-induced component which it has in common with type 2 DPN, and an additional insulin/C-peptide deficiency component specific for type 1 DPN (Fig. 2), which hence shows a more severe overall NCV defect.

Sensory nerve conduction velocity (SNCV) deficits in the two models show slower progression rates with a significant deficit only after 6 weeks of diabetes in the BB/Wor-rat and only after 8 months of diabetes in the type 2 BBZDR/Wor-rat (Fig. 3). Like MNCV, SNCV shows a relatively steep decline during the first 2 months in the BB/Wor-rat, which levels off to be followed by a further progressive decline after 6 months of diabetes. The initial decline in SNCV occurs only after 6 months of diabetes in the type 2 model (Fig. 3). The more severe deficits under type 1 diabetic conditions are ameliorated with replenishment of C-peptide, analogous to the deficits in MNCV. Therefore, distinct differences exist in the progression and severity of both MNCV and SNCV between the two models despite the same exposure to hyperglycemia (Figs. 2 and 3).

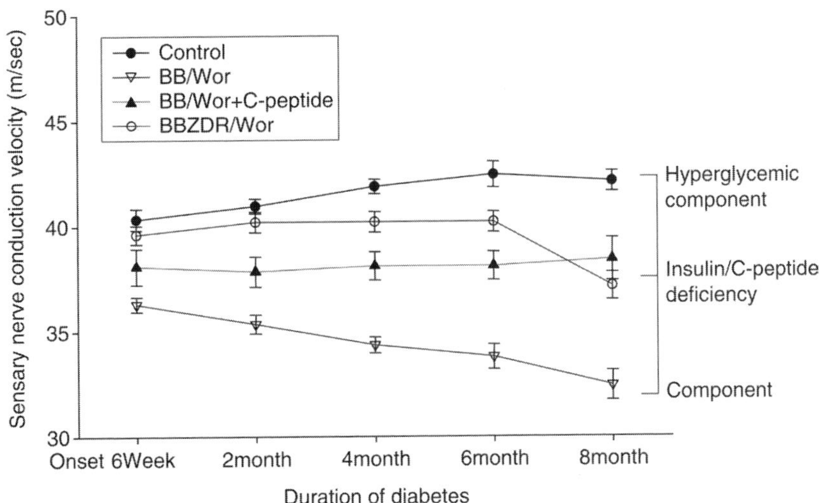

Fig. 3. Sensory nerve conduction velocity (SNCV) profiles in type 1 BB/Wor-rats with and without C-peptide replacement and in type 2 BBZDR/Wor-rats. Note in BB/Wor-rats an acute significant decline in SNCV like that seen in MNCV (Fig. 2). However, this is only evident after 6 weeks of diabetes. SNCV then stabilizes to show a further decline starting at 6 months. In contrast BBZDR/Wor-rats show only a significant decline in SNCV beyond 6 months of diabetes (Fig. 3). C-peptide replacement showed a significant effect on SNCV, although this is not completely prevented, again suggesting a hyperglycemic and an insulin/C-peptide deficiency component. Data points represent means ± SEM's for clarity of at least eight animals.

As alluded to, these differences can be partly abolished by replenishment of insulinomimetic C-peptide, thereby confirming the role of default insulin signaling in the genesis of nerve dysfunction in type 1 diabetes.

Unmyelinated Fiber Function

Painful diabetic neuropathy is a common and often debilitating symptom in DPN *(62)*. The underlying mechanisms are multiple and have not been fully elucidated *(63)*. However, it is clear that damage to unmyelinated and small myelinated fibers play a prominent role *(64)* along with remodeling of afferent large myelinated Aβ fibers to secondary nociceptive neurons in the spinal cord, so-called central sensitization *(65)*.

Perturbed nociception is associated with degenerative damage to C-fibers giving rise to an increase in Na^+-channels and α-adrenergic receptors *(63)* lending them hyperexcitable *(66)*, with a high-frequency spontaneous firing pattern *(67–69)*, which also sensitizes and maximizes spinal nociceptive circuits *(68)*.

The unmyelinated fiber populations in peripheral nerve are made up of nociceptive C-fibers and the axons of secondary sympathetic ganglia. The most common modes of measuring somatic C-fiber function is through thresholds to mechanical or thermal nociceptive stimulation.

Measurements of the latencies of hind paw withdrawal to a thermal noxious stimulus are an established technique for measurements of hyperalgesia or hyperexcitability of C-fibers. In control rats the latencies to thermal stimuli remain fairly constant over a 10-month

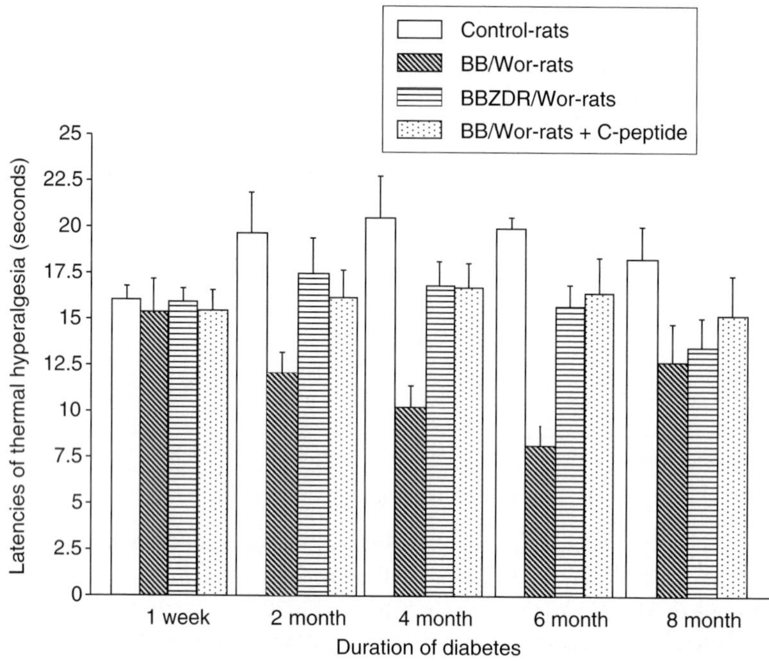

Fig. 4. Latencies of hind paw withdrawal after a noxious thermal stimulus reflecting C-fiber function. In type 1 BB/Wor-rats the latencies decreased significantly to less than half of that in control rats. Hyperalgesia reflects hyperexcitability of damaged C-fibers (*see* text). This decrease was followed by a recovery of the latencies most likely reflecting loss of hyperexcitable C-fibers (*see* Fig. 6). In the type 2 BBZDR/Wor-rat the decrease in latency to thermal stimuli was slower and was only significantly different from that in control rats after 6 months of diabetes consistent with the near normal morphometric parameters of C-fibers in this model (Fig. 6). C-peptide replacement in BB/Wor-rat significantly prevented hyperalgesia resulting in a profile similar to that in BBZDR/Wor-rat. The data points represent the means ± SD's of at least eight animals.

period (Fig. 4). However, in type 1 BB/Wor-rats, there is a rapid and progressive decline in the latencies during the first 6 months of diabetes, followed by an increase from 6 to 10 months of diabetes, representing increasing relative analgesia *(47)*. The hyperalgesia in type 1 BB/Wor-rats can be significantly, but not completely prevented by insulinomimetic C-peptide (Fig. 4) *(47)*. In contrast the type 2 BBZDR/Wor-rat shows a significantly slower progression of hyperalgesia (Fig. 4) *(46)*.

Nociceptive C-fibers emanate from small nociceptive SP and CGRP dorsal root ganglion cells, which are dependent on neurotrophic support by NGF, insulin, and IGF-1 *(10,44,70)*. In the BB/Wor-rat both systemic insulin and IGF-1 are significantly diminished as is endogenous IGF-1, abnormalities which are coupled with significantly decreased expression of the insulin and IGF-1 receptors in dorsal root ganglia *(46)*. These changes are either milder or nonexistent even in chronically diabetic BBZDR/Wor-rat *(46)*. Added to these deficiencies, sciatic nerve NGF as well as the expression of NGF-TrkA in dorsal root ganglion cells are more severely affected in the type 1 model *(46)*. Hence, as would be expected, these deficiencies lead to impaired expression of SP and CGRP in type 1 but not in type 2 BB-rats *(46)*. The underlying molecular abnormalities in the type 1 BB/Wor-rat are almost totally prevented by replenishment of insulinomimetic C-peptide that is associated with prevention of hyperalgesia *(47,71)*, which suggests that nociceptive sensory neuropathy is mainly an insulin/C-peptide deficiency-mediated phenomenon rather than a hyperglycemia-induced entity. This is further supported by the frequent occurrence of "idiopathic" painful neuropathy in patients *(72,73)* and animals *(70)* with prediabetes or impaired glucose tolerance and β-cell dysfunction.

STRUCTURAL ABNORMALITIES IN TYPE 1 AND TYPE 2 DPN

Myelinated Sensory Fibers

One of the earliest detectable structural changes in sensory myelinated fibers is the conspicuous enlargement or swelling of the nodal and paranodal axon, which correlates with the early Na^+/K^+-ATPase defect and increased axonal $[Na^+]^i$ *(30,33)* and is reversible after metabolic corrections. This abnormality is less frequent in early type 2 DPN in the BBZDR/Wor-rat, probably related to the milder defect in the Na^+/K^+-ATPase activity *(31,56)*. Other early ultrastructural abnormalities observed in sensory nerves consist of glycogen accumulation in axonal mitochondria, so called glycogenosomes, and misalignment of neuroskeletal structures *(74,75)*. These structural changes are likely to reflect impaired axonal energy metabolism *(74,76)* and aberrant phosphorylation and nonalignment of particularly neurofilaments, respectively *(75,77–79)*. Maligned neuroskeletal elements appear to induce phagocytotic activities by the Schwann cell that extends cytoplasmic loops engulfing abnormal axoplasm leading to so-called honeycombing of the axon *(75)*. These early changes are associated with perturbed phosphorylation and synthesis of neurofilaments and decreased slow axonal transport leading to progressive axonal atrophy evident in the BB/Wor-rat already after 4 months of diabetes (Table 1) *(45,80,81)*. Axonal atrophy leads to decreased circularity of axons associated with excessive myelin wrinkling best assessed in teased fiber preparations. The ultimate fate of these changes is axonal degeneration with secondary myelin breakdown and fiber loss. Significant fiber loss of 10% is already detectable in the sural nerve after 4 months of diabetes and increases to 33% after 11 months in the BB/Wor-rat (Table 1). Fiber loss in the tibial nerve at 11 months of diabetes is 12% and in the dorsal root 0% *(81)*. Therefore, the degenerative processes progress in a proximal direction both in the peripheral as well as the central sensory axons, hence the characterization of DPN as a *central-peripheral axonopathy of dying back type (81,82)*.

Primary demyelination is rare in type 1 DPN of the BB/Wor-rat, but somewhat more common in both human and experimental type 2 DPN *(1,31)*. The reason for this is not well known, although more common comorbidities in both human and experimental type 2 diabetes such as hypercholesterolemia and triglyceridemia have to be considered.

In the BBZDR/Wor-rat the structural changes progress at a slower pace. So for instance, nodal/paranodal axonal swelling is only evident in 14-month diabetic rats, reflecting the milder Na^+/K^+-ATPase defect. Myelinated fiber atrophy of the sural nerve also progresses slower, becoming significant only after 6 months of diabetes and reaching a reduction of 11% at 14 months (cf. Table 1). At this time-point there is also a 10% loss of myelinated fibers in the sural nerve. On the other hand, segmental demyelination

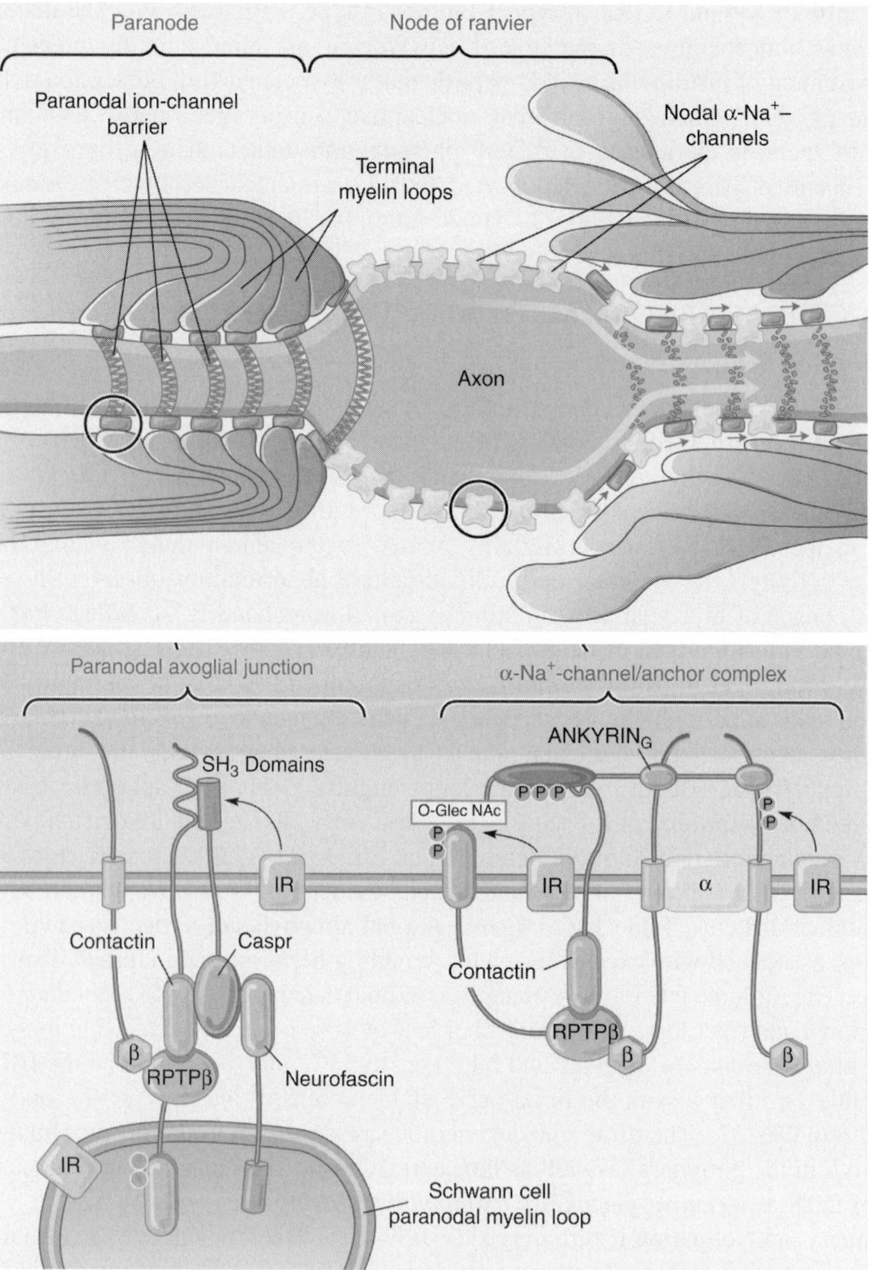

Fig. 5. Axoglial dysjunction is a characteristic degenerative change of type 1 DPN. As the disease progresses (left to right, top panel), it results in a breach of the paranodal ion-channel barrier (red in the top panel), which connects the terminal myelin loops with the axolemma. This defect allows the nodal α-Na^+-channels (yellow) to diffuse away from the node, resulting in severe nerve conduction deficits. Insulin receptors (IR, lower panel) are particularly clustered to the nodal axolemma and paranode. In type 1 DPN the expression of key nodal molecules such, as β-Na^+-channel adhesive molecules (β), ankyrin$_G$, contactin, and RPTP$_β$ is severely suppressed. Also, their ability to interact with neighboring proteins is hampered by impaired phosphorylation. The expression of the pore forming α-Na^+-channel (a) is not altered in type 1 DPN,

is three times as frequent in comparison with the type 1 BB/Wor-rat and affects 4.2% of all fibers in chronically diabetic BBZDR/Wor-rats *(15,31)*. It is therefore obvious that the spectrum and progression of structural changes differ greatly between the two models despite the fact that cumulative hyperglycemic exposure is the same. These differences are not dissimilar from the differences previously described between human type 1 and type 2 DPN *(1)*.

Nodal and Paranodal Changes

When initially described *(1,55)* these lesions were met with some controversy, because investigators failed to identify them in biopsy material from mainly type 2 diabetic patients or in acutely diabetic BB/Wor-rat *(83–86)*. Following the recent elucidation of the longitudinal development of molecular changes underlying the nodal and paranodal abnormalities in type 1 and type 2 DPN *(48,61)*, these changes are now firmly established.

The principal ultrastructural change is the breach of the junctional complexes adhering the terminal myelin loops to the paranodal axolemma, referred to as *axoglial dysjunction* (Fig. 5). This is followed by retraction of the myelin, paranodal demyelination, a lesion which may be repaired by the lay down of small thinly myelinated intercalated internodes *(55,61)*. Axoglial dysjunction is not specific for type 1 DPN, but occurs in a variety of neuropathies summarized by Yamamoto et al. *(87)*.

The molecular compositions of the node of Ranvier and the paranodal apparatus are complex (Fig. 5) *(88,89)*. Voltage-gated Na^+ channels are concentrated to the nodal axolemma. They consist of the pore-forming Na^+ channel α-subunit and two auxiliary Na^+ channel subunits β_1 and β_2, which act as adhesive anchors *(90)* and interact with axonal ankyrin$_G$ *(91)*. The β-subunits also interact with neurofascin, Nr-CAM, N-cadherin and L1 *(89,92)* mediating contacts with Schwann cell microvilli. Post-translational modification of ankyrin$_G$ by O-linked *N*-acetyl-glycosamine, inhibits phosphorylation of serin residues and prevents interaction with the β-subunits, and its interaction with receptor protein tyrosin phosphatase (RPTP)-β, which is mediated by tyrosine phosphorylation sites *(61,93,94)*. It should be mentioned that the high affinity insulin receptor in peripheral nerve is concentrated to the nodal axolemma and colocalizes with axoglial junctions at the paranode (Fig. 5) *(95)*.

At the paranode, myelin loops adhere to the axolemma through tight junctions constituting the paranodal ion-channel barrier separating nodal Na^+ channels from juxtaparanodal K^+ channels. Caspr is the principal molecule of tight junctions and is coupled to contactin, serving as a receptor for RPTP-β (Fig. 5) *(96,97)*. The cytoplasmic tail of caspr mediates protein–protein interactions by adducts of p85 to its protein 4.1 and SH3

Fig. 5. *(Continued)* although anchoring of the channel to the axolemma is compromised by the defective β-subunits. At the paranode, the backbone molecule of the tight junctions, caspr is responsible for the ion-channel barrier function and is compromised in its expression and post-translational activity by impaired binding of p85 to intracytoplasmic SH_3 domains. Furthermore, caspr's interaction with contactin, RPTP$_\beta$ and β-Na^+-channels is impaired. These molecular abnormalities lead to the progressive degeneration of the paranodal barrier allowing the now mobile α-Na^+-channels to diffuse away from the nodal axolemma (upper panel). α: α-Na^+-channel; β: β- Na^+-channels; IR: insulin receptor. Reproduced by permission from ref. *48*.

domains. p85 is the regulatory subunit of PI3-kinase, and is probably mediated by insulin signaling (Fig. 5) *(61,97)*. Hence, the paranodal ion-channel barrier is not a static rigid structure but merely a complex of metabolically regulated protein–protein interactions.

In type 1 diabetic BB/Wor-rat the expression of ankyrin$_G$, contactin, RPTPβ, and β-Na$^+$-channel subunits are unaltered after 2 months of diabetes, a time-point at which axoglial dysjunction is undetectable. However, at 8 months of diabetes, the expression of these molecules is significantly decreased. In addition, the glycation of ankyrin$_G$ is increased coupled with decreased phosphorylation *(61)*, the socalled "yin-yang" relationship, hence compromising its protein–protein interaction. Interestingly the pore-forming α-Na$^+$ channel expression is not altered. Of the paranodal constituents, caspr is unaltered at 2 months, but shows a 25% reduction in expression at 8 months at which time there is also marked suppression of contactin and RPTPβ *(61)*. Similar changes are not detectable in 8-month BBZDR/Wor-rats *(61)*, suggesting that these aberrations in type 1 diabetes are associated with impaired insulin signaling. Indirect evidence for this construct is provided by the beneficial effects of insulinomimetic C-peptide *(48,61)*, which prevents both the impaired expression of these molecular elements and maximizes their perturbed post-translational modifications, necessary for protein–protein interaction.

However, more chronic 14-month diabetic BBZDR/Wor-rats, do show evidence of nodal and paranodal degenerative changes, such as significant paranodal demyelination and increased frequencies of intercalated internodes *(31)*.

Therefore, the progressive axoglial dysjunction first evident after 4 months of diabetes in the BB/Wor-rats has a molecular underpinning that appears to be caused by impaired insulin signaling, thereby, explaining the differences between DPN in type 1 and type 2 diabetes with respect to nodal and paranodal pathology.

Unmyelinated Fiber Pathology

The sensory C-fiber population is probably the most vulnerable anatomical component in DPN. This is evidenced by the occurrence of C-fiber related symptoms already during prediabetic conditions *(72,73)* and C-fiber atrophy in the glucose-intolerant and insulin deprived GK-rat *(70)*.

In the type 1 BB/Wor-rat, sural nerve C-fibers show profound axonal atrophy and a 50% fiber loss at 8 months of diabetes (Fig. 6), leaving behind increased frequencies of denervated Schwann cell profiles and collagen pockets. The degeneration of C-fibers is associated with loss of mesaxonal junctional complexes of supporting Schwann cells, exposing C-fibers directly to the endoneurial environment, so-called type 2 axon/Schwann cell relationship *(46)*. Interestingly, as with the paranodal ion-channel barrier, the insulin receptor colocalizes with C-fiber mesaxons *(95,98)*. Whether insulin signaling abnormalities are of pathogenetic significance here as demonstrated for axoglial dysjunction has not been explored.

The C-fiber pathologies are associated with decreased sciatic nerve content of NGF and systemic insulin with consequent effects on the expression of SP and CGRP in dorsal root ganglion (DRG) cells.

In the type 2 BBZDR/Wor-rat the C-fiber population in sensory nerve is substantially less affected with normal axonal size and number (Fig. 6) even after 8 months exposure to severe hyperglycemia. Consequently the frequencies of denervated Schwann cell profiles and type 2 axon/Schwann cell relationships are not different from nondiabetic

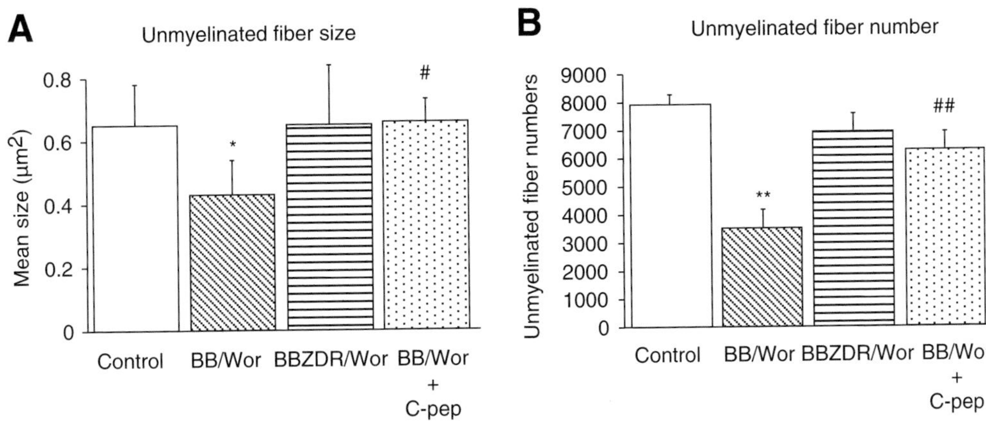

Fig. 6. C-fiber size and number in sural nerves of 8 month diabetic BB/Wor-, C-peptide-replaced BB/Wor- and type 2 BBZDR/Wor-rats. Data represent mean ± SDs of eight animals. $*p < 0.05$; $**p < 0.001$ vs control rats: $\#p < 0.05$; $\#\#p < 0.001$ vs BB/Wor-rats.

control rats *(46)*. The relative absence of significant C-fiber pathology is associated with normal expressions of neurotrophic factors and their receptors as well as normal content of SP and CGRP in dorsal root ganglia *(46)*, and substantially milder functional deficits.

Therefore, the significant differences between C-fiber involvement between the two models necessitated investigations concerning whether insulin action may have an overriding impact. Type 1 BB/Wor-rat replenished with proinsulin C-peptide *(71)* for 8 months demonstrated corrections of the DRG insulin receptor, IGF-1R, TrkA and Trk C-receptors, and normalization of peripheral NGF and NT-3. These effects resulted in normal SP and CGRP contents in DRG's and prevention of C-fiber loss and partial prevention of C-fiber atrophy (Fig. 6) *(47)*, resulting in a functionally mild C-fiber neuropathy similar to that seen in the type 2 BBZDR/Wor-rat. Hence, these data strongly suggest that C-fiber neuropathy, resulting in painful diabetic neuropathy is caused mainly by impaired insulin and C-peptide signaling mediated through its effect on the expression of neurotrophic factors with secondary effects on SP and CGRP positive neurons.

DRG apoptosis has been implied as a potential component in sensory neuropathies. In the BB/Wor-rat these data has not been confirmed. Rather apoptotic stresses occurring in DRG neurons in the BB/Wor-rat appears to be completely counter balanced by various survival factors *(99)*.

STRUCTURAL–FUNCTIONAL CORRELATIONS

Myelinated Fibers

From the above it is clear that the early defects in NCV are caused by metabolic abnormalities, most noticeably the early Na^+/K^+-ATPase defect. The type 1 diabetes model shows a more severe defect, which is likely to cause subthreshold initial Na^+ currents at the node resulting in a conduction block of large fast conducting myelinated fibers *(52,53)*. This would explain the early steep decline in NCV in this model. The early reversible NCV defect is associated with reversible paranodal and nodal axonal swellings induced by the increase in intra-axonal $[Na^+]^i$ concentration *(53)*. In contrast, the type 2 rat shows a significantly milder initial decline in NCV, which most likely reflects the

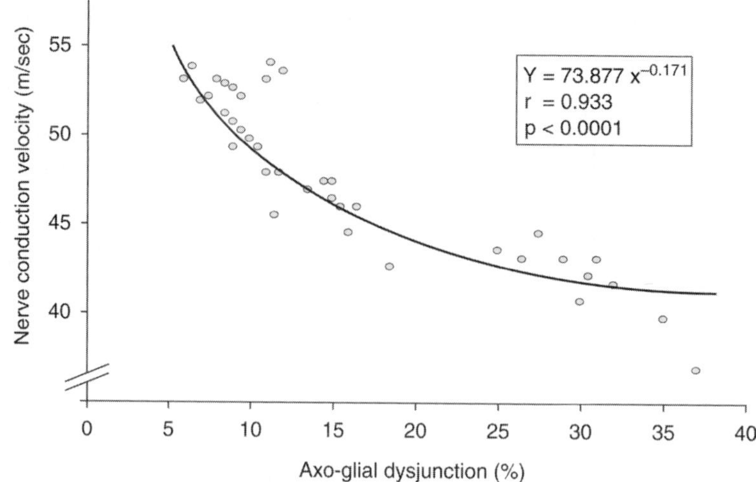

Fig. 7. Correlation between NCV and extent of axoglial dysjunction in control and type 1 diabetic BB/Wor-rats at different stages of DPN. Each data point represents one animal.

milder Na^+/K^+-ATPase defect *(31)*, which may not be sufficient to cause the same extent of large fiber conduction block, although this has not been specifically examined.

Following the initial defect in the BB/Wor-rat the NCV plateaus at a 25% deficit up to 4 to 5 months duration of diabetes, followed by a further progressive decline (Fig. 2). This second phase coincides with the progressive nodal and paranodal changes such as axoglial dysjunction and emerging axonal atrophy and loss of myelinated fibers. It is obvious that the molecular and structural changes of the node of Ranvier leading to the escape of nodal Na^+ channels *(60,61)* has a profound effect on NCV. Indeed there is a highly significant correlation between the extent of axoglial dysjunction and NCV (Fig. 7) *(55)*. In addition, it is well known that axonal caliber correlates with NCV *(100,101)*, hence adding to and propagating the NCV deficits.

As described earlier, the BBZDR/Wor-rat develops nodal pathologies only at a late stage, detectable only after 14 months of diabetes, at which point it shows an accelerated decrease in NCV *(31)*. Moreover, the magnitude and progression of axonal atrophy is substantially milder, resulting in a smoother and slower decline of NCV over time in comparison with the type 1 counterpart (Figs. 2 and 3).

Unmyelinated Fibers

The progressive degeneration of unmyelinated fibers in the sural nerve of BB/Wor-rats correlates with the increasing thermal hyperalgesia of the hind paw, reflecting the hyperexcitability of these fibers *(66,67)*. The degenerative changes are followed by progressive loss of fibers, including high frequency firing fibers *(47,48)*, which is reflected in a reversal of hyperalgesia (Figs. 4 and 6) and is likely to eventually result in progressive analgesia with duration of diabetes.

The involvement of C-fiber pathology is substantially milder in the BBZDR/Wor-rat and is reflected in a significantly milder increase in hyperalgesia, both of which are similar to those demonstrated by C-peptide replaced BB/Wor-rats with the same duration of diabetes.

CONCLUSION

It is clear from these data that the neuropathies occurring in the two BB-rat models show distinct differences in underlying metabolic and molecular changes, progression of functional deficits and the spectra of morphological changes despite the same exposure to hyperglycemia. Therefore the differences imply that hyperglycemia is only one component of the pathogenetic web underlying DPN. The other major component contributing to DPN is provided by the deficiencies in insulin and synergistically acting C-peptide, resulting in impaired insulin signaling. These latter defects appear to substantially add to the severity of the neural Na^+/K^+-ATPase defect and to be the major culprit in the perturbations of impaired neurotrophic support, and to be the sole factor in the development of nodal/paranodal dysfunction and pathology. Hence, these differences in underlying mechanisms explain the differences in the progression and severity between type 1 and type 2 DPN. Only by recognizing such differences in underlying factors and their associated dynamic consequences in the development of DPN will it be possible to approach these disorders therapeutically in biologically meaningful ways, as already documented by several successful C-peptide trials in type 1 DPN.

ACKNOWLEDGMENTS

Many studies referred to in this chapter were supported by grants from Canadian Diabetes Association, NIH, JDRF, and the Thomas Foundation.

REFERENCES

1. Sima AAF, Nathaniel V, Bril V, McEwen TAJ, Greene DA. Histopathological heterogeneity of neuropathy in insulin-dependent and non-insulin-dependent diabetes, and demonstration of axo-glial dysjunction in human diabetic neuropathy. *J Clin Invest* 1988; 81:349–364.
2. Sugimoto K, Murakawa Y, Sima AAF. Diabetic neuropathy—a continuing enigma. *Diabetes/Metab Res Rev* 2000;16(6):408–433.
3. Dyck PJ, Davies JL, Wilson DM, Service FJ, Melton LJ III, O'Brien PC. Risk factors for severity of diabetic polyneuropathy: intensive longitudinal assessment of the Rochester Diabetic Neuropathy Study Cohort. *Diabetes Care* 1999;22:1479–1486.
4. Dyck JB, Dyck PJ. Diabetic neuropathy. in *Diabetic neuropathy* (Dyck and Thomas eds.), WB Saunders Comp., Philadelphia, 1999, pp. 255–295.
5. Pirart J. Diabetes mellitus and its degenerative complications: a prospective study of 4,400 patients observed between 1947 and 1973. *Diabete Metab* 1977;3:97–107.
6. Vinik AI, Liuzze FJ, Holland MT, Stansberry KB, LeBean JM, Colen LB. Diabetic neuropathies. *Diabetes Care* 1992;15:1926–1975.
7. Sima AAF. Pathological definition and evaluation of diabetic neuropathy and clinical correlations. *Can J Neurol Sci* 1994;21(Suppl 4):S13–S17.
8. Tesfaye S, Stevens LK, Stephanson JM, et al. Prevalence of diabetic peripheral neuropathy and its relation to glycaemic control and potential risk factors: the EURODIAB IDDM Complication Study. *Diabetologia* 1996;39:1377–1384.
9. Sima AAF, Thomas PK, Ishii D, Vinik A. Diabetic Neuropathies. *Diabetologia* 1997;40: B74–B77.
10. Sima AAF. New insights into the metabolic and molecular basis for diabetic neuropathy. *Cell Mol Life Sci* 2003;60:2445–2464.
11. Greene DA, Sima AAF, Stevens MB, Feldman EL, Lattimer SA. Complications: neuropathy, pathogenetic considerations. *Diabetes Care* 1992;15:1902–1925.

12. Sima AAF. Diabetes underlies common neurological disorders. *Ann Neurol* 2004;56:459–461 (Editorial).
13. Sima AAF. Can the BB-rat help to unravel diabetic neuropathy? Annotation. *Neuropath Appl Neurobiol* 1985;11:253–264.
14. Marliss EB, Nakhooda AF, Poussier P, Sima AAF. The diabetic syndrome of the BB-Wistar rat. Possible relevance to type I (insulin dependent) diabetes in man. *Diabetologia* 1982;22:225–232.
15. Sima AAF, Merry AC, Hall DE, Grant M, Murray FT, Guberski D. The BB/Z^{DR}-rat; A model for type II diabetic neuropathy: Exp. *Clin Endocrin Diabetes* 1997;105:63–64.
16. Sima AAF, Bril V, Greene DA. Pathogenetic heterogeneity in human diabetic neuropathy. *Pediatr Adoles Endocrin* 1989;18:56–62.
17. Greene DA, Lattimer SA, Sima AAF. Perspectives in diabetes. Are disturbances of sorbitol, phosphoinositide and (Na,K)-ATP-ase regulation involved in the pathogenesis of diabetic neuropathy? *Diabetes* 1988;37:688–693.
18. Pop-Busui R, Sullivan KA, van Huysen C, et al. Depletion of taurine in experimental diabetic neuropathy: implications for nerve metabolic, vascular and functional deficits. *Exp Neurol* 2001;168:259–272.
19. Stevens MJ, Dananberg J, Feldman EL, et al. The linked roles of nitric oxide, aldose reductase and (Na^+,K^+)-ATPase in the slowing of nerve conduction in the streptozotocin diabetic rat. *Metabolism* 1996;45:865–872.
20. Requena JR, Baynes JW. Studies in animal models on the role of glycation and advanced glycation-end-products (AGE's) in the pathogenesis of diabetic complications: pitfalls and limitations. in *Chronic Complications in Diabetes* (Sima AAF ed.), Harwood Academy Publication, Amsterdam, 2000, pp. 43–70.
21. Apfel SC. Neurotrophic factors and diabetic peripheral neuropathy. *Eur Neurol* 1999;41(Suppl 1):27–34.
22. LeRoith D. The insulin-like growth factor system. *Exp Diabetes Res* 2003;4:205–212.
23. Pittinger G, Vinik A. Nerve growth factor and diabetic neuropathy. *Exp Diabetes Res* 2003;4:257–270.
24. Sima AAF, Li Z-G, Zhang W. The IGF system and neurological complications in diabetes. *Exp Diabetes Res* 2003;4:235–256.
25. Brownlee M. Biochemistry and molecular cell biology of diabetic complications. *Nature* 2001;414:813–820.
26. Cameron NE, Cotter MA, Robertson S. Rapid reversal of a motor nerve conduction deficit in streptozotocin-diabetic rats by the angiotensin converting enzyme inhibitor lisinopril. *Acta Diabetol* 1993;30:46–48.
27. Stevens MJ, Obrosova I, Pop-Busui R, Greene DA, Feldman EL. Pathogenesis of diabetic neuropathy. in *Ellenberg and Rifkin's Diabetes Mellitus* (Porte D Jr, Sherwin RS, Baron A eds.), McGraw Hill, New York, 2002, pp. 747–770.
28. Stevens MJ, Zhang W, Li F, Sima AAF. C-peptide corrects endoneurial blood flow but not oxidative stress in type 1 BB/Wor-rats. *Am J Physiol* 2004;287:E497–E505.
29. Greene DA, Lattimer SA, Sima AAF. Sorbitol, phosphoinositides and sodium-potassium ATPase in the pathogenesis of diabetic complications. *N Engl J Med* 1987;316:599–606.
30. Greene DA, Chakrabarti S, Lattimer SA, Sima AAF. Role of sorbitol accumulation and myoinositol depletion in paranodal swelling of large myelinated nerve fibers in the insulin-deficient spontaneously diabetic biobreeding rat. *J Clin Invest* 1987;79:1479–1485.
31. Sima AAF, Zhang W, Xu G, Sugimoto K, Guberski DL, Yorek MA. A comparison of diabetic polyneuropathy in type-2 diabetic BBZDR/Wor-rat and in type 1 diabetic BB/Wor-rat. *Diabetologia* 2000;43:786–793.
32. Sima AAF, Zhang W-X, Sugimoto K, et al. C-peptide prevents and improves chronic type 1 diabetic neuropathy in the BB/Wor-rat. *Diabetologia* 2001;44:889–897.

33. Zhang W, Yorek M, Pierson CR, Murakawa Y, Breidenbach A, Sima AAF. Human C-peptide dose dependently prevents early neuropathy in the BB/Wor-rat. *Intern J Exp Diabetes Res* 2001;2(3):187–194.
34. Forst T, de la Tour DD, Kunt T, et al. Effects of proinsulin C-peptide on nitric oxide, microvascular blood flow and erythrocyte Na^+, K^+-ATPase activity in diabetes mellitus type 1. *Clin Sci* 2000;98:283–290.
35. Ohtomo Y, Aperia A, Sahlgren B, Johansson B-L, Wahren J. C-peptide stimulates rat renal tubular Na^+/K^+-ATPase activity in synergism with neuropeptide Y. *Diabetologia* 1996;39:199–205.
36. Greene DA, Sima AAF, Stevens M, et al. Aldose reductase inhibitors: An approach to the treatment of the nerve damage of diabetic neuropathy. *Diabetes/Metab Rev* 1993;9(3): 189–217.
37. Kitamura T, Kimura K, Jung BD, et al. Proinsulin C-peptide activates cAMP response element-binding proteins through the p38 mitogen-activated protein kinase pathway in mouse lung capillary endothelial cells. *Biochem J* 2002;366:737–744.
38. Wahren J, Ekberg K, Johansson J, et al. Role of C-peptide in human physiology. *Am J Physiol* 2000;278:E759–E768.
39. Grunberger G, Sima AAF. The C-peptide signaling. *Exp Diabetes Res* 2004;5:25–36.
40. Pittinger GL, Liu D, Vinik AI. The apoptotic death of neuroblastoma cells caused by serum from patients with insulin-dependent diabetes and neuropathy may be Fas-mediated. *J Neuroimmunol* 1997;76:153–160.
41. Pierson CR, Zhang W, Sima AAF. Proinsulin C-peptide replacement in type 1 diabetic BB/Wor-rats prevents deficits in nerve fiber regeneration. *J Neuropath Exp Neurology* 2003;62:765–779.
42. Li Z-G, Zhang W, Sima AAF. C-peptide enhances insulin-mediated cell growth and protection against high glucose induced apoptosis in SH-SY5Y cells. *Diabetes Metab Res Rev* 2003;19:375–385.
43. Li Z-G, Zhang W, Sima AAF. The role of impaired insulin/IGF action in primary diabetic encephalopathy. *Brain Res* 2005;1037:12–24.
44. Reico-Pinto E, Lang FF, Ishii DN. Insulin and insulin-like growth factor II permit nerve growth factor binding and the neurite formation response in cultured human blastoma cells. *Proc Natl Acad Sci USA* 1984;81:2562–2566.
45. Pierson CR, Zhang W, Murakawa Y, Sima AAF. Tubulin and neurofilament expression and axonal growth differ in type 1 and type 2 diabetic polyneuropathy. *J Neuropath Exp Neurol* 2003;62:260–271.
46. Kamiya H, Murakawa Y, Zhang W, Sima AAF. Sensory nociceptive neuropathy differs in type 1 and type 2 diabetes. *Diabetes Metab Res Rev* 2005;21:448–458.
47. Kamiya H, Zhang W, Sima AAF. C-peptide prevents nociceptive sensory neuropathy in type 1 diabetes. *Ann Neurol* 2004;56:827–835.
48. Sima AAF, Kamiya H. Insulin, C-peptide and diabetic neuropathy. *Sci Med* 2004;10:308–319.
49. Johansson BL, Borg K, Fernquist-Forbes E, et al. Beneficial effects of C-peptide on incipient nephropathy and neuropathy in patients with type 1 diabetes mellitus. *Diabetes Med* 2000;17:181–189.
50. Johansson BL, Borg K, Fernquist-Forbes E, et al. C-peptide improves autonomic nerve function in IDDM patients. *Diabetologia* 1996;39:687–695.
51. Ekberg K, Brismar T, Johansson B-L, et al. Amelioration of sensory nerve dysfunction by C-peptide in patients with type 1 diabetes. *Diabetes* 2003;52:536–541.
52. Brismar T, Sima AAF. Changes in nodal function in nerve fibres of the spontaneously diabetic BB-Wistar rat. Nodal clamp analysis. *Acta Physiol Scand* 1981;113:499–506.
53. Sima AAF, Brismar T. Reversible diabetic nerve dysfunction. Structural correlates to electrophysiological abnormalities. *Ann Neurol* 1985;18:21–29.

54. Brismar T. Abnormal Na-currents in diabetic rat nerve nodal membrane. *Diabetes Med* 1993;10(Suppl 2):S110–S112.
55. Sima AAF, Lattimer SA, Yagihashi S, Greene DA. Axo-glial dysjunction: A novel structural lesion that accounts for poorly reversible slowing of nerve conduction in the spontaneously diabetic BB-rat. *J Clin Invest* 1986;77:474–484.
56. Sima AAF, Prashar A, Zhang W-X, Chakrabarti S, Greene DA. Preventive effect of long term aldose reductase inhibition (Ponalrestat) on nerve conduction and sural nerve structure in the spontaneously diabetic BB-rat. *J Clin Invest* 1990;85:1410–1420.
57. Sima AAF, Ristic H, Merry A, et al. The primary preventional and secondary interventative effects of acetyl-L-carnitine on diabetic neuropathy in the BB/W-rat. *J Clin Invest* 1996;97:1900–1907.
58. Kitano Y, Kuwabara S, Misawa S, et al. The acute effect of glycemic control on axonal excitability in human diabetics. *Ann Neurol* 2004;56:462–467.
59. Brismar T, Sima AAF, Greene DA. Reversible and irreversible nodal dysfunction in diabetic neuropathy. *Ann Neurol* 1987;21:504–507.
60. Cherian PV, Kamijo M, Angelides KJ, Sima AAF. Nodal Na+-channel displacement is associated with nerve conduction slowing in the chronically diabetic BB/W-rat. *J Diabetes Complications* 1996;10:192–200.
61. Sima AAF, Zhang W, Li Z-G, Murakawa Y, Pierson CR. Molecular alterations underlie nodal and paranodal degeneration in type 1 diabetic neuropathy and are prevented by C-peptide. *Diabetes* 2004;53:1556–1563.
62. Quattrini C, Tesfaye S. Understanding the impact of painful diabetic neuropathy. *Diabetes Metab Res Rev* 2003;19(Suppl 1):S2–S8.
63. Kapur D. Neuropathic pain and diabetes. *Diabetes Metab Res Rev* 2003;19(Suppl 1): S9–S15.
64. Dyck PJ, Lambert EH, O'Brien PC. Pain in peripheral neuropathy related to rate and kind of fiber degeneration. *Neurology* 1976;26:466–471.
65. Woolf CJ, Shortland P, Reynolds M, et al. Reorganization of central terminals of myelinated primary afferents in rat dorsal horn following peripheral axotomy. *J Comp Neurol* 1995;360:121–134.
66. Chen X, Levin JD. Altered temporal pattern of mechanically evoked C-fiber activity in a model of diabetic neuropathy in the rat. *Neuroscience* 2003;121:1007–1015.
67. Burchiel KJ, Russel LC, Lee RP, Sima AAF. Spontaneous activity of primary afferent neurons in diabetic BB-Wistar rats. A possible mechanism of chronic diabetic pain. *Diabetes* 1985;34:1210–1213.
68. Arendt-Nielsen L, Sonnenborg FA, Andersen OK. Fascilitation of the withdrawal reflex by repeated transcutaneous electrical stimulation: an experimental study on central integration in humans. *Eur J Appl Physiol* 2000;81:165–173.
69. Hirade M, Yasuda H, Omatsu-Kanbe M, et al. Tetrodotoxin resistant sodium channels of dorsal root ganglion neurons are readily activated in diabetic rats. *Neuroscience* 1999;90:933–939.
70. Murakawa Y, Zhang W, Pierson CR, et al. Impaired glucose tolerance and insulinopenia in the GK-rat causes peripheral neuropathy. *Diabetes Metab Res Rev* 2002;18:473–483.
71. Grunberger G, Qiang X, Li Z-G, et al. Molecular basis for the insulinomimetic effects of C-peptide. *Diabetologia* 2001;44:1247–1257.
72. Singleton JR, Smith AG, Bromberg MB. Increased prevalence of impaired glucose tolerance in patients with painful sensory neuropathy. *Diabetes Care* 2001;24:1448–1453.
73. Novella SP, Inzucchi SE, Goldstein JM. The frequency of undiagnosed diabetes and impaired glucose tolerance in patients with idiopathic sensory neuropathy. *Muscle Nerve* 2001;24:1229–1231.
74. Sima AAF, Hay K. Functional aspects and pathogenetic considerations of the neuropathy in the spontaneously diabetic BB-Wistar rat. *Neuropath Appl Neurobiol* 1981;7:341–350.

75. Sima AAF, Lorusso AC, Thibert P. Distal symmetric polyneuropathy in the spontaneously diabetic BB-Wistar rat. An ultrastructural and teased fiber study. *Acta Neuropath (Berl)* 1982;58:39–47.
76. Greene DA, Lattimer SA, Sima AAF. Perspectives in diabetes. Are disturbances of sorbitol, phosphoinositide and (Na,K)-ATP-ase regulation involved in the pathogenesis of diabetic neuropathy? *Diabetes* 1988;37:688–693.
77. Sima AAF, Hinton D. Hirano-bodies in the distal symmetric polyneuropathy of the spontaneously diabetic BB-Wistar rat. *Acta Neurol Scand* 1983;68:107–112.
78. Zochodne DW, Verge VMK, Cheng C, Sun H, Johnston J. Does diabetes target ganglion neurons? Progressive sensory neuron involvement in long term experimental diabetes. *Brain* 2001;124:2319–2334.
79. Medori R, Jenich H, Autilio-Gambetti L, Gambetti L, Gambetti P. Experimental diabetic neuropathy: similar changes of slow axonal transport and axonal size in different animal models. *J Neurosci* 1988;8:1814–1821.
80. Scott JN, Clark AW, Zochodne DW. Neurofilament and tubulin gene expression in progressive experimental diabetes: failure of synthesis and export by sensory neurons. *Brain* 1999;122:2109–2118.
81. Sima AAF, Bouchier M, Christensen H. Axonal atrophy in sensory nerves of the diabetic BB-Wistar rat, a possible early correlate of human diabetic neuropathy. *Ann Neurol* 1983;13:264–272.
82. Sima AAF, Yagihashi S. Central-peripheral distal axonopathy in the spontaneously diabetic BB- rat: Ultrastructural and morphometric findings. *Diabetes Res Clin Prac* 1986;1: 289–298.
83. Dyck PJ, Giannini C. Pathologic alterations in the diabetic neuropathies of humans. *J Neuropath Exp Neurol* 1996;55:1181–1193.
84. Sima AAF. Diabetic Neuropathy. (Letter to the Editor). *J Neuropath Exp Neurol* 1997;56: 458.
85. Brown AA, Xu T, Arroyo EJ, et al. Molecular organization of the nodal region is not altered in spontaneously diabetic BB-Wistar rat. *J Neurosci Res* 2001;65:1226–1277.
86. Sima AAF, Pierson CR. Diabetic neuropathy; a heterogeneous, dynamic and progressive disorder. *J Neurosci Res* 2001;66:1226–1227.
87. Yamamoto K, Merry A, Sima AAF. An orderly development of paranodal axoglial junctions and bracelets of Nageotte in the rat sural nerve. *Dev Brain Res* 1996;96:36–45.
88. Pedraza L, Huang JK, Colman DR. Organizing principles of the axoglial apparatus. *Neuron* 2001;30:335–344.
89. Davis JQ, Lambert S, Bennett V. Molecular composition of the node of Ranvier: identification of ankyrin-binding cell adhesion molecules neurofascin (micin +/– third FN III domain) on NrCAM at nodal axon segments. *J Cell Biol* 1996;135:1355–1367.
90. Isom LL. The role of sodium channels in cell adhesion. *Front Biosci* 2002;7:12–23.
91. Malhotra JD, Koopman MC, Kazen-Gillespie KA, Fettman M, Hortsch M, Isom L. Structural requirements for interaction of sodium channel β_1 subunits with ankyrin. *J Biol Chem* 2002;277:26,681–26,688.
92. Lustig H, Zanazzi G, Sakurai T, et al. Nr-CAM and neurofascin interactions regulate ankyrin G and sodium channel clustering at the node of Ranvier. *Curr Biol* 2001;11:1864–1869.
93. Hart GW. Dynamic O-linked glycosylation of nuclear and cytoskeletal proteins. *Ann Rev Biochem* 1997;66:315–335.
94. Wells L, Vosseller K, Hart GW. Glycosylation of nucleocytoplasmic proteins: signal transduction and O-GlcNAc. *Science* 2001;291:2376–2378.
95. Sugimoto K, Murakawa Y, Zhang W-X, Xu G, Sima AAF. Insulin receptor in rat peripheral nerve: its localization and alternatively spliced isoforms. *Diabetes/Metab Res Rev* 2000;16(5):354–363.

96. Einheber S, Zanazzi G, Ching W, et al. The axonal membrane Caspr, a homologue of neurorexin IV, is a component of the septate-like paranodal junctions that assemble during myelination. *J Cell Biol* 1997;139:1495–1506.
97. Peles E, Nativ M, Lustig M, et al. Identification of a novel contactin associated transmembrane receptor with multiple domains implicated in protein–protein interactions. *EMBO J* 1997;16:978–988.
98. Sugimoto K, Murakawa Y, Sima AAF. Expression and localization of insulin receptor in rat dorsal root ganglion and spinal cord. *JPNS* 2002;7:44–53.
99. Sima AAF, Kamiya H. Progressive diabetic sensory neuropathy is not apoptosis related. Peripheral Nervous System Society, Florence, Italy, 2005.
100. Yagihashi S, Kamijo M, Watanabe K. Reduced myelinated fiber size correlates with loss of axonal neurofilaments in peripheral nerve of chronically streptozotocin diabetic rats. *Am J Pathol* 1990;136:1365–1373.
101. Hoffman PN, Cleveland DW, Griffin JW, Landes PW, Cowan NJ, Price DL. Neurofilament gene expression: a major determinant of axonal caliber. *Proc Natl Acad Sci USA* 1987;84: 3472–3476.

9
Experimental Diabetic Autonomic Neuropathy

Phillip A. Low, MD

SUMMARY

Experimental diabetic autonomic neuropathy (DAN) recapitulates the pattern of physiological and pathological changes seen in human DAN albeit in milder form. Impaired vasoregulation occurs early. Cardiovagal function is impaired in both spontaneous and induced DAN in rodents. Baroreflex gain is modestly impaired in the rabbit. Cardiac noradrenergic innervation is reduced in DAN. Splanchnic-mesenteric vasoregulation is reduced, ascribed to prejunctional impairment of neurotransmission and impaired endothelial function. Excessive venous pooling is associated with reduced density of 5-hydroxytrytamine and tyrosine hydroxylase labeling of splanchnic veins. Arterial norepinephrine is reduced in DAN. Structural changes affecting sympathetic neurons are well-established in rodent DAN of 1 year duration. Sudomotor denervation is present in diabetic mouse and rat. Erectile dysfunction regularly occurs, related to impaired nitric oxide synthase activity.

Key Words: Baroreflex; erectile; ganglia; norepinephrine; splanchnic; sudomotor.

INTRODUCTION

Autonomic neurons and their preganglionic and postganglionic nerve fibers are involved as part of peripheral neuropathic process in human diabetic neuropathy. The distribution of involvement is extensive; affecting sympathetic, parasympathetic, and peptidergic fibers and involves their supply to peripheral integumental structures, splanchnic-mesenteric bed, genitourinary, sweat gland, and indeed all regions. Studies of similar involvement in experimental diabetes are not well documented compared with human and are better documented for physiological changes than for structural alterations. In this chapter, the focus is on the involvement of autonomic sympathetic nerves in the following structures:

1. Somatic nerves.
2. Autonomic regulation of cardiovascular function.
3. Splanchnic-mesenteric nerves.
4. Sudomotor fibers.
5. Autonomic and dorsal root ganglia.
6. Erectile dysfunction.

From: *Contemporary Diabetes: Diabetic Neuropathy: Clinical Management, Second Edition*
Edited by: A. Veves and R. Malik © Humana Press Inc., Totowa, NJ

Table 1
Results of Studies on Nerve Blood Flow in Experimental Diabetes

Investigator/program	Method	Results
Low, Mayo, Rochester, MN	H_2, LDF, iodo_AP	↓
Powell/Myers, San Diego, CA	LDF	↓
Greene, Michigan, MI	H_2	↓
Cameron/Cotter, Scotland, UK	H_2, LDF	↓
Gispen, Netherlands, UK	LDF	↓
Hotta, Nagoya, Japan, Japan	LDF, H_2	↓
Stevens, Michigan, MI	H_2	↓
Tomlinson, London, UK	LDF	↓
Ueno, Kanagawa, Japan	LDF	↓
Yasuda, Ohtsu, Japan	LDF	↓
Wright/Nukada, New Zealand	LDF	↓
Yorek, WI	H_2	↓
Kihara, Nagoya, Japan	H_2	↓
Nakamura, Nagoya, Japan	–	–
Schratzberger, Boston, MA	LDF, imaging	↓
Ueno, Japan	LDF	↓
Yamamoto, Osaka, Japan	LDF	↓
Van Dam, Utrect, Netherlands	LDF	↓
Van Buren, Utrect, Netherland	LDF	↓
Zochodne, Calgary Canada	LDF, H_2	?
Williamson, TX	^{3}H-desmethylimiprimine	↑

VASOREGULATION OF SOMATIC NERVE FIBERS

An early and consistent finding is impaired vasoregulation of peripheral nerve trunk. Nerve blood flow to peripheral nerve is reduced to about 50% of normal. The reduction occurs early and is sustained. In a recent review *(1)* of studies of peripheral nerve blood flow in experimental diabetic neuropathy, a reduction was demonstrated in 19/21 research programs (Table 1) and typically on multiple occasions. The two laboratories that failed to demonstrate this deficit had methodological problems such as inexperience with a label or contaminating nutritive flow with arteriovenous shunt flow. This reduction is because of impairment of nitric oxide synthase activity *(2,3)* and is initially reversible. To address the issue of whether the impaired perfusion is pathophysiologically important, Cameron et al. *(4)* regressed nerve blood flow against nerve conduction velocity. There is a close relationship between nerve blood flow and nerve conduction slowing (Fig. 1). This relationship highlights the importance of a reduction in endoneurial perfusion, either reflecting the effect of the same primary process (oxidative stress) affecting both microvessels and large somatic nerves or the primary role of nerve ischemia. The importance of oxidative stress is highlighted by correction of this perfusion deficit by the antioxidant α-lipoic acid *(5,6)*.

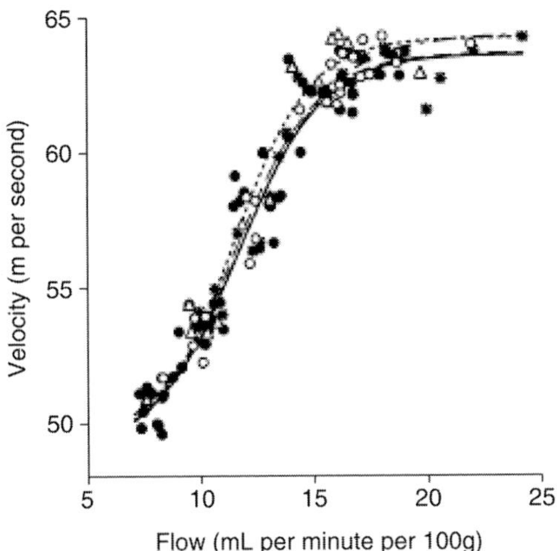

Fig. 1. Relationship between nerve conduction velocity of peripheral nerve and nerve blood flow (Reprinted with permission from ref. *4*).

AUTONOMIC REGULATION OF CARDIOVASCULAR FUNCTION

The best known manifestation of early dysautonomia in human diabetic neuropathy is a loss of cardiovagal function *(7)*. Similar abnormalities have been described after several months of diabetes in experimental diabetic neuropathy (EDN). In a study of Yucatan miniature pigs, blood pressure (BP) and heart rate where recorded telemetrically *(8)*. After 3 months of diabetes induced with streptozotocin (STZ), there was a marked reduction in respiratory sinus arrhythmia. Beyond 3 months, the impairment of cardiovagal function became more pronounced and was associated with increased resting heart rate. Similar observations were reported in spontaneous diabetes in the WBN/Kob rat *(9)*. Florid hyperglycemia was present by 8–9 months, at which time there was a loss of the circadian rhythm of the heart rate and BP with a loss of the nocturnal fall in BP. Sympathetic failure is typically preceded by evidence of sympathetic overactivity, and much of the resting tachycardia is sympathetic in origin.

Baroreflex sensitivity is typically studied in human subjects as heart period change in response to induced reduction followed by an increase in BP. The agents used are usually intravenous boluses of phenylephrine followed by nitroprusside. This has been studied in experimental diabetes using this paradigm and was found to be significantly reduced *(10)*. These workers studied baroreflex gain in alloxan diabetic rabbits after 12 and 24 weeks of diabetes *(10)*. Baroreflex control of heart rate was evaluated in conscious rabbits by measuring changes in heart rate during phenylephrine-induced increases and nitroglycerin-induced decreases in arterial pressure. In diabetic rabbits, the gain of the baroreflex-mediated bradycardia in response to transient hypertension was significantly reduced after 12 and 24 weeks of diabetes. The gain of the baroreflex-mediated tachycardia in response to induced hypotension was not altered. Baroreflex function in anesthetized STZ rat was reported to be unchanged *(11)*. These workers measured heart rate and renal sympathetic nerve activity. The effect of anesthesia in blunting baroreflex function needs to be considered because there were other changes in these rats including hypertension and resting tachycardia, suggesting that dysautonomia was present.

The neuropathological correlate to these changes in cardiovagal function has been explored *(12,13)*. STZ-induced diabetic (STZ-D) and euglycemic control rats were studied at 8- and 16-week time-points after initiation of the diabetic state. Activation of the afferent limb of the baroreceptor reflex was assessed by measuring the numbers of c-Fos-immunoreactive neurons in the brainstem site of termination of the baroreceptor afferent neurons, the nucleus of the solitary tract. Initial experiments established that baseline cardiovascular parameters and nucleus of tractus solitarius expression of c-Fos-immunoreactive neurons were not different between diabetic and control rats at either time-point. Phenylephrine-induced activation of baroreceptors resulted in a significant increase in immunoreactive neurons in this nucleus of control rats. Although diabetic rats showed similar pressor responses to phenylephrine (PE), the activation of c-Fos-positive neurons in the solitary nucleus of diabetic rats was significantly attenuated. At both 8 and 16 weeks, STZ-D rats had significantly fewer positive neurons in the commissural nucleus of solitary tract and in the caudal subpostremal region of this nucleus when in comparison with the nondiabetic control animals receiving phenylephrine. These data suggest that diabetes results in reduced activity in the afferent baroreceptor input to the nucleus of solitary tract and are consistent with diabetes-induced damage to baroreceptor afferent nerves. Oxidative injury may be involved as these authors described attenuation of these changes with α-lipoic acid treatment given during the last 4 weeks before the final experiment *(13)*.

Changes in cardiac adrenergic innervation has been described in experimental human diabetic autonomic neuropathy (DAN) *(14,15)*. Schmid et al. *(14)* evaluated myocardial sympathetic innervation scintigraphically using the sympathetic neurotransmitter analog C-11 hydroxyephedrine ($[^{11}C]$HED) and compared with regional changes in myocardial nerve growth factor protein abundance and norepinephrine content after 6 and 9 months in nondiabetic and STZ-D rats. In nondiabetic rats, no difference in $[^{11}C]$HED retention or norepinephrine content was detected in the proximal versus distal myocardium. After 6 months, compared with nondiabetic rats, myocardial $[^{11}C]$HED retention had declined in the proximal segments of diabetic rats by only 9% (NS) compared with a 33% decrease in the distal myocardium ($p < 0.05$). Myocardial norepinephrine content was similar in both groups of rats. At 6 months, left venticular myocardial nerve growth factor protein content in diabetic rats decreased by 52% in the proximal myocardial segments ($p < 0.01$ vs nondiabetic rats) and by 82% distally ($p < 0.01$ vs nondiabetic rats, $p < 0.05$ vs proximal segments). By 9 months, $[^{11}C]$HED retention had declined in both the proximal and distal myocardial segments of the diabetic rats by 42% ($p < 0.01$ vs nondiabetic rats), and left ventricular norepinephrine content and nerve growth factor protein were decreased in parallel. Therefore, 6 months of diabetes results in heterogeneous cardiac sympathetic denervation in the rat, with maximal denervation occurring distally, and is associated with a proximal-to-distal gradient of left ventricular nerve growth factor protein depletion, suggestive of heterogeneous cardiac sympathetic denervation complicating diabetes.

In a different preliminary study, cardiac adrenergic innervation was evaluated using ^{123}I-metaiodobenzylguanidine imaging in spontaneous Otsuka Long-Evans Tokushima

Fatty rats, an animal model of spontaneous noninsulin-dependent diabetes mellitus *(15)*. Male rats that were 31-week-old were maintained for 8 weeks with or without 30% sucrose solution as drinking water. Long-Evans Tokushima Otsuka rats served as controls. Plasma and cardiac tissue cathecolamine levels were also determined. Plasma glucose levels of diabetic rats with and without sucrose loading (554 ± 106 and 141 ± 1.5 mg/dL, respectively) were significantly higher than those of control rats (116 ± 3.7 mg/dL). Norepinephrine concentrations in heart and plasma tended to be lower in diabetic rats. Cardiac uptake of ^{123}I-MIBG, calculated as % dose/g of tissue, was significantly lower in diabetic rats than in control rats, indicative of reduced adrenergic innervation.

Peripheral vasoregulation has been studied in the nerves of limbs and the splanchnic-mesenteric bed. Mesenteric arterial function was assessed in constantly perfused preparations isolated from rats 12 weeks after treatment with STZ to induce diabetes *(16)*. Frequency-dependent vasoconstrictor responses to electrical field stimulation of sympathetic nerves were severely attenuated in preparations from STZ-diabetic rats. These results suggest 12 weeks after induction of STZ-diabetes in rats, there is prejunctional impairment of sympathetic neurotransmission and impaired endothelial function of the mesenteric arteries.

A major problem in DAN is excessive splanchnic mesenteric venous pooling, which reduces venous return and contributes to the development of orthostatic hypotension *(17)*. Mesenteric venous pooling may also occur in experimental diabetic neuropathy *(18)*. Veins from rats with STZ-induced diabetes were markedly dilated in vivo compared with veins from control animals. Dilation appeared to be the result of loss of smooth muscle tone. Using quantification by image analysis and double-labeling immunohistochemistry on mesenteric veins, significant reductions in the density of nerve plexuses staining for 5-hydroxytryptamine and tyrosine hydroxylase were shown in vessels from diabetic rats compared with controls. These deficits may contribute to an increase in venous pooling of blood in the splanchnic vasculature of diabetic rats and thus, to inadequate venous return to the heart *(18)*. Adrenergic innervation of vessels is reduced. For instance, 6 weeks of alloxan-induced diabetes mellitus was found to result in a neuropathy of arteries characterized by a 38% reduction in the arterial content of norepinephrine. Norepinephrine release from the nerves measured from electrically stimulated superfused arterial segments was decreased. The cocaine-sensitive accumulation of [^{3}H]-norepinephrine was also reduced, reflecting decreased neuronal uptake *(19)*.

SPLANCHNIC-MESENTERIC BED

Experimental diabetes because of STZ or other models associated with insulin deficiency results in gastric and colonic dilatation and loose stools. Schmidt et al. *(20)* described distal axonal swellings and dystrophic changes in the ileal mesentery of diabetic rats, containing a variety of normal and unusual subcellular organelles similar to those described in experimental and clinical axonal dystrophies. These alterations, consisting a distinctive distal axonopathy involving terminal axons and synapses, are particularly dense in the prevertebral superior mesenteric ganglia and celiac ganglia. These axonal alterations were seen after 6, 9, and 12 months of diabetes, apparently increasing in frequency with time. The changes were not seen at 3.5 months. An apparent proximo-distal gradient in the frequency of unmyelinated axonal lesions in this system, suggests experimental DAN may represent an example of distal axonopathy. Retrograde axonal transport of nerve growth factor was reduced *(21)*. Aldose reduction inhibition was reported to partially reduce the development of these dystrophic changes *(22)*. In a recent study, these workers reported that the changes were more prominent in the STZ-D rat and BB/Wor rat, both models of hypoinsulinemic type 1 diabetes, than in the BBZDR/Wor rat, a hyperglycemic and hyperinsulinemic type 2 diabetes model. They argued that hyperglycemia alone is not sufficient to produce sympathetic ganglionic neuroaxonal dystrophy, but rather that it may be the diabetes-induced superimposed loss of trophic support that ultimately causes these lesions *(23)*. Similar findings to the pancreas have been reported *(24)*. In a study of diabetes induced by STZ and occurring spontaneously in BB/W rats, morphometric analysis of contacts between [^{3}H]norepinephrine-labeled sympathetic nerve terminals and α-cells in pancreases from STZ-D rats revealed a 65–70% reduction in direct contacts. An 80% reduction in the number of nerve endings in direct contact with α-cells was also noted in the BB/W diabetic rats.

These structural changes tend to be well-developed only in very chronic diabetes, typically studies done on rats that had been diabetic for 1 year or more. For instance, in a study of diabetes because of STZ, for a duration of 1 year, florid pathological changes were found on light and electronmicroscopy *(25)*. The changes included changes in sympathetic neurons, with intra-axonal glycogen deposits, accumulation of large amounts of lipoid material in autonomic ganglion cells and endoneural cells. By morphometry, the cytoplasmic area and cytoplasmic to nuclear ratio were significantly reduced in the sympathetic neurons of diabetic rats. The axons demonstrated dwindling in the sympathetic preganglionic fibers of diabetic animals. Axonal glycogenosomes were absent in the vagus of control and were present in that of diabetic rats.

In a wide survey of sympathetic adrenergic innervation of nerves, adrenergic nerves were studied in nervi nervorum and perivascular nerve plexus of vasa nervorum in whole-mount nerve sheath preparations of optic, sciatic, and vagus nerves and in the paravertebral sympathetic chain in normal and STZ-treated diabetic rats. A substantial or complete loss of fluorescent adrenergic fibres around blood vessels in the optic nerves was observed 8 weeks after induction of diabetes; whereas perivascular adrenergic fibres in the sciatic, vagus, and sympathetic chain nerve trunks were increased at that early time-point.

SECRETOMOTOR FUNCTION

Kennedy et al. *(26)* has done extensive studies on sudomotor innervation in human and experiment diabetic neuropathy. Most of the experimental studies were done on experimental diabetes in the mouse. They provided detailed ultrastructural studies of the mouse sweat gland *(27)*. Many nerve fibers are entwined with the secretory tubule and contain accumulations of round, clear vesicles, some microtubules, but apparently no neurofilaments. Cholinesterase is found in the clefts between nerve fibers and their ensheathing Schwann cells. The nerve fibers tend to run parallel with capillaries, but have no close association with either the capillaries or the secretory epithelium. Capillaries provide an abundant blood supply to the sweat gland and are fenestrated. The relationships between cellular elements of the sweat gland provide no direct evidence of the mechanisms involved in neurogenic sweating, although it seems likely that effector substances are diffusely distributed. These workers described a reduction with aging, in sudomotor territories, the complement of sweat glands for individual nerves, the number of sweat glands responsive to cholinergic stimulation, as well as their capabilities for compensatory reinnervation of sweat glands by regeneration and by sprouting *(28)*.

Cardone et al. *(29)*, in a detailed and careful study of the sweat response in STZ-induced diabetes in the rat, reported decreased sweating that paralleled severity of hyperglycemia. The pilocarpine-induced sweat responses in the hind foot pads of groups of control and streptozocin diabetic rats, in good and in poor glycemic control and with a crossover design after 20 weeks of diabetes, were evaluated with the silicone mold sweat test to determine the number of sweat droplets per group of foot pads. The sweat response was dose dependent and reproducible, disappearing with denervation and reappearing with reinnervation. In the good glycemic controlled group, the sweat response was not different from that of the control group for up to 136 days. In the poor controlled group, the sweat response became reduced ($p < 0.005$) at 16 days and progressively worsened: 40% of baseline values at 14 weeks ($p < 0.001$). After restoring euglycemia in the poor control group, a normal sweat response occurred at 12 days. These results show that human neuropathic deficit, failure of sweating, can be prevented or ameliorated by good glycemic control.

Secretomotor functional impairment of parotid and submandibular glands has been reported in experimental diabetes. The right parotid ducts were cannulated and parotid salivary flow was induced by stimulating the sympathetic trunk in bursts (50 Hz, 1:10). Total protein and amylase output from the gland were reduced in diabetic animals compared with controls *(30)*. A reduction in submandibular salivary protein concentration in response to sympathetic nerve stimulation was seen in rats that had been diabetic at 3 and 6 months *(31)*. These changes were accompanied by a reduction in secretory granule release from acinar and granular duct cells.

AUTONOMIC GANGLIA

Prominent physiological and less dramatic pathological changes are present in autonomic ganglia of DAN. There is a significant reduction in blood flow in autonomic ganglia such as superior cervical ganglion *(32,33)*. This reduction by about 50% is present as early as 1 week and is persistent over 24 weeks *(4)*. Glucose uptake was reduced to 30% of control values in superior cervical ganglion in rats with DAN. α-Lipoic acid supplementation had no effect on glucose uptake in normal nerves at any dose, but reversed the deficit in DAN, with a threshold between 10 and 25 mg/kg. ATP, creatine phosphate, and lactate were measured in sciatic nerve and superior cervical ganglion. α-Lipoic acid prevented the reduction in autonomic ganglion creatine phosphate *(34)*.

In both diabetic humans and experimental animals, neuroaxonal dystrophy of autonomic nerve terminals has been found, particularly in the prevertebral superior mesenteric and celiac ganglia, which innervate the diabetic small intestine. However, NGF content, NGF receptor expression, p75 low-affinity neurotrophin receptor (NTR), and trkA (high-affinity NGF receptor) expression showed an approximate doubling of NGF content in the diabetic superior mesenteric and celiac ganglia. No change in NGF content was detected in the diabetic superior cervical ganglion *(35)*. These observations suggest that increased NGF content in sympathetic ganglia innervating the diabetic alimentary tract coupled with intact receptor expression may produce aberrant axonal sprouting and neuroaxonal dystrophy.

Treatment of STZ-diabetic rats for 2–3 months with pharmacological doses of NGF or NT-3, neurotrophic substances with known effects on the adult sympathetic nervous system, did not prevent and instead increased the frequency of neuroaxonal dystrophy in the superior mesenteric ganglion of normal rats *(36)*. The sorbitol dehydrogenase inhibitor SDI-158 resulted in a dramatically increased frequency of neuroaxonal dystrophy in ileal mesenteric nerves and superior mesenteric ganglion of SDI-treated vs untreated diabetics. The effect of SDI on diabetic ganglion was completely prevented by concomitant administration of the aldose reductase inhibitor sorbinil. Treatment of diabetic rats with sorbinil also prevented these dystrophic changes in diabetic rats not treated with SDI. These findings indicate that sorbitol pathway-linked metabolic imbalances play a critical role in the development of neuroaxonal dystrophy in this model of diabetic sympathetic autonomic neuropathy *(37)*. The morphological changes are confined to neuroaxonal dystrophy. There is no loss of neurons in either superior mesenteric or superior cervical ganglia after 10 months of severe untreated diabetes *(38)*. A role or aberrant neurofilamentous phosphorylation and its possible involvement in the impaired delivery of neurofilament to the distal axon have been suggested as the relevant mechanism *(39)*.

EXPERIMENTAL ERECTILE DYSFUNCTION

Experimental erectile dysfunction in experimental diabetes and aging has been studied in the rat *(40–42)*. Rat studies typically consist a measurement of intracavernous pressure in response to electrical stimulation of the cavernous nerve in normal and diabetic rats *(43)*. The pathophysiology of erectile dysfunction in DAN appears to mimic the human condition wherein it is vasculogenic resulting in engorgement of corpora cavernosa and is because of a deficiency of nitric oxide *(40,44–46)*. In the penile corpora cavernosa, nitric oxide is produced mainly by the activation of the neuronal nitric oxide synthase (NOS) in the nerve terminals and, to a lesser extent, by endothelial NOS in the lacunar and vascular endothelium *(40,46)*. Nitric oxide stimulates guanylate cyclase → cGMP → activation of phosphokinase G → reduction of intracellular Ca^{2+} → relaxation of the smooth muscle cells → penile engorgement. Support for this concept in the rat derives from a number of observations. Nitric oxide downregulation in the vasculature and penile corpora is associated with erectile dysfunction *(46)*. Chronic treatment with the nitric oxide inhibitor L-NAME leads to abolition of the erectile response *(46,47)*.

Structural changes in corpora are also considered important. There is impaired compliance of the corpora cavernosa and the penile arteries *(40,48)* because of alterations in the smooth muscle and an increase in collagen deposition in the corporal tissue *(40,49)*. Corporal fibrosis results in tissue stiffness and venous leakage. Smooth muscle function is important in that its relaxation results in an increase in intracorporeal pressure, sufficient to compress veins against tunica albuginea. Impaired smooth muscle relaxation results in insufficient pressure → insufficient venous compression → venous leakage *(50)*.

Urological investigators have used the rat model to develop and evaluate novel approaches to treatment *(51)*. In addition to standard approaches such as the evaluation of novel phosphodiesterase inhibitors, investigators have additionally used novel gene therapy with different genes and vectors and ex vivo gene therapy, combining gene transfer with stem cell implants *(42)*. Considerable success has been encountered using gene transfer with the large conductance, Ca-sensitive K channel subtype (i.e., hSlo). The mechanism of action was presumably related to the importance of K channel hyperpolarizing currents to relaxation of corporal smooth muscle and penile erection. A single intracavernous injection of the "naked" pcDNA-*hSlo* (100 μg), which encodes the α-subunit of the human maxi-K channel, was associated with physiologically significant increases in the magnitude of the cavernous nerve-stimulated intracorporeal pressure response that lasts for up to 6 months after a single intracavernous injection *(52)*. Gene transfer prevented an age-related decrease in resting intracavernous pressure and a physiologically relevant, significant effect on normalizing erection in vivo *(53)*. Recently, the efficacy of this gene in the treatment of experimental diabetic erectile dysfunction has been reported *(51)*. The ability of gene transfer with this pore-forming subunit of the human maxi-K channel (hSlo) to ameliorate the decline in erectile capacity commensurate with 12–24 weeks of STZ-diabetes examined in 181 Fischer-344 rats.

Erectile capacity was evaluated by measuring the intracavernous pressure response to cavernous nerve stimulation (ranging from 0.5 to 10 mA). In the first series of experiments, ANOVA revealed increased engorgement pressure in treated animals. A second series of experiments further examined the dose dependence and duration of gene transfer. The intracavernous pressure response to submaximal (0.5 mA) and maximal (10 mA) nerve stimulation was evaluated 3 or 4 months postinjection of a single dose of pcDNA–hSlo ranging from 10 to 1000 μg. ANOVA again revealed that hSlo overexpression was associated with increased nerve-stimulated pressure responses compared with responses in corresponding control animals. Histological studies revealed no immune response to the presence of hSlo. Polymerase chain reaction analysis documented that expression of both plasmid and transcript were largely confined to the corporal tissue. In the third series of pharmacological experiments, hSlo gene transfer in vivo was associated with iberiotoxin-sensitive relaxation responses to sodium nitroprusside in corporal tissue strips in vitro. The latter data indicate that gene transfer produces functional maxi-K-channels that participate in the modulation of corporal smooth muscle cell tone. Taken together, these observations suggest a fundamental diabetes-related change in corporal myocyte maxi-K-channel regulation, expression, or function that may be corrected by expression of recombinant hSlo. Another gene that has been evaluated has been through intracavernosal gene therapy with PnNOS cDNA, which is reported to correct the aging-related erectile dysfunction for at least 18 days *(54)*.

REFERENCES

1. McManis PG, Low PA, Lagerlund TD. Nerve Blood Flow and Microenvironment, in *Peripheral Neuropathy* (Dyck PJ, Thomas PK, eds.), Elsevier Saunders, Philadelphia, 2005, pp. 667–680.
2. Kihara M, Low PA. Regulation of rat nerve blood flow: role of epineurial alpha-receptors. *J Physiol* 1990;422:145–152.
3. Kihara M, Low PA. Impaired vasoreactivity to nitric oxide in experimental diabetic neuropathy. *Exp Neurol* 1995;132:180–185.

4. Cameron NE, Eaton SE, Cotter MA, Tesfaye S. Vascular factors and metabolic interactions in the pathogenesis of diabetic neuropathy. *Diabetologia* 2001;44:1973–1988.
5. Nagamatsu M, Nickander KK, Schmelzer JD, et al. Lipoic acid improves nerve blood flow, reduces oxidative stress, and improves distal nerve conduction in experimental diabetic neuropathy. *Diabetes Care* 1995;18:1160–1167.
6. Keegan A, Cotter MA, Cameron NE. Effects of diabetes and treatment with the antioxidant alpha-lipoic acid on endothelial and neurogenic responses of corpus cavernosum in rats. *Diabetologia* 1999;42:343–350.
7. Low PA, Zimmerman BR, Dyck PJ. Comparison of distal sympathetic with vagal function in diabetic neuropathy. *Muscle Nerve* 1986;9:592–596.
8. Mesangeau D, Laude D, Elghozi JL. Early detection of cardiovascular autonomic neuropathy in diabetic pigs using blood pressure and heart rate variability. *Cardiovasc Res* 2000;45:889–899.
9. Hashimoto M, Harada T, Ishikawa T, Obata M, Shibutani Y. Investigation on diabetic autonomic neuropathy assessed by power spectral analysis of heart rate variability in WBN/Kob rats. *J Electrocardiol* 2001;34:243–250.
10. McDowell TS, Chapleau MW, Hajduczok G, Abboud FM. Baroreflex dysfunction in diabetes mellitus. I. Selective impairment of parasympathetic control of heart rate. *Am J Physiol* 1994;266:H235–H243.
11. Patel KP, Zhang PL. Baroreflex function in streptozotocin (STZ) induced diabetic rats. *Diabetes Res Clin Pract* 1995;27:1–9.
12. Gouty S, Regalia J, Helke CJ. Attenuation of the afferent limb of the baroreceptor reflex in streptozotocin-induced diabetic rats. *Auton Neurosci* 2001;89:86–95.
13. Gouty S, Regalia J, Cai F, Helke CJ. Alpha-lipoic acid treatment prevents the diabetes-induced attenuation of the afferent limb of the baroreceptor reflex in rats. *Auton Neurosci* 2003;108:32–44.
14. Schmid H, Forman LA, Cao X, Sherman PS, Stevens MJ. Heterogeneous cardiac sympathetic denervation and decreased myocardial nerve growth factor in streptozotocin-induced diabetic rats: implications for cardiac sympathetic dysinnervation complicating diabetes. *Diabetes* 1999;48:603–608.
15. Togane Y. Evaluation of the cardiac autonomic nervous system in spontaneously non-insulin-dependent diabetic rats by 123I-metaiodobenzylguanidine imaging. *Ann Nucl Med* 1999;13:19–26.
16. Ralevic V, Belai A, Burnstock G. Effects of streptozotocin-diabetes on sympathetic nerve, endothelial and smooth muscle function in the rat mesenteric arterial bed. *Eur J Pharmacol* 1995;286:193–199.
17. Low PA, Walsh JC, Huang CY, McLeod JG. The sympathetic nervous system in diabetic neuropathy. A clinical and pathological study. *Brain* 1975;98:341–356.
18. Webster GJ, Petch EW, Cowen T. Streptozotocin-induced diabetes in rats causes neuronal deficits in tyrosine hydroxylase and 5-hydroxytryptamine specific to mesenteric perivascular sympathetic nerves and without loss of nerve fibers. *Exp Neurol* 1991;113:53–62.
19. Cohen RA, Tesfamariam B, Weisbrod RM, Zitnay KM. Adrenergic denervation in rabbits with diabetes mellitus. *Am J Physiol* 1990;259:H55–H61.
20. Schmidt RE, Scharp DW. Axonal dystrophy in experimental diabetic autonomic neuropathy. *Diabetes* 1982;31:761–770.
21. Schmidt RE, Modert CW, Yip HK, Johnson EM Jr. Retrograde axonal transport of intravenously administered 125I-nerve growth factor in rats with streptozotocin-induced diabetes. *Diabetes* 1983;32:654–663.
22. Schmidt RE, Plurad SB, Sherman WR, Williamson JR, Tilton RG. Effects of aldose reductase inhibitor sorbinil on neuroaxonal dystrophy and levels of myo-inositol and sorbitol in

sympathetic autonomic ganglia of streptozocin-induced diabetic rats. *Diabetes* 1989; 38:569–579.

23. Schmidt RE, Dorsey DA, Beaudet LN, Parvin CA, Zhang W, Sima AA. Experimental rat models of types 1 and 2 diabetes differ in sympathetic neuroaxonal dystrophy. *J Neuropathol Exp Neurol* 2004;63:450–460.
24. Tominaga M, Maruyama H, Vasko MR, Baetens D, Orci L, Unger RH. Morphologic and functional changes in sympathetic nerve relationships with pancreatic alpha-cells after destruction of beta-cells in rats. *Diabetes* 1987;36:365–373.
25. Kniel PC, Junker U, Perrin IV, Bestetti GE, Rossi GL. Varied effects of experimental diabetes on the autonomic nervous system of the rat. *Lab Invest* 1986;54:523–530.
26. Kennedy WR, Navarro X, Sutherland DE. Neuropathy profile of diabetic patients in a pancreas transplantation program. *Neurology* 1995;45:773–780.
27. Quick DC, Kennedy WR, Yoon KS. Ultrastructure of the secretory epithelium, nerve fibers, and capillaries in the mouse sweat gland. *Anat Rec* 1984;208:491–499.
28. Navarro X, Kennedy WR. Changes in sudomotor nerve territories with aging in the mouse. *J Auton Nerv Syst* 1990;31:101–107.
29. Cardone C, Dyck PJ. A neuropathic deficit, decreased sweating, is prevented and ameliorated by euglycemia in streptozocin diabetes in rats. *J Clin Invest* 1990;86:248–253.
30. Anderson LC, Garrett JR, Proctor GB. Morphological effects of sympathetic nerve stimulation on rat parotid glands 3–4 weeks after the induction of streptozotocin diabetes. *Arch Oral Biol* 1990;35:829–838.
31. Anderson LC, Garrett JR, Suleiman AH, Proctor GB, Chan KM, Hartley R. In vivo secretory responses of submandibular glands in streptozotocin-diabetic rats to sympathetic and parasympathetic nerve stimulation. *Cell Tissue Res* 1993;274:559–566.
32. Sasaki H, Schmelzer JD, Zollman PJ, Low PA. Neuropathology and blood flow of nerve, spinal roots and dorsal root ganglia in longstanding diabetic rats. *Acta Neuropathol* 1997;93:118–128.
33. McManis PG, Schmelzer JD, Zollman PJ, Low PA. Blood flow and autoregulation in somatic and autonomic ganglia. Comparison with sciatic nerve. *Brain* 1997;120:445–449.
34. Kishi Y, Schmelzer JD, Yao JK, et al. Alpha-lipoic acid: effect on glucose uptake, sorbitol pathway, and energy metabolism in experimental diabetic neuropathy. *Diabetes* 1999;48:2045–2051.
35. Schmidt RE, Dorsey DA, Roth KA, Parvin CA, Hounsom L, Tomlinson DR. Effect of streptozotocin-induced diabetes on NGF, P75(NTR) and TrkA content of prevertebral and paravertebral rat sympathetic ganglia. *Brain Res* 2000;867:146–156.
36. Schmidt RE, Dorsey DA, Beaudet LN, Parvin CA, Escandon E. Effect of NGF and neurotrophin-3 treatment on experimental diabetic autonomic neuropathy. *J Neuropathol Exp Neurol* 2001;60:263–273.
37. Schmidt RE, Dorsey DA, Beaudet LN, et al. Inhibition of sorbitol dehydrogenase exacerbates autonomic neuropathy in rats with streptozotocin-induced diabetes. *J Neuropathol Exp Neurol* 2001;60:1153–1169.
38. Schmidt RE. Neuronal preservation in the sympathetic ganglia of rats with chronic streptozotocin-induced diabetes. *Brain Res* 2001;921:256–259.
39. Fernyhough P, Schmidt RE. Neurofilaments in diabetic neuropathy. *Int Rev Neurobiol* 2002;50:115–144.
40. Melman A. Pathophysiologic basis of erectile dysfunction. What can we learn from animal models? *Int J Impot Res* 2001;13:140–142.
41. Melman A, Christ GJ. Integrative erectile biology. The effects of age and disease on gap junctions and ion channels and their potential value to the treatment of erectile dysfunction. *Urol Clin North Am* 2001;28:217–231.

42. Gonzalez-Cadavid NF, Rajfer J. Therapy of erectile dysfunction: potential future treatments. *Endocrine* 2004;23:167–176.
43. Rehman J, Christ G, Melman A, Fleischmann J. Intracavernous pressure responses to physical and electrical stimulation of the cavernous nerve in rats. *Urology* 1998;51:640–644.
44. Ignarro LJ, Bush PA, Buga GM, Wood KS, Fukuto JM, Rajfer J. Nitric oxide and cyclic GMP formation upon electrical field stimulation cause relaxation of corpus cavernosum smooth muscle. *Biochem Biophys Res Commun* 1990;170:843–850.
45. Vernet D, Cai L, Garban H, et al. Reduction of penile nitric oxide synthase in diabetic BB/WORdp (type I) and BBZ/WORdp (type II) rats with erectile dysfunction. *Endocrinology* 1995;136:5709–5717.
46. Gonzalez-Cadavid NF, Ignarro LJ, Rajfer J. Nitric oxide and cyclic GMP in the penis. *Mol Urol* 1999;3:51–59.
47. Li H, Forstermann U. Nitric oxide in the pathogenesis of vascular disease. *J Pathol* 2000;190:244–254.
48. Garban H, Vernet D, Freedman A, Rajfer J, Gonzalez-Cadavid N. Effect of aging on nitric oxide-mediated penile erection in rats. *Am J Physiol* 1995;268:H467–475.
49. Nehra A, Azadzoi KM, Moreland RB, et al. Cavernosal expandability is an erectile tissue mechanical property which predicts trabecular histology in an animal model of vasculogenic erectile dysfunction. *J Urol* 1998;159:2229–2236.
50. Nehra A, Goldstein I, Pabby A, et al. Mechanisms of venous leakage: a prospective clinicopathological correlation of corporeal function and structure. *J Urol* 1996;156:1320–1329.
51. Christ GJ, Day N, Santizo C, et al. Intracorporal injection of hSlo cDNA restores erectile capacity in STZ-diabetic F-344 rats in vivo. *Am J Physiol Heart Circ Physiol* 2004;287: H1544–H1553.
52. Christ GJ, Rehman J, Day N, et al. Intracorporal injection of hSlo cDNA in rats produces physiologically relevant alterations in penile function. *Am J Physiol* 1998;275: H600–H608.
53. Melman A, Zhao W, Davies KP, Bakal R, Christ GJ. The successful long-term treatment of age related erectile dysfunction with hSlo cDNA in rats in vivo. *J Urol* 2003;170:285–290.
54. Magee TR, Ferrini M, Garban HJ, et al. Gene therapy of erectile dysfunction in the rat with penile neuronal nitric oxide synthase. *Biol Reprod* 2002;67:20–28.

10
Spinal Cord
Structure and Function in Diabetes

Andrew P. Mizisin, Corinne G. Jolivalt, and Nigel A. Calcutt

SUMMARY

The spinal cord is a relatively understudied target of diabetes. In this chapter an overview of the anatomy of the spinal cord and its associated structures is presented before reviewing the published literature describing evidence for structural damage to the spinal cord reported in both diabetic patients and animal models of diabetes. Spinal cord pathology is accompanied by functional disorders and diabetic rodents are being increasingly used to investigate the neurochemical and molecular mechanisms that contribute to impaired structure and function. The aetiological mechanisms that lead from hyperglyacemia to disruption of spinal cord structure and function are only beginning to be explored. The growing appreciation of the role that the spinal cord plays in modulating sensory input to and motor output from the central nervous system should prompt wider interest in diabetes-induced spinal cord injury that will complement studies of diabetic encephalopathy and peripheral neuropathy.

Key Words: Diabetes; hyperglycemia; myelopathy; neuropathology; neuropathy; painful neuropathy radiculopathy; sensory processing; spinal cord.

INTRODUCTION

Although myelopathy was first described in the spinal cord of diabetic patients at autopsy over 100 years ago, the impact of diabetes on this portion of the nervous system has been infrequently studied compared with the peripheral nervous system (PNS). In part, this may reflect a tendency to target the regions of the nervous system from where patients perceive pain and/or loss of sensation to emanate. The greater accessibility of the peripheral nerves to biopsy and functional studies probably also contributes to the imbalance. Recent technical advances have re-emphasized that the spinal cord is subject to injury in diabetic patients *(1)* and exhibits unique structural and functional features that possess both scientific and clinical significance. For example, the spinal cord lies within the blood–brain barrier and glucose levels in the cerebrospinal fluid are substantially lower than those to which peripheral nerves are exposed, both in normal and hyperglycemic conditions. Consequently, the cell body and the peripherally projecting axon of a primary sensory neuron are exposed to higher glucose concentrations

From: *Contemporary Diabetes: Diabetic Neuropathy: Clinical Management, Second Edition*
Edited by: A. Veves and R. Malik © Humana Press Inc., Totowa, NJ

during hyperglycemia than the terminal regions of the central projection that enter the spinal cord and synapse with second-order neurons in the dorsal horn. Conversely, motor neuron cell bodies located in the ventral horn are relatively protected in comparison with the sensory cell bodies in the dorsal root ganglia and indeed relative to their own axons that leave the spinal cord and project to target organs. As hyperglycemia is widely regarded as a primary pathogenic mechanism for diabetic neuropathy, the regional variability in glucotoxic exposure may have important consequences for the manifestation of diabetic neuropathy.

There is increasing scientific interest in the spinal cord as clinical and experimental studies have revealed the extent to which it is involved in integrating and modulating both sensory input from peripheral nerves to the higher central nervous system (CNS) and also output from the CNS to peripheral organs. Phenomena such as phantom limb and some neuropathic pain states indicate that the perception and pathogenic site of a lesion do not always match. Research studies of peripheral nerve injury have also highlighted associations between the PNS and spinal cord, such that injury to the PNS can have long-acting consequences in the spinal cord that modify how future sensory input from the PNS is modulated and presented to the CNS. The extent to which the well-documented effects of diabetes on the PNS have an impact on the structure and function of the spinal cord, including its processing of sensory input, is largely unexplored. The direct effects of hyperaglycemia on spinal cord have to be incorporated into the pathogenic scheme of diabetic neuropathy.

FUNCTIONAL ANATOMY

It might be helpful if an overview of the anatomy of the spinal cord and associated structures that is a distillation of more detailed texts is provided first (*see* ref. *2*). The spinal cord, which is divided into 31 segments, is ensheathed by the spinal canal that is formed by the bodies, pedicles, and spinous processes of individual vertebra. Each spinal segment (8 cervical, 12 thoracic, 5 lumbar, 5 sacral, and 1 coccygeal) gives rise to a pair of spinal nerves that are joined to their segments by a pair of posterior (dorsal in quadrupeds) and anterior (ventral in quadrupeds) roots (Fig. 1). The spinal cord is partitioned into peripherally oriented white matter that is organized into tracts containing bundles of axons and centrally oriented gray matter with a "butterfly-shaped" appearance (Figs. 2 and 3). White matter contains myelinated and unmyelinated axons traveling to (posterior roots) and from (anterior roots) the spinal cord and to (ascending tracts) and from (descending tracts) the brain. Gray matter contains neuronal cell bodies, their dendrites and axons, as well as neuroglia, and is functionally organized into the laminae of Rexed (*see Gray Matter* and Fig. 2).

Cell bodies of sensory neurons are located in ganglia that sit on the posterior (dorsal) roots of spinal nerves. Correlations between neuronal size and electrophysiological properties of their cell bodies and axons have resulted in a classification into large clear neurons (type A) and smaller dark neurons (type B) *(3,4)*. The processes of these pseudounipolar afferent neurons conduct somatic and visceral impulses from the periphery to the spinal cord (Fig. 1). Nerve fibers of somatic afferents carry exteroceptive (pain, temperature, and touch) and proprioceptive (body position, muscle tone, and movement) input from sensory receptors in the body wall, muscle, tendons, and joints.

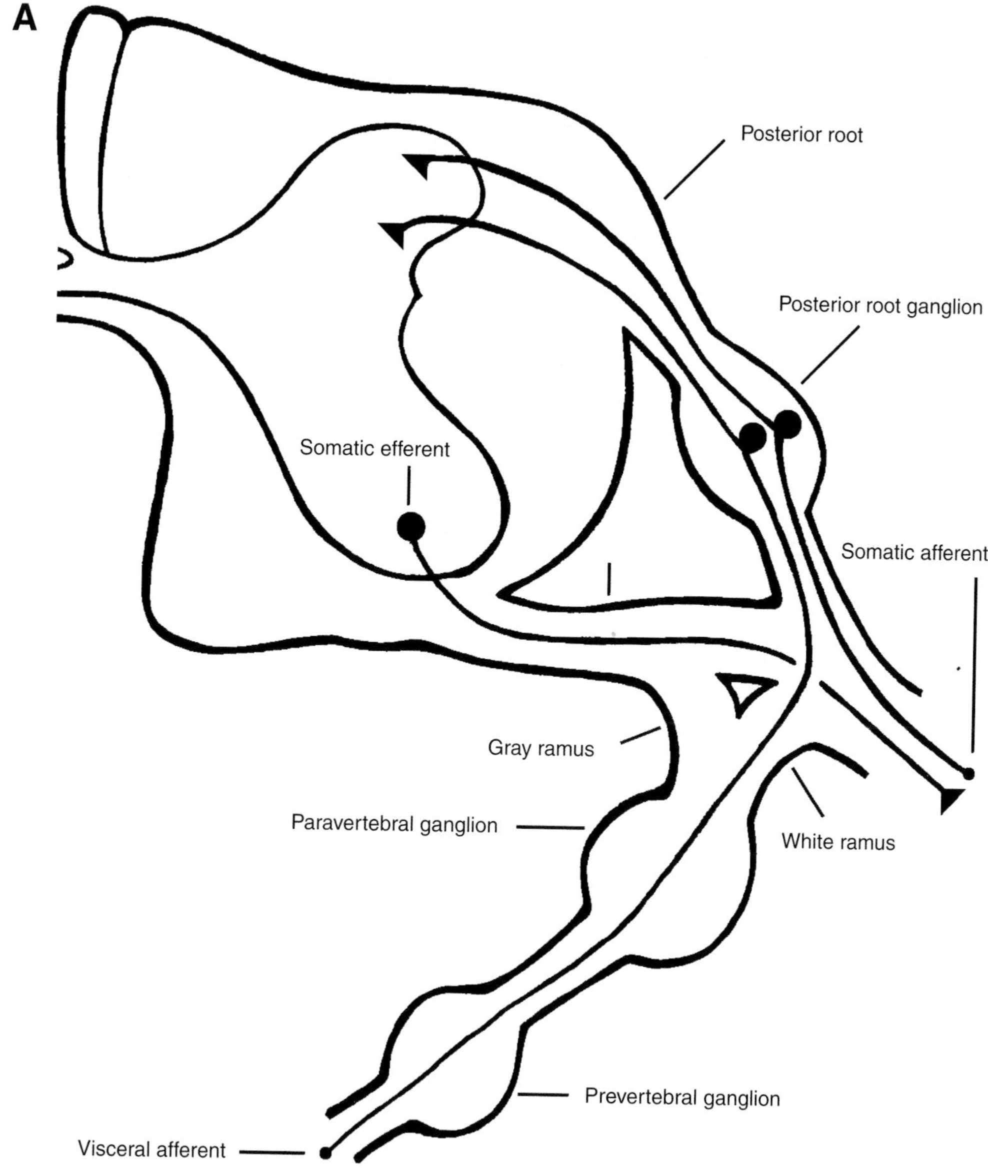

Fig. 1. *(Continued)*

Nerve fibers of visceral afferents carry enteroceptive (degree of filling or stretch of alimentary tract, bladder, and blood vessels) input from the viscera.

Cell bodies of efferent motor neurons are located in lamina IX of the anterior (ventral) horn of the spinal cord (Fig. 2) and conduct somatic impulses from the spinal cord to the periphery through myelinated axons in anterior (ventral) roots. Somatic efferents of α and γ motor neurons innervate striated muscle. Anatomically, the situation for visceral efferents is more complicated and is dependent on whether the efferents are part of the sympathetic or parasympathetic divisions of the autonomic nervous system. Cell

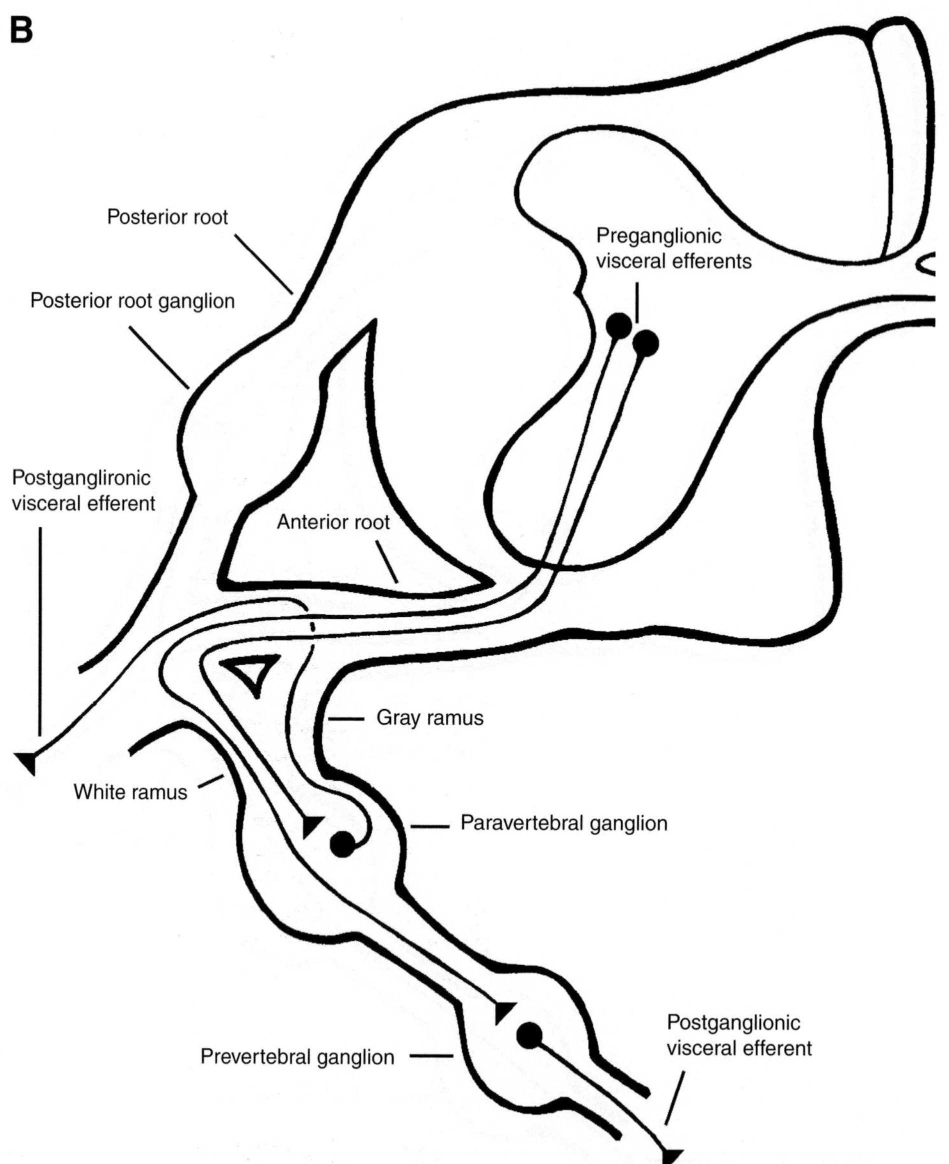

Fig. 1. Spinal nerves and roots, and sympathetic components of the autonomic nervous system in a schematic diagram of a section of thoracic spinal cord. Somatic and visceral afferent input, and somatic efferent output are illustrated in **(A)**, whereas visceral efferent output is shown in **(B)**.

bodies of efferent preganglionic autonomic neurons are located in the interomediolateral cell column of lamina VII that extends from the last cervical segment to the last lumbar segment (sympathetic) or in the midbrain, medulla, and sacral segments 2 through 4 (parasympathetic). Postganglionic autonomic cell bodies are either in paravertebral or prevertebral ganglia (Fig. 1). Myelinated preganglionic and unmyelinated postganglionic visceral efferents innervate smooth and cardiac muscle, and regulate glandular secretion.

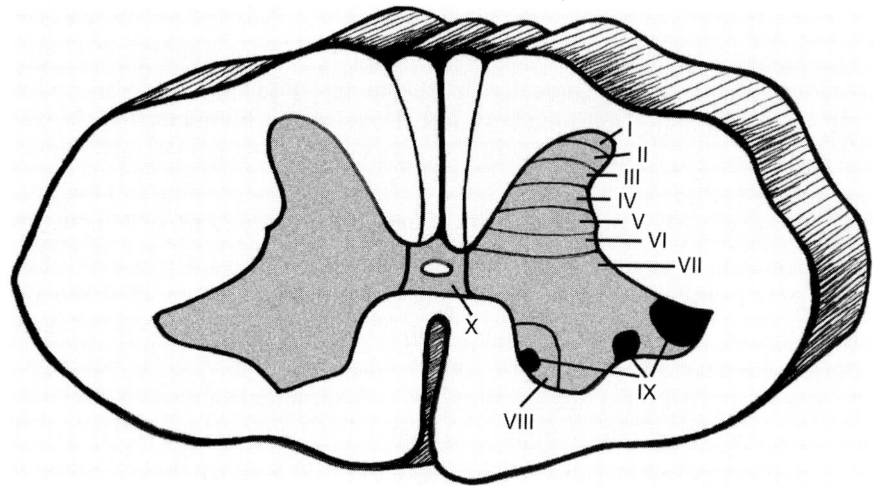

Fig. 2. Schematic representation depicting the location of the laminae of Rexed in spinal cord gray matter.

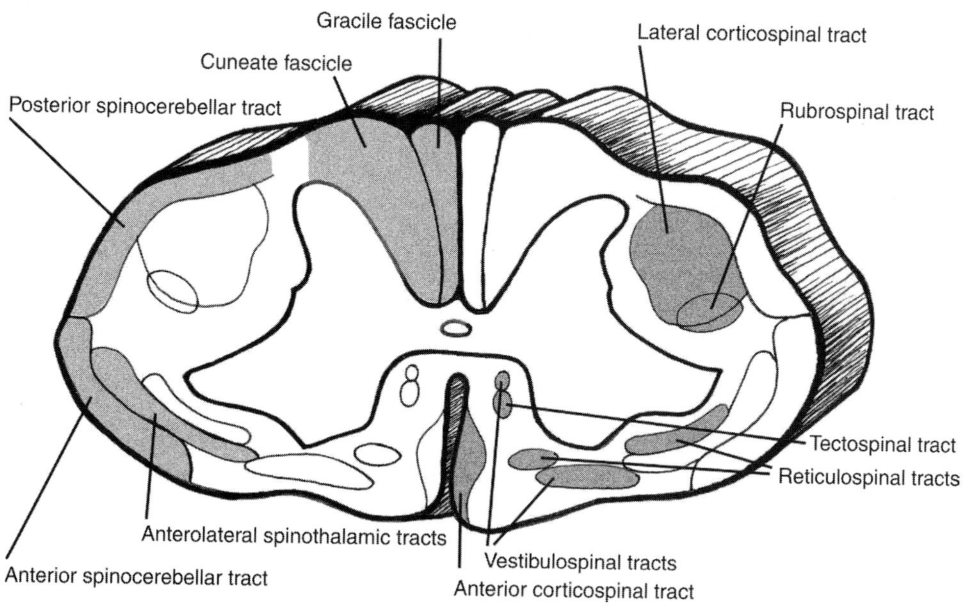

Fig. 3. Schematic representation depicting the location of the various ascending (left) and descending (right) tracts in spinal cord white matter.

Gray Matter

In the spinal cord, the "butterfly-shaped" gray matter consists of a pair of posterior (dorsal) horns and a pair of anterior (ventral) horns connected by the gray commissure that contains the central canal. The size of the gray matter and thus, the spinal cord is larger in the cervical and lumbar regions, where it contains the numerous large motor neurons that control the movements of the arms and legs. Aside from regional variation in size and the presence of large motor neurons in the anterior horn, the gray matter of the spinal cord is a microscopically homogenous mixture of neurons and their processes, neuroglia cells, and blood vessels. Despite this homogeneity, the posterior and anterior horns have been functionally subdivided into distinct regions known as the laminae of Rexed (Fig. 2).

The posterior horns contain laminae I–VI and most receive afferent input from the periphery. Lamina I, also known as the posterior marginal nucleus, contains neurons whose axons contribute to the ascending spinothalamic tract and respond to input from primary afferents that sense pain and temperature. Lamina II, the substantia gelatinosa, receives afferents from Lissauer's fasciculus that convey information about pain, temperature, and touch. Laminae III and IV, the nucleus proprius, contain interneurons that relay touch and pressure sensations. The dendrites of these neurons extend up into lamina II and their axons contribute to the contralateral spinothalamic tract. As with laminae II and IV, interneurons in lamina V supply projections to the contralateral spinothalamic tract. In addition, they receive input from afferent neurons that respond to both painful and nonpainful stimuli. Located at the base of the posterior horns in the cervical and lumbar enlargements, lamina VI receives input from central processes of primary sensory neurons.

The anterior horn contains laminae VII–IX, with the gray commissure, lamina X, surrounding the central canal and continuous with laminae VII on each side of the spinal cord. Also, known as the intermediate zone, lamina VII contains interneurons, such as those in the nucleus dorsalis of the thoracic and upper lumbar regions that are associated with the posterior spinocerebellar tract. The interneurons found at the base of the anterior horn that synapse with axons of the descending tracts include lamina VIII. Lamina IX contains cell bodies of α and γ motor neurons whose axons constitute efferent motor output to striated muscle.

White Matter

Surrounding the gray matter, the white matter of the spinal cord is a homogeneous mixture of myelinated and unmyelinated axons, neuroglia cells, and blood vessels. It can be divided into three general regions: the posterior (dorsal), lateral and anterior (ventral) funiculi. Funiculi are further functionally subdivided into tracts or fasciculi (Fig. 3). Spinal cord tracts either carries peripheral input to the brain through a sequence of primary and secondary neurons that constitute the ascending tracts, or direct central input from the brain to the spinal cord in descending tracts that modify efferent output. The white commissure carries impulses of crossed tracts from one side of the spinal cord to the other.

Ascending Tracts

In the white matter, there are three main ascending tracts: the posterior columns (tracts), the spinothalamic tracts, and the spinocerebellar tracts (Fig. 3). The posterior columns contain central processes of sensory neurons in spinal ganglia that carry input from receptors in muscles, joint capsules, and skin. These fibers ascend directly to the medulla oblongata where they synapse with secondary neurons. The posterior column contains two fasciculi: the medial fasciculus gracilis that receives central processes of primary sensory neurons in the lumbosacral region; and the lateral fasciculus cuneatus that receives central processes from neurons in the cervical and thoracic regions. Posterior tract axons convey information about well-localized touch, movement, and position senses.

The ascending spinothalamic tract is divided into the lateral and anterior components, although this division is not clearly defined. Free nerve endings throughout the body convey impulses to the sensory neurons in spinal ganglia through thinly myelinated (A δ) and unmyelinated (C) fibers. Short central processes of these neurons enter the spinal cord through Lissauer's fasciculus, ascend one segment and then synapse with secondary neurons in laminae I, IV, and V, whose axons cross the midline in the anterior white commissure before ascending to the thalamus in the contralateral spinothalamic tract. Secondary neurons of the lateral spinothalamic tract convey sensations of pain and temperature that are subject to modification by emotion and experience. Secondary neurons of the anterior spinothalamic tract receive input from central processes of sensory neurons with peripheral receptors in hairless skin that project throughout laminae IV–VII. These secondary neurons also cross through the anterior white commissure before ascending and conveying sensations of light, poorly localized touch.

The ascending spinocerebellar tracts have posterior and anterior components. In the posterior spinocerebellar and cuneocerebellar tracts, myelinated fibers carry input from muscle spindles (Ia), golgi tendon organs (Ib), and skin (II) in the lower and upper body, respectively. It is conveyed by central processes of neurons in spinal ganglia, which ultimately synapse with neurons in the nucleus dorsalis of lamina VII or the cuneate nucleus of the medulla. Axons of these secondary neurons consist the posterior spinocerebellar and cuneocerebellar tracts and terminate on mossy fibers in the cerebellar cortex. These tracts convey muscle-spindle or tendon-organ related information with resolution to the level of a single muscle fiber of a muscle-tendon complex. The anterior and rostral spinocerebellar tracts convey similar input from the lower and upper body, respectively, to the cerebellum, whereas secondary neurons in lamina VII cross to contralateral tracts through the gray commissure before ascending with postural information relating to an entire limb.

Descending Tracts

The main descending tracts of spinal cord white matter are the corticospinal, rubrospinal, tectospinal, reticulospinal, and vestibular tracts (Fig. 3). These tracts carry information from neurons originating in the cerebral cortex, midbrain, medulla, and vestibular apparatus, respectively. As a portion of the upper motor neuron pool, axons of neurons in the cerebral cortex contribute to the corticospinal tracts. They descend directly to terminate on interneurons at the base of the posterior horn and modify sensory input on anterior motor horn neurons in lamina IX or on adjacent interneurons. Cortical and subcortical neurons decussate at the level of the medullary pyramids and then travel in the lateral and anterior corticospinal tracts. Corticospinal tract function concerns voluntary control relating to manipulation of objects (upper limbs) and locomotion (lower limbs). Neurons of the rubrospinal tract originate in the red nucleus of the midbrain and their axons descend in the spinal cord where they intermingle with corticospinal tracts as far as the thoracic level. Rubrospinal terminal fibers synapse with interneurons in laminae V, VI, and VIII that project to α and γ motor neurons.

Rubrospinal tract activity is regulated by sensory input provided to the cerebellum through the spinocerebellar tracts and controls the tone of flexor muscle groups.

The remaining descending tracts run in the anterior funiculus. The tectospinal tract originates in the superior colliculus of the midbrain, crosses the midline in the periaqueductal gray area and descends in the anterior funiculus, where it intermingles with the medial longitudinal fasciculus. Tectospinal terminal fibers project to interneurons in laminae VI, VII, and VIII that synapse on motor neurons of the anterior horn to help blend the interaction of visual and auditory stimuli with postural reflex movements. Axons of the vestibulospinal tract are derived from neurons in the lateral vestibular nucleus that receive afferent input from both the vestibular apparatus of the inner ear and the cerebellum. Vestibulospinal fibers descend ipsilaterally through the anterolateral spinal cord, where they synapse with interneurons in laminae VII and VIII that project to motor neurons in the anterior horn. The vestibulospinal tract helps control basic posture or stance by facilitating activity in all extensor muscles. The axons of the two uncrossed reticulospinal tracts originate from several levels in the reticular core of the brainstem and terminate on interneurons in laminae VII and VIII that project to α and γ neurons of the anterior horn. Reticulospinal tracts modify motor and sensory functions of the spinal cord and facilitate motor and cardiovascular responses (pontine reticulospinal tract) or inhibit motor and cardiovascular responses (medullary reticulospinal tract).

DIABETES-INDUCED NEUROPATHOLOGY

While there are earlier reports of spinal cord lesions associated with diabetes mellitus (refs. *5–7*), the publication of a series of key *(8–12)* and other *(13–16)* neuropathological studies in the latter half of the 20th century established the histological nature of this injury. These reports helped promote the concept that myelopathy is a part of the diabetic process and remain the definitive neuropathological studies. Unlike myelopathy, the existence of peripheral neuropathy and radiculopathy is not disputed and the pathology has been well documented. The following section will first consider morphological evidence from autopsy material for diabetes-induced injury to the spinal cord, associated ganglia and roots, and then available evidence from studies using experimental models of diabetes.

Human Studies

Among the earliest observations of spinal cord lesions in diabetes mellitus are those of Williamson *(5,6)*, who described macroscopic changes evident in the posterior columns of the cervical and thoracic regions after hardening in Müller's fluid. In sections from the affected regions of celloidin-embedded spinal cords of three patients, swollen axis cylinders surrounded by distended or thin myelin sheaths and scattered degenerated fibers were evident. These early observations suggest that both demyelination and axonal degeneration occur in lesions of the posterior column white matter. Later, distension and/or thinning of myelin sheaths and axonal loss in the white matter of paraffin-embedded autopsy material from patients with diabetes mellitus were also described *(8,11)*, whereas others have simply noted degeneration of the long tracts *(9,10,13)*. The most comprehensive autopsy investigation of diabetic myelopathy is that reported by Slager *(12)*, who expanded an earlier series of 37 patients *(16)* to 75 unselected diabetic patients and reported posterior column demyelination with relative sparing of axons in 27% of spinal cords. A subsequent report quantitatively documented a decrease in myelinated fiber density in the fasciculus gracilis of the cervical posterior columns *(17)*. Although the posterior columns are the most commonly reported site of injury in diabetes mellitus, lesions have also been documented in the lateral (spinocerebellar tracts) and ventral columns *(8,9)*, with the lower segments of all regions affected more than the upper segments.

Diabetes-associated injury to the gray matter of the spinal cord is not as commonly reported as that in the white matter and, where reported, involves neuron shrinkage and loss, chromatolysis, and gliosis. Dolman described a slight loss of anterior horn cells in three patients and chromatolysis in four others *(8)*. Similarly, neuron loss in the anterior horn was reported in a single patient in each of two studies *(9,13)* where surviving cells appeared shrunken. In contrast, Reske-Nielsen and Lunbaek documented mild-to-moderate loss of neurons in both the posterior and anterior horns that was associated with mild gliosis in their series of 15 long-term juvenile diabetic patients *(11)*. In this study, the remaining neurons had swollen or displaced nuclei and cytoplasmic PAS- and fat-positive accumulations. Similar to lesions in the white matter, neuronal loss in the gray matter has been reported to be more severe in the lower spinal cord segments *(13)*.

As with motor neurons in the anterior horn, diabetes-associated injury to primary sensory neurons in spinal ganglia has only been sporadically documented. Dolman *(8)* and Greenbaum et al. *(13)* observed some loss of neurons, particularly in lumbar ganglia, accompanied by proliferation of satellite cells. In a clinically uniform series of nine patients dying after early-onset diabetes of long duration, Olsson and colleagues *(9)* reported heavy loss of neurons and formation of noduli of Nageotte in ganglia from all levels, with chromatolysis in some of the remaining neurons. In a morphometric analysis of posterior spinal ganglia, Ohnishi et al. *(17)* documented a decrease in the relative frequency of large size (type A) cell bodies, but no loss of neurons. More recently, neuroaxonal dystrophy has been described in the posterior spinal ganglia *(18)*. The swollen axon terminals and enlarged initial segments were usually located within the satellite cell sheath, where they compressed and distorted adjacent sensory neuronal cell bodies. These dystrophic accumulations, consisting of hyperphosphorylated neurofilaments or collections of tubulovesicular bodies with intermingled neurotransmitter granules, occurred in calcitonin gene related peptide (CGRP)-containing axons, but not in sympathetic noradrenergic axons, which appeared earlier and with greater frequency in diabetic patients than in aged human subjects, and are also a structural hallmark of diabetic autonomic neuropathy (reviewed in ref. *19*).

Similar to peripheral neuropathy, radiculopathy is a frequently described manifestation of diabetes mellitus and is well documented in the literature. Williamson described degenerated nerve fibers in the intramedullary course of posterior roots in Lissauer's fasciculus of lumbar and cervical spinal segments and noted that generally roots external to the spinal cord in these regions lacked degenerated fibers *(5)*. Others *(9,11,13)* have also documented varying degrees of loss and degeneration of myelin sheaths and axons in spinal roots. In these studies, the extramedullary portions of both posterior and anterior roots were affected, although injury to the anterior roots was usually less advanced. In contrast to these observations are reports of widespread demyelination without extensive axonal degeneration in spinal roots *(8,12,17)*. The presence of segmental demyelination and remyelination in both posterior and anterior roots with and without myelinated fiber loss, respectively *(17)*, argues that this Schwann cell response is not secondary to axonal atrophy and/or degeneration.

In summary, there is unequivocal histological evidence of radiculopathy and degeneration of the long tracts in studies with diabetic patients that range from clinically uniform to unselected. Lesions at both sites are more frequent in the posterior roots and columns, and with the exception of microinfarcts, may well be independent of vascular lesions in these sites. Neuronal degeneration is less commonly observed in sensory ganglia and spinal cord gray matter. Much of the debate related to diabetes-induced spinal cord injury has centered on whether myelopathy is an independent lesion or a secondary consequence of peripheral neuropathy and/or radiculopathy, the most frequently described neurological manifestations of diabetes mellitus. Indeed, many symptoms and clinical signs considered indicative of myelopathy can be attributed to involvement of the peripheral neuraxis. For example, abnormal cutaneous sensation, paresthesia, and ataxia clearly involve lesions in peripheral nerves and roots. However, alterations in proprioceptive sensation and lack of muscle coordination without profound changes in cutaneous sensation point to an independent lesion in the ascending tracts of the posterior column *(20)*. Further, the dissociation of histological changes in the posterior columns from posterior radiculopathy or clinical signs of sensory neuropathy in some of the cases reported by Slager *(12)* argue that myelopathy is an independent lesion.

Experimental Studies

Although there is structural evidence for spinal lesions in human diabetes mellitus, little support is present in the literature for comparable injury in experimental animal studies. There is better documentation of radiculopathy in animal studies and some reports of neuronal degeneration and loss in the dorsal root ganglia. Lack of evidence for myelopathy in animal, particularly rodent, studies is perhaps not surprising, given that there are relatively few pathological abnormalities in peripheral nerves from diabetic animals. The majority of animal studies concerned with structural injury to the spinal cord, dorsal root ganglia, and roots involve rats and mice with streptozotocin-induced diabetes, with an occasional report concerned with alloxan-induced diabetes or genetic models. Unlike the paraffin-embedded autopsy material of human studies noted earlier, most animal studies are based on plastic-embedded material and appear in the literature after the definitive human reports.

The earliest report of diabetes-induced structural abnormalities in the spinal cord is a morphometric study of lower motor and primary sensory neurons in rats with streptozotocin-induced diabetes of 4 weeks duration *(21)*. Although no histological signs of neuronal degeneration or loss were identified, diabetes was associated with a significant reduction in perikaryal volume of both motor and sensory neurons of the same magnitude as the atrophy previously reported for axons in the peroneal nerve *(22,23)*. Aside from preliminary observations of α motor neuron loss throughout the anterior horn in streptozotocin- and alloxan-diabetic rats and db/db mice that have not been subsequently published *(24)* there are no reports of neuronal loss in spinal cord gray matter. Regarding structural injury in the spinal cord, Yagihashi et al. *(25)* observed neuroaxonal dystrophy in neurons of the sensory ganglia and in the myelinated axons constituting the tracts of the posterior columns in spontaneously diabetic BB/Wor rats. As described by Schmidt et al. *(18)* in human studies, the dystrophic accumulations consisted of tubulovesicles, tubular rings, layered and electron-dense membranes and neurofilaments, and increased with increasing duration of diabetes.

Unlike the spinal cord, the literature concerned with structural injury to sensory ganglia and roots in experimental diabetes is more extensive but also more controversial, particularly with respect to the ganglia. Points of contention include whether there is neuronal loss in sensory ganglia and whether there is histological evidence of neuronal degeneration. As noted above, Sidenius and Jakobsen *(21)* reported no cell loss in the lumbar dorsal root ganglia of streptozotocin-diabetic rats, with abnormalities restricted to decreases in perikaryal volume and the relative number of large type-A neurons. Using systematic dissector counting approaches, Russell et al. *(26)* and Zochodne et al. *(27)* report neuronal atrophy but with a relative preservation of neurons in lumbar dorsal root ganglia from rats with streptozotocin-induced diabetes of 3 or 12 months duration, respectively. Using less rigorous profile counts of lumbar dorsal root ganglia from streptozotocin-diabetic rats after 12 months of diabetes, Kishi et al. *(28)* were also unable to detect neuronal loss but did confirm an increase in the ratio of small type-B neurons to large type-A neurons reported earlier *(21,29)*. At this point, overt sensory neuron loss in experimental diabetes has only been observed in a recent study *(30)* using long-term streptozotocin-diabetic mice, which do not show the neuronal atrophy reported in rats except when overexpressing human aldose reductase *(31)*.

In spite of morphometric evidence documenting preservation of neuron number, neuronal apoptosis has been claimed in several experimental reports using streptozotocin-diabetic rats with diabetes ranging from 1 to 12 months duration *(26,32)*. TUNEL-positive neurons in the dorsal root ganglia, considered indicative of apoptosis, consisted of 7–34% of the total and was concomitant with markers of oxidative stress and activation of caspase-3. It is worth noting that apoptosis in experimental diabetic neuropathy is not supported by morphometric determination of neuronal or peripheral myelinated fiber loss, suggesting DNA strand damage does not necessarily equate to neuronal loss. Further, sensory neurons with activated caspase-3 survive long-term streptozotocin-induced diabetes *(33)*, again indicating that expression of apoptotic markers does not always correspond to cell death.

Regarding structural injury in the dorsal root ganglia in experimental diabetes, Sidenius and Jakobsen *(21)* report that neuronal degeneration was not evident in rats with short-term streptozotocin-induced diabetes. As noted earlier, neuroaxonal dystrophy has been observed in sensory ganglia from diabetic BB rats *(25)*. Several studies have documented degenerative changes in the dorsal root ganglia neurons from short-term *(26)* and long-term *(28,34)* streptozotocin-diabetic rats. Neuronal vacuolation is the most prominent change described, with vacuoles evenly distributed throughout the perikaryon in diabetic animals *(28)*. In some instances, vacuoles appear to contain remnants of mitochondrial cristae or to be associated with lipofuscin granules *(34)*. Vacuoles, condensed chromatin, and ballooned mitochondria with disrupted cristae were observed in neurons and dorsal root Schwann cells in short-term experimental diabetes by Russell et al. *(26)*. Although neuronal vacuolation and mitochondrial disruption have been suggested to result from hyperglycemia-induced oxidative stress *(26,28,34)*, these changes may be a feature of poor fixation. Moreover, aging-associated oxidative mitochondrial damage involves effaced cristae in an otherwise intact, not ballooned, organelle *(35)*.

Radicular pathology in experimental diabetes was first reported by Tamura and Parry *(36)* and has subsequently been confirmed with remarkable agreement by others in both streptozotocin-diabetic and galactose-fed rats *(28,34,37–39)*. The structural abnormality is focused on the myelin sheath and occurs in the context of marked interstitial oedema in both roots, although it is more frequent in the dorsal root. The earliest change consists of myelin splitting at the intraperiod line progressing to often-spectacular myelin ballooning. At this stage, strands of tubulovesicular myelin debris span the intramyelinic space and intratubal macrophages are sometimes observed stripping away myelin lamellae. There is minimal axonal degeneration associated with this myelin defect, suggesting that this lesion is a primary Schwann cell defect. Similar radicular pathology has been described in aged rodents *(40)*, leading to the suggestion that its earlier appearance in experimental diabetes represents an acceleration of the aging process in this disease *(41)*. However, myelin splitting and ballooning is prevented by aldose reductase inhibition and is present in several toxic neuropathies, pointing to other aetiologies *(38)*.

In summary, whether there is neuronal loss and degeneration in dorsal root ganglia remains an unresolved issue in experimental diabetes. Presently, neuronal loss has only been documented in a murine model of long-term streptozotocin diabetes. In spite of claims of programmed cell death based on various markers of apoptosis, pathological evidence of neuronal loss and degenerative changes has not yet been convincingly demonstrated in the streptozotocin-diabetic rat. Radiculopathy is the most striking and consistently observed pathology in experimental diabetes and provides a stark contrast to the more modest injury present in peripheral nerves in rodent models of diabetes. As for spinal cord injury, there is a distinct paucity of evidence, with a single mention in the literature of neuroaxonal dystrophy in the posterior columns. With the possible exception of radiculopathy, there is discordance between the neuropathology present in diabetic animals and humans. The short life-span and small size of rats and mice, the most frequently used species in animal studies, may preclude the full development of the diabetic neuropathy that develops over time with a "stocking and glove" distribution in the longer nerves of humans. Also, particularly with reference to the spinal cord, it is possible that lesions have been overlooked because this tissue has not been as routinely studied as the peripheral nerves and spinal roots. Careful evaluation of longer-term rat and mouse models, while controlling for age-related confounds, might help reconcile the differences in structural injury between human and experimental diabetic neuropathy, as might the development and characterization of new animal models.

SPINAL ELECTROPHYSIOLOGY IN DIABETES

Conduction Velocity

Slowing of large motor and sensory fiber conduction velocity has long been recognized as an early indicator of neuropathy in the PNS *(41,42)* and these deficits are widely used to follow progression of neuropathy and assess efficacy of therapeutic interventions. In contrast, there have been relatively few evaluations of spinal electrophysiology in diabetic subjects and such measurements are rarely included in global assessments of neuropathy. Increased latencies, indicative of conduction slowing are described in diabetic subjects *(43–45),* but it is not definitively established that this disorder shares a common presentation or aetiology with peripheral conduction slowing. For example, evaluation of a series of diabetic subjects indicated that relatively few showed both spinal and PNS conduction slowing, with many cases of either PNS or CNS dysfunction *(46)* and there is not a strong correlation between conduction slowing in the PNS and CNS *(47)*. It had also been reported that slowing in sensory (ascending) tracts precedes that of motor (descending) tracts *(48)*. The aetiology of CNS conduction slowing is poorly understood and the extent to which it precedes or reflects the pathological changes that occur in the spinal cord described earlier is not known.

There have been occasional reports of conduction slowing in the spinal cord of diabetic rats as early as 2 weeks after onset of hyperglycemia *(49)*, although others reported that months of diabetes were required to show slowing in both ascending and descending tracts *(50,51)*. Again, little is known about the pathogenesis of the disorder and the extent to which it mirrors the early metabolic and later structurally mediated aetiology of PNS conduction slowing has not been established, although conduction slowing in the PNS does appear to precede that in the CNS *(51)*. It may be worth noting that glucose levels in spinal cerebrospinal fluid of diabetic rats are markedly lower than in plasma of the same animals *(52)*, so that spinal axons and lower motor neuron cell bodies are exposed to less glycemic stress than their PNS counterparts.

Response Properties

Characterization of the response properties of spinal neurons that are triggered by peripheral sensory stimuli have been studied only in rats with short-term diabetes. There is agreement that spontaneous activity of the second order neurons that respond to a broad range of sensory stimuli (wide dynamic range or WDR neurons) is increased in spinal cord of diabetic rats *(53,54)*. This could reflect diverse mechanisms including ectopic primary afferent input to the cord, rewiring of spinal synapses or altered post-synaptic signal transduction properties. Increased spontaneous activity of WDR neurons that project to the brain through the spinothalamic tract has been proposed to underlie spontaneous pain and hyperalgesia in diabetes. There is less agreement on other parameters, with a report of increased receptive field size, lower activation thresholds, and augmented responses to mechanical stimulation in ascending (sensory) spinothalamic tract neurons *(54)* being balanced by another showing no change in these parameters *(53)*. Most recently, the phenomenon of spinal wind-up, where repeated electrical stimulation of C fibers leads to a frequency-dependent increase in the excitability of spinal neurons has been reported to be enhanced in short-term diabetic mice *(55)*, further supporting the idea that spinal mediation of sensory processing is altered by diabetes.

SPINAL NEUROCHEMISTRY IN DIABETES

Neurotransmitter Release

The structural and electrophysiological properties of the spinal cord during diabetes described earlier present a picture that resembles the paradox often noted in studies of the peripheral nerve, namely structural and electrophysiological indices of progressive degeneration and functional loss that are accompanied by increased activity in some sensory fibers and associated with hyperalgesia, allodynia, or spontaneous pain. There has been speculation that the spontaneous or enhanced activity of spinal sensory pathways is responsible for diabetic neuropathic pain and is secondary to enhanced excitatory input from peripheral nerve primary afferent fibers. This is difficult to verify in clinical studies, whereas evidence of spontaneous or exaggerated evoked activity of primary afferents in animal models of diabetes has been reported in some studies *(56–59)* but also discounted in others *(60,61)*. Of course, electrical activity of sensory fibers is only one component of any altered input to the spinal cord and other factors, such as the amount of available neurotransmitters and patency of vesicular release mechanisms, must also be considered. To date, few studies have addressed spinal neurotransmitter release properties during diabetes. Current evidence obtained using in vitro perfusion and in vivo spinal microdialysis techniques indicates that evoked release of the excitatory amino acid neurotransmitter glutamate that drives nociception and of neuropeptides that modulate nociceptive processing are diminished, rather than exaggerated, in diabetic animals *(62–65)*. Such depression of sensory input is consistent with the general view of peripheral nerve as developing a degenerative phenotype during prolonged diabetes where, even if overt degenerative pathology is not observed in rodents, loss of neurotrophic support leads to decreased synthesis, axonal transport and therefore evoked release of neuropeptides (*see* ref. *66*). While the stimulus-evoked release of excitatory neurotransmitters is reduced in diabetic rats, the appearance of prostaglandin E_2 (PGE_2) in spinal dialysates after paw stimulation is prolonged and accompanied by an increase in paw flinching behavior indicative of hyperalgesia *(67)*. The release of PGE_2 in the spinal cord is triggered by primary afferent input and is responsible for the subsequent sensitization of spinal sensory processing systems that contributes to hyperalgesia in a number of models of neuropathic pain *(68,69)*. Increased PGE_2 release in the cord of diabetic rats after paw stimulation with formalin is accompanied by an increase in the amount of protein for the enzyme cyclooxygenase-2 (COX-2), which converts arachidonate to prostaglandins *(67)*. Moreover, spinal delivery of inhibitors of cyclooxygenase prevents the increase in formalin-evoked flinching of diabetic rats. Together, these data suggest that a diabetes-induced increase in spinal COX-2 may underlie spinal sensitization and hyperalgesia in rats, although presently it is not clear how diabetes causes the increase in COX-2 or which cells of the spinal cord are involved in modifying spinal sensory processing.

Receptors

The complexities of the distribution and actions of neurotransmitter receptors in the spinal cord and their role in spinal pain processing are still being unravelled for many neuropathic pain conditions, including diabetes. Models of simple synaptic transmission involving excitatory postsynaptic receptors have been augmented by including consideration of the role of descending inhibitory systems that can act on both pre- and postsynaptic receptors and by the growing appreciation that modulation of synaptic function can also occur through both the postsynaptic neuron and other cells, such as astrocytes and microglia (reviewed in refs. *70,71*). A thorough appreciation of the involvement of a particular receptor in diabetic neuropathy requires understanding of a number of parameters including: the amount of receptor protein; location of the receptor (both within the cell and in different cell types); receptor turn-over patterns; ligand binding and channel activation properties, and the function of downstream signaling cascades. At present, the literature offers some interesting snapshots of the effects of diabetes on spinal receptors (*see* Table 1) but a detailed evaluation of spinal sensory processing mechanisms is lacking.

It has been previously speculated that decreased excitatory neurotransmitter input to the spinal cord as a result of a hyperglycemia-induced shift in the phenotype of primary afferents could lead to a sensitized postsynapse through upregulation of receptors for the excitatory neurotransmitter glutamate and the modulating neuropeptides substance P and CGRP. This hypothesis was prompted by the observation that whereas peripherally-evoked spinal release of substance P is reduced in diabetic rats, direct delivery of substance P to the spinal cord of diabetic rats elicits a protracted hyperalgesic response *(52,65)*. The biological precedent for such a mechanism is seen in skeletal muscle, which responds to denervation and loss of cholinergic excitatory input by increasing the amount of ACH receptor protein and progressing to a state of denervation hypersensitivity (*see* ref. *72*). Of the few studies published to date, ligand binding experiments have reported increased binding of substance P in the spinal cord of diabetic rats *(73)* and of ligands for both the AMPA and NMDA glutamate receptors in genetically diabetic ob/ob mice *(74)*. Increased ligand binding could reflect elevated protein production, as mRNA levels for the glutamatergic AMPA receptor, the R2 subunit of the glutamatergic NMDA receptor and assorted metabotropic glutamate receptors are also increased in the dorsal horn of the spinal cord from diabetic rats *(75)*, although the own studies have been unable to detect increased protein for either the NK-1 substance P receptor or the NMDA R1 subunit in the cord of diabetic rats (Jolivalt and Calcutt, unpublished observations).

A variety of neurotransmitters regulate spinal synaptic activity after release from descending inhibitory systems, interneurons or glial cells. Opiates have long been known to have a spinal site of analgesic action. Although there appears to be no change in the amount of protein for the μ-opioid receptor in the cord of diabetic rats *(76)*, receptor functions, as indicated by measuring downstream signaling activity, is reduced *(77)*. Suppression of opioid receptor function could account for reports of reduced efficacy of agents, such as morphine, against pain in diabetic subjects and perhaps also impede any tonic inhibitory tone acting through this mechanism. Other plausible contributors to inhibitory tone in the spinal cord include adrenergic and GABAergic systems. Both mRNA for the α2-adrenoceptor sub-type and ligand binding to the α2-adrenoceptor are reduced in the cord of diabetic rats *(78)* so that a loss of inhibitory tone could well contribute to spinal sensitization. In contrast, there have been reports suggesting increased number or activity of spinal muscarinic ACH receptors *(79)*, bradykinin B1 receptors *(80)*, and serotonin receptors (Jolivalt and Calcutt, unpublished), although the significance of these findings to spinal sensory processing remains to be established.

Pharmacology

Many studies have used receptor agonists or antagonists in attempts to address the effects of diabetes on spinal sensory processing and to develop treatments for neuropathic pain (reviewed in ref. *81*). However, there are a number of caveats that prompt caution

Table 1
Effects of Diabetes on Spinal Cord Receptors

Ligand	Receptor	Diabetes effect	What measured	Model	Reference
Glutamate	NMDA R1	Increased	Ligand binding	ob/ob mouse	*74*
		Unchanged	Protein	STZ rat	Jolivalt and Calcutt (unpublished)
	NMDA R2	Increased	mRNA	STZ rat	*75*
	M Glu R	Increased mGlu 1,2,3,5	mRNA	STZ rat	*76*
	AMPA	Increased	Ligand binding	ob/ob mouse	*74*
		Increased	mRNA	STZ rat	*75*
Substance P	NK-1	Increased	Ligand binding	STZ rat	*73*
		Unchanged	Protein	STZ rat	Jolivalt and Calcutt (unpublished)
Opiates	μ	Unchanged	Ligand binding	STZ rat	*76*
		Reduced	Signal pathway activation	STZ rat	*77*
	κ	Unchanged	Protein	STZ rat	Jolivalt and Calcutt (unpublished)
Noradrenaline	α1	Unchanged	mRNA/ ligand binding	STZ rat	*85*
	α2	Reduced	mRNA/ ligand binding	STZ rat	*78*
Acetylcholine	mACHr	Increased	Ligand binding/ signal pathway activation	STZ rat	*79*
Serotonin	5HT 2a	Increased	Protein	STZ rat	Jolivalt and Calcutt (unpublished)
Bradykinin	Kinin B1	Increased	mRNA/ ligand binding	STZ rat	*80*
IGF-1	IGF-1	Reduced	mRNA	STZ rat	*86*

when interpreting these findings, particularly when drugs are delivered systemically. The extreme metabolic profile of diabetic rodents, with raging polydypsia, polyphagia, polyuria, and attendant changes to the digestive and urinary systems and the blood–brain and blood–nerve barriers can alter many aspects of pharmacokinetics and drug distribution, so that simplistic interpretations of shifts in dose-effect curves of systemically delivered drugs between control and diabetic animals can be misleading and need not reflect changes in receptor number or function *(82,83)*. Direct intrathecal delivery of drugs overcomes some of these issues, but agents delivered in this manner still distribute to the higher CNS *(84)* and can be subject to altered access and clearance mechanisms. Although pharmacological studies have value for assessing potential efficacy of drugs in altering behavioral indices of nociception and neuropathic pain in animals, their value for investigating aetiological mechanisms is tied to concurrent use of other techniques for assessing spinal receptor number and function.

CONCLUSION

Though understudied when compared with peripheral nerve, it is clear that the spinal cord is not protected from diabetes-induced injury and that structural and functional damage is discernable in diabetic subjects. Animal models of diabetes show a number of disorders similar to those seen in humans and these changes are accompanied by neurochemical changes, which may have functional significance. Because the spinal cord is the first site of integration of sensory input from the periphery and the last site of descending control of sensory and motor systems, disruption of spinal cord function has the capacity to impede appropriate CNS control systems and contribute to apparent peripheral neuropathy. The extent to which aberrant spinal cord processing is evoked by direct metabolic consequences of diabetes or is secondary to peripheral neuropathy, is an intriguing question that has not yet been widely addressed.

ACKNOWLEDGMENTS

The authors would like to thank Daniel P. Mizisin for his skilful rendition of the line drawings used in Figs. 1–3. Supported by NIH grant DK57629 (NAC).

REFERENCES

1. Eaton SE, Harris ND, Rajbhandarim SM, et al. Spinal-cord involvement in diabetic peripheral neuropathy. *Lancet* 2001;358:35–36.
2. Diamond MC, Scheibel AB, Elson LM. *The Human Brain Coloring Book*. Harper Collins, New York, NY, 1985.
3. Harper AA, Lawson SN. Conduction velocity is related to morphological cell type in rat dorsal root ganglion neurons. *J Physiol* 1985;359:31–46.
4. Lee KH, Chung K, Chung JM, Coggeshall RE. Correlation of cell body size, axon size, and signal conduction velocity for individually labeled dorsal root ganglion cells in the cat. *J Comp Neurol* 1986;243:335–346.
5. Williamson RT. Changes in the posterior columns of the spinal cord in diabetes mellitus. *Brit Med J* 1894;1:398–399.
6. Williamson RT. Changes in the spinal cord in diabetes mellitus. *Brit Med J* 1904;1:122–123.
7. Woltman HW, Wilder RM. Pathologic changes in the spinal cord and peripheral nerves. *Arch Intern Med* 1929;44:576–603.

8. Dolman CL. The morbid anatomy of diabetic neuropathy. *Neurology* 1963;13:135–142.
9. Olsson Y, Säve-Söderbergh J, Sourander P, Angervall L. A patho-anatomical study of the central and peripheral nervous system in diabetes of early onset and long duration. *Path Europ* 1968;3:62–79.
10. Olsson Y, Sourander P. Changes in the sympathetic nervous system in diabetes mellitus. A preliminary report. *J Neurovisc Relat* 1968;31:86–95.
11. Reske-Nielsen E, Lundbaek K. Pathological changes in the central and peripheral nervous system of young long-term diabetics. *Diabetologia* 1968;4:34–43.
12. Slager U. Diabetic myelopathy. *Arch Pathol Lab Med* 1978;102:467–469.
13. Greenbaum D, Richardson PC, Salmon MV, Urich H. Pathological observations on six cases of diabetic neuropathy. *Brain* 1964;87:201–214.
14. Reidel H. Systematische morphologische untersuchungen am rückenmark von diabetikern. *Zbl Allg Path* 1965;107:506–513.
15. Kott E, Bechar M, Bornstein B, Sandbank U. Demyelination of the posterior and anterior columns of the spinal cord in association with metabolic disturbances. *Israel J Med Sci* 1971;7:577–580.
16. Slager UT, Webb AT. Pathologic findings in the spinal cord. *Arch Pathol* 1973;96:388–394.
17. Ohnishi A, Harada M, Tateishi J, Ogata J, Kawanami S. Segmental demyelination and remyelination in lumbar spinal roots of patients dying with diabetes mellitus. *Ann Neurol* 1983;13:541–548.
18. Schmidt RE, Dorsey D, Parvin CA, Beaudet LN, Plurad SB, Roth KA. Dystrophic axonal swellings develop as a function of age and diabetes in human dorsal root ganglia. *J Neuropathol Exp Neurol* 1997;56:1028–1043.
19. Schmidt RE. Neuropathology and pathogenesis of diabetic autonomic neuropathy. *Int Rev Neurobiol* 2002;50:257–292.
20. De Jong RN. CNS manifestations of diabetes mellitus. *Postgrad Med* 1977;61:101–107.
21. Sidenius P, Jakobsen J. reduced perikaryal volume of lower motor and primary sensory neurons in early experimental diabetes. *Diabetes* 1980;29:182–186.
22. Jakobsen J. Axonal dwindling in early experimental diabetes. I. A study of cross sectioned nerves. *Diabetologia* 1976;12:539–546.
23. Jakobsen J. Earlyt and preventable changes of peripheral nerve structure and function in insulin-deficient diabetic rats. *J Neurol Neurosurg Psychiatr* 1979;42:509–518.
24. Felton DL. Spinal cord alterations in streptozotocin-induced diabetes. *Anat Rec* 1979;193:741–742.
25. Yagihashi S, Zhang WX, Sima AA. Neuroaxonal dystrophy in distal symmetric sensory polyneuropathy of the diabetic BB-rat. *J Diabet Complications* 1989;3:202–210.
26. Russell JW, Sullivan KA, Windebank AJ, Herrman DN, Feldman EL. Neurons undergo apoptosis in animal and cell culture models of diabetes. *Neurobiol Dis* 1999;6:347–363.
27. Zochodne DW, Verge VM, Cheng C, Sun H, Johnston J. Does diabetes target ganglion neurones? Progressive sensory neurone involvement in long-term experimental diabetes. *Brain* 2001;124:2319–2334.
28. Kishi M, Tanabe J, Schmelzer JD, Low PA. Morphometry of dorsal root ganglion in chronic experimental diabetic neuropathy. *Diabetes* 2002;51:819–824.
29. Noorafshan A, Ebrahimpoor MR, Sadeghi Y. Stereological study of the cells if dorsal root ganglia in male diabetic rats. *APMIS* 2001;109:762–766.
30. Kennedy JM, Zochodne DW. Experimental diabetic neuropathy with spontaneous recovery: Is there irreparable damage? *Diabetes* 2005;54:830–837.
31. Uehara K, Yamagishi S, Otsuki S, Chin S, Yagihashi S. Effects of polyol pathway hyperactivity on protein kinase C activity, nociceptive peptide expression, and neuronal structure in dorsal root ganglia in diabetic mice. *Diabetes* 2004;53:3239–3247.
32. Schmeichel AM, Schmelzer JD, Low PA. Oxidative injury and apoptosis of dorsal root ganglion neurons in chronic experimental diabetic neuropathy. *Diabetes* 2003;52:165–171.

33. Cheng C, Zochodne DW. Sensory neurons with activated caspase-3 survive long-term experimental diabetes. *Diabetes* 2003;52:2363–2371.
34. Sasaki H, Schmelzer JD, Zollman PJ, Low PA. Neuropathology and blood flow of nerve, spinal roots and dorsal root ganglia in longstanding diabetic rats. *Acta Neuropathol* 1997;93:118–128.
35. Lui J, Atamna H, Kuratsuune H, Ames BN. Delaying brain mitochondrial decay and aging with mitochondrial antioxidants and metabolites. *Ann NY Acad Sci* 2002;959:133–166.
36. Tamura E, Parry GJ. Severe radicular pathology in rats with longstanding diabetes. *J Neurol Sci* 1994;127:29–35.
37. Mizisin AP, Bache M, DiStefano PS, Acheson A, Lindsay RM, Calcutt NA. BDNF attenuates functional and structural disorders in nerves of galactose-fed rats. *J Neuropathol Exp Neurol* 1997;56:1290–1301.
38. Mizisin AP, Kalichman MW, Bache M, Dines KC, DiStefano PS. NT-3 attenuates functional and structural disorders in sensory nerves of galactose-fed rats. *J Neuropathol Exp Neurol* 1998;57:803–813.
39. Mizisin AP, Steinhardt RC, O'Brien JS, Calcutt NA. TX14(A), a prosaposin-derived peptide, reverses established nerve disorders in streptozotocin-diabetic rats and prevents them in galactose-fed rats. *J Neuropathol Exp Neurol* 2001;60:953–960.
40. Berge BN, Wolf A, Simms HS. Degenerative lesions of spinal roots and peripheral nerves in aging rats. *Gerontologia* 1962;6:72–80.
41. Downie AW, Newell DJ. Sensory nerve conduction in patients with diabetes mellitus and controls. *Neurology* 1961;11:876–882.
42. Lawrence DG, Locke S. Motor nerve conduction velocity in diabetes. *Arch Neurol* 1961;5: 483–489.
43. Gupta PR, Dorfman LJ. Spinal somatosensory conduction in diabetes. *Neurology* 1981;31: 841–845.
44. Nakamura R, Noritake M, Hosoda Y, Kamakura K, Nagata N, Shibasaki H. Somatosensory conduction delay in central and peripheral nervous system of diabetic patients. *Diabetes Care* 1992;5:532–535.
45. Varsik P, Kucera P, Buranova D, Balaz M. Is the spinal cord lesion rare in diabetes mellitus? Somatosensory evoked potentials and central conduction time in diabetes mellitus. *Med Sci Monit* 2001;5:712–715.
46. Cracco J, Castells S, Mark E. Spinal somatosensory evoked potentials in juvenile diabetes. *Ann Neurol* 1984;15:55–58.
47. Suzuki C, Ozaki I, Tanosaki M, Sudam T, Baba M, Matsunaga M. Peripheral and central conduction abnormalities in diabetes mellitus. *Neurology* 2000;54:1932–1937.
48. Maetzu C, Villoslada C, Cruz Martinez A. Somatosensory evoked potentials and central motor pathways conduction after magnetic stimulation of the brain in diabetes. *Electromyogr Clin Neurophysiol* 1995;35:443–448.
49. Carsten RE, Whalen LR, Ishii DN. Impairment of spinal cord conduction velocity in diabetic rats. *Diabetes* 1989;38:730–736.
50. Terada M, Yasuda H, Kikkawa R, Koyama N, Yokota T, Shigeta Y. Electrophysiological study of dorsal column function in streptozocin-induced diabetic rats: comparison with 2,5-hexanedione intoxication. *J Neurol Sci* 1993;115:58–66.
51. Biessels GJ, Cristino NA, Rutten GJ, Hamers FP, Erkelens DW, Gispen WH. Neurophysiological changes in the central and peripheral nervous system of streptozotocin-diabetic rats. Course of development and effects of insulin treatment. *Brain* 1999;122: 757–768.
52. Calcutt NA, Freshwater JD, O'Brien JS. Protection of sensory function and antihyperalgesic properties of a prosaposin-derived peptide in diabetic rats. *Anesthesiology* 2000;93:1271–1278.

53. Pertovaara A, Wei H, Kalmari J, Ruotsalainen M. Pain behavior and response properties of spinal dorsal horn neurons following experimental diabetic neuropathy in the rat: modulation by nitecapone, a COMT inhibitor with antioxidant properties. *Exp Neurol* 2001; 167:25–34.
54. Chen SR, Pan HL. Hypersensitivity of spinothalamic tract neurons associated with diabetic neuropathic pain in rats. *J Neurophysiol* 2002;87:2726–2733.
55. Kimura S, Taname M, Honda M, Ono H. Enhanced wind up of the c-fiber-mediated nociceptive flexor movement following painful diabetic neuropathy in mice. *J Pharmacol Sci* 2005;97:195–202.
56. Burchiel KJ, Russell LC, Lee RP, Sima AA. Spontaneous activity of primary afferent neurons in diabetic BB/Wistar rats. A possible mechanism of chronic diabetic neuropathic pain. *Diabetes* 1985;34:1210–1213.
57. Ahlgren SC, Levine JD. Protein kinase C inhibitors decrease hyperalgesia and C-fiber hyperexcitability in the streptozotocin-diabetic rat. *J Neurophysiol* 1994;72:684–692.
58. Chen X, Levine JD. Hyper-responsivity in a subset of C-fiber nociceptors in a model of painful diabetic neuropathy in the rat. *Neuroscience* 2001;102:185–192.
59. Khan GM, Chen SR, Pan HL. Role of primary afferent nerves in allodynia caused by diabetic neuropathy in rats. *Neuroscience* 2002;114:291–299.
60. Ahlgren SC, White DM, Levine JD. Increased responsiveness of sensory neurons in the saphenous nerve of the streptozotocin-diabetic rat. *J Neurophysiol* 1992;68:2077–2085.
61. Russell LC, Burchiel KJ. Abnormal activity in diabetic rat saphenous nerve. *Diabetes* 1993;42:814–819.
62. Calcutt NA, Malmberg AB. Basal and formalin-evoked spinal levels of amino acids in conscious diabetic rats. *Soc Neurosci Abs* 1995;21:650.
63. Garrett NE, Malcangio M, Dewhurst M, Tomlinson DR. alpha-Lipoic acid corrects neuropeptide deficits in diabetic rats via induction of trophic support. *Neurosci Lett* 1997;222:191–194.
64. Calcutt NA, Chen P, Hua XY. Effects of diabetes on tissue content and evoked release of calcitonin gene-related peptide-like immunoreactivity from rat sensory nerves. *Neurosci Lett* 1998;254:129–132.
65. Calcutt NA, Stiller C, Gustafsson H, Malmberg AB. Elevated substance-P-like immunoreactivity levels in spinal dialysates during the formalin test in normal and diabetic rats. *Brain Res* 2000;856:20–27.
66. Tomlinson DR, Fernyhough P, Diemel LT, Maeda K. Deficient neurotrophic support in the aetiology of diabetic neuropathy. *Diabetes Med* 1996;13:679–681.
67. Freshwater JD, Svensson CI, Malmberg AB, Calcutt NA. Elevated spinal cyclooxygenase and prostaglandin release during hyperalgesia in diabetic rats. *Diabetes* 2002;51: 2249–2255.
68. Malmberg AB, Yaksh TL. Hyperalgesia mediated by spinal glutamate or substance P receptor blocked by spinal cyclooxygenase inhibition. *Science* 1992;257:1276–1279.
69. Svensson CI, Yaksh TL. The spinal phospholipase-cyclooxygenase-prostanoid cascade in nociceptive processing. *Annu Rev Pharmacol Toxicol* 2002;42:553–583.
70. Miller G. The dark side of glia. *Science* 2005;305:778–781.
71. Tsuda M, Inoue K, Salter MW. Neuropathic pain and spinal microglia: a big problem from molecules in "small" glia. *Trends Neurosci* 2005;28:101–107.
72. Fambrough DM. Control of acetylcholine receptors in skeletal muscle. *Physiol Rev* 1979;59:165–227.
73. Kamei J, Ogawa M, Kasuya Y. Development of supersensitivity to substance P in the spinal cord of the streptozotocin-induced diabetic rats. *Pharmacol Biochem Behav* 1990;35: 473–475.

74. Li N, Young MM, Bailey CJ, Smith ME. NMDA and AMPA glutamate receptor subtypes in the thoracic spinal cord in lean and obese-diabetic ob/ob mice. *Brain Res* 1999;849: 34–44.
75. Tomiyama M, Furusawa K, Kamijo M, Kimura T, Matsunaga M, Baba M. Upregulation of mRNAs coding for AMPA and NMDA receptor subunits and metabotropic glutamate receptors in the dorsal horn of the spinal cord in a rat model of diabetes mellitus. *Mol Brain Res* 2005;136:275–281.
76. Chen SR, Pan HL. Antinociceptive effect of morphine, but not mu opioid receptor number, is attenuated in the spinal cord of diabetic rats. *Anesthesiology* 2003;99:1409–1414.
77. Chen SR, Sweigart KL, Lakoski JM, Pan HL. Functional mu opioid receptors are reduced in the spinal cord dorsal horn of diabetic rats. *Anesthesiology* 2002;97:1602–1608.
78. Bitar MS, Bajic KT, Farook T, Thomas MI, Pilcher CW. Spinal cord noradrenergic dynamics in diabetic and hypercortisolaemic states. *Brain Res* 1999;830:1–9.
79. Chen SR, Pan HL. Up-regulation of spinal muscarinic receptors and increased antinociceptive effect of intrathecal muscarine in diabetic rats. *J Pharmacol Exp Ther* 2003; 307:676–681.
80. Ongali B, Campos MM, Petcu M, et al. Expression of kinin B1 receptors in the spinal cord of streptozotocin-diabetic rat. *Neuroreport* 2004;15:2463–2466.
81. Calcutt NA. Potential mechanisms of neuropathic pain in diabetes. *Int Rev Neurobiol* 2002;50:205–228.
82. Malcangio M, Tomlinson DR. A pharmacologic analysis of mechanical hyperalgesia in streptozotocin/diabetic rats. *Pain* 1998;76:151–157.
83. Courteix C, Bourget P, Caussade F, et al. Is the reduced efficacy of morphine in diabetic rats caused by alterations of opiate receptors or of morphine pharmacokinetics? *J Pharmacol Exp Ther* 1998;285:63–70.
84. Yaksh TL, Rudy TA. Chronic catheterization of the spinal subarachnoid space. *Physiol Behav* 1976;17:1031–1036.
85. Lee YH, Ryu TG, Park SJ, et al. Alpha1-adrenoceptors involvement in painful diabetic neuropathy: a role in allodynia. *Neuroreport* 2000;11:1417–1420.
86. Bitar MS, Pilcher CW. Attenuation of IGF-1 antinociceptive action and a reduction in spinal cord gene expression of its receptor in experimental diabetes. *Pain* 1998;75:69–74.

11
Diabetic Encephalopathy

Geert Jan Biessels, MD, PhD

SUMMARY

Diabetes and its treatment are associated with functional and structural disturbances in the brain. Acute disturbances are related to acute hypoglycemia or severe hyperglycemia and stroke. These acute metabolic and vascular insults to the brain are well known and beyond the scope of this chapter, which will focus on changes in cerebral function and structure that develop more insidiously. These changes are referred to as diabetic encephalopathy, a term that encompasses functional impairment of cognition, cerebral signal conduction, neurotransmission and synaptic plasticity, and underlying structural pathology associated with diabetes. The first section addresses animal studies, and focuses on the cellular and molecular events that underlie changes in cognition. The second section deals with studies in man and provides an overview of the nature and severity of the changes in cognition, and identifies groups of diabetic patients that are at particular risk of developing cognitive impairments (i.e., the very young and the old). In addition, neurophysiological and neuroimaging studies of diabetic patients will be considered. The final section of this chapter provides a practical guide to the clinical approach of a diabetic patient with complaints of cognitive dysfunction.

Key Words: Brain MRI; cognition; dementia; evoked potentials; hippocampus; learning.

Diabetes and its treatment are associated with functional and structural disturbances in the brain. Acute disturbances are related to acute hypoglycemia or severe hyperglycemia and stroke. These acute metabolic and vascular insults to the brain are well known and beyond the scope of this chapter, which will focus on changes in cerebral function and structure that develop more insidiously, referred to as diabetic encephalopathy.

STUDIES IN ANIMALS

Outside the field of diabetes research, animal models are widely used to explore the mechanisms of learning and memory. Although many questions remain unanswered, much progress has been made in identifying the cellular and molecular events that underlie the storage of information in specific brain areas. In this respect, the hippocampus, a structure in the medial temporal lobe, has attracted particular attention. Within the hippocampus, activity-dependent plastic changes in the strength of synaptic connections between neurons can be studied in vivo and in vitro and serve as a model for information storage at the cellular level *(1)*. Long-term potentiation (LTP) and depression (LTD) are two such forms of synaptic plasticity. In LTP, brief high-frequency

From: *Contemporary Diabetes: Diabetic Neuropathy: Clinical Management, Second Edition*
Edited by: A. Veves and R. Malik © Humana Press Inc., Totowa, NJ

afferent activity leads to a long-lasting increase in the strength of synaptic transmission, whereas in LTD prolonged low-frequency activity results in a persistent reduction in synaptic strength. Both processes depend on glutamatergic neurotransmission and are triggered by an increase in the level of postsynaptic intracellular calcium concentration $[Ca^{2+}]_i$ *(1)*. Experimental manipulations that disturb hippocampal synaptic plasticity, typically also disturb behavioral learning tasks, such as spatial learning in a water maze.

Several aspects of hippocampal function and structure have been studied in diabetic rodents to increase our understanding of the effects of diabetes on the brain. The majority of these studies have been performed in streptozotocin (STZ) diabetic rats, although the number of studies in spontaneously diabetic rodent models is increasing.

Behavioral Findings

Studies of behavioral learning in STZ-diabetic rodents have used several learning tasks *(2)*. Whereas performance on relatively simple passive or active avoidance tasks is generally preserved, performance on more complex learning tasks, such as an active avoidance T-maze, or a Morris water maze, is impaired *(3,4)*. The development of learning deficits in the water maze is dependent on the duration of STZ-diabetes and the level of hyperglycemia *(4,5)*. Subcutaneous implantation of insulin pellets at the onset of diabetes, leading to near normalization of blood glucose levels, completely prevents the learning deficit *(5)*. If, however, insulin-treatment is started 10 weeks after diabetes onset, when learning is already impaired, there is only partial improvement *(5)*. Control experiments show that these performance deficits are not because of sensorimotor impairment *(4,5)*. Studies on water maze learning in spontaneously diabetic BB/Wor rats, or OLETF rats, produced similar results *(6,7)*.

Hippocampal Synaptic Plasticity

Learning deficits in STZ-diabetic rats develop in association with distinct changes in synaptic plasticity in hippocampal slices, which also appear to be dependent on diabetes duration and severity *(2)*. A deficit in the expression of N-methyl-D-aspartate (NMDA)-dependent LTP in the Cornu Ammonis(CA)1 field of the hippocampus develops gradually and reaches a maximum at 12 weeks after diabetes induction *(4,8,9)*. At this time-point, NMDA-dependent LTP in the dentate gyrus and NMDA-independent LTP in the CA3 field are also impaired *(9)*. Insulin treatment prevents the development of the changes in LTP, but only partially reverses existing deficits *(5)*. In contrast to LTP, expression of LTD is enhanced in the CA1 field following low-frequency stimulation of slices from diabetic rats *(9)*.

A number of studies have tried to pinpoint the mechanisms underlying these alterations in hippocampal synaptic plasticity. In presynaptic fibers, subtle changes are detected, including reduced impulse conduction velocity *(10)*. However, as paired-pulse facilitation in the CA1-field is unaffected *(4)*, presynaptic function appears to be largely preserved. Therefore, it is likely that the plasticity deficit is mainly postsynaptic in nature, involving glutamate receptors, membrane excitability, and/or the intracellular signaling cascade involved in LTP and LTD induction *(2)*. The effects of diabetes on postsynaptic glutamate receptors in the hippocampus have been the subject of several studies *(11)*. In Sprague-Dawley rats, after 6–8 weeks STZ-diabetes, the affinity of glutamate for a-amino-3-hydroxy-5-methyl-4-isoxazole propionic acid (AMPA), but not for NMDA-receptors, is decreased *(12)*. The reduced affinity for AMPA is associated with reduced levels of the GluR1 subunit of the AMPA receptor *(12)*, whereas the level of GluR2 and 3 in the hippocampus and cortex is unaffected *(12)*. After 12 weeks of STZ-diabetes the levels of the NMDA receptor subunits NMDA receptor (NR)1 and NR2A are not changed, but there is a marked decrease (–40%) in NR2B *(13)*. Furthermore, the phosphorylation of the NR2A/B subunits by Ca^{2+}/calmodulin-dependent protein kinase II is reduced in diabetes *(13)*. These NMDA receptor related changes are likely to be involved in the LTP deficits.

Neurophysiological Changes

Evoked potentials are electrical field potentials as recorded on the scalp that are generated by specific brain structures in response to visual, auditory, or somatosensory stimuli. Measurements of the latencies of these evoked potentials can be used to study the efficiency of signal conduction in the brain, as a central equivalent of peripheral nerve conduction studies. As might be expected, in both STZ- and spontaneously diabetic rats the latencies of visual, auditory, and somatosensory evoked potentials are increased *(14,15)*. However, unlike peripheral nerve conduction deficits, increases in evoked potential latencies take months, rather than weeks, to develop *(14)*.

Structural Abnormalities

Long-term STZ-diabetes is associated with loss of neocortical neurons *(16,17)*. In BB/Wor rats, loss of hippocampal neurons is observed after 8, but not after 2 months of diabetes duration *(6)*. However, ultrastructural changes may occur much earlier, as retraction and simplification of apical dendrites of hippocampal CA3 pyramidal neurons can be demonstrated within 9 days of untreated STZ-diabetes *(18)*.

Microvascular changes, not unlike those observed in other organ systems, have also been observed in the brain of diabetic rodents, including decreased capillary density *(16)* and thickening of capillary basement membrane *(17)*.

Pathogenetic Mechansims

Several of the metabolic and vascular disturbances that are implicated in peripheral neuropathy also appear to affect the brain *(2,19)*. As in the periphery, excess glucose is converted to sorbitol and fructose, leading to increased levels of these molecules in the brain *(20,21)*. In contrast to observations in peripheral nerves, cerebral *myo*-inositol levels are increased despite the increase in sorbitol level *(21)*. The amounts of advanced glycation end products (AGEs) are also increased in the brain and spinal cord of diabetic rats *(22,23)*, as are the byproducts of lipid peroxidation, indicative of oxidative damage *(24,25)*. Furthermore, the activities of superoxide dismutase and catalase, enzymes involved in the antioxidant defence of the brain, are decreased *(26,27)*.

In the light of the changes in synaptic plasticity it is of particular interest to note that diabetes also affects the levels of second messengers and the activity of protein kinases in the brain. In diabetic rats cerebral phosphoinositide and diacylglycerol levels appear to be decreased whereas the activities of protein kinases A and C are increased *(28)* and the activity of calcium/calmodulin dependent protein kinase II is decreased *(13)*.

In addition to the aforementioned structural alterations in the cerebral microvasculature, functional vascular changes such as a reduction in cerebral blood flow also occur *(29,30)*. Interestingly, treatment of diabetic rats with the angiotensin enzyme inhibitor enalapril not only prevents deficits in blood flow, but also in water maze learning and hippocampal synaptic plasticity *(30)*, indicating that vascular disturbances may indeed play a role in the aetiology of cerebral dysfunction.

Insulin itself may also be involved. The brain has long been considered an "insulin-insensitive organ." However, insulin and its receptor are now known to be widely distributed throughout the brain, with particular abundance in defined areas, such as the hippocampus. Insulin appears to affect cerebral glucose utilization, and plays a role in the regulation of food intake and body weight *(31)*. In addition insulin acts as a "neuromodulator," influencing the release and reuptake of neurotransmitters and learning and memory *(32)*. Disturbances in insulin signaling pathways in the periphery and in the brain have recently been implicated in Alzheimer's disease (AD) and brain ageing *(2,33)*. Ageing is associated with reductions in the level of insulin and the number of its receptors in the brain *(34)*. In AD this age-related reduction in cerebral insulin levels appears to be accompanied by disturbances of insulin receptor signaling in the brain *(34)*, leading to the suggestion that AD is an "insulin-resistant brain state" *(35)*. Insulin also regulates the metabolism of β-amyloid and tau, two proteins that represent the building blocks of amyloid plaques and neurofibrillary tangles, the neuropathological hallmarks of AD *(33)*. The significance of these recent insights for diabetes is yet unknown.

STUDIES IN MAN: COGNITION AND DEMENTIA

Studies into the effects of diabetes on cognitive functioning in man can be broadly divided in two categories: case–control studies, which are mostly cross-sectional, and population-based surveys, which are often longitudinal. The case–control studies usually involved selected populations of patients and matched nondiabetic controls, using performance on a battery of neuropsychological tests as an outcome measure. Population-based surveys mostly involved elderly subjects, and used either relatively crude cognitive screening tests or a clinical diagnosis of dementia as a primary outcome measure.

Type 1 Diabetes in Children

Although quite a few studies have looked at neuropsychological test performance and school achievement in children with diabetes, this remains an area of some controversy *(36)*. Some studies report that children with type 1 diabetes perform more poorly than control subjects on measures of intelligence, attention, processing speed, long-term memory, and executive skills *(37,38)*, whereas other studies report that test performances are within the normal range *(39)*. However, the observation that children with an early onset of diabetes (e.g., before the age of 6) are at increased risk for slowing of intellectual development is quite consistent *(36,40)*. This increased vulnerability of younger children may be attributable to an increased sensitivity of the developing brain to the adverse effects of both hypo- and hyperglycemia *(40,41)*.

Importantly, a recent study, involving a large population of patients and controls, reports that for most children, type 1 diabetes is not associated with lower academic performance compared with either siblings or classmates, although increased behavioral concerns are reported by parents *(42)*. Apparently, the aforementioned subtle cognitive changes in children with type 1 diabetes do not significantly limit their functional academic abilities over time.

Type 1 Diabetes in Adults

All but a few studies on cognition in adult patients with type 1 diabetes have a cross-sectional case–control design. A recent meta-analysis of these studies shows that cognitive performance in patients with type 1 diabetes is characterized by a mild-to-moderate slowing of mental speed and a diminished mental flexibility, whereas learning and memory are spared *(43)*.

However, uncertainty remains as to the disease variables that are related to impaired cognitive performance *(43)*. This is likely to be largely because of methodological limitations of the studies that addressed this issue. Many factors other than diabetes, such as education, and genetic and socio-economic background, are important determinants of cognitive performance. This results in marked interindividual variation, which can easily obscure the effects of different diabetes-related variables in cross-sectional studies, particularly when sample sizes are relatively small, as is the case in the majority of the studies that have been published thus far. Longitudinal studies in which intraindividual changes in cognition over time can be related to specific diabetes-related variables, would resolve this issue. Nevertheless, in cross-sectional studies lowered cognitive performance in diabetic patients appears to be associated with the presence of microvascular complications *(44–46)*. Although cross-sectional studies generally report no consistent relation between diabetes duration and the severity of performance impairments *(43)*, there are clear indications that the impairments are progressive over time (Fig. 1). Taken together, these data suggest that at least part of the cognitive changes observed in type 1 diabetic patients are because of chronic exposure to hyperglycemia, despite the fact that a relation between impaired cognition and increased HbA1 levels has not been reported *(43)*.

In this context, the effect of hypoglycemia also needs to be addressed. The occurrence of episodes of severe hypoglycemia is an unwanted side effect of intensified insulin therapy *(47)*. Several case reports and small case–control series indicate that repeated severe hypoglycemia may have permanent cognitive sequelae *(43)*. In contrast, the largest available prospective survey on the consequences of severe hypoglycemic episodes on cognition in subjects receiving intensified insulin therapy does not show important negative effects *(48)*. A recent meta-analysis of studies that compared type 1 diabetic patients with and without severe hypoglycemic episodes reached the same conclusion *(43)*. Still, this issue warrants further investigation, as specific subgroups of patients, such as young children or subjects with advanced microvascular complications may be more susceptible to the adverse effects of hypoglycemia.

Type 2 Diabetes

Neuropsychological studies in type 2 diabetic patients report moderate degrees of cognitive impairment, particularly in tasks involving verbal memory or complex information processing *(49,50)*. Tasks that assess basic attentional processes, motor reaction time, and immediate memory appear to be unaffected. This pattern of cognitive impairments is quite

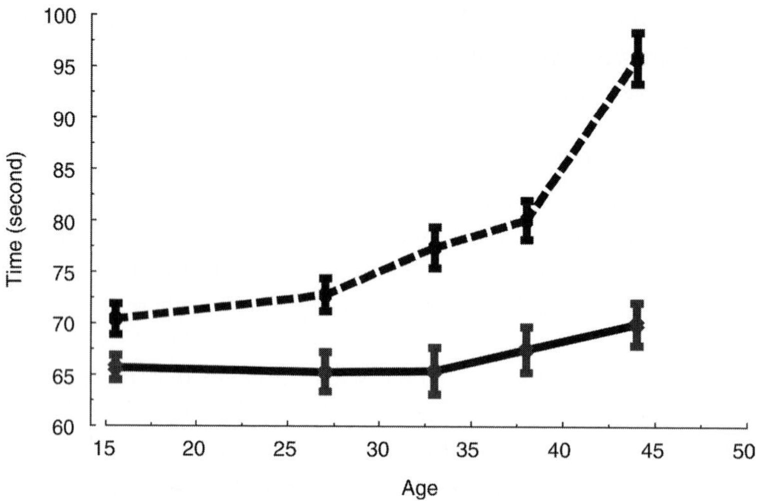

Fig. 1. Psychomotor efficiency as measured with the Grooved Pegboard test *(114)* in patients with childhood onset type 1 diabetes. The curves are comprised of data that were collected in a number of cross-sectional studies of patients with diabeties (125 children and 189 adults) and demographically similar comparison subjects without diabeties (83 children and 184 adults). Data are presented as means ± SEM. Note that with increasing duration of diabetes (and increasing age) the relative difference between the two groups increases. Courtesy of Dr CM Ryan and coworkers (Western Psychiatric Institute and Clinic,University of Pittsburgh School of Medicine, Pittsburgh, PA), who conducted these studies. Part of these data has been published previously, i.e., refs. *44, 115.*

different from that observed in type 1 diabetes. Moreover, the magnitude of the performance deficit, relative to age-matched controls, appears to be somewhat larger (Table 1).

Although, the risk of cognitive impairment in type 2 diabetes is well established, the underlying mechanisms remain largely unidentified. Type 2 diabetes typically develops in the context of a cluster of vascular and metabolic risk factors (including hypertension, dyslipidemia, and obesity), referred to as the "metabolic syndrome." The metabolic syndrome itself, with or without hyperglycemia, is associated with atherosclerotic cardiovascular disease, ischaemic stroke, and with cognitive decline and dementia *(51)*. A key question is whether hyperglycemia *per se* or other factors from the metabolic syndrome lead to impaired cognition in type 2 diabetes. Previous studies indicate that increased HbA1 or fasting plasma glucose levels appear to be risk factors for cognitive dysfunction in type 2 diabetic patients *(52)*. However, factors related to the metabolic syndrome are also likely to play a role, as elevated serum triglyceride levels are related to lower cognitive performance in type 2 diabetic subjects *(53)*. Some investigators even suggest that cognitive dysfunction in type 2 diabetic patients is primarily because of concomitant hypertension *(50)*. However, in the own cross-sectional survey on cognition in a population of 125 type 2 diabetic patients, hypertension had little effect on the nature and magnitude of cognitive impairment *(54)*.

Age is probably a key factor in cognitive impairment in type 2 diabetic patients *(54,55)*. In the above mentioned survey *(54)*, age proved to be a strong predictor of impaired cognitive performance, much more so than in nondiabetic aged controls.

Table 1
An Overview of Changes in Cognition in Type 1 and Type 2 Diabetes

Cognitive domain	Type 1	Type 2
General intelligence	0.4–0.8	0–0.4
Attention	0–0.3	0–0.3
Psychomotor speed	0.3–0.6	0.3–0.6
Verbal memory	0–0.2	0.5–1
Nonverbal memory	0–0.2	0.3–1
Mental flexibility-executive function	0.4–0.6	0.5–1
Visuospatial	0.4	0–0.4
Language	0–0.2	0–0.2

Estimates of the severity of impairments in cognition per domain expressed in standardized effect sizes (Cohen's *d*) based on meta-analyses by Brands *(43)*, Awad *(49)*, Stewart *(50)* and their coworkers. The Cohen's *d* is defined as the difference between the means of two groups divided by the pooled standard deviation of the two groups. By expressing test performances of an experimental group relative to controls in Cohen's *d* standardized effect sizes, the results of different test that access the same domain can be pooled. It also facilitates comparison across different studies. In neuropsychological studies an effect size of 0.2 is generally considered to correspond to small effects, 0.5 to medium, and 0.8 to large effects *(106)*.

Indeed several studies in elderly subjects with type 2 diabetes or "prediabetic" conditions such as impaired glucose tolerance, have detected cognitive impairment with relatively crude tests, such as a mini mental state examination, suggesting that the impairments may be more pronounced than in younger individuals *(56,57)*. In a study of 400 type 2 diabetic patients and 400 nondiabetic controls with an average age of 75, for example, 29% of diabetic subjects scored below a mini mental state examination cut-of point of 24, compared with 12% of the controls *(57)*. In the diabetic subjects a score lower than this cut-of point proved to have an impact on diabetes self-care and monitoring, and was also associated with higher hospitalisation, reduced ADL (activities of daily living) ability, and increased need for assistance in personal care.

Dementia

During the past decade several large longitudinal population based studies have provided clear evidence that the incidence of dementia is increased among elderly patients with diabetes (Table 2). This appears to be related to both AD (relative risk 1.5–2) and vascular dementia (relative risk 2–2.5), although it can be difficult to distinguish between these types of dementia based on the clinical criteria that were used in these studies.

Depression

The next section of this chapter will address structural and neurophysiological changes in the brain that are likely to underlie changes in cognition. However, it should be noted that other factors can also influence cognitive function in diabetic patients. For example, the prevalence of psychiatric disorders in particular depressive and anxiety disorders, is increased in both type 1 and type 2 diabetes *(58,59)*. A recent systematic review showed that the odds for the prevalence of depression among type 1 and type 2 diabetic patients are twice as high as in nondiabetic subjects (odds ratio [OR] 2, 95% CI 1.8–2.2) odd rate *(59)*. The significance of clinical depression in diabetic patients should not be underestimated.

Table 2
The Relative Risk of Incident Dementia in Diabetic Patients

References	Follow-up (years)	n Tot/DM[a]	Diagnosis[b]	Relative risk dementia[c]
107 (Japan)	7	826/ND	AD	2.2 (1–4.9)
			VaD	2.8 (2.6–3)
108 (USA)	6.9	ND/1455	All dem	1.6 (1.3–2)
			AD	1.6 (1.3–2)
109 (The Netherlands)	2.1	6370/ND	All dem	1.9 (1.3–2.8)
			AD	1.9 (1.2–3.1)
			VaD	2.0 (0.7–5.6)
68 (Hawaii)	2.9	2574/900	All dem	1.5 (1–2.2)[e]
			AD	1.8 (1.1–2.9)
			VaD	2.3 (1.1–5)
110 (Canada)	5	5574/503	All Dem	1.3 (0.9–1.8)[e]
			AD	1.3 (0.8–2)
			VaD	2.0 (1.2–3.6)
111 (Swedan)	6	702/108	All Dem	1.2 (0.8–1.7)[e]
			AD	0.8 (0.5–1.5)
			VaD	2.5 (1.4–4.8)
112 (USA)	5.5	824/127	AD	1.7 (1.1–2.5)[d]
113 (Swedan)	4.7	1301/ND	All dem	1.5 (1–2.1)[e]
			AD	1.3 (0.9–2.1)
			VaD	2.6 (1.2–6.1)

[a]The number of nondiabetic and diabetic participants from which follow-up was obtained.

[b]dementia diagnosis: All Dem: all subtypes of dementia combined, AD,Alzheimer's disease; VaD, vascular dementia.

[c]The relative risk of the different dementia diagnoses in diabetic subjects in comparison to the nondiabetic subjects is indicated.

[d]Relative risks are adjusted for demographics.

[e]In studies additionally adjusted for vascular risk factors, such as hypertension.

Depression is a debilitating disorder that typically impairs all aspects of an individual's functioning. Moreover, there appears to be significant and consistent association between depressive symptoms, diabetic complications *(60)*, and glycemic control *(61)*, although a causal relationship has not yet been established. It is evident that the recognition of depression in diabetic patients is important, as it is a potentially treatable condition.

STUDIES IN MAN: NEUROPATHOLOGY AND BRAIN IMAGING

Up till two decades ago, studies on the structural basis of impaired cognition in man largely depended on neuropathology. Much has changed since the introduction of powerful neuroimaging techniques, such as computed tomography, and even more so Magnetic resonance imaging (MRI). Neuroimaging now plays a key role both in daily clinical practice and in cognition and dementia research. In patients suspected of dementia, MR in particular not only serves to exclude (rare) treatable causes of dementia, but increasingly adds to a more accurate diagnosis of dementia syndromes, also in the early stages *(62)*. For research purposes structural and functional brain changes are evaluated

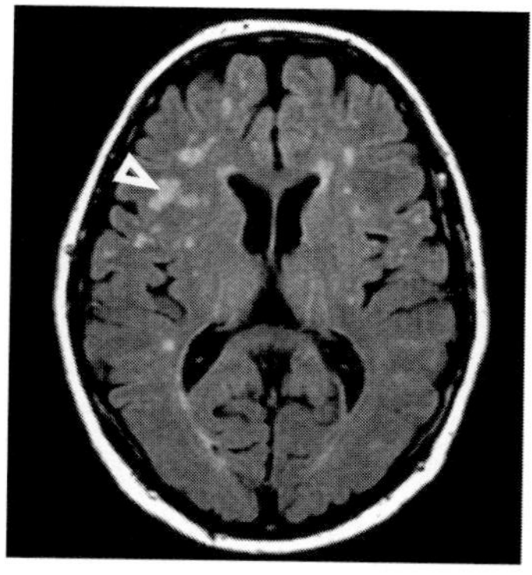
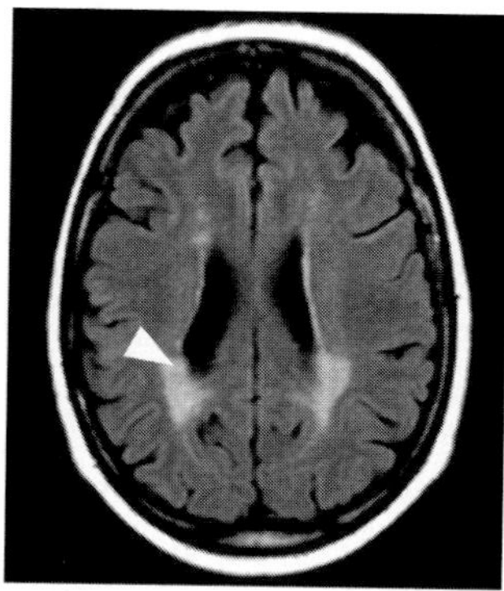
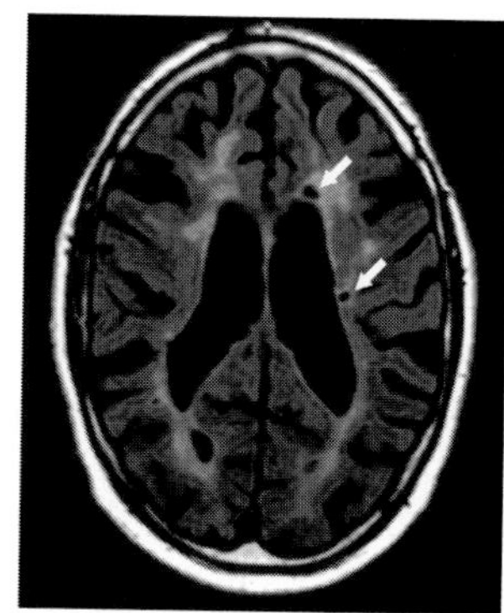

Fig. 2. Examples of white matter lesions and lacunar infarcts on magnetic resonance imaging scans obtained from type 2 patients with diabetes. The images have been acquired with fluid attenuated inversion recovery sequences. Two types of white matter lesions can be distinguished, based on their location. Periventricular lesions are located directly adjacent to the cerebral ventricles (middle, closed triangle), whereas deep subcortical lesions are patchy lesions located in the deep white matter (left, open triangle). White matter lesions can be distinguished from lacunar infarcts (right, arrow) because the latter are hypointense on fluid attenuated inversion recovery and T1-weighted images.

using a variety of methods, ranging from very simple semiquantitative visual scales to highly sophisticated computerized tools *(63)*. These methods allow the assessment of cortical and subcortical atrophy, of "silent" or symptomatic brain infarcts, and of so-called white matter lesions (Fig. 2). These white matter lesions are a common finding in aged subjects with vascular risk factors or ischaemic vascular disease. Their direct role in causing cognitive deterioration has not been established, although their frequency is higher in demented subjects than in normal controls, and they are associated with specific cognitive deficits, particularly those related to impairment of frontal lobe functions *(64)*.

Neuropathological Studies

Neuropathological studies of diabetic patients are relatively limited in number. In the mid-sixties a case series was published, involving 16 type 1 patients with diabetes widespread macro and microvascular disease, half of whom also showed "mental disturbances"*(65)*. Macroscopic examination revealed moderate to severe atrophy in five cases. Microscopic examination revealed gliosis in the cerebral cortex, and subependymal gliosis of the periventricular regions. Atherosclerosis was observed in large arteries, and basement membrane thickening in capillaries. These microvascular changes were also reported in another autopsy study *(66)*.

In a large retrospective study of 7579 necropsies, including 935 subjects with diabetes, macroscopic brain infarcts were more prevalent in subjects with diabetes than in controls, for all ages studied *(67)*. In subjects older than 70 the percent of diabetic subjects with ischemic lesions was 40–50%, vs 30% in controls.

More recent studies have assessed the relation between diabetes and the occurrence of neuropathological lesions that are common in AD, such as neurofibrillary tangles and amyloid plaques *(68–70)*, but the results are inconclusive. Possibly, diabetes in interaction with the APOE ε4 genotype leads to accelerated Alzheimer-type pathology *(68)*.

Neuroimaging Studies

A number of studies have assessed atrophy or white matter lesions in type 1 patients with diabetes. Some of these studies included a direct comparison with nondiabetic controls *(71–73)*, but sample sizes were small (generally <20 per group). Other studies compared type 1 patients diabetes with microvascular complications (e.g., retinopathy) *(45)* or a history of repeated severe hypoglycemia *(74)* to patients without these complications. Taken together, these studies suggest that there may be some degree of cerebral atrophy in type 1 patients diabetes *(73,74)*, which may be linked to the occurrence of hypoglycemia *(74)* (but *see* ref. *45*), but not to the presence of microvascular complications such as retinopathy *(45)*. In addition, white matter lesions may be more common in type 1 diabetic patients than in controls *(71)*. Additional studies on the brain MRI features of type 1 diabetes are necessary before solid conclusions can be drawn. Given the relatively modest changes in cognition in type 1 diabetes, these studies should apply MR rating methods that are sensitive enough to pick up subtle differences, and should have adequate statistical power.

Data on the brain imaging features of type 2 diabetes can be extracted from a number of large population based surveys on risk factors for cerebrovascular disease and on age-related MR changes. These studies indicate that type 2 diabetes is a risk factor for (lacunar) infarcts *(75,76)*, cortical, and subcortical atrophy *(77)* and possibly white matter lesions *(77,78)*. Studies with a case–control design provide more detailed information *(79–82)*. These latter studies show that type 2 diabetes is associated with both cortical and subcortical atrophy, relative to age-matched nondiabetic controls *(79,82,54)*. Atrophy has also been reported in the medial temporal lobe *(80)*, and may already be present in prediabetic stages *(83)*. These latter observations are of particular interest, as atrophy in this region of the brain is also one of the early manifestations of AD. Schmidt et al. *(79)* reported a nonsignificant increase in the severity of white matter lesions in type 2 diabetic patients relative to controls *(79)*, using a relatively insensitive interval scale. In our own cross-sectional survey on MRI and cognition in a population of 125 type 2 patients with diabetes and 65 matched controls *(54)*, an evident increase is observed in white matter lesion load in patients compared with controls (Fig. 3).

The amount of data on the relation of these MR changes in type 2 diabetes to different disease variables is still limited. It has been suggested that hypertension is an important determinant of cerebral atrophy in type 2 diabetes *(79)*, but in our own study hypertension had only modest effects on atrophy and white matter lesions (*54*; Fig. 3).

STUDIES IN MAN: NEUROPHYSIOLOGICAL CHANGES

Evoked Potentials

In the brainstem, auditory evoked potential five waves can be distinguished. Wave I, III, and V are considered to reflect activity in the acoustic nerve, the pons, and the midbrain, respectively. In both type 1 and type 2 patients diabetes the latency of wave I as well as the interpeak latencies I–III and III–V are prolonged *(84,85)*. The latency of the P100 wave of the visual evoked potential, which is thought to be generated in the visual cortex, is increased both in type 1 and type 2 diabetes *(86–88)*. P100 latencies correlate

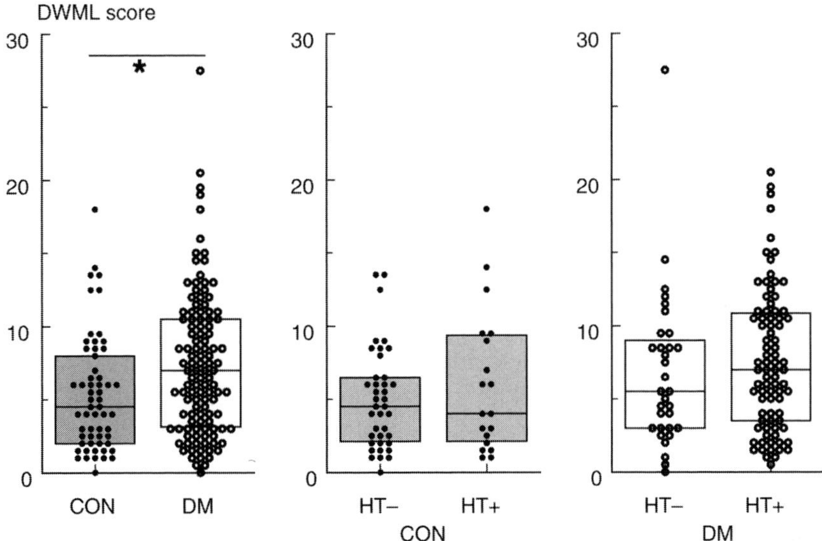

Fig. 3. Deep white matter lesions (DWML) in type 2 diabetic patients (n = 115) and age and sex-matched nondiabetic controls. The severity of DWML was assessed semi-quantitatively using the "Scheltens scale" *(116)*, a scale that takes both the number and the size of the lesions into account. Boxes represent quartiles and median scores. The DWML score is significantly ($p < 0.01$) higher in the diabetic patients. After adjustment for the presence of hypertension (HT; defined as a systolic blood pressure ≥160 mmHg and/or diastolic blood pressure ≥95 mmHg and/or self reported use of antihypertensive medication) the difference between the diabetic and nondiabetic group remains statistically significant. Data are derived from the Utrecht Diabetic Encephalopathy Study *(54)*.

positively with the duration of diabetes and HbA1 levels *(86)* and can be improved by intensive insulin treatment *(87)*.

Studies on somatosensory evoked potentials in diabetic patients have provided more variable results. Increased latencies of the central components of the somatosensory evoked potential have been reported *(89)*, although other studies have only found significant conduction delays in peripheral components of the somatosensory pathways *(90,91)*.

Event-Related Potentials

The latency of the so-called P300 wave is also increased in type 1 as well as in type 2 diabetic patients *(92,93)*. This P300 wave is a positive deflection in the human event-related potential that is considered to reflect the speed of neuronal events underlying information processing *(94)*. It is most commonly elicited with an "oddball" paradigm in which a subject is instructed to detect an occasional target stimulus in a regular train of standard stimuli *(94)*. The increased latency of the P300 wave in diabetes may thus be a neurophysiological manifestation of impairment of higher brain functions.

STUDIES IN MAN: THERAPIES

To date the only published studies that have evaluated the effects of different treatment modalities on cognition in type 1 diabetes, are the intensive insulin treatment trials

(48,95). In these trials cognition was monitored primarily in order to detect possible unwanted side effects of an increased incidence of hypoglycemic episodes. Neither study detected a deterioration of cognitive function in relation to the occurrence of hypoglycemic episodes, but they also failed to show an improvement of cognition with improved glycemic control.

In type 2 diabetes some studies suggest that intensified glycemic control may improve cognition *(96–99*; but *see* ref. *100*). However, the methodological quality of the studies is insufficient to draw firm conclusions *(101)*. Alternative treatment modalities are also being considered. There is some evidence that treatment with the lipid-lowering drug atorvastatin has beneficial effects on learning in type 2 diabetes *(102)*. Moreover, a recent randomized, double-blind, placebo-controlled crossover study showed that administration of the 11β-hydroxysteroid dehydrogenase inhibitor carbenoxolone improved verbal memory after 6 weeks in 12 patients with type 2 diabetes *(103)*. The rationale behind this treatment was that the compound might protect hippocampal cells from glucocorticoid-mediated damage that occurs in association with ageing *(103)*.

Another interesting development, outside the field of diabetes, is the observation from a recent exploratory placebo-controlled trial in nondiabetic subjects with early AD that rosiglitazone, an insulin-sensitizing compound from the thiazolidinedione class, ameliorated cognitive decline *(104)*. The effects of this compound on cognition were accompanied by an improvement of cerebrospinal fluid β-amyloid levels. Future studies should determine whether these compounds are superior than other classes of antihyperglycemic agents in preventing cognitive deterioration in patients with type 2 diabetes.

A CLINICAL APPROACH TO COMPLAINTS OF COGNITIVE DYSFUNCTION IN DIABETIC PATIENTS

The data that are reviewed in this chapter clearly show that diabetes is associated with changes in cerebral function and structure. However, it should be noted that the diagnosis "diabetic encephalopathy" cannot be readily established in individual patients. This is because of the fact that the changes in cognition and in brain structure, as observed on computed tomography or MRI, are not specific to diabetes. There is, for example, considerable overlap with functional and structural changes in the brain that occur with brain ageing, or cerebral changes that occur in association with other vascular risk factors such as hypertension. Because clinically significant cognitive impairments mainly occur in elderly diabetic patients it will be evident that it is difficult to distinguish between the effects of diabetes, ageing, and comorbidity. However, this should not lead to a nihilistic diagnostic approach. The main task of the clinician who is faced with a diabetic patient with cognitive complaints is to assess the severity and nature of the cognitive impairments, to try and classify these impairments and to exclude other (potentially treatable) causes of cognitive deterioration. The next paragraph serves as an illustration of a possible diagnostic approach.

A full disease history should be obtained, focussing on the cognitive and behavioral changes in the patient, their evolution over time, and symptoms suggestive of other medical, neurological, or psychiatric illnesses. The possibility of depression should be considered, as depression may manifest itself primarily in complaints of concentration and/or memory disturbances, particularly in the elderly. Attention should be paid to the assessment of the impact of changes in cognition on day-to-day functioning (for example: problems with such activities as cooking, shopping, managing ones financial affairs, progressive dependence on spouse, social withdrawal, problems with self care, and medication use). Helpful screening lists have been developed to this end *(105)*. Information on the presence of other diabetic complications and vascular risk factors, including blood pressure, is required. Prescription and nonprescription drugs, in particular analgesic, anticholinergic, antihypertensive, psychotropic, and sedative-hypnotic agents, should be reviewed carefully as potential causes of cognitive impairment. Alcohol use should be assessed. Laboratory tests can include a blood count, tests of liver, kidney and thyroid function, vitamin B_{12} levels, HbA1, and blood lipids. Brain imaging can be used to detect structural lesions (for example, infarction, neoplasm, subdural haematoma, and hydrocephalus), but can also contribute to the classification of dementia syndromes in their early stages *(62)*. A neuropsychological examination can help to qualify and quantify the cognitive disturbances, and can help to differentiate between early dementia and depression.

As has been stated in the previous section of this chapter, there are no specific treatments with proven efficacy in preventing cognitive decline in diabetic patients. Still, analogous to the prevention of other diabetic complications, the maintenance of adequate glycemic control while avoiding hypoglycemia, and the treatment of vascular risk factors, appear to be the main targets for the prevention of end-organ damage to the brain.

REFERENCES

1. Malenka RC, Nicoll RA. Long-term potentiation—a decade of progress? *Science* 1999;285:1870–1874.
2. Gispen WH, Biessels GJ. Cognition and synaptic plasticity in diabetes mellitus. *Trends Neurosci* 2000;23:542–549.
3. Flood JF, Mooradian AD, Morley JE. Characteristics of learning and memory in streptozocin-induced diabetic mice. *Diabetes* 1990;39:1391–1398.
4. Biessels GJ, Kamal A, Ramakers GM, et al. Place learning and hippocampal synaptic plasticity in streptozotocin-induced diabetic rats. *Diabetes* 1996;45:1259–1266.
5. Biessels GJ, Kamal A, Urban IJ, Spruijt BM, Erkelens DW, Gispen WH. Water maze learning and hippocampal synaptic plasticity in streptozotocin-diabetic rats: effects of insulin treatment. *Brain Res* 1998;800:125–135.
6. Li ZG, Zhang W, Grunberger G, Sima AA. Hippocampal neuronal apoptosis in type 1 diabetes. *Brain Res* 2002;946:221–231.
7. Li XL, Aou S, Hori T, Oomura Y. Spatial memory deficit and emotional abnormality in OLETF rats. *Physiol Behav* 2002;75:15–23.
8. Chabot C, Massicotte G, Milot M, Trudeau F, Gagne J. Impaired modulation of AMPA receptors by calcium-dependent processes in streptozotocin-induced diabetic rats. *Brain Res* 1997;768:249–256.
9. Kamal A, Biessels GJ, Urban IJA, Gispen WH. Hippocampal synaptic plasticity in streptozotocin-diabetic rats: impairment of long-term potentiation and facilitation of long-term depression. *Neuroscience* 1999;90:737–745.
10. Candy SM, Szatkowski MS. Neuronal excitability and conduction velocity changes in hippocampal slices from streptozotocin-treated diabetic rats. *Brain Res* 2000;863:298–301.
11. Trudeau F, Gagnon S, Massicotte G. Hippocampal synaptic plasticity and glutamate receptor regulation: influences of diabetes mellitus. *Eur J Pharmacol* 2004;490:177–186.

12. Gagne J, Milot M, Gelinas S, et al. Binding properties of glutamate receptors in streptozotocin-induced diabetes in rats. *Diabetes* 1997;46:841–846.
13. Di Luca M, Ruts L, Gardoni F, Cattabeni F, Biessels GJ, Gispen WH. NMDA receptor subunits are modified transcriptionally and post-translationally in the brain of streptozotocin-diabetic rats. *Diabetologia* 1999;42:693–701.
14. Biessels GJ, Cristino NA, Rutten G, Hamers FPT, Erkelens DW, Gispen WH. Neurophysiological changes in the central and peripheral nervous system of streptozotocin-diabetic rats: course of development and effects of insulin treatment. *Brain* 1999; 122:757–768.
15. Sima AA, Zhang WX, Cherian PV, Chakrabarti S. Impaired visual evoked potential and primary axonopathy of the optic nerve in the diabetic BB/W-rat. *Diabetologia* 1992;35: 602–607.
16. Jakobsen J, Sidenius P, Gundersen HJ, Osterby R. Quantitative changes of cerebral neocortical structure in insulin-treated long-term streptozocin-induced diabetes in rats. *Diabetes* 1987;36:597–601.
17. Mukai N, Hori S, Pomeroy M. Cerebral lesions in rats with streptozotocin-induced diabetes. *Acta Neuropathol (Berl)* 1980;51:79–84.
18. Magarinos AM, Mcewen BS. Experimental diabetes in rats causes hippocampal dendritic and synaptic reorganization and increased glucocorticoid reactivity to stress. *Proc Natl Acad Sci USA* 2000;97:11,056–11,061.
19. Sima AAF, Kamiya H, Li ZG. Insulin, C-peptide, hyperglycemia, and central nervous system complications in diabetes. *Eur J Pharmacol* 2004;490:187–197.
20. Sredy J, Sawicki DR, Notvest RR. Polyol pathway activity in nervous tissues of diabetic and galactose-fed rats: effect of dietary galactose withdrawal or tolrestat intervention therapy. *J Diabetes Complications* 1991;5:42–47.
21. Knudsen GM, Jakobsen J, Barry DI, Compton AM, Tomlinson DR. Myo-inositol normalizes decreased sodium permeability of the blood-brain barrier in streptozotocin diabetes. *Neuroscience* 1989;29:773–777.
22. Vlassara H, Brownlee M, Cerami A. Excessive non enzymatic glycosylation of peripheral and central nervous system myelin components in diabetic rats. *Diabetes* 1983;32: 670–674.
23. Ryle C, Leow CK, Donaghy M. Nonenzymatic glycation of peripheral and central nervous system proteins in experimental diabetes mellitus. *Muscle Nerve* 1997;20:577–584.
24. Mooradian AD. The antioxidative potential of cerebral microvessels in experimental diabetes mellitus. *Brain Res* 1995;671:164–169.
25. Reagan LP, Magarinos AM, Yee DK, et al. Oxidative stress and HNE conjugation of GLUT3 are increased in the hippocampus of diabetic rats subjected to stress. *Brain Res* 2000;862:292–300.
26. Kumar JS, Menon VP. Effect of diabetes on levels of lipid peroxides and glycolipids in rat brain. *Metabolism* 1993;42:1435–1439.
27. Makar TK, Rimpel-Lamhaouar K, Abraham DG, Gokhale VS, Cooper AJL. Antioxidant defense systems in the brains of type II diabetic mice. *J Neurochem* 1995;65:287–291.
28. Bhardwaj SK, Sandhu SK, Sharma P, Kaur G. Impact of diabetes on CNS: role of signal transduction cascade. *Brain Res Bull* 1999;49:155–162.
29. Jakobsen J, Nedergaard M, Aarslew Jensen M, Diemer NH. Regional brain glucose metabolism and blood flow in streptozocin- induced diabetic rats. *Diabetes* 1990;39:437–440.
30. Manschot SM, Biessels GJ, Cameron NE, et al. Angiotensin converting enzyme inhibition partially prevents deficits in water maze performance, hippocampal synaptic plasticity and cerebral blood flow in streptozotocin-diabetic rats. *Brain Res* 2003;966:274–282.
31. Schulingkamp RJ, Pagano TC, Hung D, Raffa RB. Insulin receptors and insulin action in the brain: review and clinical implications. *Neurosci Biobehav Rev* 2000;24:855–872.
32. Zhao W, Alkon DL. Role of insulin and insulin receptor in learning and memory. *Mol Cell Endocrinol* 2001;177:125–134.

33. Gasparini L, Netzer WJ, Greengard P, Xu H. Does insulin dysfunction play a role in Alzheimer's disease? *Trends Pharmacol Sci* 2002;23:288–293.
34. Frolich L, Blum-Degen D, Bernstein HG, et al. Brain insulin and insulin receptors in aging and sporadic Alzheimer's disease. *J Neural Transm* 1998;105:423–438.
35. Hoyer S. Is sporadic Alzheimer disease the brain type of non-insulin dependent diabetes mellitus? A challenging hypothesis. *J Neural Transm* 1998;105:415–422.
36. Ryan CM. Memory and metabolic control in children. *Diabetes Care* 1999;22:1239–1241.
37. Northam EA, Anderson PJ, Jacobs R, Hughes M, Warne GL, Werther GA. Neuropsychological profiles of children with type 1 diabetes 6 years after disease onset. *Diabetes Care* 2001;24:1541–1546.
38. Bjorgaas M, Gimse R, Vik T, Sand T. Cognitive function in Type 1 diabetic children with and without episodes of severe hypoglycaemia. *Acta Paediatr* 1997;86:148–153.
39. Kaufman FR, Epport K, Engilman R, Halvorson M. Neurocognitive functioning in children diagnosed with diabetes before age 10 years. *J Diabetes Complications* 1999;13: 31–38.
40. Schoenle EJ, Schoenle D, Molinari L, Largo RH. Impaired intellectual development in children with Type I diabetes: association with HbA(1c), age at diagnosis and sex. *Diabetologia* 2002;45:108–114.
41. Hershey T, Bhargava N, Sadler M, White NH, Craft S. Conventional versus intensive diabetes therapy in children with type 1 diabetes: effects on memory and motor speed. *Diabetes Care* 1999;22:1318–1324.
42. McCarthy AM, Lindgren S, Mengeling MA, Tsalikian E, Engvall JC. Effects of diabetes on learning in children. *Pediatrics* 2002;109:E9.
43. Brands AMA, Biessels GJ, De Haan EHF, Kappelle LJ, Kessels RPC. The effects of Type 1 diabetes on cognitive performance: a meta-analysis. *Diabetes Care* 2005;28:726–735.
44. Ryan CM, Williams TM, Finegold DN, Orchard TJ. Cognitive dysfunction in adults with type 1 (insulin-dependent) diabetes mellitus of long duration: effects of recurrent hypoglycaemia and other chronic complications. *Diabetologia* 1993;36:329–334.
45. Ferguson SC, Blane A, Perros P, et al. Cognitive ability and brain structure in type 1 diabetes: relation to microangiopathy and preceding severe hypoglycemia. *Diabetes* 2003;52:149–156.
46. Ryan CM, Geckle MO, Orchard TJ. Cognitive efficiency declines over time in adults with Type 1 diabetes: effects of micro- and macrovascular complications. *Diabetologia* 2003;46: 940–948.
47. The Diabetes Control and Complications Study Group. The effect of intensive treatment of diabetes on the development and progression of long-term complications in insulin-dependent diabetes mellitus. *N Engl J Med* 1993;329:977–986.
48. Austin EJ, Deary IJ. Effects of repeated hypoglycemia on cognitive function: a psychometrically validated reanalysis of the Diabetes Control and Complications Trial data. *Diabetes Care* 1999;22:1273–1277.
49. Awad N, Gagnon M, Messier C. The relationship between impaired glucose tolerance, type 2 diabetes, and cognitive function. *J Clin Exp Neuropsychol* 2004;26:1044–1080.
50. Stewart R, Liolitsa D. Type 2 diabetes mellitus, cognitive impairment and dementia. *Diabet Med* 1999;16:93–112.
51. Kalmijn S, Foley D, White L, et al. Metabolic cardiovascular syndrome and risk of dementia in Japanese-American elderly men. The Honolulu-Asia aging study. *Arterioscler Thromb Vasc Biol* 2000;20:2255–2260.
52. Strachan MWJ, Deary IJ, Ewing FME, Frier BM. Is type II diabetes associated with an increased risk of cognitive dysfunction? A critical review of published studies. *Diabetes Care* 1997;20:438–445.
53. Perlmuter LC, Nathan DM, Goldfinger SH, Russo PA, Yates J, Larkin M. Triglyceride levels affect cognitive function in noninsulin-dependent diabetics. *J Diabet Complications* 1988;2:210–213.

54. Manschot SM, Brands AM, van der GJ, Kessels RP, Algra A, Kapppelle LJ, Biessels GJ. Brain magnetic resonance imaging correlates of impaired cognition in patients with type 2 diabetes. *Diabetes* 2006;55:1106–1113.
55. Biessels GJ, Van der Heide LP, Kamal A, Bleys RL, Gispen WH. Ageing and diabetes: implications for brain function. *Eur J Pharmacol* 2002;441:1–14.
56. Kalmijn S, Feskens EJM, Launer LJ, Stijnen T, Kromhout D. Glucose intolerance, hyperinsulinaemia and cognitive function in a general population of elderly men. *Diabetologia* 1995;38:1096–1102.
57. Sinclair AJ, Girling AJ, Bayer AJ. Cognitive dysfunction in older subjects with diabetes mellitus: impact on diabetes self-management and use of care services. All Wales Research into Elderly (AWARE) Study. *Diabetes Res Clin Pract* 2000;50:203–212.
58. Grigsby AB, Anderson RJ, Freedland KE, Clouse RE, Lustman PJ. Prevalence of anxiety in adults with diabetes. A systematic review. *J Psychosom Res* 2002;53:1053–1060.
59. Anderson RJ, Freedland KE, Clouse RE, Lustman PJ. The prevalence of comorbid depression in adults with diabetes: a meta-analysis. *Diabetes Care* 2001;24:1069–1078.
60. de Groot M, Anderson R, Freedland KE, Clouse RE, Lustman PJ. Association of depression and diabetes complications: a meta-analysis. *Psychosom Med* 2001;63:619–630.
61. Lustman PJ, Anderson RJ, Freedland KE, de Groot M, Carney RM, Clouse RE. Depression and poor glycemic control: a meta-analytic review of the literature. *Diabetes Care* 2000; 23:934–942.
62. Scheltens P, Fox N, Barkhof F, De Carli C. Structural magnetic resonance imaging in the practical assessment of dementia: beyond exclusion. *Lancet Neurol* 2002;1:13–21.
63. Frisoni GB, Scheltens P, Galluzzi S, et al. Neuroimaging tools to rate regional atrophy, subcortical cerebrovascular disease, and regional cerebral blood flow and metabolism: consensus paper of the EADC. *J Neurol Neurosurg Psychiatry* 2003:74:1371–1381.
64. Pantoni L, Leys D, Fazekas F, et al. Role of white matter lesions in cognitive impairment of vascular origin. *Alzheimer Dis Assoc Disord* 1999;13(Suppl 3):S49–S54.
65. Reske-Nielsen E, Lundbaek K, Rafaelsen OJ. Pathological changes in the central and peripheral nervous system of young long-term diabetics. *Diabetologia* 1965;1:233–241.
66. Johnson PC, Brenedel K, Meezan E. Thickened cerebral cortical capillary basement membranes in diabetics. *Arch Pathol Lab Med* 1982;106:214–217.
67. Peress NS, Kane WC, Aronson SM. Central nervous system findings in a tenth decade autopsy population. *Prog Brain Res* 1973;40:473–483.
68. Peila R, Rodriguez BL, Launer LJ. Type 2 diabetes, APOE gene, and the risk for dementia and related pathologies: The Honolulu-Asia Aging Study. *Diabetes* 2002;51:1256–1262.
69. Janson J, Laedtke T, Parisi JE, O'Brien P, Petersen RC, Butler PC. Increased risk of type 2 diabetes in Alzheimer disease. *Diabetes* 2004;53:474–481.
70. Heitner J, Dickson D. Diabetics do not have increased Alzheimer-type pathology compared with age-matched control subjects. A retrospective postmortem immunocytochemical and histofluorescent study. *Neurology* 1997;49:1306–1311.
71. Dejgaard A, Gade A, Larsson H, Balle V, Parving A, Parving HH. Evidence for diabetic encephalopathy. *Diabetic Med* 1991;8:162–167.
72. Yousem DM, Tasman WS, Grossman RI. Proliferative retinopathy: absence of white matter lesions at MR imaging. *Radiology* 1991;179:229–230.
73. Lunetta M, Damanti AR, Fabbri G, Lombardo M, Di Mauro M, Mughini L. Evidence by magnetic resonance imaging of cerebral alterations of atrophy type in young insulin-dependent diabetic patients. *J Endocrinol Invest* 1994;17:241–245.
74. Perros P, Best JJK, Deary IJ, Frier BM, Sellar RJ. Brain abnormalities demonstrated by magnetic resonance imaging in adult IDDM patients with and without a history of recurrent severe hypoglycemia. *Diabetes Care* 1997;20:1013–1018.

75. Vermeer SE, den Heijer T, Koudstaal PJ, Oudkerk M, Hofman A, Breteler MM. Incidence and risk factors of silent brain infarcts in the population-based Rotterdam Scan Study. *Stroke* 2003;34:392–396.
76. Arauz A, Murillo L, Cantu C, Barinagarrementeria F, Higuera J. Prospective study of single and multiple lacunar infarcts using magnetic resonance imaging: risk factors, recurrence, and outcome in 175 consecutive cases. *Stroke* 2003;34:2453–2458.
77. Manolio TA, Kronmal RA, Burke GL, et al. Magnetic resonance abnormalities and cardiovascular disease in older adults. The Cardiovascular Health Study. *Stroke* 1994;25:318–327.
78. Schmidt R, Fazekas F, Kleinert G, et al. Magnetic resonance imaging signal hyperintensities in the deep and subcortical white matter. A comparative study between stroke patients and normal volunteers. *Arch Neurol* 1992;49:825–827.
79. Schmidt R, Launer LJ, Nilsson LG, et al. Magnetic resonance imaging of the brain in diabetes: the Cardiovascular Determinants of Dementia (CASCADE) Study. *Diabetes* 2004;53:687–692.
80. den Heijer T, Vermeer SE, van Dijk EJ, et al. Type 2 diabetes and atrophy of medial temporal lobe structures on brain MRI. *Diabetologia* 2003;46:1604–1610.
81. Soininen H, Puranen M, Helkala EL, Laakso M, Riekkinen PJ. Diabetes mellitus and brain atrophy: a computed tomography study in an elderly population. *Neurobiol Aging* 1992;13:717–721.
82. Biessels GJ, Manschot SM. The diabetic encephalopathy study group. Vascular risk factors for cognitive dysfunction in type 2 diabetes mellitus: study design and preliminary data. *J Neurol* 2003;250(S2):P718. Abstract.
83. Convit A, Wolf OT, Tarshish C, de Leon MJ. Reduced glucose tolerance is associated with poor memory performance and hippocampal atrophy among normal elderly. *Proc Natl Acad Sci USA* 2003;100:2019–2022.
84. Donald MW, Williams Erdahl DL, Surridge DHC, et al. Functional correlates of reduced central conduction velocity in diabetic subjects. *Diabetes* 1984;33:627–633.
85. Di Mario U, Morano S, Valle E, Pozzessere G. Electrophysiological alterations of the central nervous system in diabetes mellitus. *Diabetes Metab Rev* 1995;11:259–278.
86. Moreo G, Mariani E, Pizzamiglio G, Colucci GB. Visual evoked potentials in NIDDM: A longitudinal study. *Diabetologia* 1995;38:573–576.
87. Ziegler O, Guerci B, Algan M, Lonchamp P, Weber M, Drouin P. Improved visual evoked potential latencies in poorly controlled diabetic patients after short-term strict metabolic control. *Diabetes Care* 1994;17:1141–1147.
88. Parisi V, Uccioli L. Visual electrophysiological responses in persons with type 1 diabetes. *Diabetes Metab Res Rev* 2001;17:12–18.
89. Nakamura R, Noritake M, Hosoda Y, Kamakura K, Nagata N, Shibasaki H. Somatosensory conduction delay in central and peripheral nervous system of diabetic patients. *Diabetes Care* 1992;15:532–535.
90. Gupta PR, Dorfman LJ. Spinal somatosensory conduction in diabetes. *Neurology* 1981;31:841–845.
91. Bax G, Lelli S, Grandis U, Cospite AM, Paolo N, Fedele D. Early involvement of central nervous system type I diabetic patients. *Diabetes Care* 1995;18:559–562.
92. Mooradian AD, Perryman K, Fitten J, Kavonian GD, Morley JE. Cortical function in elderly non-insulin dependent diabetic patients. Behavioral and electrophysiologic studies. *Arch Intern Med* 1988;148:2369–2372.
93. Pozzessere G, Valle E, de-Crignis S, et al. Abnormalities of cognitive functions in IDDM revealed by P300 event-related potential analysis. Comparison with short-latency evoked potentials and psychometric tests. *Diabetes* 1991;40:952–958.

94. Picton TW. The P300 wave of the human event-related potential. *J Clin Neurophysiol* 1992;9:456–479.
95. Reichard P, Britz A, Rosenqvist U. Intensified conventional insulin treatment and neuropsychological impairment. *BMJ* 1991;303:1439–1442.
96. Naor M, Steingruber HJ, Westhoff K, Schottenfeld-Naor Y, Gries AF. Cognitive function in elderly non-insulin-dependent diabetic patients before and after inpatient treatment for metabolic control. *J Diabetes Complications* 1997;11:40–46.
97. Gradman TJ, Laws A, Thompson LW, Reaven GM. Verbal learning and/or memory improves with glycemic control in older subjects with non-insulin-dependent diabetes mellitus. *J Am Geriatr Soc* 1993;41:1305–1312.
98. Meneilly GS, Cheung E, Tessier D, Yakura C, Tuokko H. The effect of improved glycemic control on cognitive functions in the elderly patient with diabetes. *J Gerontol* 1993;48: M117–M121.
99. Wu JH, Haan MN, Liang J, Ghosh D, Gonzalez HM, Herman WH. Impact of antidiabetic medications on physical and cognitive functioning of older Mexican Americans with diabetes mellitus: a population-based cohort study. *Ann Epidemiol* 2003;13:369–376.
100. Mussell M, Hewer W, Kulzer B, Bergis K, Rist F. Effects of improved glycaemic control maintained for 3 months on cognitive function in patients with Type 2 diabetes. *Diabet Med* 2004;21:1253–1256.
101. Areosa Sastre A, Grimley Evans V. Effect of the treatment of Type II diabetes mellitus on the development of cognitive impairment and dementia. *Cochrane Database Syst Rev* 2003;CD003804.
102. Berk-Planken I, de K, I Stolk R, Jansen H, Hoogerbrugge N. Atorvastatin, diabetic dyslipidemia, and cognitive functioning. *Diabetes Care* 2002;25:1250–1251.
103. Sandeep TC, Yau JL, MacLullich AM, et al. 11Beta-hydroxysteroid dehydrogenase inhibition improves cognitive function in healthy elderly men and type 2 diabetics. *Proc Natl Acad Sci USA* 2004;101:6734–6739.
104. Watson GS, Reger MA, Cholerton BA, et al. Rosiglitazone preserves cognitive functions in patients with early Alzheimer's disease. *Neurobiol Aging* 2004;25(S2):S83 Abstract.
105. Lawton MP, Brody EM. Assessment of older people: self-maintaining and instrumental activities of daily living. *Gerontologist* 1969;9:179–186.
106. Zakzanis KK. Statistics to tell the truth, the whole truth, and nothing but the truth. Formulae, illustrative numerical examples, and heuristic interpretation of effect size analyses for neuropsychological researchers. *Arch Clin Neuropsychol* 2001;16:653–667.
107. Yoshitake T, Kiyohara Y, Kato I, et al. Incidence and risk factors of vascular dementia and Alzheimer's disease in a defined elderly Japanese population: the Hisayama Study. *Neurology* 1995;45:1161–1168.
108. Leibson CL, Rocca WA, Hanson VA, et al. Risk of dementia among persons with diabetes mellitus: a population-based cohort study. *Am J Epidemiol* 1997;145:301–308.
109. Ott A, Stolk RP, Van Harskamp F, Pols HA, Hofman A, Breteler MM. Diabetes mellitus and the risk of dementia: The Rotterdam Study. *Neurology* 1999;53:1937–1942.
110. MacKnight C, Rockwood K, Awalt E, McDowell I. Diabetes mellitus and the risk of dementia, Alzheimer's disease and vascular cognitive impairment in the Canadian Study of Health and Aging. *Dement Geriatr Cogn Disord* 2002;14:77–83.
111. Hassing LB, Johansson B, Nilsson SE, et al. Diabetes mellitus is a risk factor for vascular dementia, but not for Alzheimer's disease: a population-based study of the oldest old. *Int Psychogeriatr* 2002;14:239–248.
112. Arvanitakis Z, Wilson RS, Bienias JL, Evans DA, Bennett DA. Diabetes mellitus and risk of Alzheimer disease and decline in cognitive function. *Arch Neurol* 2004;61:661–666.
113. Xu WL, Qiu CX, Wahlin A, Winblad B, Fratiglioni L. Diabetes mellitus and risk of dementia in the Kungsholmen project: a 6-year follow-up study. *Neurology* 2004;63:1181–1186.

114. Lezak MD, Howieson DB, Loring DW. *Neuropsychological Assessment.* New York: Oxford Press, 2004.
115. Ryan C, Vega A, Drash A. Cognitive deficits in adolescents who developed diabetes early in life. *Pediatrics* 1985;75:921–927.
116. Scheltens P, Barkhof F, Leys D, et al. A semiquantative rating scale for the assessment of signal hyperintensities on magnetic resonance imaging. *J Neurol Sci* 1993;114:7–12.

12

Microangiopathy, Diabetes, and the Peripheral Nervous System

Douglas W. Zochodne, MD (FRCPC)

SUMMARY

This chapter reviews how disease of small nerve and ganglia microvessels, or microangiopathy, relates to the development of diabetic peripheral neuropathy. Microangiopathy involving vessels of the nerve trunk and those of dorsal root ganglia (that house sensory neuron cell bodies), does develop in parallel with neuropathy and is likely to eventually contribute to it. It is debatable whether early polyneuropathy in models or in humans can be exclusively linked to reductions in the blood supply of nerves. More likely, diabetes targets neural structures and vessels concurrently. There might be chronic ganglion ischemia altering neuronal function such that terminal branches of the nerve can no longer be properly supported. Downregulation, in turn, of critical structural and survival proteins in the sensory (or autonomic) neuron tree might account for early sensory dysfunction and pain (or autonomic abnormalities). There might also be exquisite sensitivity of vessels to vasoconstriction as an early functional abnormality. Rises in local endothelin levels, for example, might trigger acute nerve trunk and ganglion ischemia, and damage. Finally, failed upregulation of blood flow to injured nerves after acute injury might impair their ability to regenerate. Future therapy of diabetic polyneuropathy will require attention toward both direct neuronal degeneration and superimposed microangiopathy.

Key Words: Diabetic neuropathy; ganglion blood flow; ischemia; microangiopathy; nerve blood flow; nerve injury; regeneration; vasa nervorum.

INTRODUCTION

Microangiopathy, or dysfunction of small blood vessels, is closely linked to diabetic complications, such as nephropathy and retinopathy. Microangiopathy is also closely associated with the third complication of this triad, polyneuropathy, but its exact role in the development of nerve disease is uncertain. It is probably incorrect to conclude that microvascular disease is the primary trigger of neuropathic complications, an assumption that ignores direct neuronal damage. Instead, there is significant evidence that a unique neuroscience of diabetic neuropathy exists. The evidence that diabetes has direct impacts on sensory neuron structure and function independently of microangiopathy is reviewed in depth elsewhere *(1)*. Overall, it might be more accurate to depict chronic diabetes as involving nerve trunks, ganglion, and their respective microvessels in parallel, a process that can eventually lead to a vicious interacting cycle of damage. In some situations, such as focal nerve trunk ischemic insults or

From: *Contemporary Diabetes: Diabetic Neuropathy: Clinical Management, Second Edition*
Edited by: A. Veves and R. Malik © Humana Press Inc., Totowa, NJ

mechanical nerve injury, the relative contribution of microangiopathy might be higher. Although, a detailed technical appraisal of relationships between nerve blood flow in published work and experimental neuropathy has been recently published separately, this review will highlight and summarize some of this controversy *(2)*. In this work, aspects of nerve and ganglion blood flow and its measurement, models of ischemia, and evidence for diabetic peripheral nerve and ganglion microangiopathy are emphasized and reviewed.

BLOOD FLOW OF NERVE TRUNKS AND GANGLIA

The characteristics of the blood flow in nerve trunks and ganglia are unique and are distinguished from those of the central nervous system. Nerve trunks are supplied upstream by arterial branches of major limb vessels that share their supply with other limb tissues. At some sites, the overlapping vascular supply from several parent vessels renders zones of susceptibility to ischemia, or watershed zones. In the rat, and probably human sciatic nerve, a watershed zone can be found in the proximal tibial nerve *(3)*. In some nerve trunks, the centrofascicular portion of the nerve trunk might be the most vulnerable to ischemia, accounting for corresponding centrofascicular patterns of axon damage. However, ischemic damage of large multifascicular nerve trunks is more commonly multifocal, with irregular zones of axon damage that depend on specific features of their perfusion and the exact vessels that are involved in causing ischemia *(4,5)*. In general, nerve trunks are well-perfused from multiple anastamosing parent arteries that ultimately form a rich epineurial vascular plexus on it. Such a rich vascular supply explains why long segments of nerves can be "mobilized" by surgeons without major sequellae. Arteriovenous anastamoses are common in the epineurial plexus, but some might also exist in the endoneurium *(6)*. Because of this rich complex of vessels, it can be surprisingly difficult to distinguish arterioles from venules in the epineurial plexus when they are directly visualized in vivo.

Spinal dorsal root ganglia are supplied from segmental radicular arteries and anastamoses with branches of spinal arteries *(7)*. Unlike the peripheral nerve trunk, they do not have a prominent extracapsular plexus. Neuron perikarya that entrain higher metabolic requirements are most often located in the subcapsular space, whereas axons eventually entering roots are more frequently found in the core of the ganglia. Given this structure, microanatomic susceptibility of the ganglia to ischemia is probably even less predictable than that of nerve trunks.

Peripheral nerve trunks are supplied by blood vessels from two distinct compartments: the epineurial vascular plexus and the intrinsic endoneurial blood supply. Although, extrinsic epineurial blood flow is ultimately responsible for "downstream" blood flow in the endoneurial compartment, each compartment has distinct physiological and morphological characteristics. The epineurial plexus, as discussed, is well-perfused by arterioles, has prominent arteriovenous shunting, has innervation of its arterioles, discussed further below, and has a leaky blood–nerve barrier. This plexus supplies segmental arterioles that penetrate into the endoneurium directly or that arrive there from a remote origin traveling in a longitudinal centrofascicular pattern. Although not an absolute rule, the endoneurium is largely supplied by noninnervated capillaries that respond passively to changes in blood flow. Pericytes, smooth muscle-like contractile cells, are associated with some endoneurial capillary segments, but how they influence local blood flow is uncertain. Endoneurial capillaries might also be somewhat larger than those of other tissue beds *(8)*.

Epineurial arterioles are innervated by sympathetic adrenergic unmyelinated axons that mediate local vasoconstriction and peptidergic (Substance P, calcitonin gene-related peptide [CGRP]) sensory axons that in turn mediate local vasodilatation *(9,10)*. CGRP is a highly potent vasodilator, capable of relaxing vascular smooth muscle through both nitric oxide (NO)-dependent and -independent pathways *(11,12)*. An interesting feature of both the adrenergic and peptidergic vascular innervation is that both types of axons appear to arise from their parent nerve trunk *(13)*. Moreover, there is evidence that this innervation is tonically active, influencing the ambient caliber of arterioles of the epineurial plexus. Ongoing sympathetic and concurrent peptidergic "tone" of the epineurial vascular plexus, thus, can direct downstream endoneurial capillary blood flow. Sympathetic blockade or sympathectomy to block ongoing adrenergic tone in the normal vasa nervorum consequently is associated with rises in endoneurial nerve blood flow, whereas blockade of peptidergic innervation is associated with declines in nerve blood flow *(14–16)*. Among neuropeptides that influence vascular caliber, CGRP is likely the most potent candidate identified, although it has been observed that both Substance P (SP) and CGRP antagonists were associated with constriction of vasa nervorum *(16)*. Although not explored in peptidergic perivascular axons, the adrenergic innervation of epineurial arterioles is probably nonuniform and segmental, suggesting the presence of discrete zones of vascular regulation that might control "downstream" endoneurial capillary flow *(14)*. Hypercarbia might be associated with mild rises in epineurial plexus blood flow, but appears to have less impact on endoneurial blood flow *(17,18)*. There is very little evidence of autoregulation in peripheral nerve trunks, but instead there is a near linear passive relationship between mean arterial pressure and endoneurial blood flow *(18)*.

Quantitative hydrogen clearance (HC) or autoradiographic [^{14}C] iodoantipyrene measures of normal endoneurial blood flow yield values in the range of 15–20 mL/100 g per minute *(18,19)*.

Dorsal root ganglia, and probably sympathetic ganglia have higher levels of blood flow measuring approximately 30–40 mL/100 g per minute *(20,21)*. These higher values likely reflect higher metabolic demands of perikarya in ganglia than stable axons and Schwann cells in the nerve trunk. Similarly, oxygen tension values measured in ganglia are shifted to lower values, implying increased oxygen extraction. Such measures have been carried out using oxygen sensitive microelectrodes and polarography, an approach that constructs histograms of oxygen tension values in tissues to circumvent the variability of single estimates of oxygen tension *(22,23)*. Neither nerve trunks nor ganglia are as well perfused as spinal cord gray matter that ranges approximately 50–60 mL/100 g per minute or cortex ranging more than 100 mL/100 g per minute depending on the measurement approach *(24)*. Unlike peripheral nerve trunks, there is some evidence of partial autoregulation of ganglion blood flow, but a lesser influence of adrenergic input *(25)*. Hypercarbia does not appear to influence ganglion blood flow *(20)*.

Although newer imaging approaches might be capable of providing blood flow measures within nerve, published measures have concentrated on a few approaches: quantitative microelectrode HC polarography, laser doppler flowmetry (LDF), [^{14}C] idioantipyrene distribution or autoradiography, and microsphere embolization. Detailed appraisal of the methodology and its pitfalls is given elsewhere *(2,26)* and is only briefly highlighted here. Ancillary approaches have included direct live videoangiographic imaging of epineurial vessels *(14)*, morphometric measures of fixed or unfixed peripheral nerves *(27,28)*, and measures of indicator transit times *(29)*. Combining approaches to address primarily the epineurial plexus (LDF) and the endoneurium (HC) is a powerful way to confirm and supplement findings as both compartments have strong linkages as discussed earlier. HC requires rigorous physiological support and characterization, and locally manufactured linearly sensitive hydrogen microelectrodes with small diameter tips of 3–5 μm. Some publications have used very large microelectrodes that might excessively disrupt sampled nerves *(30–34)*. HC and autoradiographic [^{14}C] idioantipyrene distribution both offer quantitative measures of selective endoneurial blood flow, but only the former can offer serial studies. LDF is sensitive to real time changes in erythrocyte flux, but vigorous care and controls in its use are required: lighting conditions, multiple sampling, micromanipulator use, and (like all techniques) strict control of near nerve temperature. Because LDF measures can vary widely depending on the exact placement of the sampling probe, single measures are likely to be highly unreliable. For instance a small movement of the probe might shift its sampling sphere to a nearby superficial vessel, substantially altering the read out. Kalichman and Lalonde *(35)* pointed out the importance of obtaining multiple samples of LDF along the nerve trunk to provide meaningful measures. Microsphere embolization measures have yielded somewhat lower blood flow values in peripheral nerve trunks, and this might be a technical limitation of the approach *(36–38)*. Arteriovenous (AV) shunts might allow passage rather than capture of indicator microsphere, underestimating their distribution. Other isotope distribution techniques have used [^{3}H] desmethylimipramine and [^{14}C] butanol *(39,40)*.

ACUTE NERVE ISCHEMIA

It is important when considering some types of neuropathy in diabetes to ask whether ischemia plays a role. Peripheral nerve trunks are resistant to acute ischemia in part because of their rich anastamotic vascular supply and their limited metabolic demands. Several models of experimental ischemic neuropathy have been developed ranging from multiple arterial ligation, embolization by microspheres or other agents, and the topical application of the potent vasoconstrictor endothelin *(3,41–50)*. Chronic constriction injury, a model of neuropathic pain *(51)* likely develops from ischemia generated by the placement of four loose ligatures applied around a nerve trunk with gradual swelling and “strangulation” *(52)*. To irreversibly damage axons acutely, ischemia must be severe and continuous for approximately 3 hours in nondiabetic peripheral nerves *(50)*.

Several important observations have emerged from these studies that are of relevance to the understanding of localized, or focal diabetic neuropathies. It is clear that focal compressive types of nerve injury, such as ulnar neuropathy at the elbow or carpal tunnel syndrome, are unlikely to be ischemic in origin; it is unlikely that a single compressive lesion would disrupt the rich nerve vascular supply. Direct investigations of blood flow at sites of nerve crush or transection have not identified ischemia *(53,54)*. Instead, blood flow is well maintained even immediately after injury at crush sites, and tends to rise with time. However, as discussed later, it is possible that diabetic microangiopathy might impair reactive changes in local blood flow that support regeneration after injury.

Some forms of focal diabetic nerve injury at "nonentrapment" sites might have an ischemic origin. For example, diabetic lumbosacral plexopathy is thought to be a consequence of focal plexus ischemia either from microangiopathy or superimposed vascular inflammation *(55,56)*. As demonstrated in work by Nukada *(57,58)*, experimental diabetic nerves rendered even mildly ischemic develop more severe axonal damage than nondiabetic nerve. Similar findings were encountered in nerve trunks exposed to the potent vasoconstrictor endothelin *(5,59)*. Rat diabetic sciatic nerves exposed to topical endothelin experienced more prolonged and severe vasoconstriction leading to focal axon nerve conduction block followed by local axonal degeneration. Axonal damage in diabetic nerves exposed to epineurial topical endothelin also had a striking multifocal distribution, resembling changes in human diabetic sural nerve biopsies. Rises in serum endothelin levels have been reported in some human studies, but not others, and it is not certain whether transient or acute localized rises might damage human peripheral nerves *(60–62)*.

Models of sensory ganglion ischemia might be relevant in considering acute focal exacerbations of sensory neuropathy in diabetes. This possibility has had less attention, but as in nerve trunks, ganglia also appear more sensitive in diabetes to ischemic damage from exposure to local endothelin vasoconstriction. Ischemia generated ischemic necrosis of some sensory neurons, intraganglionic axon damage, and downstream degeneration of the distal sural nerve axon branches of the targeted perikarya *(63)* (Fig. 1). Neurons disappeared and were replaced by nests of Nageotte, had peripheral displacement of their nuclei, loss of neurofilaments, nuclear disruption, and had nuclear Terminal transferase dUTP nick end labeling (TUNEL). Interestingly, ischemia of diabetic ganglia thus resulted in three separate pathological reactions among neuron perikarya: ischemic necrosis of neurons, probable apoptosis of sensory neurons, and a retrograde cell body response to axonal damage.

MICROANGIOPATHY, DIABETES, AND THE PERIPHERAL NERVOUS SYSTEM: EXPERIMENTAL STUDIES

Tuck and colleagues *(22)* initially reported that experimental diabetes of rats was associated with a decline of sciatic nerve blood flow and endoneurial hypoxia. Several other laboratories have reported similar findings and a variety of interventions have been reported to both correct nerve blood flow and diabetic electrophysiological abnormalities in tandem (*see* review *[2]*). A large number of such studies through their findings have consequently implied that reductions in nerve blood flow initiate the changes of diabetic neuropathy. Although this body of work has undoubtedly provided evidence of a linkage, cause and effect has not been proven. A number of the reports have arisen from relatively few experimental laboratories *(33,34,64–97)*. Similarly, the spectrum of agents reported to correct blood flow and conduction slowing has been very wide. As such, this range of apparently beneficial interventions raises the strong possibility that they exert parallel benefits on separate, but not necessarily linked changes from diabetes. Most such studies have also not addressed the impact of interventional agents at the level of ganglia rather than nerve trunk.

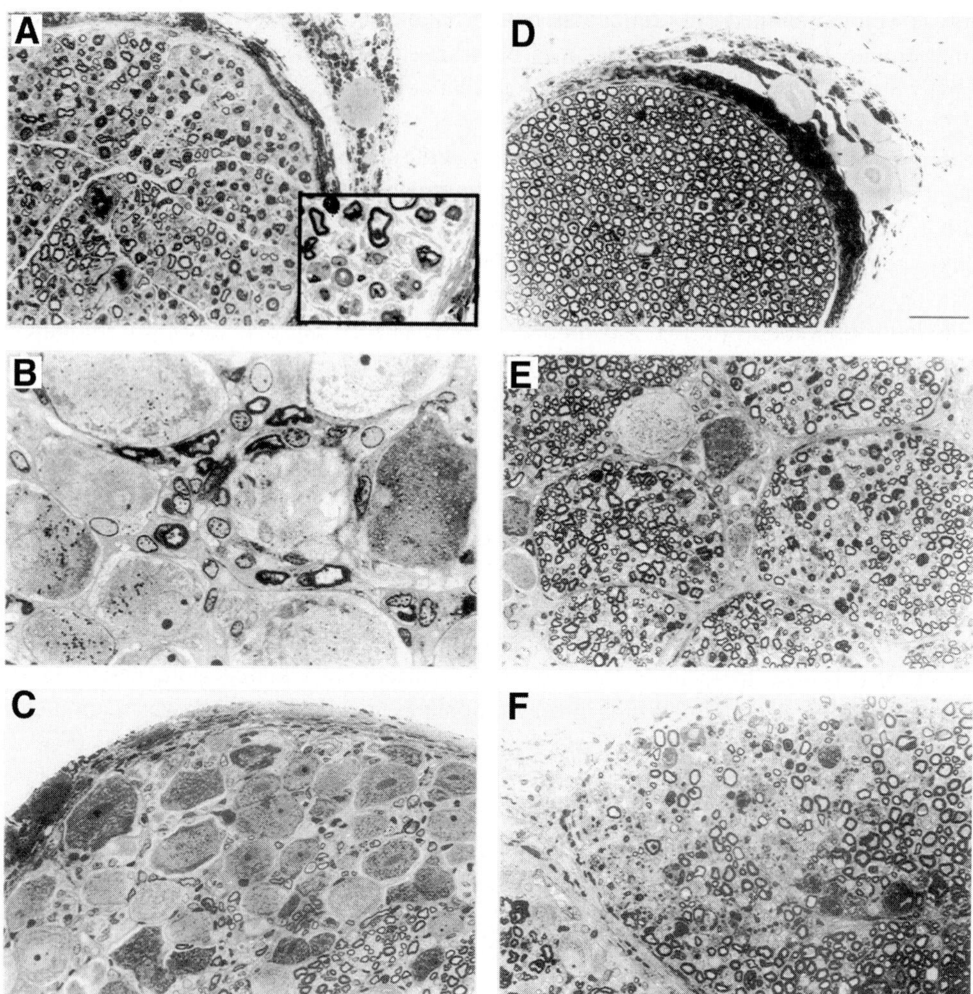

Fig. 1. Images of a L5 lumbar dorsal root ganglion and sural nerve from diabetic and nondiabetic rats exposed 2 weeks earlier to local endothelin: **(A)** Vasoconstriction in diabetics resulted in downstream sural nerve axonal degeneration (inset shows higher power). **(B)** Karyoylsis and early formation of a nest of Nageotte from a dying neuron (below it is an intact neuron with a displaced nucleus, illustrating a cell body response to axotomy). **(E,F)** Intranganglionic axonal degeneration. In contrast there is relatively little damage in a nondiabetic ganglion and sural nerve (**C,D** respectively). Bar = 50 μm for **A**, **C–F** and 20 μm for **B**. (Reproduced with permission from ref. *63*.)

Several experimental interventions have corrected electrophysiological and structural abnormalities of diabetic axons without an action on microvessels. For example, both intermittent near nerve and chronic neuron perikaryal exposure to intrathecal insulin infusion that provided low subhypoglycemic doses, corrected axon conduction slowing in experimental diabetes *(98,99)*. A direct receptor-mediated neuron cell support pathway is mediated by insulin that is unrelated to microvessels. In addition, intrathecal insulin reversed axon atrophy, whereas sequestration of endogenous intrathecal insulin by an anti-insulin antibody in nondiabetic rats generated abnormalities of conduction and caliber resembling those of diabetes *(99)*. In another example, transgenic mice lacking axon neurofilaments, (but without vascular abnormalities) had electrophysiological and structural features of neuropathy that were accelerated *(100)*.

Some of the studies examining nerve blood flow in experimental diabetes have had methodological weaknesses, such as failure to strictly maintain near nerve temperature, incorrectly described hydrogen microelectrodes, excessively large microelectrodes, and single uncontrolled LDF measures. Other laboratories, including ours, have failed to identify declines in nerve blood flow, using rigorously controlled HC or LDF in Streptozotocin (STZ) or BioBreeding Wistar (BBW) rat models of diabetes of varying durations *(23,101–103)*. One laboratory consistently described contrary rises in nerve blood flow in their diabetes models *(36–38,104)*. Moreover, despite more consistent findings of shifts toward lower levels of endoneurial oxygen in the very few studies that have addressed this change, these findings do not necessarily imply that blood flow need be reduced. Changes in erythrocyte oxygen delivery might develop in diabetes, depending on changes in perfusion. Careful morphometric studies, including those using unfixed tissues, have not identified reduced vessel calibers or numbers *(27,28,105)*, excepting one study criticized for using nonvalidated measures of nerve perfusion (whole nerve laser doppler imaging and counts of fluorescein perfused vessels of whole nerve *[106]*). Morphological changes of axons, an expected consequence of ischemia, are usually very mild in diabetic rat models indicating axonal atrophy. In contrast, there might be loss of epidermal axons in the skin (without tissue breakdown or damage otherwise), a finding similarly difficult to link with nerve trunk or skin microangiopathy. Accurate measures of nerve and ganglion blood flow in mouse models of diabetes have also not been available to date for technical reasons.

Four separate studies have identified reductions in lumbar dorsal root ganglion blood flow in experimental diabetes in rats: three in STZ rats using HC or [^{14}C] iodoantipyrene distribution and one in BBW rats *(63,102,103,107)*. In two of the studies, ganglion, but not nerve blood flow was reduced by diabetes. In the studies of BBW spontaneously diabetic female rats blood flow was normal in ganglia and nerve 2–3 months after the onset of diabetes, then declined to values less than nondiabetics by 4–6 months (Fig. 2). Oxygen tension measures trended toward lower values in nerve and ganglia (Fig. 3). In ganglia it might be that changes in blood flow and oxygen tension do not occur in parallel because there might also be decreases in oxygen extraction as blood flow declines.

A distinct feature of diabetic microangiopathy is its selective impact on vasodilation. The consequence of this alteration has been unopposed vasoconstrictor sensitivity both in large macrovessels and the microcirculatory bed (Fig. 4). Loss of vasodilation in diabetes might be secondary to vascular unresponsiveneness to NO *(108–113)*, accelerated "quenching" of intraluminal NO by advanced glycosylation end products *(114)*, or endothelial damage that fails to normally elaborate it *(115,116)*. NO synthase isoforms (NOS) protein or messenger RNA (mRNA) were not altered by experimental diabetes in our laboratory beyond a slight decline in iNOS. Thus, deficits in NO vascular actions in diabetic nerves likely reflect failed action rather than a decline in its synthesis in diabetes.

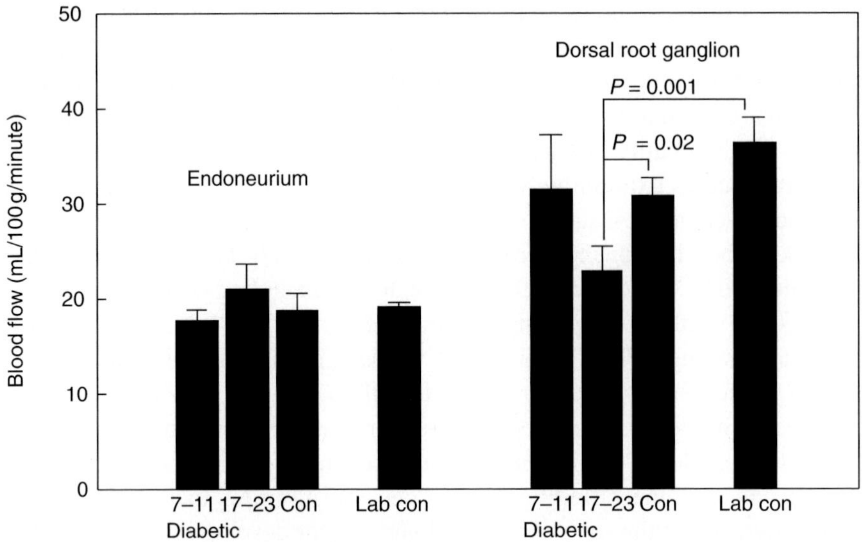

Fig. 2. Local measurements of nerve and ganglion blood flow using microelectrode HC polarography. On the left side of the bar chart, note that endoneurial blood flow measures were unaltered in BBW diabetic rats after 7–11 weeks of diabetes or 17–23 weeks of diabetes compared with nondiabetic littermates Control (Con). In L5 dorsal root ganglia, however, older diabetics did have a reduction in ganglion blood flow. Results are also compared with pooled values from normal rats (Lab con). (Reproduced with permission from ref. *103*.)

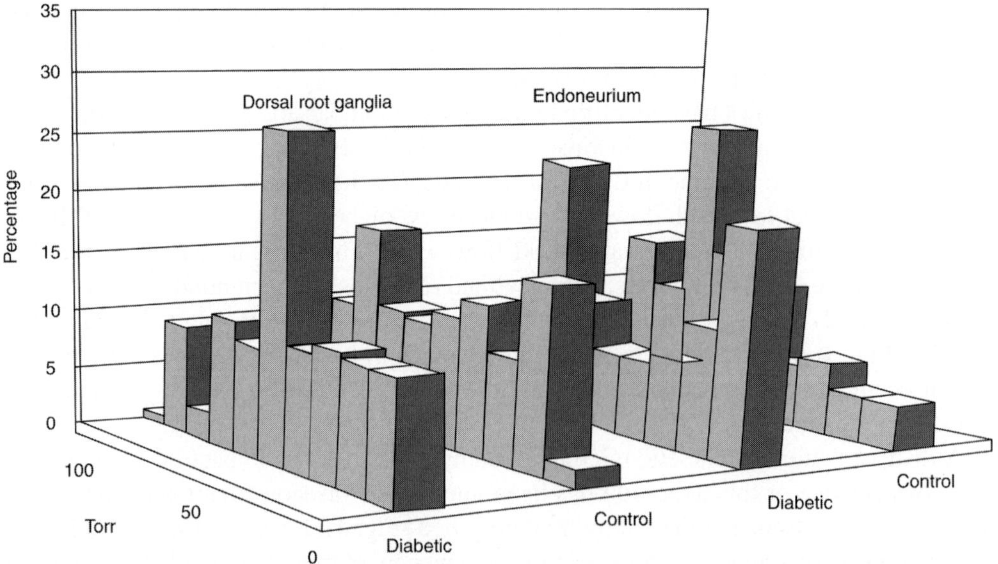

Fig. 3. Composite bar charts showing pooled oxygen tension histograms from experimental diabetes work carried out in the Zochodne lab. The values are constructed from multiple sampling in groups of diabetic rats (STZ or BBW) of diabetes duration 4 months or longer and nondiabetic littermates. Note that there are shifts toward lower oxygen tension levels in both the endoneurium and dorsal root ganglia of diabetic rats and that there are more lower level oxygen tension values in ganglia than endoneurium from nondiabetic rats.

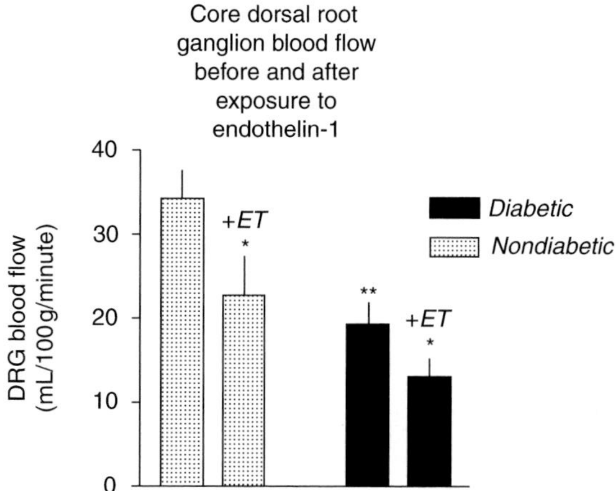

Fig. 4. Local measurements of L5 ganglion blood flow using microelectrode HC polarography in diabetic rats and nondiabetic littermates before and after exposure to local endothelin. Baseline blood flow was reduced in diabetics. With endothelin exposure, diabetic ganglion blood flow declined to lower values and had a prolonged action (not shown) rendering ischemic damage (Fig. 1). (Reproduced with permission from ref. *63.*)

Indeed, overall NOS enzyme activity was increased, perhaps indicating a compensatory rise in its production in the setting of accelerated consumption *(117)*. Diabetes might also be associated with unresponsiveness to peptide vasodilatation *(118)*, loss of perivascular peptidergic axons innervating vasa nervorum *(119)*, increased sensitivity to angiotensin II *(120)*, increased adrenergic tone *(121)*, or decreased vasodilation from prostacyclin *(122)* (Fig. 5).

If not a "triggering" event in the development of diabetic polyneuropathy, microangiopathy does account for some unique properties of diabetic nerves. As discussed earlier, diabetic peripheral nerve trunks exposed to a mild ischemic insult unexpectedly develop severe damage to axons. Such damage can occur in spite of axon resistance to ischemic conduction failure (RICF), a property whereby ischemic axons have a delayed loss of excitability. RICF is an invariable, though not exclusive, electrophysiological property of diabetic axons that is linked to chronic hypoxia and excess glucose substrate *(123)*. RICF might be thought of as a mechanism of protecting diabetic axons, yet it fails to protect them from ischemia lasting longer than the duration of even prolonged RICF (its duration is approximately 25–35 minutes after complete ischemia and is defined most often as the time for a 50% decline in motor axon excitability). For longer durations of ischemia, diabetic axons are more likely to undergo axonal degeneration than nondiabetic axons when exposed to ischemia. In nondiabetic nerves, complete ischemia of 1–3 hours is required to damage axons. In diabetic nerves, pre-existing hypoxia and loss of compensatory vasodilation are both likely to contribute to their vulnerability.

DIABETES, REGENERATION, AND THE MICROCIRCULATION

Microangiopathy likely impacts the regenerative microenvironment of an injured diabetic peripheral nerve trunk. Focal lesions or mononeuropathies are common and

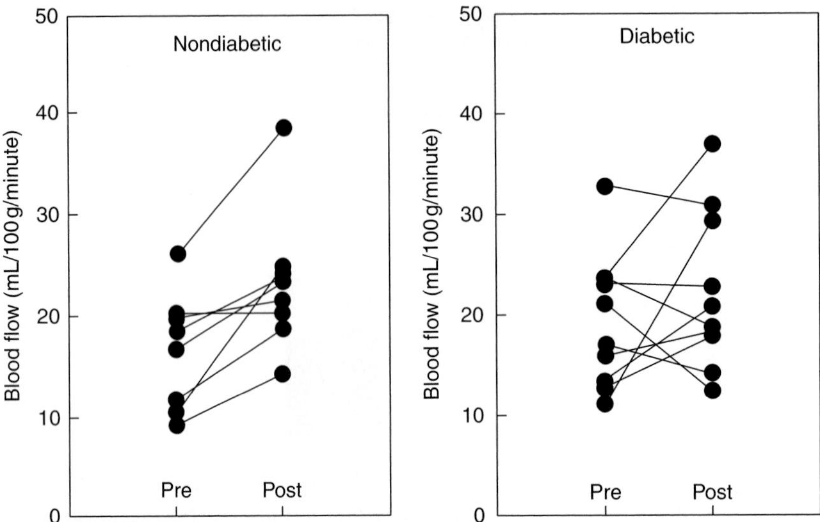

Fig. 5. Local measurements of sciatic nerve blood flow using microelectrode HC polarography in nondiabetic rats (left) and diabetic rats (right) before (pre) and after (post) exposure to topical capsaicin. Capsaicin generates acute release of vasoactive peptides from perivascular sensory terminals after topical application. In nondiabetic rats, there are prompt rises in endoneurial blood flow from acute activation of peptidergic epineurial vasodilatation. The rise was inconsistent and insignificant in diabetic rats.

disabling in diabetes. Examples are carpal tunnel syndrome, intercostal neuropathies, and lumbosacral plexopathies. These focal peripheral nerve lesions regenerate more slowly in diabetics than nondiabetics *(124,125)* and regeneration from them might be incapable of restoring function in many patients. If clinical therapy to arrest polyneuropathy is developed, attention will shift toward understanding how diabetic nerves with failed regeneration might be resurrected.

Ischemic peripheral nerve lesions also have impaired regeneration *(126)*. What level of perfusion is required to sustain or enhance regenerative activity involving axons, Schwann cells, and other cellular constituents is unknown. "Normal" rises in local blood flow, that develop when peripheral nerves are injured, are robust, persistent, and probably important in supporting nerve repair. Despite early work suggesting otherwise, most focal injuries of peripheral nerves do not involve ischemia. For example, at the site of an acute nerve crush, there might be expectations of local vessel disruption, local microthrombosis, and endoneurial edema. However, direct blood flow measures of blood flow at the site of experimental crush in rats, indicate that injured nerve trunks compensate for such microvascular disruptions with preserved and enhanced local blood flow *(53,54)*. Moreover, by 24–48 hours, endoneurial and epineurial blood flow rises substantially after peripheral nerve injury, a development linked to local actions of CGRP and NO *(54,127,128)*. Their elaboration within this microenvironment is part of an interesting and complex story involving the formation of axonal endbulbs and accumulation of peptides and enzymes within them. In the case of NO, accumulation of NOS within endbulbs allows diffusion of the vasodilator to nearby microvessels. Within a few days following nerve injury, angiogenesis, especially prominent in the epineurial plexus, ensues and is associated with local rises in vascular endothelial growth factor (VEGF) mRNA *(129,130)*. Neovascularization develops concurrently with other events within the nerve trunk involving axon outgrowth and Schwann cell (SC) proliferation.

Distal stumps of severed peripheral nerves eventually, become inhospitable to new axon entry. Several factors contribute to the hostility of long-term denervated nerve stumps including changes in their microvascular supply. Distal nerve stumps that remained unconnected for 6 months had a decline in their epineurial (LDF) and endoneurial (HC) blood flow by more than 50% *(129)*. Although new blood vessels formed soon after injury were retained in these stumps, their caliber and number gradually declined as did VEGF mRNA levels. Overall the remodeling of the microvascular supply with prolonged denervation is interesting and highlights a close relationship between axons and microvessels in the peripheral nerve. These changes also render an unsuitable ischemic microenvironment for late regeneration, should the nerve be reconnected. In injured diabetic nerves, distal nerve stumps that have not been reinnervated because of slowed regeneration suffer such problems that then impose further barriers to regrowth. In addition to ischemia, long-term denervated nerve trunks undergo other changes that make them less hospitable including Schwann cell atrophy, loss of growth factor synthesis (e.g., Glial cell line-derived neurotrophic factor [GDNF]), and perhaps excessive collagen elaboration with fibrosis *(131–133)*.

In diabetic nerve trunks that are transected, rises in local blood flow in both the proximal and distal stumps of the nerve are attenuated and angiogenesis is dampened. Kennedy and Zochodne *(134)* described microvascular changes associated with transected sciatic peripheral nerve trunks in rats with experimental diabetes (STZ) of 8 month duration using quantitative HC measures of endoneurial flow and multiple LDF epineurial plexus sampling. The findings were correlated with quantitation of endoneurial and epineurial vessels by India ink perfusion using unfixed tissues. As described earlier, nondiabetic rats exhibit substantial rises in local nerve blood flow, or hyperemia in both proximal and distal nerve stumps that is evident at both 48 hours and 2 weeks after injury. Although diabetic nerve trunks had normal, unaltered blood flow after sham exposure without injury, epineurial rises in blood flow following injury were almost completely dampened. Rises in blood flow within the endoneurium also failed to develop in diabetic nerves at 48 hours, but began to rise by 2 weeks (Fig. 6). There were rises in the numbers of epineurial vascular profiles in nondiabetic, but not in diabetic rats in the distal and proximal stumps. Similarly, there were substantial rises in mean vascular luminal areas of both endoneurial and epineurial vessels of the proximal and distal stumps after transection that were almost completely attenuated in diabetic vessels (Figs. 7 and 8). Overall the findings suggested that diabetic functional microangiopathy imposes severe limitations on the capability of vasa nervorum to respond to injury. These limitations involve both failed epineurial and endoneurial vascular dilatation and a somewhat later failure of compensatory angiogenesis.

Additional work indicates that diabetic nerves also fail to upregulate NOS activity at the site of a peripheral nerve injury. Normally, iNOS expression and activity rise following peripheral nerve injury concomitant with SC phagocytic activity and macrophage invasion. Both SCs and macrophages express iNOS *(135)*. Rises of iNOS activity in turn, are important in facilitating the process of Wallerian degeneration through clearance of axon and probably more importantly, myelin components that inhibit regeneration. As such, effective clearance is a prerequisite for later successful axonal ingrowth. Nondiabetic

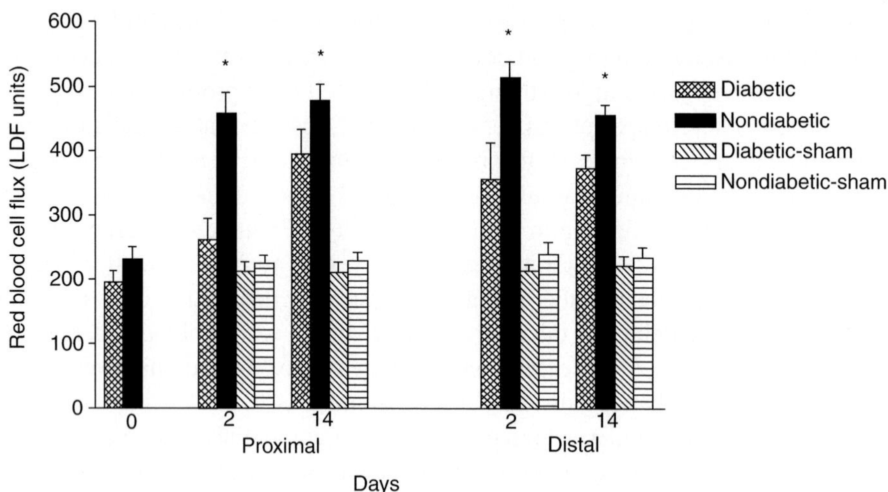

Fig. 6. Local measurements of erythrocyte flux (LDF) made in rats with experimental diabetes of 8 months duration and littermates, proximal and distal to a sciatic nerve transection. Note the prominent rises in blood flow after injury in nondiabetic sciatic nerves that are attenuated in diabetics. There are no changes in flux of intact nerves in diabetic rats (sham surgery). (*$p < 0.05$ between diabetics and nondiabetics). (Reproduced with modifications and permission from ref. *134.*)

mice lacking iNOS have delays in the progress of Wallerian degeneration and subsequent regeneration *(136)*.

MICROANGIOPATHY, DIABETES, AND THE PERIPHERAL NERVOUS SYSTEM

Human Investigations

There have been a limited number of human investigations of nerve trunk microangiopathy in diabetes. The earliest and most convincing data are rigorous morphological studies of epineurial and endoneurial blood vessels in human sural nerve biopsies. These have identified microthrombosis and microvessel occlusion in diabetic nerves, endothelial duplication, smooth muscle proliferation, endoneurial capillary closure, basement membrane thickening, pericyte degeneration, and other changes *(105,137–146)*. The loss of axons in a multifocal pattern in such biopsies has also suggested an ischemic or microvascular etiology *(4,140,141,147)*. However, it is difficult to ascribe cause and effect to morphological changes of peripheral nerve biopsies because they cannot tell us whether the changes in vessels parallel or follow loss of axons or other abnormalities. In earlier investigations, such biopsies were harvested from older patients with already existing neuropathy. More recently, however, Malik and colleagues *(148)* have demonstrated that microvascular changes might develop early in patients with only mild neuropathy, findings that suggest a role in promoting axonal damage. Similarly recent work by Tesfaye and colleagues *(149)* has linked the development of neuropathy with risk factors for cardiovascular disease, as well as implying a close relationship between macrovessels and neuropathy.

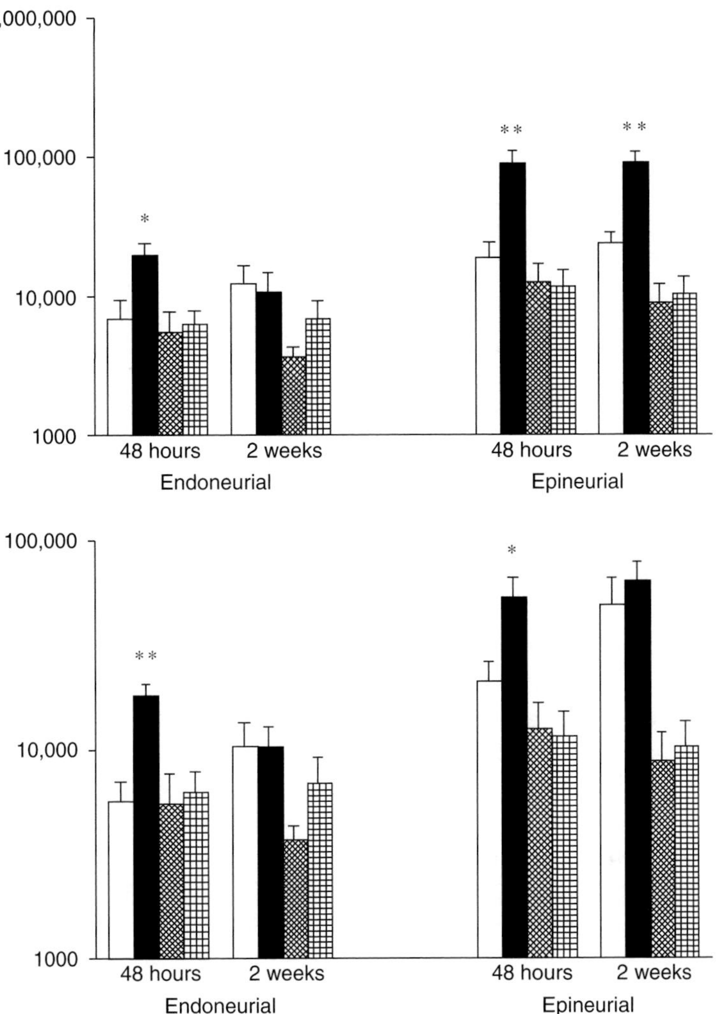

Fig. 7. Total vascular luminal areas of vasa nervorum from nerves of 8 month diabetic rats or littermates proximal (above) or distal (below) to a sciatic nerve transection. The rats were perfused with India ink and both endoneurial and epineurial vascular profiles were counted and sized using unfixed tissues. (Units are in μm^2. Bars are diabetics [open], nondiabetics [solid], diabetic sham [hatched], and nondiabetic sham [squares]). Note that in nondiabetics there is a rise in endoneurial vascular area at the early 48 hour time-point but a more prominent rise in the epineurium at both time-points. These rises are attenuated in diabetics. (Reproduced with permission from ref. *134*.)

Direct approaches to measure blood flow in human nerve have been fewer and less definitive. Such approaches have included fluorescein transit times that are delayed in patients with diabetes with advanced neuropathy *(29,150)*. Endoneurial oxygen tensions in patients with established neuropathy were reduced when measured with direct microelectrode recordings *(151)*. Theriault et al. *(152)* measured human sural nerve blood flow using multiple epineurial LDF measures of erythrocyte flux in patients in the operating room (with a micromanipulator and theater lights turned off) undergoing sural

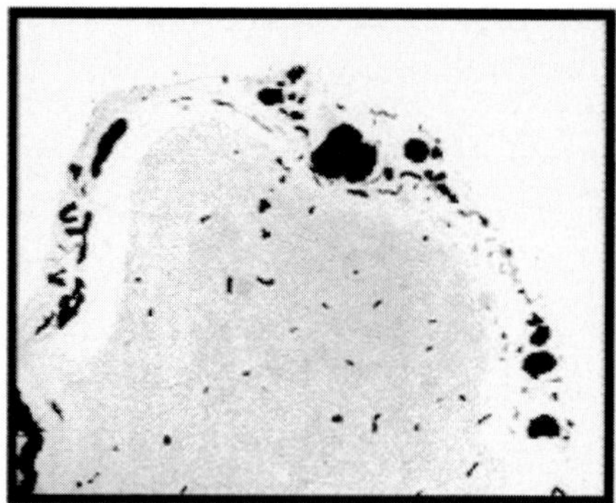
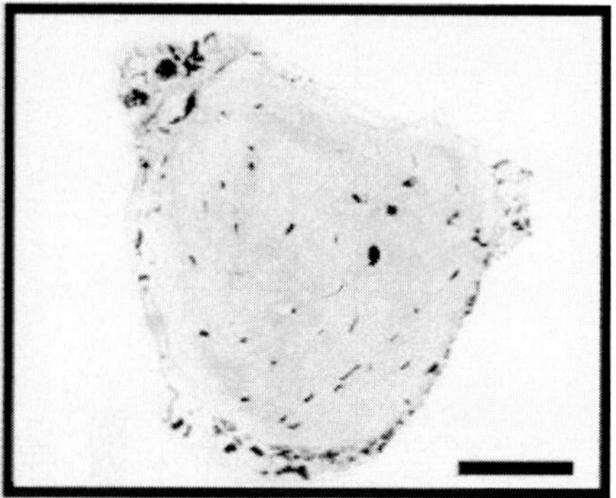

Fig. 8. Examples of sciatic nerves from nondiabetic (left) and diabetic (right) rats perfused with India ink to outline vasa nervorum in the distal nerve stump 2 weeks following transection. Note the large number of perfused vessels in epineurial area of the nondiabetics, but fewer in diabetics. (Bar = 1 mm) (Reproduced with permission from ref. *134.*)

nerve biopsy as part of a clinical trial for therapy in diabetic neuropathy. In the trial, subjects with relatively mild diabetic polyneuropathy (presence of a sural nerve sensory nerve action potential) underwent a biopsy on one leg at the outset of the trial then on the contralateral leg one year later. Ultimately, the trial agent (acetyl-L-carnitine) did not improve neuropathy, but the LDF measures yielded interesting insights. Measures were compared with results from "disease control" subjects with nondiabetic neuropathies. These controls provided proof of principal, because patients with necrotizing vasculitis of nerve had expected reductions in blood flow as did one subject in whom the surgeon applied the vasoconstrictor epinephrine over the epineurial plexus before biopsy. Overall diabetic subjects had no evidence of lowered blood flow, but trends toward higher values (Fig. 9). Interestingly, there were similar trends toward higher blood flow values in the same subjects when studied serially after one year, and patients with lower sural nerve sensory nerve action potentials (that correlated very closely with lowered myelinated fiber density) also trended toward higher, rather than lower blood flow values. These findings therefore did not link alterations in blood flow, as assessed using an epineurial LDF probe, with progressive diabetic axon loss and neuropathy.

CONCLUSION: LINKING MICROVESSELS, DIABETES, AND NEUROPATHY

Compelling experimental and human work, as summarized here, has highlighted the intimate connection between microangiopathy and diabetic polyneuropathy. Epidemiological work has similarly suggested that patients with macrovascular risk factors are at greater risk of developing polyneuropathy. A number of experimental and human studies have suggested that there is a direct cause and effect relationship between diabetic microangiopathy and polyneuropathy. These have identified reduced nerve blood flow in diabetic models and possibly humans, correction of flow and nerve conduction in tandem with agents that can modify vessels, and changes of vessels in human biopsy material. However, other evidence should caution against overinterpreting such a connection. This evidence has pointed out that rigorous experimental blood flow measures and

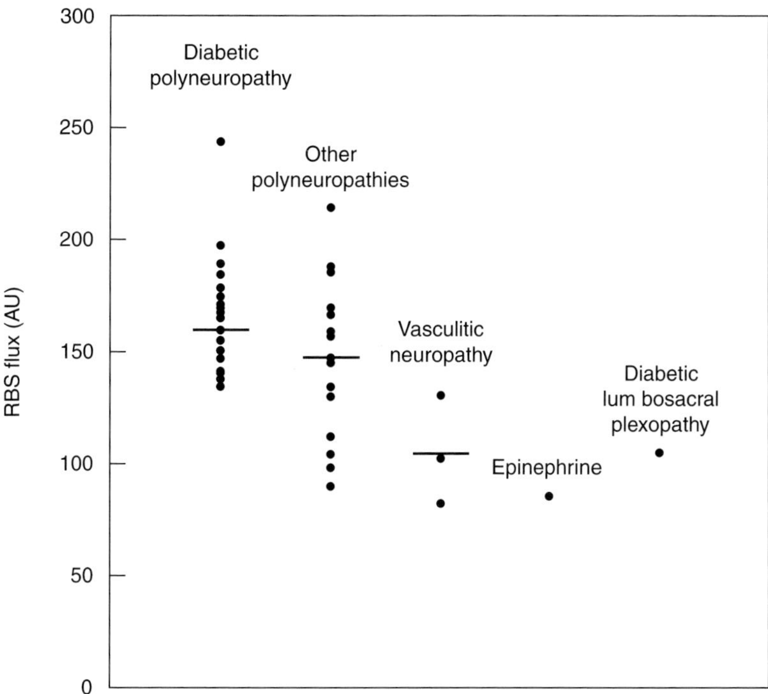

Fig. 9. Local measurements of erythrocyte flux (LDF) made in patients with mild diabetic polyneuropathy before a sural nerve biopsy in comparison with patients without diabetes with other polyneuropathies or with vasculitic polyneuropathy. Note that patients with diabetes had trends toward higher flux whereas patients with vasculitis had significant reductions in local blood flow. One patient with a sural nerve that was treated with epinephrine had reduced flux whereas a patient with diabetes with severe lumbosacral plexopathy had significantly reduced local blood flow. (Reproduced with permission from ref. *152.*)

morphological work have not identified such alterations in a variety of models or in a human study. Very few interventional studies have gone beyond short-term rat models, where structural evidence of axon damage is very limited. Indeed the sheer numbers and varieties of agents proposed for human therapy based on some of the experimental work is so large as to question specificity of the corrections they have identified and proposed. Similarly, few studies have explored the possibility that interventions directed primarily toward microvessels might more importantly target events in ganglia, rather than nerve trunks. Many human diabetic subjects already undergo chronic therapy for a number of macrovascular complications and hypertension, yet it is unclear if they are protected from polyneuropathy by these agents. Other interventions without vascular actions have substantially altered the development of neuropathy or reversed it through mechanisms that directly target neurons, rather than blood vessels.

Future work should likely de-emphasize exclusive attention toward microvessels in the pathogenesis of diabetic neuropathy. Thinking about diabetic polyneuropathy needs to be flexible, multidisciplinary, and not exclusive. It should emphasize rigorous, long-term models in more than one species, several clinically relevant end points beyond changes in nerve conduction, and should consider the range of potential actions of pharmacological interventions applied. It might be that shared molecular mechanisms, not yet thoroughly worked out, of microvessel dysfunction and direct neuron targeting, best explains the development of this complex and intractable problem.

ACKNOWLEDGMENTS

D.W. Z. is a Scientist of the Alberta Heritage Foundation for Medical Research. Brenda Boake provided expert secretarial assistance.

REFERENCES

1. Toth C, Brussee V, Cheng C, Zochodne DW. Diabetes mellitus and the sensory neuron. *J Neuropathol Exp Neurol* 2004;63:561–573.
2. Zochodne DW. Nerve and ganglion blood flow in diabetes: an appraisal, in *Neurobiology of diabetic neuropathy* (Tomlinson D, eds.), Academic Press, San Diego, 2002, pp. 161–202.
3. McManis PG, Low PA. Factors affecting the relative viability of centrifascicular and subperineurial axons in acute peripheral nerve ischemia. *Exp Neurol* 988;99:84–95.
4. Dyck PJ, Karnes J, O'Brien P, Nukada H, Lais A, Low P. Spatial pattern of nerve fiber abnormality indicative of pathologic mechanism. *Am J Pathol* 1984;117:225–238.
5. Zochodne DW, Cheng C. Diabetic peripheral nerves are susceptible to multifocal ischemic damage from endothelin. *Brain Res* 1999;838:11–17.
6. Lagerlund TD, Low PA. Mathematical modeling of hydrogen clearance blood flow measurements in peripheral nerve. *Comput Biol Med* 1994;24:77–89.
7. Adams WE. The blood supply of nerves. I. Historical review. *J Anat* 1942;76:323–341.
8. Bell MA, Weddell AG. A morphometric study of intrafascicular vessels of mammalian sciatic nerve. *Muscle Nerve* 1984;7:524–534.
9. Appenzeller O, Dhital KK, Cowen T, Burnstock G. The nerves to blood vessels supplying blood to nerves: the innervation of vasa nervorum. *Brain Res* 1984;304:383–386.
10. Dhital KK, Appenzeller O. Innervation of Vasa Nervorum, in *Nonadrenergic innervation of blood vessels* (Burnstock G, Griffith SG, eds.), CRC Press, Boca Raton, FL, 1988, pp. 191–211.
11. Brain SD, Williams TJ, Tippins JR, Morris HR, MacIntyre I. Calcitonin gene-related peptide is a potent vasodilator. *Nature* 1985;313:54–56.
12. Quayle JM, Bonev AD, Brayden JE, Nelson MT. Calcitonin gene-related peptide activated ATP-sensitive K+ currents in rabbit arterial smooth muscle via protein kinase A. *J Physiol* 1994;475(1):9–13.
13. Rechthand E, Hervonen A, Sato S, Rapoport SI. Distribution of adrenergic innervation of blood vessels in peripheral nerve. *Brain Res* 1986;374:185–189.
14. Zochodne DW, Low PA. Adrenergic control of nerve blood flow. *Exp Neurol* 1990; 109:300–307.
15. Zochodne DW, Huang ZX, Ward KK, Low PA. Guanethidine-induced adrenergic sympathectomy augments endoneurial perfusion and lowers endoneurial microvascular resistance. *Brain Res* 1990;519:112–117.
16. Zochodne DW, Ho LT. Vasa nervorum constriction from substance P and calcitonin gene- related peptide antagonists: sensitivity to phentolamine and nimodipine. *Regul Pept* 1993;47:285–290.
17. Rechthand E, Sato S, Oberg PA, Rapoport SI. Sciatic nerve blood flow response to carbon dioxide. *Brain Res* 1988;446:61–66.
18. Low PA, Tuck RR. Effects of changes of blood pressure, respiratory acidosis and hypoxia on blood flow in the sciatic nerve of the rat. *J Physiol* 1984;347:513–524.
19. Rundquist I, Smith QR, Michel ME, Ask P, Oberg PA, Rapoport SI. Sciatic nerve blood flow measured by laser Doppler flowmetry and [^{14}C]iodoantipyrine. *Am J Physiol* 1985; 248:H311–H317.

20. Zochodne DW, Ho LT. Unique microvascular characteristics of the dorsal root ganglion in the rat. *Brain Res* 1991;559:89–93.
21. McManis PG, Schmelzer JD, Zollman PJ, Low PA. Blood flow and autoregulation in somatic and autonomic ganglia. Comparison with sciatic nerve. *Brain* 1997;120(Pt 3):445–449.
22. Tuck RR, Schmelzer JD, Low PA. Endoneurial blood flow and oxygen tension in the sciatic nerves of rats with experimental diabetic neuropathy. *Brain* 1984;107:935–950.
23. Zochodne DW, Ho LT. Normal blood flow but lower oxygen tension in diabetes of young rats: microenvironment and the influence of sympathectomy. *Can J Physiol Pharmacol* 1992;70:651–659.
24. Zochodne DW, Sun H, Li XQ. Evidence that nitric oxide and opioid containing interneurons innerate vessels in the dorsal horn of the spinal cord of rats. J Physiol 2001;532:749–758.
25. Zochodne DW, Ho LT. Neonatal guanethidine treatment alters endoneurial but not dorsal root ganglion perfusion in the rat. *Brain Res* 1994;649:147–150.
26. Low PA, Lagerlund TD, McManis PG. Nerve blood flow and oxygen delivery in normal, diabetic, and ischemic neuropathy. *Int Rev Neurobiol* 1989;31:355–438.
27. Sugimoto K, Yagihashi S. Effects of aminoguanidine on structural alterations of microvessels in peripheral nerve of streptozotocin diabetic rats. *Microvasc Res* 1997; 53:105–112.
28. Zochodne DW, Nguyen C. Increased peripheral nerve microvessels in early experimental diabetic neuropathy: quantitative studies of nerve and dorsal root ganglia. *J Neurol Sci* 1999;166:40–46.
29. Tesfaye S, Harris N, Jakubowski JJ, et al. Impaired blood flow and arterior-venous shunting in human diabetic neuropathy: a novel technique of nerve photography and fluorescein angiography. *Diabetologia* 1993;36:1266–1274.
30. Hotta N, Koh N, Sakakibara F, et al. Effects of beraprost sodium and insulin on the electroretinogram, nerve conduction, and nerve blood flow in rats with streptozotocin-induced diabetes. *Diabetes* 1996;45:361–366.
31. Hotta N, Koh N, Sakakibara F, et al. Effect of propionyl-L-carnitine on motor nerve conduction, autonomic cardiac function, and nerve blood flow in rats with streptozotocin-induced diabetes: comparison with an aldose reductase inhibitor. *J Pharmacol Exp Ther* 1996;276:49–55.
32. Hotta N, Koh N, Sakakibara F, et al. Prevention of abnormalities in motor nerve conduction and nerve blood-flow by a prostacyclin analog, beraprost sodium, in streptozotocin-induced diabetic rats. *Prostaglandins* 1995;49:339–349.
33. Obrosova IG, Van Huysen C, Fathallah L, Cao X, Stevens MJ, Greene DA. Evaluation of alpha(1)-adrenoceptor antagonist on diabetes-induced changes in peripheral nerve function, metabolism, and antioxidative defense. *FASEB J* 2000;14:1548–1558.
34. Stevens MJ, Obrosova I, Cao X, Van Huysen C, Greene DA. Effects of DL-alpha-lipoic acid on peripheral nerve conduction, blood flow, energy metabolism, and oxidative stress in experimental diabetic neuropathy. *Diabetes* 2000;49:1006–1015.
35. Kalichman MW, Lalonde AW. Experimental nerve ischemia and injury produced by cocaine and procaine. *Brain Res* 1991;565:34–41.
36. Pugliese G, Tilton RG, Speedy A, et al. Effects of very mild versus overt diabetes on vascular haemodynamics and barrier function in rats. *Diabetologia* 1989;32:845–857.
37. Tilton RG, Chang K, Nyengaard JR, Van Den Enden M, Ido Y, Williamson JR. Inhibition of sorbitol dehydrogenase. Effects on vascular and neural dysfunction in streptozocin-induced diabetic rats. *Diabetes* 1995;44:234–242.
38. Sutera SP, Chang K, Marvel J, Williamson JR. Concurrent increases in regional hematocrit and blood flow in diabetic rats: prevention by sorbinil. *Am J Physiol* 1992;263:H945–H950.
39. Sugimoto H, Monafo WW, Eliasson SG. Regional sciatic nerve and muscle blood flow in conscious and anesthetized rats. *Am J Physiol* 1986;251:H1211–H1216.

40. Chang K, Ido Y, LeJeune W, Williamson JR, Tilton RG. Increased sciatic nerve blood flow in diabetic rats: assessment by "molecular" vs. particulate microspheres. *Am J Physiol* 1997;273:E164–E173.
41. Korthals JK, Korthals MA. Distribution of nerve lesions in serotonin-induced acute ischemic neuropathy. *Acta Neuropathol* 1990;81:20–24.
42. Korthals JK, Korthals MA, Wisniewski HM. Peripheral nerve ischemia: Part 2. Accumulation of organelles. *Ann Neurol* 1978;4:487–498.
43. Korthals JK, Maki T, Gieron MA. Nerve and muscle vulnerability to ischemia. *J Neurol Sci* 1985;71:283–290.
44. Korthals JK, Maki T, Korthals MA, Prockop LD. Nerve and muscle damage after experimental thrombosis of large artery. Electrophysiology and morphology. *J Neurol Sci* 1996; 136:24–30.
45. Korthals JK, Wisniewski HM. Peripheral nerve ischemia. Part 1. Experimental model. *J Neurol Sci* 1975;24:65–76.
46. Parry GJ, Brown MJ. Arachidonate-induced experimental nerve infarction. *J Neurol Sci* 1981;50:123–133.
47. Kihara M, Zollman PJ, Schmelzer JD, Low PA. The influence of dose of microspheres on nerve blood flow, electrophysiology and fiber degeneration of rat peripheral nerve. *Muscle Nerve* 1993;16:1383–1389.
48. Kihara M, McManis PG, Schmelzer JD, Kihara Y, Low PA. Experimental ischemic neuropathy: salvage with hyperbaric oxygenation. *Ann Neurol* 1995;37:89–94.
49. Day TJ, Schmelzer JD, Low PA. Aortic occlusion and reperfusion and conduction, blood flow and the blood-nerve barrier of rat sciatic nerve. *Exp Neurol* 1989;103:173–178.
50. Schmelzer JD, Zochodne DW, Low PA. Ischemic and reperfusion injury of rat peripheral nerve. *Proc Natl Acad Sci USA* 1989;86:1639–1642.
51. Bennett GJ, Xie YK. A peripheral mononeuropathy in rat that produces disorders of pain sensation like those seen in man. *Pain* 1988;33:87–107.
52. Sommer C, Myers RR. Vascular pathology in CCI neuropathy: a quantitative temporal study. *Exp Neurol* 1996;141:113–119.
53. Zochodne DW, Ho LT. Endoneurial microenvironment and acute nerve crush injury in the rat sciatic nerve. *Brain Res* 1990;535:43–48.
54. Zochodne DW, Ho LT. Hyperemia of injured peripheral nerve: sensitivity to CGRP antagonism. *Brain Res* 1992;598:59–66.
55. Raff MC, Sangalang V, Asbury AK. Ischemic mononeuropathy multiplex associated with diabetes mellitus. *Arch Neurol* 1968;18:487–499.
56. Dyck PJ, Norell JE. Microvasculitis and ischemia in diabetic lumbosacral radiculoplexus neuropathy. *Neurology* 1999;53:2113–2121.
57. Nukada H. Increased susceptibility to ischemic damage in steptozocin diabetic nerve. *Diabetes* 1986;35:1058–1061.
58. Nukada H. Mild Ischemia Causes Severe Pathological Changes in Experimental Diabetic Nerve. *Muscle Nerve* 1992;15(10):1116–1122.
59. Zochodne DW, Cheng C, Sun H. Diabetes increases sciatic nerve susceptibility to endothelin- induced ischemia. *Diabetes* 1996;45:627–632.
60. Takahashi K, Ghatei MA, Lam H-C, O'Halloran DJ, Bloom SR. Elevated plasma endothelin in patients with diabetes mellitus. *Diabetologia* 1990;33:306–310.
61. Ak G, Buyukberber S, Sevinc A, et al. The relation between plasma endothelin-1 levels and metabolic control, risk factors, treatment modalities, and diabetic microangiopathy in patients with Type 2 diabetes mellitus. *J Diab Comp* 2001;15:150–157.
62. Bertello P, Veglio F, Pinna G, et al. Plasma endothelin in NIDDM patients with and without complications. *Diabetes Care* 1994;17:574–577.
63. Xu Q-G, Cheng C, Sun H, Thomsen K, Zochodne DW. Local sensory ganglion ischemia induced by endothelin vasoconstriction. *Neuroscience* 2003;122:897–905.

64. Cameron NE, Cotter MA. Comparison of the effects of ascorbyl gamma-linolenic acid and gamma-linolenic acid in the correction of neurovascular deficits in diabetic rats. *Diabetologia* 1996;39:1047–1054.
65. Cameron NE, Cotter MA. Diabetes causes an early reduction in autonomic ganglion blood flow in rats. *J Diab Comp* 2001;15:198–202.
66. Cameron NE, Cotter MA. Effects of a nonpeptide endothelin-1 ETA antagonist on neurovascular function in diabetic rats: interaction with the renin-angiotensin system. *J Pharmacol Exp Ther* 1996;278:1262–1268.
67. Cameron NE, Cotter MA. Effects of an extracellular metal chelator on neurovascular function in diabetic rats. *Diabetologia* 2001;44:621–628.
68. Cameron NE, Cotter MA. Effects of chronic treatment with a nitric oxide donor on nerve conduction abnormalities and endoneurial blood flow in streptozotocin-diabetic rats. *Eur J Clin Invest* 1995;25:19–24.
69. Cameron NE, Cotter MA. Effects of evening primrose oil treatment on sciatic nerve blood flow and endoneurial oxygen tension in streptozotocin-diabetic rats. *Acta Diabetol* 1994;31:220–225.
70. Cameron NE, Cotter MA. Impaired contraction and relaxation in aorta from streptozotocin- diabetic rats: role of polyol pathway. *Diabetologia* 1992;35:1011–1019.
71. Cameron NE, Cotter MA. Interaction between oxidative stress and gamma-linolenic acid in impaired neurovascular function of diabetic rats. *Am J Physiol* 1996;271: E471–E476.
72. Cameron NE, Cotter MA. Potential therapeutic approaches to the treatment or prevention of diabetic neuropathy: evidence from experimental studies. *Diabet Med* 1993;10: 593–605.
73. Cameron NE, Cotter MA. Rapid reversal by aminoguanidine of the neurovascular effects of diabetes in rats: modulation by nitric oxide synthase inhibition. *Metabolism* 1996;45: 1147–1152.
74. Cameron NE, Cotter MA, Archibald V, Dines KC, Maxfield EK. Anti-oxidant and pro-oxidant effects on nerve conduction velocity, endoneurial blood flow and oxygen tension in non- diabetic and streptozotocin-diabetic rats. *Diabetologia* 1994;37:449–459.
75. Cameron NE, Cotter MA, Basso M, Hohman TC. Comparison of the effects of inhibitors of aldose reductase and sorbitol dehydrogenase on neurovascular function, nerve conduction and tissue polyol pathway metabolites in streptozotocin-diabetic rats. *Diabetologia* 1997;40:271–281.
76. Cameron NE, Cotter MA, Dines K, Love A. Effects of aminoguanidine on peripheral nerve function and polyol pathway metabolites in streptozotocin-diabetic rats. *Diabetologia* 1992;35:946–950.
77. Cameron NE, Cotter MA, Dines KC, Maxfield EK. Pharmacological manipulation of vascular endothelium function in non-diabetic and streptozotocin-diabetic rats: effects on nerve conduction, hypoxic resistance and endoneurial capillarization. *Diabetologia* 1993;36:516–522.
78. Cameron NE, Cotter MA, Dines KC, Maxfield EK, Carey F, Mirrlees DJ. Aldose reductase inhibition, nerve perfusion, oxygenation and function in streptozotocin-diabetic rats: dose-response considerations and independence from a myo-inositol mechanism. *Diabetologia* 1994;37:651–663.
79. Cameron NE, Cotter MA, Dines KC, Robertson S, Cox D. The effects of evening primrose oil on nerve function and capillarization in streptozotocin-diabetic rats: modulation by the cyclo-oxygenase inhibitor flurbiprofen. *Br J Pharmacol* 1993;109:972–979.
80. Cameron NE, Cotter MA, Ferguson K, Robertson S, Radcliffe MA. Effects of chronic alpha-adrenergic receptor blockade on peripheral nerve conduction, hypoxic resistance, polyols, Na+-k+- ATPase activity, and vascular supply in STZ-D rats. *Diabetes* 1991;40: 1652–1658.

81. Cameron NE, Cotter MA, Hohman TC. Interactions between essential fatty acid, prostanoid, polyol pathway and nitric oxide mechanisms in the neurovascular deficit of diabetic rats. *Diabetologia* 1996;39:172–182.
82. Cameron NE, Cotter MA, Horrobin DH, Tritschler HJ. Effects of alpha-lipoic acid on neurovascular function in diabetic rats: interaction with essential fatty acids. *Diabetologia* 1998;41:390–399.
83. Cameron NE, Cotter MA, Jack AM, Basso MD, Hohman TC. Protein kinase C effects on nerve function, perfusion, Na(+), K(+)-ATPase activity and glutathione content in diabetic rats. *Diabetologia* 1999;42:1120–1130.
84. Cameron NE, Cotter MA, Low PA. Nerve blood flow in early experimental diabetes in rats: relation to conduction deficits. *Am J Physiol* 1991;261:E1–E8.
85. Cameron NE, Cotter MA, Maxfield EK. Anti-oxidant treatment prevents the development of peripheral nerve dysfunction in streptozotocin-diabetic rats. *Diabetologia* 1993;36: 299–304.
86. Cameron NE, Cotter MA, Robertson S. Chronic low frequency electrical activation for one week corrects nerve conduction velocity deficits in rats with diabetes of three months duration. *Diabetologia* 1989;32:759–761.
87. Cameron NE, Cotter MA, Robertson S. Rapid reversal of a motor nerve conduction deficit in streptozotocin-diabetic rats by the angiotensin converting enzyme inhibitor lisinopril. *Acta Diabetol* 1993;30:46–48.
88. Cameron NE, Cotter MA, Robertson S. The effect of aldose reductase inhibition on the pattern of nerve conduction deficits in diabetic rats. *Q J Exp Physiol* 1989;74:917–926.
89. Cameron NE, Cotter MA, Robertson S, Maxfield EK. Nerve function in experimental diabetes in rats: effects of electrical stimulation. *Am J Physiol* 1993;264:E161–E166.
90. Cameron NE, Dines KC, Cotter MA. The potential contribution of endothelin-1 to neurovascular abnormalities in streptozotocin-diabetic rats. *Diabetologia* 1994;37:1209–1215.
91. Cotter MA, Cameron NE. Correction of neurovascular deficits in diabetic rats by beta2-adrenoceptor agonist and alpha1-adrenoceptor antagonist treatment: interactions with the nitric oxide system. *Eur J Pharmacol* 1998;343:217–223.
92. Cotter MA, Cameron NE. Neuroprotective effects of carvedilol in diabetic rats: prevention of defective peripheral nerve perfusion and conduction velocity. *Naunyn Schmiedebergs Arch Pharmacol* 1995;351:630–635.
93. Cotter MA, Cameron NE, Hohman TC. Correction of nerve conduction and endoneurial blood flow deficits by the aldose reductase inhibitor, tolrestat, in diabetic rats. *J Peripher Nerv Syst* 1998;3:217–223.
94. Cotter MA, Love A, Watt MJ, Cameron NE, Dines KC. Effects of natural free radical scavengers on peripheral nerve and neurovascular function in diabetic rats. *Diabetologia* 1995;38:1285–1294.
95. Obrosova IG, Van Huysen C, Fathallah L, Cao XC, Greene DA, Stevens MJ. An aldose reductase inhibitor reverses early diabetes-induced changes in peripheral nerve function, metabolism, and antioxidative defense. *FASEB J* 2002;16:123–125.
96. Hotta N, Koh N, Sakakibara F, et al. Nerve function and blood flow in Otsuka Long-Evans Tokushima Fatty rats with sucrose feeding: effect of an anticoagulant. *Eur J Pharmacol* 1996;313:201–209.
97. Kihara M, Schmelzer JD, Low PA. Effect of cilostazol on experimental diabetic neuropathy in the rat. *Diabetologia* 1995;38:914–918.
98. Singhal A, Cheng C, Sun H, Zochodne DW. Near nerve local insulin prevents conduction slowing in experimental diabetes. *Brain Res* 1997;763:209–214.
99. Brussee V, Cunningham FA, Zochodne DW. Direct insulin signaling of neurons reverses diabetic neuropathy. *Diabetes* 2004;53:1824–1830.
100. Zochodne DW, Sun H-S, Cheng C, Eyer J. Accelerated diabetic neuropathy in axons without neurofilaments. *Brain* 2004;127:2193–2200.

101. Zochodne DW, Ho LT. The influence of indomethacin and guanethidine on experimental streptozotocin diabetic neuropathy. *Can J Neurol Sci* 1992;19:433–441.
102. Zochodne DW, Ho LT. The influence of sulindac on experimental streptozotocin-induced diabetic neuropathy. *Can J Neurol Sci* 1994;21:194–202.
103. Zochodne DW, Ho LT, Allison JA. Dorsal root ganglia microenvironment of female BB Wistar diabetic rats with mild neuropathy. *J Neurol Sci* 1994;127:36–42.
104. Chang K, Ido Y, LeJeune W, Williamson JR, Tilton RG. Increased sciatic nerve blood flow in diabetic rats: assessment by "molecular" vs. particulate microspheres. *Am J Physiol* 1997;273:E164–E173.
105. Yasuda H, Dyck PJ. Abnormalities of endoneurial microvessels and sural nerve pathology in diabetic neuropathy. *Neurology* 1987;37:20–28.
106. Schratzberger P, Walter DH, Rittig K, et al. Reversal of experimental diabetic neuropathy by VEGF gene transfer. *J Clin Invest* 2001;107:1083–1092.
107. Sasaki H, Schmelzer JD, Zollman PJ, Low PA. Neuropathology and blood flow of nerve, spinal roots and dorsal root ganglia in longstanding diabetic rats. *Acta Neuropathol* 1997;93:118–128.
108. Calver A, Collier J, Vallance P. Inhibition and stimulation of nitric oxide synthesis in the human forearm arterial bed of patients with insulin-dependent diabetes. *J Clin Invest* 1992;90:2548–2554.
109. Elliott TG, Cockcroft JR, Groop PH, Viberti GC, Ritter JM. Inhibition of nitric oxide synthesis in forearm vasculature of insulin-dependent diabetic patients: blunted vasoconstriction in patients with microalbuminuria. *Clin Sci* 1993;85:687–693.
110. Durante W, Sen AK, Sunahara FA. Impairment of endothelium-dependent relaxation in aortae from spontaneously diabetic rats. *Br J Pharmacol* 1988;94:463–468.
111. Kihara M, Low PA. Impaired vasoreactivity to nitric oxide in experimental diabetic neuropathy. *Exp Neurol* 1995;132:180–185.
112. Lawrence E, Brain SD. Altered microvascular reactivity to endothelin-1, endothelin-3 and NG-nitro-L-arginine methyl ester in streptozotocin-induced diabetes mellitus. *Br J Pharmacol* 1992;106:1035–1040.
113. Tolins JP, Schultz PJ, Raij L, Brown DM, Mauer SM. Abnormal renal hemodynamic response to reduced renal perfusion pressure in diabetic rats: role of NO. *Am J Physiol* 1993;265:F886–F895.
114. Bucala R, Tracey KJ, Cerami A. Advanced glycosylation products quench nitric oxide and mediate defective endothelium-dependent vasodilatation in experimental diabetes. *J Clin Invest* 1991;87:432–438.
115. Diederich D, Skopec J, Diederich A, Dai FX. Endothelial dysfunction in mesenteric resistance arteries of diabetic rats: role of free radicals. *Am J Physiol* 1994;266: H1153–H1161.
116. Hill MA, Meininger GA, Larkins RG. Alterations in microvascular reactivity in experimental diabetes mellitus: contribution of the endothelium?, in *Endothelial cell function in diabetic microangiopathy: problems in methodology and clinical aspects* (Molinatti GM, Bar RS, Belfiore F, Porta M, eds.), Karger, Basel, 1990, pp.118–126.
117. Zochodne DW, Verge VM, Cheng C, et al. Nitric oxide synthase activity and expression in experimental diabetic neuropathy. *J Neuropathol Exp Neurol* 2000;59:798–807.
118. Zochodne DW, Ho LT. Diabetes mellitus prevents capsaicin from inducing hyperaemia in the rat sciatic nerve. *Diabetologia* 1993;36:493–496.
119. Willars GB, Calcutt NA, Compton AM, Tomlinson DR, Keen P. Substance P levels in peripheral nerve, skin, atrial myocardium and gastrointestinal tract of rats with long-term diabetes mellitus. Effects of aldose reductase inhibition. *J Neurol Sci* 1989;91:153–164.
120. Kihara M, Mitsui MK, Mitsui Y, et al. Altered vasoreactivity to angiotension II in experimental diabetic neuropathy: role of nitric oxide. *Muscle Nerve* 1999;22:920–925.

121. White RE, Carrier GO. Enhanced vascular alpha-adrenergic neuroeffector system in diabetes: importance of calcium. *Am J Physiol* 1988;255:H1036–H1042.
122. Ward KK, Low PA, Schmelzer JD, Zochodne DW. Prostacyclin and noradrenaline in peripheral nerve of chronic experimental diabetes in rats. *Brain* 1989;112:197–208.
123. Parry GJ, Kohzu H. Studies of resistance to ischemic nerve conduction failure in normal and diabetic rats. *J Neurol Sci* 1989;93:61–67.
124. Kennedy JM, Zochodne D. Impaired peripheral nerve regeneration in diabetes mellitus. *J Peripher Nerv Syst* 2005;10(2):144–157.
125. Kennedy JM, Zochodne DW. The regenerative deficit of peripheral nerves in experimental diabetes: its extent, timing and possible mechanisms. *Brain* 2000;123:2118–2129.
126. Nukada H. Post-traumatic endoneurial neovascularization and nerve regeneration: a morphometric study. *Brain Res* 1988;449:89–96.
127. Zochodne DW, Levy D, Zwiers H, et al. Evidence for nitric oxide and nitric oxide synthase activity in proximal stumps of transected peripheral nerves. *Neuroscience* 1999;91: 1515–1527.
128. Zochodne DW, Allison JA, Ho W, Ho LT, Hargreaves K, Sharkey KA. Evidence for CGRP accumulation and activity in experimental neuromas. *Am J Physiol* 1995;268:H584–H590.
129. Hoke A, Sun H, Gordon T, Zochodne DW. Do denevated peripheral nerve trunks become ischomic? *Exp Neurol* 2001;172(2):398–406.
130. Zochodne DW, Nguyen C. Angiogenesis at the site of neuroma formation in transected peripheral nerve. *J Anat* 1997;191:23–30.
131. Hoke A, Gordon T, Zochodne DW, Sulaiman OA. A decline in glial cell-line-derived neurotrophic factor expression is associated with impaired regeneration after long-term Schwann cell denervation. *Exp Neurol* 2002;173:77–85.
132. Roytta M, Salonen V. Long-term endoneurial changes after nerve transection. *Acta Neuropathol* 1988;76:35–45.
133. Siironen J, Vuorinen V, Taskinen HS, Roytta M. Axonal regeneration into chronically denervated distal stump. 2. Active expression of type I collagen mRNA in epineurium. *Acta Neuropathol* 1995;89:219–226.
134. Kennedy JM, Zochodne DW. Influence of experimental diabetes on the microcirculation of injured peripheral nerve. Functional and morphological aspects. *Diabetes* 2002;51: 2233–2240.
135. Kennedy JM, Rubin I, Lauritzen M, Zochodne DW. Injury-induced nitric oxide synthase activity in regenerating diabetic peripheral nerves. *Soc Neurosci Abs* 2002;31:449(Abstract).
136. Levy D, Kubes P, Zochodne DW. Delayed peripheral nerve degeneration, regeneration, and pain in mice lacking inducible nitric oxide synthase. *J Neuropathol Exp Neurol* 2001;60:411–421.
137. Dyck PJ, Giannini C. Pathologic alterations in the diabetic neuropathies of humans: a review. *J Neuropathol Exp Neurol* 1996;55:1181–1193.
138. Dyck PJ, Hansen S, Karnes J, et al. Capillary number and percentage closed in human diabetic sural nerve. *Proc Natl Acad Sci USA* 1985;82:2513–2517.
139. Korthals JK, Gieron MA, Dyck PJ. Intima of epineurial arterioles is increased in diabetic polyneuropathy. *Neurology* 1988;38:1582–1586.
140. Dyck PJ, Karnes JL, O'Brien P, Okazaki H, Lais A, Engelstad J. The spatial distribution of fiber loss in diabetic polyneuropathy suggests ischemia. *Ann Neurol* 1986;19:440–449.
141. Dyck PJ, Lais A, Karnes JL, O'Brien P, Rizza R. Fiber loss is primary and multifocal in sural nerves in diabetic polyneuropathy. *Ann Neurol* 1986;19:425–439.
142. Dyck PJ. Hypoxic neuropathy: Does hypoxia play a role in diabetic neuropathy? The 1988 Robert Wartenberg lecture. *Neurology* 1989;39:111–118.
143. Malik RA. The pathology of human diabetic neuropathy. *Diabetes* 1997;46:S50–S53.
144. Malik RA, Newrick PG, Sharma AK, et al. Microangiopathy in human diabetic neuropathy: relationship between capillary abnormalities and the severity of neuropathy. *Diabetologia* 1989;32:92–102.

145. Malik RA, Tesfaye S, Thompson SD, et al. Endoneurial localisation of microvascular damage in human diabetic neuropathy. *Diabetologia* 1993;36:454–459.
146. Malik RA, Veves A, Masson EA, et al. Endoneurial capillary abnormalities in mild human diabetic neuropathy. *J Neurol Neurosurg Psychiatry* 1992;55:557–561.
147. Johnson PC, Doll SC, Cromey DW. Pathogenesis of diabetic neuropathy. *Ann Neurol* 1986; 19:450–457.
148. Thrainsdottir S, Malik RA, Dahlin LB, et al. Endoneurial capillary abnormalities presage deterioration of glucose tolerance and accompany peripheral neuropathy in man. *Diabetes* 2003;52:2615–2622.
149. Tesfaye S, Chaturvedi N, Eaton SE, et al. Vascular risk factors and diabetic neuropathy. *N Engl J Med* 2005;352:341–350.
150. Ibrahim S, Harris ND, Radatz M, et al. A new minimally invasive technique to show nerve ischaemia in diabetic neuropathy. *Diabetologia* 1999;42:737–742.
151. Newrick PG, Wilson AJ, Jakubowski J, Boulton AJ, Ward JD. Sural nerve oxygen tension in diabetes. *Br Med J* 1986;293:1053–1054.
152. Theriault M, Dort J, Sutherland G, Zochodne DW. Local human sural nerve blood flow in diabetic and other polyneuropathies. *Brain* 1997;120:1131–1138.

13
Pathogenesis of Human Diabetic Neuropathy

Rayaz Ahmed Malik and Aristides Veves

SUMMARY

Experimental studies have provided multiple mechanisms for the development of diabetic neuropathy, yet very few findings have been replicated in patients. Hyperglycemia mediated nerve damage may begin very early even prior to overt diabetes as evidenced by several recent studies in patients with impaired glucose tolerance. Polyol pathway abnormalities have been exhaustively explored in animals, but studies in man are limited and inconsistent and hence not surprisingly, clinical trials with aldose reductase inhibitors have consistently failed. Glycation is widespread and may induce a range of structural and functional changes and glycation inhibitors are being actively developed. Both large and small vessel disease have been implicated in diabetic neuropathy and treatment with ACE inhibitors has shown some benefit. Growth factors may be important in maintaining both the vascular and neuronal phenotype. Thus a range of neurotrophic and vascular growth factors have entered phase III clinical trials for human diabetic neuropathy recently.

Key Words: Neuropathy; aldose reductasef; glycation; vascular; neurotrophins.

PATHOGENESIS

Studies in animal models and cultured cells provide a conceptual framework for the cause, and potentially, the treatment of diabetic neuropathy *(1)* (Fig. 1). Each of these putative pathways has been discussed in detail in several other chapters.

Although, experimental evidence in vivo suggests that these paradigms provide a novel basis for research and drug development, limited translational work in patients with diabetes continues to generate much debate and controversy about their relevance to human diabetic neuropathy. This chapter will therefore focus entirely on the changes, which have been reported in man.

Hyperglycemia

The role of even minor and intermittent episodes of hyperglycemia has been explored recently in patients with impaired glucose tolerance (IGT). Thus, 25% of patients with apparent "idiopathic painful neuropathy" and electrodiagnostic evidence of axonal injury with loss of epidermal nerve fibers have been shown to have IGT *(2)*. The

From: *Contemporary Diabetes: Diabetic Neuropathy: Clinical Management, Second Edition*
Edited by: A. Veves and R. Malik © Humana Press Inc., Totowa, NJ

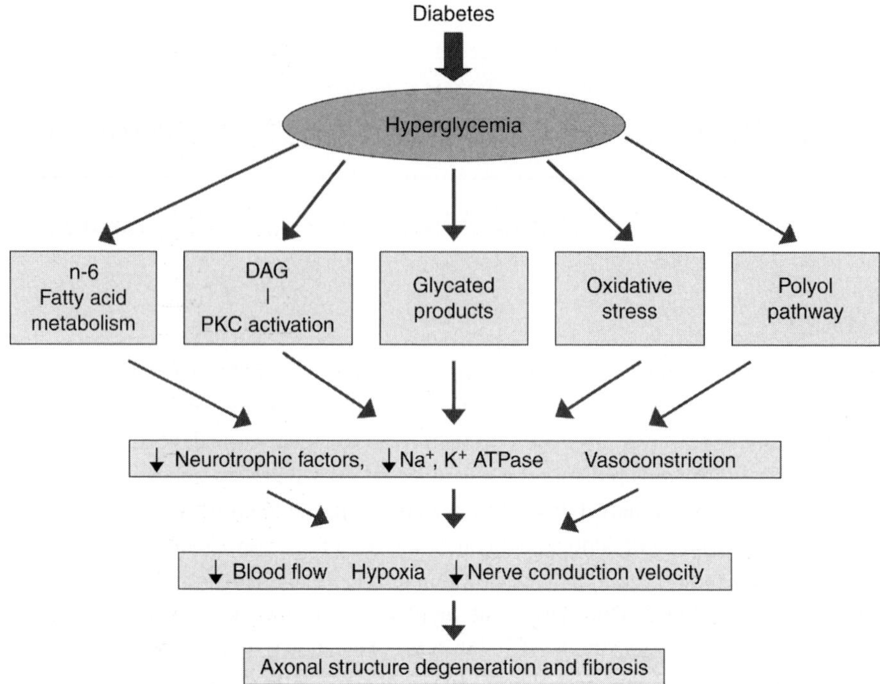

Fig. 1. Pathogenesis of diabetic neuropathy. Factors implicated in the pathogenesis of diabetic neuropathy include the activation of the polyol pathway, the activation of PKC, increased oxidative stress, the impaired *n*-6 fatty acid metabolism, auto-oxidation of glucose and the formation of advanced glycation end products, and the reduced bioavailability of neurotrophic factors. All these mechanisms are interrelated and can potentiate each other's detrimental effects. Although the exact mechanisms of their action are not well understood, it is currently believed that these factors lead to reduced Na^+, K^+ ATPase activity and vasoconstriction, reduced endoneurial blood flow, and nerve hypoxia. All these changes initially result in reduced nerve conduction velocity and demyelination with later axonal loss *(75)*.

neuropathy in patients with IGT appears milder than the neuropathy associated with newly diagnosed diabetes and it may particularly affect the small nerve fibers *(3)*. They have not demonstrated a reduction in sural nerve amplitude or myelinated fiber density *(4)*. However, a recent study has shown a decrease in distal sural conduction velocity in IGT subjects with normal distal and proximal amplitudes and proximal sural sensory conduction velocity, suggestive of distal demyelination *(5)*. Regarding the mechanistic basis for IGT neuropathy a small nerve biopsy study has shown increased expression of the ligand N epsilon-carboxymethyl lysine and the receptor for advanced glycation end products (RAGE) as well as the transcription factor nuclear factor (NF)-κB in the perineurium, epineurial, and endoneurial vessels in subjects with IGT *(6)*.

In patients with predominantly type 2 diabetes, longitudinal data from the Rochester cohort has suggested that the duration and severity of exposure to hyperglycemia are related to the severity of neuropathy *(7)*. Improvement of glycemic control in type 1 diabetes by intensified insulin as in the Diabetes Control and Complications trial (DCCT) *(8)*, pancreatic transplantation *(9)*, or recently with islet cell transplantation *(10)* improves neuropathy. However, similar results have not been achieved in patients with type 2 diabetes either in the United Kingdom Prospective Diabetes Study (UKPDS) *(11)*, Veterans Affairs Cooperative Study on Glycemic Control and Complication in NIDDM (VACSDM) study *(12)*, or the Steno-2 study *(13)*, suggesting that either hyperglycemia is not the major driving factor for neuropathy in type 2 diabetes, or that other factors such as hypertension or hyperlipidemia might play more important roles.

Polyol Pathway

Animal models consistently demonstrate an association between increased polyol pathway flux and a reduction in nerve conduction velocity (NCV), which can be ameliorated with aldose reductase inhibitors (ARI's) *(14,15)*. In man, perhaps the potential role of the polyol pathway has been oversimplified and oversold. Thus, in patients with diabetes, considerable heterogeneity has been observed in the level of polyol pathway metabolites in different studies *(16–19)* and subjects with IGT do not demonstrate an elevated nerve sorbitol, suggestive of a glycemic threshold for activation of this pathway *(4)*. Only one study has shown a significant inverse correlation between the levels of nerve sorbitol and myelinated fiber density *(19)*. Although a careful and detailed study using neurophysiology has shown that subjects with diabetes with the T allele of the C-106T polymorphism had lower peroneal, sural, and radial sensory response amplitudes at baseline and a higher decrease in peroneal motor NCV than those with the C-106C genotype *(20)*. It also appears that those at the highest risk of developing the complications are those with a higher set-point for AR activity *(21)*, which may be further modulated by the activity of Sorbitol dehydrogenase *(22)*. Despite the disappointing results in somatic neuropathy of a meta-analysis of 19 randomized ARI trials which demonstrated only a small reduction in decline of median (0.66 m/second) and peroneal (0.53 m/second) motor NCV *(23)*, several other interventional studies have been more positive and suggest there might be a dose response relationship between the degree of AR inhibition and peripheral nerve regeneration *(24–26)*. Furthermore, recently ARI's have been shown to benefit autonomic dysfunction by showing improvements in esophageal dysfunction *(27)*, gastroparesis *(28)*, and left ventricular ejection fraction *(29)*.

Glycation

Glycation induces a range of cellular and subcellular alterations, which have far reaching effects on tissue biology *(30)*. It might affect the function of matrix metalloproteinase's, their tissue inhibitors -1 and -2, transforming growth factor-β *(31)*, epidermal growth factor induced autophosphorylation, and activation of extra cellular signal-regulated kinases *(32)*. Sural nerves obtained from patients with diabetes at amputation demonstrate significantly elevated pentosidine levels in both cytoskeletal and myelin protein *(33)*. In a recent biopsy study of eight patients with diabetes with polyneuropathy and proximal neuropathy, advanced glycation end product (AGE) was localized to the endoneurium, perineurium, and microvessels and the intensity of axonal AGE expression correlated with the loss of axons *(34)*. Pyrraline, an AGE, is also increased in postmortem samples of optic nerve from patients with diabetes *(35)*. The RAGE and its

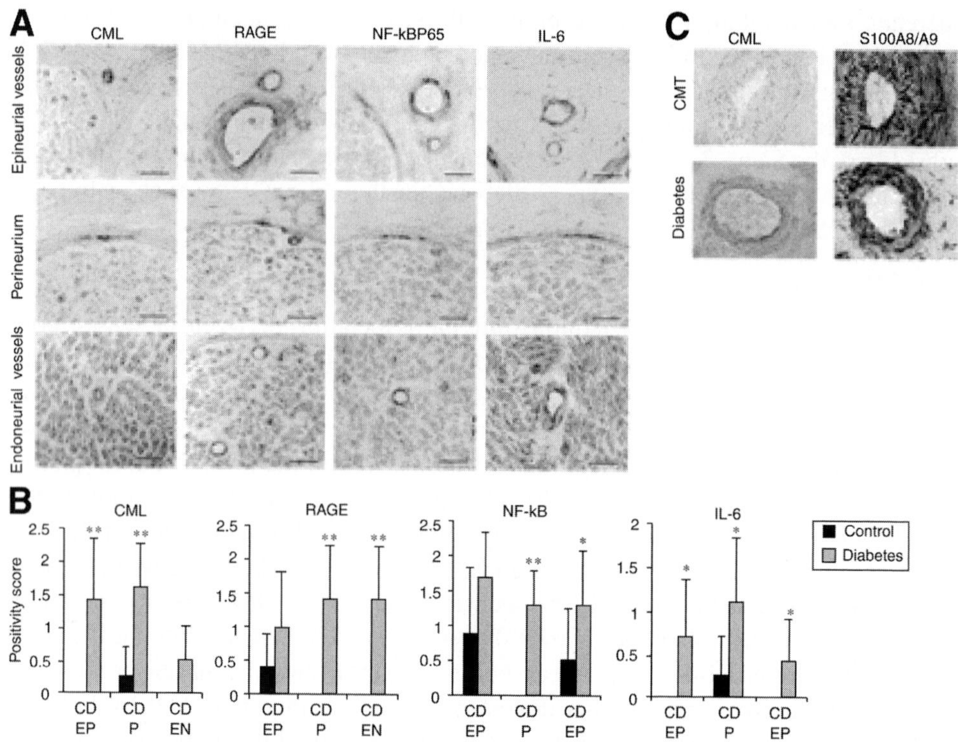

Fig. 2. **(A)** Localization of carboxymethyl lysine, receptor for advanced glycation end products, activated nuclear factor-κBp65, and interleukin-6 antigens in epineurial vessels (top), perineurium (middle), and endoneurial vessels (bottom) of sural nerve biopsies from a representative patient with diabetes mellitus and Charcot-Marie-Tooth disease (Scale bars: 100 μm). **(B)** Quantification of staining intensities of epineurial vessels, perineurium, and endoneurial vessels in nondiabetic ($n = 8$) and diabetic ($n = 10$) patients (mean ± SD, $*p < 0.05$, $**p < 0.005$). **(C)** Comparison of the staining intensity for carboxymethyl lysine and the receptor for advanced glycation end products ligand S100A8/A9 on epineurial vessels ×400 ref. *36*.

primary ligands (activated NF-κB, and interleukin-6) have been colocalized in the sural nerve microvasculature of patients with diabetic neuropathy *(36)* (Fig. 2). The formation of AGE's can be limited by inhibitors such as pyridoxamine, tenilsetam, 2, 3-diaminophenazone and aminoguanidine, or recombinant RAGE may hinder the AGE–RAGE interaction *(37)*. However, no agents are currently in clinical trials for human diabetic neuropathy.

Oxidative Stress

Oxidative stress has been implicated strongly in the pathogenesis of diabetic neuropathy in animal models *(38)*, but to a lesser extent for somatic and autonomic diabetic neuropathy in patients *(39)*. Benefits have been observed with α-lipoic acid (LA), a powerful antioxidant that scavenges hydroxyl radicals, superoxide and peroxyl radicals and regenerates glutathione *(40)*. The Alpha Lipoic Acid in Diabetic Neuropathy (ALADIN) study demonstrated that 3 weeks of intravenous LA improved neuropathic symptoms *(41)* and in the oral pilot (ORPIL) study, oral LA improved the total symptom score and surprisingly the neuropathy disability score *(42)*. In ALADIN-II, 5 days of intravenous LA followed by 2 years of oral treatment led to a significant improvement in sural sensory nerve conduction velocity (SNCV), sensory nerve action potential (SNAP), and tibial motor nerve conduction velocity (MNCV) but not neuropathy disability score (NDS) *(43)*. Finally, the SYDNEY study has demonstrated a significant improvement in the neuropathy symptom score, neuropathy impairment score, and one attribute of nerve conduction after 14 (5 days/week) intravenous treatments with racemic LA *(44)*.

Vascular Factors

A substantial body of data implicates vascular disease in the pathogenesis of diabetic neuropathy *(45)*. Large vessel revascularization improved NCV in one study *(46)*, prevented worsening in another study *(47)*, but failed to show any benefit in another study *(48)*. It was also shown to improve, but not totally correct microvascular perfusion *(49)*. In 55 type 2 patients with diabetes, independent of traditional risk factors, systolic blood pressure and pulse pressure were related strongly to the severity of diabetic neuropathy *(50)*. Whereas in 1172 type 1 patients with diabetes in the European Diabetes (EURODIAB) prospective complications study, apart from glycemic control, the incidence of neuropathy was associated with potentially modifiable cardiovascular risk factors, including a raised triglyceride level, body-mass index, smoking, and hypertension *(51)*. The recent nerve biopsy studies demonstrate the early occurrence of a significant diabetic microangiopathy in patients with IGT *(52)* and minimal neuropathy *(53)* (Fig. 3). In diabetic patients it has been previously shown that resistance vessel endothelial function is worse in those with hypertension *(54)*, but can improve markedly even with short-term treatment with an angiotensin II receptor blocker *(55)*. Thus, in a 12-week open label dose escalation study with lisinopril, a significant improvement was observed in electrophysiology and quantitative sensory testing *(56)*. A larger double-blind placebo-controlled clinical trial with Trandalopril showed an improvement in peroneal motor NCV, M-wave amplitude F-wave latency, and sural nerve amplitude *(57)*. However, in the appropriate blood pressure control in diabetes trial although a significant reduction in blood pressure was achieved, neuropathy did not improve with Enalapril *(58)*.

1,2-diacylglycerol induced activation of protein kinase C (PKC)-β, has been proposed to play a major role in diabetic neuropathy *(59)*. Although a fall in 1,2-diacylglycerol levels and a consistent pattern of change in PKC activity has not been observed in diabetic animal models, inhibition of PKC-β in diabetic rats appears to correct reduced nerve blood flow and NCV *(60)*. In a multinational, randomized, phase II, double-blind, placebo-controlled parallel-group trial comparing 32 mg/d or 64 mg/d of the PKC-β inhibitor ruboxistaurin with placebo for 1 year, 205 diabetic patients were enrolled. The primary analysis failed to show an improvement in VDT and NTSS-6 scores, although an improvement was seen in a posthoc analysis of patients with less severe symptomatic DPN *(61)*. Indeed two phase II trials with ruboxistaurin have recently failed to show an improvement in symptoms, although a larger randomized double-blind placebo-controlled trial assessing an effect on neurological deficits is currently underway and is due for report in 2007.

As noted previously, abnormal lipids also appear to be important in the pathogenesis and progression of human diabetic neuropathy *(51)*. Thus, the statins and fibrates may

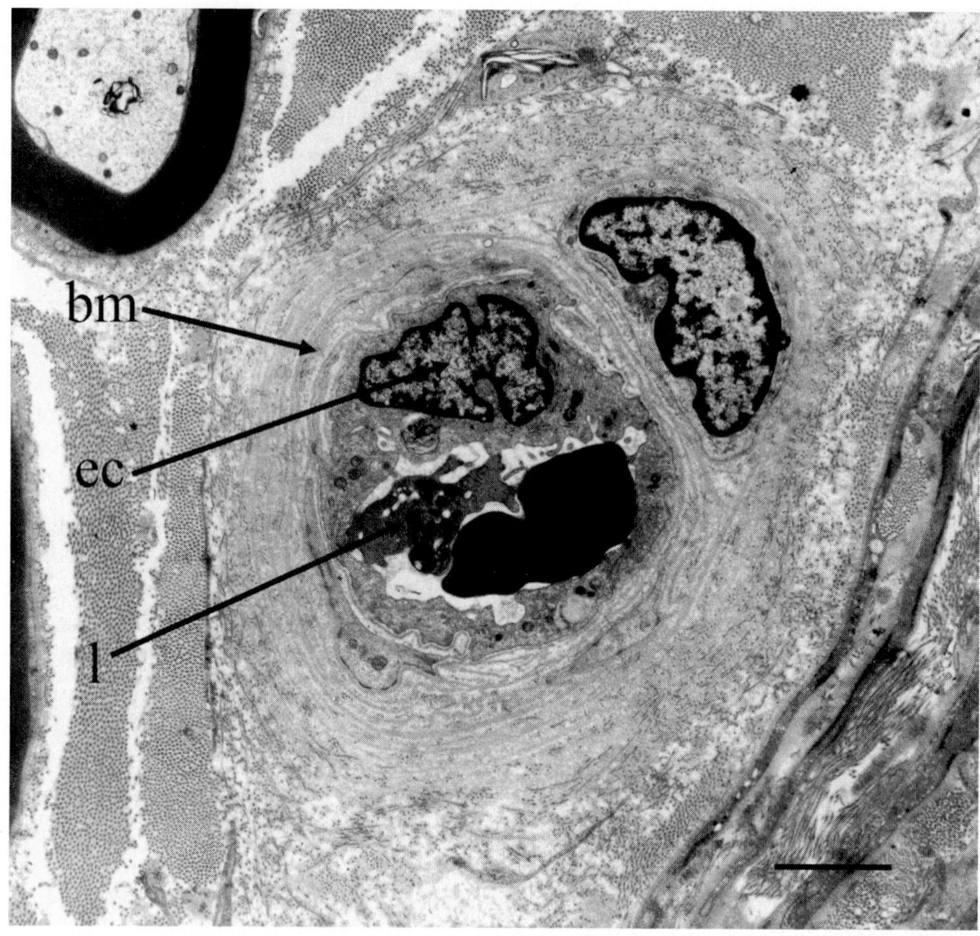

Fig. 3. Electronmicrograph of endoneurial capillary from a diabetic patient with minimal neuropathy demonstrating basement membrane (bm) thickening, endothelial cell (e) hyperplasia and luminal (l) narrowing bar = 2 μm *(53)*.

well be expected to benefit the patients by reducing low-density lipoproteins and triglycerides, respectively and improving endothelial function *(62)*. In addition statins can completely prevent AGE-induced NF-κβ induced protein-1 activation and upregulation of vascular endothelial growth factor (VEGF) mRNA, in microvascular endothelial cells *(63)*. Thus simvastatin has shown a trend toward slower progression of neuropathy assessed using vibration perception threshold, but no change in clinical neuropathy *(64)*.

GROWTH FACTORS

Insulin-Like Growth Factors

A deficiency of insulin like growth factors (IGF's) has been proposed to lead to cell death. Neuroaxonal dystrophy occurs in the nerve terminals of the prevertebral sympathetic ganglia and ileal mesenteric nerves of the streptozotocin (STZ)-diabetic and biobreeding/Worcester rat, and has been related to hyperglycemia and a deficiency of circulating IGF-I levels. In contrast, although the Zucker diabetic fatty rat is hyperglycemic it does not develop neuroaxonal dystrophy because it is claimed it has normal levels of plasma IGF-I *(65)*. In cultured Schwann cells and the STZ-diabetic rat, IGF-1 administration prevents apoptosis through PI 3-kinase *(66)*. However, again translational studies in man have failed to show any differences in the expression of Insulin-like growth factor I and IGF-I receptor mRNA levels in the sural nerve of patients with diabetes compared with control subjects *(67)*.

C-Peptide

C-peptide deficiency has emerged as a prominent factor in the pathogenesis of the microvascular complications in type 1 diabetes *(68)*. In neuropathy it has been shown to have effects on Na(+)/K(+)-ATPase activity, expression of neurotrophical factors, regulation of molecular species underlying the degeneration of the nodal apparatus as well as DNA binding of transcription factors leading to apoptosis *(69)*. Administration of C-peptide in the STZ rat improves NCV through enhanced activity of endothelial nitric oxide synthase and an improvement in nerve blood flow *(70)*. In a small randomized double-blind placebo-controlled study of 46 patients with type 1 diabetes and excellent glycemic control (HbA1c-7%), a significant improvement in sural sensory NCV and vibration perception, without a benefit in either cold or heat perception was observed after 12 weeks of daily subcutaneous C-peptide treatment *(71)*. More recently, a larger randomized double-blind placebo-controlled study of 139 patients has also demonstrated a significant improvement in sensory NCV and a clinical score of neurological deficits after 6 months of daily C-peptide *(72)*.

Vascular Endothelial Growth Factor

VEGF was originally discovered as an endothelial-specific growth factor with a predominant role in angiogenesis and retinopathy *(73)*. However, recent observations indicate that VEGF also has direct effects on neurons and glial cells stimulating their growth, survival, and axonal outgrowth *(74)*. Thus with its potential for a dual impact on both the vasculature and neurones it could represent an important therapeutic intervention in diabetic neuropathy *(75)*. A transient increase in the transcriptional regulator hypoxia-inducible factor-1α and a number of its target genes including VEGF and erythropoietin has been demonstrated recently in diabetic rats *(76)*. Similarly in the STZ-diabetic rat intense VEGF staining has been shown in cell bodies and nerve fibers compared with no or very little VEGF in controls and animals treated with insulin or NGF *(77)*. After 4-week intramuscular gene transfer of plasmid DNA encoding VEGF-1/2 nerve vascularity, blood flow, and both large and small fiber dysfunction were restored in the STZ-diabetic rat and the alloxan-induced diabetic rabbit *(78)*. Thus, although there is an intrinsic capacity to upregulate hypoxia-inducible factor-1α and hence VEGF, this appears insufficient and may require exogenous delivery possibly through gene therapy. In 29 patients with angiographically proven critical leg ischemia (six patients with diabetes), injections of phVEGF165 in the muscles of the ischemic limb resulted in a significant improvement in the sensory examination score, peroneal nerve motor amplitude, and vibration perception threshold *(79)*. The improvement in the vascular ankle-brachial index corresponded to the improvement in neuropathy and four of six patients with diabetes also showed an improvement in neurological deficits.

A phase I/II double-blind, placebo-controlled study evaluating the impact of VEGF165 gene transfer on diabetic sensory neuropathy is currently underway *(80)*.

Neurotrophins

Neurotrophins promote neuronal survival by inducing morphological differentiation, enhancing nerve regeneration, and stimulating neurotransmitter expression *(81)*. Although the data implicating deranged neurotrophical support is compelling in animal models, in diabetic patients results are somewhat contradictory. Thus, although dermal NGF protein levels are reduced in patients with diabetes, sensory fiber dysfunction *(82)*, skin mRNA NGF *(83)*, and NT-3 *(84)* are increased and sciatic nerve ciliary neurotrophic factor levels remain unchanged *(85)*. Furthermore, *in situ* hybridization studies demonstrate increased expression of TrkA (NGF-receptor) and trkC (NT-3 receptor) in the skin of patients with diabetes *(86)*, whereas a phase II clinical trial of recombinant human nerve growth factor demonstrated a significant improvement in neuropathy *(87)*, a phase III trial failed to demonstrate a significant benefit *(88)*. More recently brain-derived neurotrophic factor has demonstrated no significant improvement in nerve conduction, quantitative sensory, and autonomic function tests, including the cutaneous axon-reflex *(89)*.

REFERENCES

1. Nishikawa T, Edelstein D, Du XL, et al. Normalizing mitochondrial superoxide production blocks three pathways of hyperglycemic damage. *Nature* 2000;404:787–790.
2. Smith AG, Ramachandran P, Tripp S, Singleton JR. Epidermal nerve innervation in impaired glucose tolerance and diabetes-associated neuropathy. *Neurology* 2001;13:1701–1704.
3. Sumner CJ, Sheth S, Griffin JW, Cornblath DR, Polydefkis M. The spectrum of neuropathy in diabetes and impaired glucose tolerance. *Neurology* 2003;60:108–111.
4. Sundkvist G, Dahlin LB, Nilsson H, et al. Sorbitol and myo-inositol levels and morphology of sural nerve in relation to peripheral nerve function and clinical neuropathy in men with diabetic, impaired, and normal glucose tolerance. *Diabetic Med* 2000;17:259–268.
5. Cappellari A, Airaghi L, Capra R, et al. Early peripheral nerve abnormalities in impaired glucose tolerance. *Electromyogr Clin Neurophysiol* 2005;45:241–244.
6. Haslbeck KM, Schleicher E, Bierhaus A, et al. The AGE/RAGE/NF-(kappa) B pathway may contribute to the pathogenesis of polyneuropathy in impaired glucose tolerance (IGT). *Exp Clin Endocrinol Diabetes* 2005;113:288–291.
7. Dyck PJ, Kratz KM, Karnes JZ, et al. The prevalence by staged severity of various types of diabetic neuropathy, retinopathy and nephropathy in a population-based cohort: the Rochester Diabetic Neuropathy Study. *Neurology* 1993;43:817–824.
8. DCCT Trial Research Group. The effect of intensive diabetes therapy on the development and progression of neuropathy. *Ann Int Med* 1995;122:561–568.
9. Navarro X, Sutherland DE, Kennedy WR. Long-term effects of pancreatic transplantation on diabetic neuropathy. *Ann Neurol* 1997;42:727–736.
10. Lee TC, Barshes NR, O'Mahony CA, et al. The effect of pancreatic islet transplantation on progression of diabetic retinopathy and neuropathy. *Transplant Proc* 2005;37:2263–2265.
11. UKPDS. Intensive blood glucose control with sulphonylureas or insulin compared with conventional treatment and risk of complications in patients with Type 2 diabetes. *Lancet* 1998;352:837–853.
12. Azad N, Emanuele NV, Abraira C, et al. The effects of intensive glycemic control on neuropathy in the VA cooperative study on type II diabetes mellitus (VA CSDM). *J Diabetes Complications* 1999;13:307–313.

13. Gaede P, Vedel P, Larsen N, Jensen GV, Parving HH, Pedersen O. Multifactorial intervention and cardiovascular disease in patients with type 2 diabetes. *N Engl J Med* 2003; 348:383–393.
14. Oates PJ. Polyol pathway and diabetic peripheral neuropathy. *Int Rev Neurobiol* 2002;50:325–392.
15. Chung SS, Chung SK. Aldose reductase in diabetic microvascular complications. *Curr Drug Targets* 2005;6:475–486.
16. Dyck PJ, Sherman WR, Hallcher LM, et al. Human diabetic endoneurial sorbitol, fructose, and myo-inositol related to sural nerve morphometry. *Ann Neurol* 1980;8:590–596.
17. Mayhew JA, Gillon KR, Hawthorne JN. Free and lipid inositol, sorbitol and sugars in sciatic nerve obtained post-mortem from diabetic patients and control subjects. *Diabetologia* 1983;24:13–15.
18. Hale PJ, Nattrass M, Silverman SH, et al. Peripheral nerve concentrations of glucose, fructose, sorbitol and myoinositol in diabetic and non-diabetic patients. *Diabetologia* 1987;30:464–467.
19. Dyck PJ, Zimmerman BR, Vilen TH, et al. Nerve glucose, fructose, sorbitol, myo-inositol, and fiber degeneration and regeneration in diabetic neuropathy. *N Engl J Med* 1988;319:542–548.
20. Sivenius K, Pihlajamaki J, Partanen J, Niskanen L, Laakso M, Uusitupa M. Aldose reductase gene polymorphisms and peripheral nerve function in patients with type 2 diabetes. *Diabetes Care* 2004;27:2021–2026.
21. Kasajima H, Yamagishi S, Sugai S, Yagihashi N, Yagihashi S. Enhanced in situ expression of aldose reductase in peripheral nerve and renal glomeruli in diabetic patients. *Virchows Arch* 2001;439:46–54.
22. Shimizu H, Ohtani KI, Tsuchiya T, et al. Aldose reductase mRNA expression is associated with rapid development of diabetic microangiopathy in Japanese Type 2 diabetic (T2DM) patients. *Diabetes Nutr Metab* 2000;13:75–79.
23. Airey M, Bennett C, Nicolucci A, Williams R. Aldose reductase inhibitors for the prevention and treatment of diabetic peripheral neuropathy. *Cochrane Database Syst Rev* 2000;(2): CD002182.
24. Sima AA, Bril V, Nathaniel V, et al. Regeneration and repair of myelinated fibers in sural-nerve biopsy specimens from patients with diabetic neuropathy treated with sorbinil. *N Engl J Med* 1988;319:548–555.
25. Greene DA, Arezzo JC, Brown MB. Effect of aldose reductase inhibition on nerve conduction and morphometry in diabetic neuropathy. Zenarestat Study Group. *Neurology* 1999;53:580–591.
26. Hotta N, Toyota T, Matsuoka K, et al. The SNK-860 Diabetic Neuropathy Study Group. Clinical efficacy of fidarestat, a novel aldose reductase inhibitor, for diabetic peripheral neuropathy: a 52-week multicentre placebo-controlled double-blind parallel group study. *Diabetes Care* 2001;24:1776–1782.
27. Kinekawa F, Kubo F, Matsuda K, et al. Effect of an aldose reductase inhibitor on esophageal dysfunction in diabetic patients. *Hepatogastroenterology* 2005;52:471–474.
28. Okamoto H, Nomura M, Nakaya Y, et al. Effects of epalrestat, an aldose reductase inhibitor, on diabetic neuropathy and gastroparesis. *Intern Med* 2003;42:655–664.
29. Johnson BF, Nesto RW, Pfeifer MA, et al. Cardiac abnormalities in diabetic patients with neuropathy: effects of aldose reductase inhibitor administration. *Diabetes Care* 2004;27: 448–454.
30. Wada R, Yagihashi S. Role of advanced glycation end products and their receptors in development of diabetic neuropathy. *Ann NY Acad Sci* 2005;1043:598–604.
31. McLennan SV, Martell SK, Yue DK. Effects of mesangium glycation on matrix metalloproteinase activities: possible role in diabetic nephropathy. *Diabetes* 2002;51:2612–2618.

32. Portero-Otin M, Pamplona R, Bellmunt MJ, et al. Advanced glycation end product precursors impair epidermal growth factor receptor signaling. *Diabetes* 2002;51:1535–1542.
33. Sugimoto K, Nishizawa Y, Horiuchi S, Yagihashi S. Localization in human diabetic peripheral nerve of N (epsilon)-carboxymethyllysine-protein adducts, an advanced glycation end product. *Diabetologia* 1997;40:1380–1387.
34. Misur I, Zarkovic K, Barada A, Batelja L, Milicevic Z, Turk Z. Advanced glycation end products in peripheral nerve in type 2 diabetes with neuropathy. *Acta Diabetol* 2004;41: 158–166.
35. Amano S, Kaji Y, Oshika T, et al. Advanced glycation end products in human optic nerve head. *Br J Ophthalmol* 2001;85:52–55.
36. Bierhaus A, Haslbeck KM, Humpert PM, et al. Loss of pain perception in diabetes is dependent on a receptor of the immunoglobulin superfamily. *J Clin Invest* 2004;114: 1741–1751.
37. Cameron NE, Gibson TM, Nangle MR, Cotter MA. Inhibitors of advanced glycation end product formation and neurovascular dysfunction in experimental diabetes. *Ann NY Acad Sci* 2005;1043:784–792.
38. Vincent AM, Russell JW, Low P, Feldman EL. Oxidative stress in the pathogenesis of diabetic neuropathy. *Endocr Rev* 2004;25:612–628.
39. Ziegler D, Sohr CG, Nourooz-Zadeh J. Oxidative stress and antioxidant defense in relation to the severity of diabetic polyneuropathy and cardiovascular autonomic neuropathy. *Diabetes Care* 2004;27:2178–2183.
40. Ziegler D, Hanefeld M, Ruhnau KJ, et al. Treatment of symptomatic diabetic peripheral neuropathy with the anti-oxidant alpha-lipoic acid. A 3-week multicentre randomized controlled trial (ALADIN Study). *Diabetologia* 1995;38:1425–1433.
41. Ruhnau KJ, Meissner HP, Finn JR, et al. Effects of 3-week oral treatment with the antioxidant thioctic acid (alpha-lipoic acid) in symptomatic diabetic polyneuropathy. *Diabetic Med* 1999;16:1040–1043.
42. Reljanovic M, Reichel G, Rett K, et al. Treatment of diabetic polyneuropathy with the antioxidant thioctic acid (alpha-lipoic acid): a two year multicentre randomized double-blind placebo-controlled trial (ALADIN II). *Free Radic Res* 1999;31:171–179.
43. Ziegler D, Hanefeld M, Ruhnau KJ, et al. Treatment of symptomatic diabetic polyneuropathy with the antioxidant alpha-lipoic acid: a 7-month multicentre randomized controlled trial (ALADIN III Study). ALADIN III Study Group. *Diabetes Care* 1999;22: 1296–1301.
44. Ametov AS, Barinov A, Dyck PJ, et al. SYDNEY Trial Study Group. The sensory symptoms of diabetic polyneuropathy are improved with alpha-lipoic acid: the SYDNEY trial. *Diabetes Care* 2003;26:770–776.
45. Malik RA, Tomlinson DR. Angiotensin-converting enzyme inhibitors: are there credible mechanisms for beneficial effects in diabetic neuropathy? *Int Rev Neurobiol* 2002;50: 415–430.
46. Young MJ, Veves A, Walker MG, Boulton AJM. Correlations between nerve function and tissue oxygenation in diabetic patients: further clues to the etiology of diabetic neuropathy? *Diabetologia* 1992;35:1146–1150.
47. Akbari CM, Gibbons GW, Habershaw GM, LoGerfo FW, Veves A. The effect of arterial reconstruction on the natural history of diabetic neuropathy. *Arch Surg* 1997;132:148–152.
48. Veves A, Donaghue VM, Sarnow MR, Giurini JM, Campbell DR, LoGerfo FW. The impact of reversal of hypoxia by revascularization on the peripheral nerve function of diabetic patients. *Diabetologia* 1996;39:344–348.
49. Arora S, Pomposelli F, LoGerfo FW, Veves A. Cutaneous microcirculation in the neuropathic diabetic foot improves significantly but not completely after successful lower extremity revascularization. *J Vasc Surg* 2002;35:501–505.

50. Jarmuzewska EA, Mangoni AA. Pulse pressure is independently associated with sensorimotor peripheral neuropathy in patients with type 2 diabetes. *J Intern Med* 2005;258: 38–44.
51. Tesfaye S, Chaturvedi N, Eaton SE, et al. EURODIAB Prospective Complications Study Group. Vascular risk factors and diabetic neuropathy. *N Engl J Med* 2005;352:341–350.
52. Thrainsdottir S, Malik RA, Dahlin LB, et al. Endoneurial capillary abnormalities presage deterioration of glucose tolerance and accompany peripheral neuropathy in man. *Diabetes* 2003;52:2615–2622.
53. Malik RA, Tesfaye S, Newrick PG, et al. Sural nerve pathology in diabetic patients with minimal but progressive neuropathy. *Diabetologia* 2005;48:578–585.
54. Schofield I, Malik R, Izzard A, Austin C, Heagerty A. Vascular structural and functional changes in type 2 diabetes mellitus: evidence for the roles of abnormal myogenic responsiveness and dyslipidemia. *Circulation* 2002;106:3037–3043.
55. Malik RA, Schofield IJ, Izzard A, Austin C, Bermann G, Heagerty AM. Effects of angiotensin type-1 receptor antagonism on small artery function in patients with type 2 diabetes mellitus. *Hypertension* 2005;45:264–269.
56. Reja A, Tesfaye S, Harris N, Ward JD. Improvement in nerve conduction and quantitative sensory tests after treatment with lisinopril. *Diabetic Med* 1995;12:307–309.
57. Malik RA, Williamson S, Abbott CA, et al. Effect of angiotensin-converting enzyme (ACE) inhibitor trandalopril on human diabetic neuropathy: randomised double-blind controlled trial. *Lancet* 1998;352:1978–1981.
58. Estaci RO, Jeffers BW, Gifford N, Schrier RW. Effect of blood pressure control on diabetic microvascular complications in patients with hypertension and type 2 diabetes. *Diabetes Care* 2000;23:B54–B64.
59. Eichberg J. Protein kinase C changes in diabetes: is the concept relevant to neuropathy? *Int Rev Neurobiol* 2002;50:61–82.
60. Cameron NE, Cotter MA. Effects of protein kinase C beta inhibition on neurovascular dysfunction in diabetic rats: interaction with oxidative stress and essential fatty acid dysmetabolism. *Diabetes Metab Res Rev* 2002;18:315–323.
61. Vinik AI, Bril V, Kempler P, et al. the MBBQ Study Group. Treatment of symptomatic diabetic peripheral neuropathy with the protein kinase C beta-inhibitor ruboxistaurin mesylate during a 1-year, randomized, placebo-controlled, double-blind clinical trial. *Clin Ther* 2005;27:1164–1180.
62. Economides PA, Caselli A, Tiani E, Khaodhiar L, Horton ES, Veves A. The effects of atorvastatin on endothelial function in diabetic patients and subjects at risk for type 2 diabetes. *J Clin Endocrinol Metab* 2004;89:740–747.
63. Okamoto T, Yamagishi SI, Inagaki Y, et al. Angiogenesis induced by advanced glycation end products and its prevention by cerivastatin. *FASEB J* 2002;16:1928–1930.
64. Fried LF, Forrest KY, Ellis D, Chang Y, Silvers N, Orchard TJ. Lipid modulation in insulin-dependent diabetes mellitus: effect on microvascular outcomes. *J Diabetes Complications* 2001;15:113–119.
65. Schmidt RE, Dorsey DA, Beaudet LN, Peterson RG. Analysis of the Zucker Diabetic Fatty (ZDF) type 2 diabetic rat model suggests a neurotrophic role for insulin/IGF-I in diabetic autonomic neuropathy. *Am J Pathol* 2003;163:21–28.
66. Delaney CL, Russell JW, Cheng HL, Feldman EL. Insulin-like growth factor-I and over-expression of Bcl-xL prevent glucose-mediated apoptosis in Schwann cells. *J Neuropathol Exp Neurol* 2001;60:147–160.
67. Grandis M, Nobbio L, Abbruzzese M, et al. Insulin treatment enhances expression of IGF-I in sural nerves of diabetic patients. *Muscle Nerve* 2001;24:622–629.
68. Wahren J, Shafqat J, Johansson J, Chibalin A, Ekberg K, Jornvall H. Molecular and cellular effects of C-peptide—new perspectives on an old peptide. *Exp Diabesity Res* 2004;5: 15–23.

69. Sima AA. C-peptide and diabetic neuropathy. *Expert Opin Investig Drugs* 2003;12: 1471–1488.
70. Cotter MA, Ekberg K, Wahren J, Cameron NE. Effects of proinsulin C-peptide in experimental diabetic neuropathy: vascular actions and modulation by nitric oxide synthase inhibition. *Diabetes* 2003;52:1812–1817.
71. Ekberg K, Brismar T, Johansson BL, Jonsson B, Lindstrom P, Wahren J. Amelioration of sensory nerve dysfunction by C-Peptide in patients with type 1 diabetes. *Diabetes* 2003;52:536–541.
72. Ekberg K, Juntti-Berggren L, Norrby A, et al. C-peptide improves sensory nerve function in type 1 diabetes and neuropathy. *Diabetologia* 2005;48:A81.
73. Malik RA, Li C, Aziz W, et al. Elevated plasma CD105 and vitreous VEGF levels in diabetic retinopathy. *J Cell Mol Med* 2005;9:692–697.
74. Carmeliet P, Storkebaum E. Vascular and neuronal effects of VEGF in the nervous system: implications for neurological disorders. *Semin Cell Dev Biol* 2002;13:39–53.
75. Veves A, King GL. Can VEGF reverse diabetic neuropathy in human subjects? *J Clin Invest* 2001;107:1215–1218.
76. Chavez JC, Almhanna K, Berti-Mattera LN. Transient expression of hypoxia-inducible factor-1 alpha and target genes in peripheral nerves from diabetic rats. *Neurosci Lett* 2005;374:179–182.
77. Samii A, Unger J, Lange W. Vascular endothelial growth factor expression in peripheral nerves and dorsal root ganglia in diabetic neuropathy in rats. *Neurosci Lett* 1999;262:159–162.
78. Schratzberger P, Walter DH, Rittig K, et al. Reversal of experimental diabetic neuropathy by VEGF gene transfer. *J Clin Invest* 2001;107:1083–1092.
79. Simovic D, Isner JM, Ropper AH, Pieczek A, Weinberg DH. Improvement in chronic ischemic neuropathy after intramuscular phVEGF165 gene transfer in patients with critical limb ischemia. *Arch Neurol* 2001;8:761–768.
80. Isner JM, Ropper A, Hirst K. VEGF gene transfer for diabetic neuropathy. *Hum Gene Ther* 2001;12:1593–1594.
81. Apfel SC. Neurotrophic factors in peripheral neuropathies: therapeutic implications. *Brain Pathol* 1999;9:393–413.
82. Anand P, Terenghi G, Warner G, Kopelman P, Williams-Chestnut RE, Sinicropi DV. The role of endogenous nerve growth factor in human diabetic neuropathy. *Nat Med* 1996;2:703–707.
83. Diemel LT, Cai F, Anand P, et al. Increased nerve growth factor mRNA in lateral calf skin biopsies from diabetic patients. *Diabetic Med* 1999;16:113–118.
84. Kennedy AJ, Wellmer A, Facer P, et al. Neurotrophin-3 is increased in skin in human diabetic neuropathy. *J Neurol Neurosurg Psychiatry* 1998;65:393–395.
85. Lee DA, Gross L, Wittrock DA, Windebank AJ. Localization and expression of ciliary neurotrophic factor (CNTF) in postmortem sciatic nerve from patients with motor neuron disease and diabetic neuropathy. *J Neuropathol Exp Neurol* 1996;55:915–923.
86. Terenghi G, Mann D, Kopelman PG, Anand P. trkA and trkC expression is increased in human diabetic skin. *Neurosci Lett* 1997;228:33–36.
87. Apfel SC, Kessler JA, Adornato BT, Litchy WJ, Sanders C, Rask CA. Recombinant human nerve growth factor in the treatment of diabetic polyneuropathy. NGF Study Group. *Neurology* 1998;51:695–702.
88. Apfel SC, Schwartz S, Adornato BT, et al. Efficacy and safety of recombinant human nerve growth factor in patients with diabetic polyneuropathy: a randomized controlled trial. *JAMA* 2000;284:2215–2221.
89. Wellmer A, Misra VP, Sharief MK, Kopelman PG, Anand P. A double-blind placebo-controlled clinical trial of recombinant human brain-derived neurotrophic factor (rhBDNF) in diabetic polyneuropathy. *J Peripher Nerv Syst* 2001;6:204–210.

14
Clinical Features of Diabetic Polyneuropathy

Solomon Tesfaye MD, FRCP

SUMMARY

Neuropathy affects approximately 30–50% of all diabetic patients and is the commonest form of neuropathy in the developed world. It encompasses several neuropathic syndromes including focal and symmetrical neuropathies, by far the commonest of which is distal symmetrical neuropathy. The two main clinical consequences, foot ulceration sometimes leading to amputation and painful neuropathy, are associated with much patient morbidity and mortality. There is now little doubt that glycaemic control and duration of diabetes are major determinants of distal symmetrical neuropathy. In addition potentially modifiable, traditional markers of macrovascular disease such as hypertension, hyperlipidaemia and smoking are also independent risk factors.

There is now increasing evidence that the cause of distal symmetrical neuropathy may be nerve ischaemia, though metabolic factors may be important early. Pain is the most distressing symptom of neuropathy and the main factor that prompts the patient to seek medical advice. Pain may also occur within the context of all neuropathic syndromes associated with diabetes, including focal neuropathies. In acute painful neuropathies the pain indeed the neuropathy is self-limiting and usually subsides within a year.

Abnormalities of autonomic function are very common in subjects with longstanding diabetes; however, clinically significant autonomic dysfunction is uncommon. Several systems including the cardiovascular, gastrointestinal and genitor-urinary systems may be affected. Focal (asymmetrical) neuropathies including diabetic amyotrophy are well-recognised complications of diabetes. They have a relatively rapid onset and cause major disability, but there may be complete recovery.

Key Words: Diabetes; diabetic polyneuropathy; diabetic peripheral neuropathy; focal neuropathies; entrapment neuropathies; painful diabetic neuropathy.

INTRODUCTION

Diabetic polyneuropathy is one of the most common complications of the diabetes and the most common form of neuropathy in the developed World. It encompasses several neuropathic syndromes the most common of which is distal symmetrical neuropathy, the main initiating factor for foot ulceration. The epidemiology of diabetic neuropathy has been reviewed in reasonable detail *(1)*. Several clinic- *(2,3)* and population-based studies *(4,5)* show surprisingly similar prevalence rates for distal symmetrical neuropathy, affecting about 30% of all diabetic people. The EURODIAB Prospective Complications Study, which involved the examination of 3250 type I patients, from 16 European countries, found a prevalence rate of 28% for distal symmetrical neuropathy *(2)*. After

From: *Contemporary Diabetes: Diabetic Neuropathy: Clinical Management, Second Edition*
Edited by: A. Veves and R. Malik © Humana Press Inc., Totowa, NJ

Table 1
Differential Diagnosis of Distal Symmetrical Neuropathy

Metabolic
Diabetes
Amyloidosis
Uremia
Myxedema
Porphyria
Vitamin deficiency (thiamin, B12, B6, pyridoxine)
Drugs and chemicals
Alcohol
Cytotoxic drugs e.g., Vincristine
Chlorambucil
Nitrofurantoin
Isoniazid
Neoplastic disorders
Bronchial or gastric carcinoma
Lymphoma
Infective or inflammatory
Leprosy
Guillain-Barre syndrome
Lyme borreliosis
Chronic inflammatory demyelinating polyneuropathy
Polyarteritis nodosa
Genetic
Charcot-Marie-Tooth disease
Hereditary sensory neuropathies

excluding those with neuropathy at baseline, the study showed that over a 7-year period, about one quarter of type 1 diabetic patients developed distal symmetrical neuropathy; age, duration of diabetes and poor glycamic control being major determinants *(6)*. The development of neuropathy was also associated with potentially modifiable cardiovascular risk factors such as hyperlipidaemia, hypertension, body mass index, and cigarette smoking *(6)*. Furthermore, cardiovascular disease at baseline carried a twofold risk of neuropathy, independent of cardiovascular risk factors *(6)*. Based on recent epidemiological studies, correlates of diabetic neuropathy include increasing age, increasing duration of diabetes, poor glycemic control, retinopathy, albuminuria, and vascular risk factors *(1,2,4,6)*. The differing clinical presentation of the several neuropathic syndromes in diabetes suggests varied etiological factors.

The clinical consequences of diabetic neuropathy are also varied. Some may have minor complaints, such as tingling in one or two toes; others may be affected with the devastating complications such as "the numb diabetic foot," or severe painful neuropathy that does not respond to drug therapy *(7)*. Moreover, diabetic neuropathy is a major contributor to male erectile dysfunction and other autonomic symptoms that are thankfully rare.

Diabetic peripheral neuropathy presents in a similar way to neuropathies of other causes, and thus, the physician needs to carefully exclude other common causes before attributing the neuropathy to diabetes (Table 1). Absence of other complications of diabetes, rapid

Table 2
Classification of Diabetic Neuropathy Based on Natural History

1. Progressive neuropathies. These are associated with increasing duration of diabetes and with other microvascular complications. Sensory disturbance predominates and autonomic involvement is common. The onset is gradual and there is no recovery.
2. Reversible neuropathies. These have an acute onset, often occurring at the presentation of diabetes itself, and are not related to the duration of diabetes or other microvascular complications. There is spontaneous recovery of these acute neuropathies.
3. Pressure palsies. Although, these are not specific to diabetes only, they tend to occur more frequently in patients with diabetes than the general population. There is no association with duration of diabetes or other microvascular complications of diabetes.

Table 3
The Varied Presentations of the Neuropathic Syndromes Associated With Diabetes

1. Chronic insidious sensory neuropathy
2. Acute painful neuropathy
3. Proximal motor neuropathy
4. Diffuse symmetrical motor neuropathy
5. The neuropathic foot
6. Pressure neuropathy
7. Focal vascular neuropathy
8. Neuropathy present at diagnosis
9. Treatment induced neuropathy
10. Hypoglycemic neuropathy

Adapted from ref. *9*.

weight loss, excessive alcohol intake, and other atypical features in either the history or clinical examination should alert the physician to search for other causes of neuropathy *(8)*.

CLINICAL CLASSIFICATION OF DIABETIC POLYNEUROPATHY

Although clinical classification of the various syndromes of diabetic peripheral neuropathy are often difficult because of the very considerable overlap in the mixture of clinical features, attempts at classification stimulate thought as to the etiology of the various syndromes and also assist in the planning of management strategy for the patient. Watkins and Edmonds *(9)* have suggested a classification for diabetic polyneuropathy based on the natural history of the various syndromes, which clearly separates them into three distinct groups (Table 2).

Based on the various distinct clinical presentations to the physician, Ward recommended a classification of diabetic polyneuropathy depicted in Table 3 *(10)*. This practical approach to the classification of diabetic neuropathies provides the clinician to have workable, crude definitions for the various neuropathic syndromes, and also assists in the management of the patient.

Another method of classifying diabetic polyneuropathy is by considering whether the clinical involvement is symmetrical or assymetrical. However, the separation to symmetrical and asymmetrical neuropathies, although useful in identifying distinct

Table 4
Classification of Diabetic Neuropathy

Symmetrical neuropathies
Distal sensory and sensori-motor neuropathy
Large-fiber type of diabetic neuropathy
Small-fiber type of diabetic neuropathy
Distal small-fiber neuropathy
"Insulin neuropathy"
Chronic inflammatory demyelinating polyradiculoneuropathy
Asymmetrical neuropathies
Mononeuropathy
Mononeuropathy multiplex
Radiculopathies
Lumbar plexopathy or radiculoplexopathy
Chronic inflammatory demyelinating polyradiculoneuropathy

Adapted from ref. *13*.

entities and perhaps providing clues to the varied aetiologies, is an oversimplification of the truth as there is a great overlapping of the syndromes. This method was originally suggested by Bruyn and Garland *(11)*, and later modified by Thomas *(12)*. More recently, Low and Suarez *(13)* have further modified this classification (Table 4).

SYMMETRICAL NEUROPATHIES

Chronic Distal Symmetrical Neuropathy

This is the most common neuropathic syndrome and what is meant in clinical practice by the phrase "diabetic neuropathy." Clinical manifestations *(14)* and measurements *(15,16)* of distal symmetrical neuropathy have recently been reviewed. There is a "length-related" pattern of sensory loss, with sensory symptoms starting in the toes and then extending to involve the feet and legs in a stocking distribution. In more severe cases, there is often upper limb involvement, with a similar progression proximally starting in the fingers. Although the nerve damage can extend over the entire body including the head and face, this is exceptional. Subclinical neuropathy detectable by autonomic function tests is usually present. However, clinical autonomic neuropathy is less common. Autonomic neuropathy is considered in more detail in Chapter 24. As the disease advances, overt motor manifestations, such as wasting of the small muscles of the hands and limb weakness become apparent. However, subclinical motor involvement detected by magnetic resonance imaging appears to be common, and thus, motor disturbance is clearly part of the functional impairment caused by distal symmetrical neuropathy *(17)*.

Symptoms

The main clinical presentation of distal symmetrical neuropathy is sensory loss, which the patient may not be aware of, or may be described as "numbness" or "dead feeling." However, some may experience a progressive buildup of unpleasant sensory symptoms including tingling (paraesthesae); burning pain; shooting pains down the legs; lancinating pains; contact pain often with day-time clothes and bedclothes (allodynia); pain on walking often described as "walking barefoot on marbles," or "walking barefoot on hot sand," sensations of heat or cold in the feet; persistent achy feeling in the feet; and cramp-like sensations in the legs. Occasionally, pain can extend above the feet and may involve the whole of the legs, and when this is the case there is usually upper limb involvement also. There is a large spectrum of severity of these symptoms. Some may have minor complaints such as tingling in one or two toes; others may be affected with the devastating complications, such as "the numb diabetic foot," or severe painful neuropathy that does not respond to drug therapy.

Diabetic neuropathic pain is characteristically more severe at night, and often prevents sleep *(18,19)*. Some patients may be in a constant state of tiredness because of sleep deprivation *(18,19)*. Others are unable to maintain full employment *(18–21)*. Severe painful neuropathy can occasionally cause marked reduction in exercise threshold thus interfere with daily activities *(20)*. This is particularly the case when there is an associated disabling, severe postural hypotension because of autonomic involvement *(9)*. Not surprisingly therefore, depressive, symptoms are not uncommon *(21)*. Although, subclinical autonomic neuropathy is commonly found in patients with distal symmetrical neuropathy *(22)*, symptomatic autonomic neuropathy is uncommon.

It is important to appreciate that many subjects with distal symmetrical neuropathy may not have any of the above symptoms, and their first presentation may be with a foot ulcer *(7)*. This underpins the need for carefully examining and screening the feet of all people with diabetes, in order to identify those at risk of developing foot ulceration *(7)*. The insensate foot is at risk of developing mechanical and thermal injuries, and patients must therefore be warned about these and given appropriate advice regarding foot care *(7,23)*. A curious feature of the neuropathic foot is that both numbness and pain may occur, the so called "painful, painless" leg *(23)*. It is indeed a paradox that the patient with a large foot ulcer may also have severe neuropathic pain. In those with advanced neuropathy, there may be sensory ataxia. The unfortunate sufferer is affected by unsteadiness on walking, and even falls particularly if there is associated visual impairment because of retinopathy.

Signs

Neuropathy is usually easily detected by simple clinical examination *(15,16,23)*. Shoes and socks should be removed and the feet examined at least annually and more often if neuropathy is present. The most common presenting abnormality is a reduction or absence of vibration sense in the toes. As the disease progresses there is sensory loss in a "stocking" and sometimes in a "glove" distribution involving all modalities. When there is severe sensory loss, proprioception may also be impaired, leading to a positive Romberg's sign. Ankle tendon reflexes are lost and with more advanced neuropathy, knee reflexes are often reduced or absent.

Muscle strength is usually normal during the early course of the disease, although mild weakness may be found in toe extensors. However, with progressive disease there is significant generalized muscular wasting, particularly in the small muscles of the hand and feet. The fine movements of fingers would then be affected, and there is difficulty in handling small objects. However, wasting of dorsal interossei is usually because of entrapment of the ulnar nerve at the elbow. The clawing of the toes is believed to be as a result of unopposed (because of wasting of the small muscles of the foot) pulling of the long extensor and flexor tendons. This scenario results in elevated plantar pressure points at the metatarsal heads that are prone to callus formation and foot ulceration *(7)*. Deformities such as a bunion can form the focus of ulceration and with more extreme deformities, such as those associated with Charcot arthropathy, the risk is further increased *(24)*. As one of the most common precipitants to foot ulceration is inappropriate footwear, a thorough assessment should also include examination of shoes for poor fit, abnormal wear, and internal pressure areas or foreign bodies *(7)*.

Autonomic neuropathy affecting the feet can cause a reduction in sweating and consequently dry the skin that is likely to crack easily, predisposing the patient to the risk of infection *(7)*. The "purely" neuropathic foot is also warm because of artero/venous shunting first described by Ward *(25)*. This results in the distension of foot veins that fail to collapse even when the foot is elevated. It is not unusual to observe a gangrenous toe in a foot that has bounding arterial pulses, as there is impairment of the nutritive capillary circulation because of arterio-venous shunting. The oxygen tension of the blood in these veins is typically raised *(26)*. The increasing blood flow brought about by autonomic neuropathy can sometimes result in neuropathic oedema, which is resistant to treatment with diuretics, but may respond to treatment with ephedrine *(27)*.

Small-Fiber Neuropathy

Some authorities have advocated the existence of "small-fiber neuropathy" as a distinct entity *(28,29)*, usually within the context of young type 1 patients. A prominent feature of this syndrome is neuropathic pain, which may be very severe, with relative sparing of large-fiber functions (vibration and proprioception). The pain is described as burning, deep, and aching. The sensation of pins and needles (paraesthesae) is also often experienced and contact hypersensitivity may be present. Rarely, patients with small-fiber neuropathy might not have neuropathic pain, and some might occasionally have foot ulceration. Autonomic involvement is common, and severely affected patients may be disabled by postural hypotension and/or gastrointestinal symptoms. The syndrome tends to develop within a few years of diabetes as a relatively early complication.

On clinical examination there is little evidence of objective signs of nerve damage, apart from a reduction in pinprick and temperature sensation, which are reduced in a "stocking" and "glove" distribution. There is relative sparing of vibration and position sense (because of relative sparing of the large diameter Aβ fibers). Muscle strength is usually normal and reflexes are also usually normal. However, autonomic function tests are frequently abnormal and affected male patients usually have erectile dysfunction. Electrophysiological tests support small-fiber dysfunction. Sural sensory conduction velocity may be normal, although the amplitude may be reduced. Motor nerves appear to be less affected. Controversy still exists regarding whether small-fiber neuropathy is a distinct entity or an earlier manifestation of chronic sensory motor neuropathy *(28,29)*. Said et al. *(28)* studied a small series of subjects with this syndrome and showed that small-fiber degeneration predominated morphometrically. Veves et al. *(30)* found a varying degree of early small-fiber involvement in all diabetic polyneuropathies, which was confirmed by detailed sensory and autonomic function tests. Therefore it is unclear, whether this syndrome is in fact distinct or merely represents the early stages of distal symmetrical neuropathy that has been detected by the prominence of early symptoms.

Natural History of Distal Symmetrical Neuropathy

The natural history of chronic distal symmetrical neuropathy remains poorly understood. This is mainly because there is paucity of well conducted prospective studies that have sought to examine this *(6)*. In addition, the inadequate knowledge regarding the pathogenesis of distal symmetrical neuropathy is also a contributory factor, although several mechanisms have been suggested *(31–35)*, and the list of potential mechanisms is constantly growing. Unlike in diabetic retinopathy and nephropathy, the scarcity of simple, accurate, and readily reproduciable methods of measuring neuropathy further complicates the problem *(15,16)*. One study *(36)* reported that neuropathic symptoms remain or get worse over a 5-year period in patients with chronic distal symmetrical neuropathy. A major drawback of this study was that it involved highly selected patients from a hospital base. A more recent study reported improvements in painful symptoms with worsening of quantitative measures of nerve function for a duration of 3.5 years *(37)*. Neuropathic pain was assessed using a visual analog scale, and small-fiber function by thermal limen, heat pain threshold, and weighted pinprick threshold. At follow-up, 3.5 years later one third of the 50 patients at baseline had died or were lost to follow-up. Clearly, this is a major drawback. There was symptomatic improvement in painful neuropathy in the majority of the remaining patients. It should be noted that many of the subjects were being treated with pain relieving drugs that may have influenced the findings. However, despite this symptomatic improvement, small fiber function as measured by the aforementioned tests deteriorated significantly. Thus, there was a dichotomy in the evolution of neuropathic symptoms and neurophysiological measures.

Are Painful and Painless Neuropathies Distinct Entities?

One of the complexities of distal symmetrical neuropathy is the variety of presentation to the clinician. A relative minority present with pain as the predominant symptom *(38)*. There is controversy as to whether the clinical, neurophysiological, peripheral nerve haemodynamic/morphometric findings are distinctly different in subjects with painful and painless diabetic neuropathy. Young et al. *(39)* reported that patients with painful neuropathy had a higher ratio of autonomic (small-fiber) abnormality to electrophysiological (large-fiber) abnormality. In contrast, they found that electrophysiological parameters were significantly worse in patients with foot ulceration compared with those with painful neuropathy. They concluded that in distal symmetrical neuropathy, the relationship between large-fiber and small-fibre damage is not uniform, and that there may be different etiological influences on large- and small-fibre neuropathy in diabetic subjects, with the predominant type of fibre damage determining the form of the presenting clinical syndrome *(39)*. This view is supported by the study of Tsigos et al. *(40)* who also suggested that painful and painless neuropathies represent two distinct clinical entities with little overlap. However, a contrary view was expressed by Veves et al. *(41)* who found that painful symptoms were frequent in diabetic neuropathy, irrespective of the presence or absence of foot ulceration, and that these symptoms may occur at any stage of the disease. They concluded that there is a spectrum of presentations from varying degrees of painful neuropathy to predominantly painless neuropathy associated with foot ulceration, and that much overlap is present *(41)*. The author's clinical observations support this view, as painful symptoms are often similarly present in patients with and without foot ulceration, suggesting that painless and painful neuropathy represent extreme forms of the same syndrome. Thus, an important clinical point is that the neuropathic foot with painful symptoms is just as vulnerable to foot ulceration as the foot with absence of painful neuropathic symptoms. The crucial determining factor is elevation of vibration perception threshold *(42)* and not the presence or absence of painful symptoms. Indeed, the "painful–painless" foot with ulceration, is frequently observed in the diabetic foot clinic, a phenomenon first described by Ward *(23)*.

ACUTE PAINFUL NEUROPATHIES

These are transient neuropathic syndromes characterized by an acute onset of pain in the lower limbs. Acute neuropathies present in a symmetrical fashion are relatively uncommon. Pain is invariably present and is usually distressing to the patient, and can sometimes be incapacitating. There are two distinct syndromes, the first of which occurs within the context of poor glycemic control, and the second with rapid improvements in metabolic control *(43)*.

Acute Painful Neuropathy of Poor Glycemic Control

This may occur in the context of type 1 or type 2 diabetic subjects with poor glycemic control. There is no relationship to the presence of other chronic diabetic complications. There is often an associated severe weight loss *(44)*. Ellenberg coined the description of this condition as "neuropathic cachexia" *(45)*. Patients typically develop persistent burning pain associated with allodynia (contact pain). The pain is most marked in the feet, but often affects the whole of the lower extremities. As in chronic distal symmetrical neuropathy, the pain is typically worse at night although persistent pain during day time is also common. The pain is likened to "walking on burning sand" and there may be a subjective feeling of the feet being "swollen." Patients also describe intermittent bouts of stabbing pain that shoot up the legs from the feet (peak pain), superimposed on the background of burning pain (background pain). Not surprisingly therefore, these disabling symptoms often lead to depression *(21,43)*.

On examination, sensory loss is usually surprisingly mild or even absent. There are usually no motor signs, although ankle jerks may be absent. Nerve conduction studies are also usually normal or mildly abnormal. However, temperature discrimination threshold (small-fibre function) is affected more commonly than vibration perception threshold (large-fibre function) *(46)*. There is usually complete resolution of symptoms within 12 months, and weight gain is usual with continued improvement in glycemic control with the use of insulin. The lack of objective signs should not raise the doubt that these painful symptoms are not real. Many patients feel that people including health care professionals do not fully appreciate their predicament.

Acute Painful Neuropathy of Rapid Glycemic Control (Insulin Neuritis)

The term "insulin neuritis" was coined by Caravati *(47)* who first described the syndrome of acute painful neuropathy of rapid glycemic control. The term is a misnomer as the condition can follow rapid improvement in glycemic control with oral hypoglycemic agents, and "neuritis" implies a neural inflammatory process for which there is no evidence. The author has therefore recommended that the term "acute painful neuropathy of rapid glycemic control" be used to describe this condition *(48)*.

The natural history of acute painful neuropathies is an almost guaranteed improvement *(49)* in contrast to chronic distal symmetrical neuropathy *(36)*. The patient presents with burning pain, paraesthesiae, allodynia, often with a nocturnal exacerbation of symptoms; and depression may be a feature. There is no associated weight loss, unlike acute painful neuropathy of poor glycemic control. Sensory loss is often mild or absent, and there are no motor signs. There is little or no abnormality on nerve conduction studies, but there is impaired exercise induced conduction velocity increment *(48,50)*. There is usually complete resolution of symptoms within 12 months.

On sural nerve biopsy, typical morphometric changes of chronic distal symmetrical neuropathy but with active regeneration, were observed *(49)*. In contrast, degeneration of both myelinated and unmyelinated fibres was found in acute painful neuropathy of poor glycemic control *(44)*. A recent study looking into the epineurial vessels of sural nerves in patients with acute painful neuropathy of rapid glycemic control demonstrated marked arterio/venous abnormality including the presence of proliferating new vessels, similar to those found in the retina *(48)*. The study suggested that the presence of this fine network of epineural vessels may lead to a "steal" effect rendering the endoneurium ischaemic, and the authors also suggested that this process may be important in the genesis of neuropathic pain *(48)*. These findings were also supported by studies in experimental diabetes, which demonstrated that insulin administration led to acute endoneurial hypoxia, by increasing nerve arterio-venous flow, and reducing the nutritive flow of normal nerves *(51)*. Further work needs to address whether these observed sural nerve vessel changes resolve with the resolution of painful symptoms.

ASYMMETRICAL NEUROPATHIES

The diabetic state can also affect single nerves (mononeuropathy), multiple nerves (mononeuropathy multiplex), or groups of nerve roots. These asymmetrical or focal neuropathies have a relatively rapid onset, and complete recovery is usual. This contrasts with chronic distal symmetrical neuropathy, where there is usually no improvement in symptoms 5 years after onset *(36)*. Unlike chronic distal symmetrical neuropathy they are often unrelated to the presence of other diabetic complications *(9,15,16)*. Asymmetrical neuropathies are more common in men and tend to predominantly affect older patients *(52)*. A careful history is therefore mandatory in order to identify any associated symptoms that might point to another cause for the neuropathy. A vascular etiology has been suggested by virtue of the rapid onset of symptoms and the focal nature of the neuropathic syndromes *(53)*.

Proximal Motor Neuropathy (Femoral Neuropathy, Amyotrophy, and Plexopathy)

The syndrome of progressive asymmetrical proximal leg weakness and atrophy was first described by Garland *(54)*, who coined the term "diabetic amyotrophy." This condition has also been named as "proximal motor neuropathy," "femoral neuropathy" or "plexopathy." The patient presents with severe pain, which is felt deep in the thigh, but can sometimes be of burning quality and extend lower than the knee. The pain is usually continuous and often causes insomnia and depression *(55)*. Both type 1 and type 2 patients more than the age of 50 are affected *(54–57)*. There is an associated weight loss, which can sometimes be very severe, and can raise the possibility of an occult malignancy.

On examination there is profound wasting of the quadriceps with marked weakness in these muscle groups, although hip flexors and hip abductors can also be affected *(58)*. Thigh adductors, glutei, and hamstring muscles may also be involved. The knee jerk is usually reduced or absent. The profound weakness can lead to difficulty from getting out of a low chair or climbing stairs. Sensory loss is unusual, and if present indicates a coexistent distal sensory neuropathy.

It is important to carefully exclude other causes of quadriceps wasting, such as nerve root and cauda equina lesions, and the possibility of occult malignancy causing proximal myopathy syndromes such as polymyocytis. Magnetic resonance imaging (MRI) of the lumbo-sacral spine is now mandatory in order to exclude focal nerve root intrapment and other pathologies. An erythrocyte sedimentation rate, an X-ray of the lumbar/sacral spine, a chest X-ray, and ultrasound of the abdomen may also be required. CSF protein is often elevated. Electrophysiological studies may demonstrate increased femoral nerve latency and active denervation of affected muscles.

The cause of diabetic proximal motor neuropathy is not known. It tends to occur within the background of diabetic distal symmetrical neuropathy *(59)*. It has been suggested that the combination of focal features superimposed on diffuse peripheral neuropathy may suggest vascular damage to the femoral nerve roots, as a cause of this condition *(60)*.

As in distal symmetrical neuropathy there is scarcity of prospective studies that have looked at the natural history of proximal motor neuropathy. Coppack and Watkins *(55)* have reported that pain usually starts to settle after about 3 months, and usually settles by 1 year, while the knee jerk is restored in 50% of the patients after 2 years. Recurrence on the other side is a rare event. Management is largely symptomatic and supportive. Patients should be encouraged and reassured that this condition is likely to resolve. There is still controversy as to whether the use of insulin therapy influences the natural history of this syndrome as there are no controlled trials. Some patients benefit from physiotherapy that involves extension exercises aimed at strengthening the quadriceps. The management of pain in proximal motor neuropathy is similar to that of chronic or acute distal symmetrical neuropathies (*see* Chapter 21).

Chronic Inflammatory Demyelinating Polyradiculopathy

Chronic inflammatory demyelinating polyradiculopathy (CIDP) occurs more commonly among patients with diabetes, creating diagnostic and management challenges *(61)*. Patients with diabetes may develop clinical and electrodiagnostic features similar to that of CIDP *(62)*. Clearly, it is vital to recognize these patients as unlike diabetic polyneuropathy, CIDP is treatable *(63)*. One should particularly be alerted when an unusually severe, rapid, and progressive polyneuropathy develops in a diabetic patient.

Nerve conduction studies show features of demyelination. The presence of 3 of the following criteria for demyelination is required: partial motor nerve conduction block, reduced motor nerve conduction velocity, prolonged distal motor latencies, and prolonged F-wave latencies *(64)*. Although, electrophysiological parameters are important, these alone cannot be entirely relied on to differentiate CIDP from diabetic polyneuropathy *(65)*.

Most experts recommend CSF analysis in order to demonstrate the typical findings in this condition: increased protein and a normal or only slightly elevated cell count *(63)*. However, spinal taps are not mandatory *(63)*.

The diagnostic value of nerve biopsy, usually of the sural nerve has been debated recently. Some authorities assert that nerve biopsy is of no value *(66),* whereas others consider it essential for the diagnosis and management of upto 60% patients with CIDP *(67)*. The diagnostic yield of sural nerve biopsies may be limited as the most prominent abnormalities may lie in the proximal segments of the nerve roots or in the motor nerves, which are areas not accessible to biopsy. Typical appearances include segmental demyelination and remyelination, anion bulbs, and inflammatory infiltrates, but these may also be found in diabetic polyneuropathy *(68)*. A defining feature of CIDP not found in diabetic polyneuropathy is the presence of macrophages in biopsy specimens in association with demyelination *(68)*.

Treatments for CIDP include intravenous immunoglobulin, plasma exchange, and corticosteroids *(63)*. Therapy should be started early in order to prevent continuing demyelination and also as it results in rapid and significant reversal of neurological disability *(69,70)*.

Mononeuropathies

The most common cranial mononeuropathy is the third cranial nerve palsy. The patient presents with pain in the orbit, or sometimes with a frontal headache *(53,71)*. There is typically ptosis and ophthalmoplegia, although the pupil is usually spared *(72,73)*. Recovery occurs usually over three months. The clinical onset and time-scale for recovery, and the focal nature of the lesions on the third cranial nerve, on post-mortem studies suggested an ischaemic etiology *(53,74)*. It is important to exclude any other cause of third cranial nerve palsy (aneurysm or tumour) by computed tomography or MRI scanning, where the diagnosis is in doubt. Fourth, sixth, and seventh cranial nerve palsies have also been described in diabetic subjects, but the association with diabetes is not as strong as that with third cranial nerve palsy.

Truncal Radiculopathy

Truncal radiculopathy is well recognized to occur in diabetes. It is characterized by an acute onset pain in a dermatomal distribution over the thorax or the abdomen *(75)*. The pain is usually asymmetrical, and can cause local bulging of the muscle *(76)*. There may be patchy sensory loss detected by pin prick and light touch examination. It is important to exclude other causes of nerve root compression and occasionally, MRI of the spine may be required. Some patients presenting with abdominal pain have undergone unnecessary investigations, such as barium enema, colonoscopy, and even laparotomy, when the diagnosis could easily have been made by careful clinical history and examination. Recovery is usually the rule within several months, although symptoms can sometimes persist for a few years.

Pressure Neuropathies

Carpal Tunnel Syndrome

A number of nerves are vulnerable to pressure damage in diabetes. In the Rochester Diabetic Neuropathy Study, which was a population-based epidemiological study, Dyck et al. *(77)*, found electrophysiological evidence of median nerve lesions at the wrist in about 30% of diabetic subjects, although the typical symptoms of carpel tunnel syndrome occurred in less than 10%. The patient typically has pain and paraesthesia in the hands, which sometimes radiate to the forearm and are particularly marked at night. In severe cases clinical examination may reveal a reduction in sensation in the median territory in the hands, and wasting of the muscle bulk in the thenar eminence. The clinical diagnosis is easily confirmed by median nerve conduction studies and treatment involves surgical decompression at the carpel tunnel in the wrist. There is generally good response to surgery, although painful symptoms appear to relapse more commonly than in the nondiabetic population *(78)*.

Ulnar Nerve and Other Isolated Nerve Entrapments

The ulnar nerve is also vulnerable to pressure damage at the elbow in the ulnar groove. This results in wasting of the dorsal interossei, particularly the first dorsal interossius. This is easily confirmed by ulnar electrophysiological studies which localize the lesion to the elbow. Rarely, the patients may present with wrist drop because of radial nerve palsy after prolonged sitting (with pressure on the radial nerve in the back of the arms) while unconscious during hypoglycaemia or asleep after an alcohol binge.

In the lower limbs the common peroneal (lateral popliteal) is the most commonly affected nerve. The compression is at the level of the head of the fibula and causes foot drop. Unfortunately, complete recovery is not usual. The lateral cutaneous nerve of the thigh is occasionally also affected with entrapment neuropathy in diabetes. Phrenic nerve involvement in association with diabetes has also been described, although the possibility of a pressure lesion could not be excluded *(79)*.

REFERENFCES

1. Shaw JE, Zimmet PZ. The epidemiology of diabetic neuropathy. *Diabetes Rev* 1999; 7:245–252.
2. Tesfaye S, Stephens L, Stephenson J, et al. The prevalence of diabetic neuropathy and its relation to glycaemic control and potential risk factors: the EURODIAB IDDM Complications Study. *Diabetologia* 1996;39:1377–1384.
3. Young MJ, Boulton AJM, Macleod AF, Williams DRR, Sonksen PH. A multicentre study of the prevalence of diabetic peripheral neuropathy in the United Kingdom hospital clinic population. *Diabetologia* 1993;36:150–154.
4. Maser RE, Steenkiste AR, Dorman JS, et al. Epidemiological correlates of diabetic neuropathy. Report from Pittsburgh Epidemiology of Diabetes Complications Study. *Diabetes* 1989;38:1456–1461.
5. Ziegler D. Diagnosis, staging and epidemiology of diabetic peripheral neuropathy. *Diab Nutr Metab* 1994;7:342–348.
6. Tesfaye S, Chaturvedi N, Eaton SEM, Witte D, Ward JD, Fuller J. Vascular risk factors and diabetic neuropathy. *N Engl J Med* 2005;352:341–350.
7. Boulton AJM, Kirsner RS, Viliekyte L. Neuropathic diabetic foot ulcers. *N Engl J Med* 2004;351:48–55.
8. Tesfaye S. Diabetic neuropathy: achieving best practice. *Br J Vasc Dis* 2003;3:112–117.
9. Watkins PJ, Edmonds ME. Clinical features of diabetic neuropathy, in *Textbook of Diabetes* (Pickup J, Williams G, eds.), 1997, Vol. 2, pp. 50.1–50.20.
10. Ward JD. Clinical features of diabetic neuropathy. in *Diabetic Neuropathy* (Ward JD, Goto Y, eds.), Chichester, UK., Wiley, 1990, pp. 281–296.

11. Bruyn GW, Garland H. Neuropathies of endocrine origin. in *Handbook of clinical neurology* (Vinken PJ, Bruyn GW, eds.), Amsterdam, North-Holland Publishing Co., 1970, Vol. 8, 29p.
12. Thomas PK. Metabolic neuropathy. *J Roy Coll Phys* (*Lond*) 1973;7:154–160.
13. Low PA, Suarez GA. Diabetic neuropathies. in *Bailliere's Clinical Neurology* 1995;4(3):401–425.
14. Boulton AJM, Malik RA, Arezzo JC, Sosenko JM. Diabetic Somatic neuropathies. *Diabetes Care* 2004;27:1458–1486.
15. Eaton SEM, Tesfaye S. Clinical manifestations and measurement of somatic neuropathy. *Diabetes Rev* 1999;7:312–325.
16. Scott LA, Tesfaye S. Measurement of somatic neuropathy for clinical practice and clinical trials. *Curr Diabetes Rep* 2001;1:208–215.
17. Andersen H, Jakobsen J. Motor function in diabetes. *Diabetes Rev* 1999;7:326–341.
18. Watkins PJ. Pain and diabetic neuropathy. *Br Med J* 1984;288:168–169.
19. Tesfaye S, Price D. Therapeutic approaches in diabetic neuropathy and neuropathic pain. in *Diabetic Neuropathy*. (Boulton AJM, ed.), 1997;159–181.
20. Tesfaye S, Watt J, Benbow SJ, Pang KA, Miles J, MacFarlane IA. Electrical spinal cord stimulation for painful diabetic peripheral neuropathy. *Lancet* 1996;348:1696–1701.
21. Quattrini C, Tesfaye S. Understanding the impact of painful diabetic neuropathy. *Diabetes Metab Res Rev* 2003;(Suppl 1):S1–S8.
22. Ewing DJ, Borsey DQ, Bellavere F, Clarke BF. Cardiac autonomic neuropathy in diabetes: comparison of measures of R-R interval variation. *Diabetologia* 1981;21:18–24.
23. Ward JD. The diabetic leg. *Diabetologia* 1982;22:141–147.
24. Rajbhandari SM, Jenkins R, Davies C, Tesfaye S. Charcot neuroarthropathy in diabetes mellitus. *Diabetologia* 2002;1085–1096.
25. Ward JD, Simms JM, Knight G, Boulton AJM, Sandler DA. Venous distension in the diabetic neuropathic foot (physical sign of arterio-venous shunting). *J Roy Soc Med* 1983;76:1011–1014.
26. Boulton AJM, Scarpello JHB, Ward JD. Venous oxygenation in the diabetic neuropathic foot: evidence of arterial venous shunting? *Diabetologia* 1982;22:6–8.
27. Edmonds ME, Archer AG, Watkins PJ. Ephedrine: a new treatment for diabetic neuropathic oedema. *Lancet* 1983;1(8324):548–551.
28. Said G, Slama G, Selva J. Progressive centripital degeneration of of axons in small-fibre type diabetic polyneuropathy. A clinical and pathological study. *Brain* 1983;106:791.
29. Vinik AI, Park TS, Stansberry KB, Pittenger GL. Diabetic neuropathies. *Diabetologia* 2000;43:957–973.
30. Veves A, Young MJ, Manes C, et al. Differences in peripheral and autonomic nerve function measurements in painful and painless neuropathy: a Clinical study. *Diabetes Care* 1994;17:1200–1202.
31. Ward JD, Tesfaye S. Pathogenesis of diabetic neuropathy. in *Textbook of Diabetes* (Pickup J, Williams G, eds.), 1997, Vol. 2, pp. 49.1– 49.19.
32. Cameron NE, Eaton SE, Cotter MA, Tesfaye S.Vascular factors and metabolic interactions in the pathogenesis of diabetic neuropathy. *Diabetologia* 2001;44:1973–1988.
33. Tesfaye S, Harris N, Jakubowski J, et al. Impaired blood flow and arterio-venous shunting in human diabetic neuropathy: a novel technique of nerve photography and fluorescein angiography. *Diabetologia* 1993;36:1266–1274.
34. Eaton SE, Harris ND, Ibrahim S, et al. Differnces insural nerve haemodynamics in painful and painless neuropathy. *Diabetologia* 2003;934–939.
35. Malik RA, Tesfaye S, Newrick PG, et al. Sural nerve pathology in diabetic patients with minimal but progressive neuropathy. *Diabetologia* 2005;48:578–585.
36. Boulton AJM, Armstrong WD, Scarpello JHB, Ward JD. The natural history of painful diabetic neuropathy - a 4 year study. *Postgrad Med J* 1983;59:556–559.

37. Benbow SJ, Chan AW, Bowsher D, McFarlane IA, Williams G. A prospective study of painful symptoms, small fibre function and peripheral vascular disease in chronic painful diabetic neuropathy. *Diabetic Med* 1994;11:17–21.
38. Chan AW, MacFarlane IA, Bowsher DR, Wells JC, Bessex C, Griffiths K. Chronic pain in patients with diabetes mellitus: comparison with non-diabetic population. *Pain Clin* 3 1990;147–159.
39. Young RJ, Zhou YQ, Rodriguez E, Prescott RJ, Ewing DJ, Clarke BF. Variable relationship between peripheral somatic and autonomic neuropathy in patients with different syndromes of diabetic polyneuropathy. *Diabetes* 1986;35:192–197.
40. Tsigos C, White A, Young RJ. Discrimination between painful and painless diabetic neuropathy based on testing of large somatic nerve and sympathetic nerve function. *Diabetic Med* 1992;9:359–365.
41. Veves A, Manes C, Murray HJ, Young MJ, Boulton AJM. Painful neuropathy and foot ulceration in diabetic patients. *Diabetes Care* 1993;16:1187–1189.
42. Young MJ, Manes C, Boulton AJM. Vibration perception threshold predicts foot ulceration: a prospective study (Abstract). *Diabetic Med* 1992;9(Suppl 2):542.
43. Tesfaye S, Kempler P. Painful diabetic neuropathy. *Diabetologia* 2005;48:805–807.
44. Archer AG, Watkins PJ, Thomas PJ, Sharma AK, Payan J. The natural history of acute painful neuropathy in diabetes mellitus. *J Neurol Neorosurg Psychiatr* 1983;46:491–496.
45. Ellenberg M. Diabetic neuropathic cachexia. *Diabetes* 1974;23:418–423.
46. Guy RJC, Clark CA, Malcolm PN, Watkins PJ. Evaluation of thermal and vibration sensation in diabetic neuropathy. *Diabetologia*, 1985;28:131.
47. Caravati CM. Insulin neuritis: a case report. *Va Med Mon* 1933;59:745–746.
48. Tesfaye S, Malik R, Harris N, et al. Arteriovenous shunting and proliferating new vessels in acute painful neuropathy of rapid glycaemic control (insulin neuritis). *Diabetologia* 1996;39:329–335.
49. Llewelyn JG, Thomas PK, Fonseca V, King RHM, Dandona P. Acute painful diabetic neuropathy precipitated by strict glycaemic control. *Acta Neuropathol* (*Berl*) 1986;72: 157–163.
50. Tesfaye S, Harris N, Wilson RM, Ward JD. Exercise induced conduction veolcity increment: a marker of impaired nerve blood flow in diabetic neuropathy. *Diabetologia* 1992;35:155–159.
51. Kihara M, Zollman PJ, Smithson IL, et al. Hypoxic effect of endogenous insulin on normal and diabetic peripheral nerve. *Am J Physiol* 1994;266:E980–E985.
52. Matikainen E, Juntunen J. Diabetic neuropathy: Epidemiological, pathogenetic, and clinical aspects with special emphasis on type 2 diabetes mellitus. *Acta Endocrinol Suppl* (*Copenh*) 1984;262:89–94.
53. Asbury AK, Aldredge H, Hershberg R, Fisher CM. Oculomotor palsy in diabetes mellitus: a clinicopathological study. *Brain* 1970;93:555–557.
54. Garland H. Diabetic amyotrophy. *Br Med J* 1955;2:1287–1290.
55. Coppack SW, Watkins PJ. The natural history of femoral neuropathy. *Q J Med* 1991; 79:307–313.
56. Casey EB, Harrison MJG. Diabetic amyotrophy: a follow-up study. *Br Med J* 1972;1:656.
57. Garland H, Taverner D. Diabetic myelopathy. *Br Med J* 1953;1:1405.
58. Subramony SH, Willbourn AJ. Diabetic proximal neuropathy. Clinical and electromyographic studies. *J Neurol Sci* 1982;53:293–304.
59. Bastron JA, Thomas JE. Diabetic polyradiculoneuropathy: clinical and electromyographic findings in 105 patients. *Mayo Clinic Proc* 1981;56:725–732.
60. Said G, Goulon-Goeau C, Lacroix C, Moulonguet A. Nerve biopsy findings in different patterns of proximal diabetic neuropathy. *Ann Neurol* 1994;33:559–569.
61. Haq RU, Pendlebury WW, Fries TJ, Tandan R. Chronic inflammatory demyelinating polyradiculoneuropathy in diabetic patients. *Muscle Nerve* 2003;27:465–470.

62. Steward JD, McKelvey R, Durcan L, Carpenter S, Karpati G. Chronic inflammatory demyelinating polyneuropathy (CIPD) in diabetes. *J Neurol Sci* 1996;142:59–64.
63. Koller H, Kieseier BC, Jander S, Hartung H. Chronic Inflammatory Demyelinating Polyneuropathy. *NEJM* 2005;352:1343–1356.
64. Research criteria for diagnosis of chronic inflammatory demyelinating polyneuropathy (CIDP): report from an ad hoc sub-committee of the America Academy of Neurology AIDS Task Force. *Neurology* 1991;41:617–618.
65. Wilson JR, Park Y, Fisher MA. Electrodiagnostic criteria in CIDP: comparison with diabetic neuropathy. *Electromyogr Clin Neurophsiol* 2000;40:181–185.
66. Molenaar DS, Vermeulen M, de Haan R. Diagnostic value of sural nerve biopsy in chronic inflammatory demyelinating polyneuropathy. *J Neurol Neurosurg Psychiatry* 1998;64: 84–89.
67. Gabriel CM, Howard R, Kinsella N, et al. Prospective study of the usefulness of sural nerve biopsy. *J Neurol Neurosurg Psychiatry* 2000;69:442–446.
68. Vital C, Vital A, Lagueny A, et al. Chronic inflammatory demyelinating polyneuropathy; immunopathological and ultrastructural study of peripheral nerve biopsy in 42 cases. *Ultrastruct Pathol* 2000;24:363–369.
69. Cocito D, Ciaramitaro P, Isoardo G, et al. Intravenous immunoglobulin as first treatment in diabetics with concomitant distal symmetric axonal polyneuropathy and CIDP. *J Neurol* 2002;249:719–722.
70. Sharma KR, Cross J, Ayyar DR, Martinez-Arizala A, Bradley WG. Diabetic demyelinating polyneuropathy responsive to intravenous immunoglobulin therapy. *Arch Neurol* 2002; 59:751–757.
71. Zorilla E, Kozak GP. Ophthalmoplegia in diabetes mellitus. *Ann Internal Med* 1967;67:968–976.
72. Goldstein JE, Cogan DG. Diabetic ophthalmoplegia with special reference to the pupil. *Arch Ophthalmol* 1960;64:592–600.
73. Leslie RDG, Ellis C. Clinical course following diabetic ocular palsy. *Postgrad Med J* 1978;54:791–792.
74. Dreyfuss PM, Hakim S, Adams RD. Diabetic ophthalmoplegia. *Arch Neurol Psychiatry* 1957;77:337–349.
75. Ellenberg M. Diabetic truncal mononeuropathy—a new clincal syndrome. *Diabetes Care* 1978;1:10–13.
76. Boulton AJM, Angus E, Ayyar DR, Weiss R. Diabetic thoracic polyradiculopathy presenting as abdominal swelling. *BMJ* 1984;289:798–799.
77. Dyck PJ, Kratz KM, Karnes JL, et al. The prevalence by staged severity of various types of diabetic neuropathy, retinopathy, and nephropathy in a population-based cohort: the Rochester Diabetic Neuropathy Study. *Neurology* 1993;43:817–824.
78. Clayburgh RH, Beckenbaugh RD, Dobyns JH. Carp[el tunnel release in patients with diffuse peripheral neuropathy. *J Hand Surg* 1987;12A:380–383.
79. White JES, Bullock RF, Hudgson P, Home PD, Gibson GJ. Phrenic neuropathy in association with diabetes. *Diabet Med* 1992;9:954–956.

15
Micro- and Macrovascular Disease in Diabetic Neuropathy

Aristidis Veves, MD and Antonella Caselli, MD, PhD

SUMMARY

Diabetes is often defined a "vascular disease" because of the early and extensive involvement of the vascular-tree observed in patients with diabetes and even in those at risk of developing diabetes. Both the micro- and macrocirculation are affected. Changes in the micro- and macrocirculation, both anatomical and functional, contribute to the development of diabetic neuropathy. On the other hand, the development of diabetic neuropathy also affects the vasodilatory capacity of the microcirculation. Thus, the interaction between changes in the vasculature and peripheral nerves is bidirectional and results in changes in both blood flow and neuronal function. The possible links between diabetic micro- and macrovascular alterations and nerve damage will be the focus of this chapter.

Key Words: Blood flow; endothelial dysfunction; micro- and macrocirculation; neuronal function; vascular smooth muscle cell; iontophoresis.

INTRODUCTION

Diabetes is often defined a "vascular disease" because of the early and extensive involvement of the vascular tree observed in patients with diabetes and even in those at risk of developing diabetes. Both the micro- and macrocirculation are affected, though the pathophysiology, histology, clinical history, and clinical sequelae at the two vascular levels appear to be quite different. It is recently believed that a common pathway causes precocious vascular damage at both vascular districts in diabetes leading to the development of diabetic chronic complications, if not of diabetes itself. Chronic diabetic complications are mostly ascribed to small vessel disease. Diabetic microangiopathy has been considered the main anatomic alteration leading to the development of retinopathy, nephropathy, and neuropathy. Nevertheless, macroangiopathy, i.e., atherosclerosis of peripheral arteries, is also a peculiar feature of long-lasting diabetes and is characterized for being precocious, involving predominantly distal arteries and having inadequate collateral development. The possible links between diabetic micro- and macrovascular alterations and nerve damage will be the focus of this chapter.

MICROVASCULAR DISEASE: OVERVIEW AND ANATOMIC CHANGES

Lesions specific for diabetes have been observed in the arterioles and capillaries of the foot and other organs that are the typical targets of diabetic chronic complications.

From: *Contemporary Diabetes: Diabetic Neuropathy: Clinical Management, Second Edition*
Edited by: A. Veves and R. Malik © Humana Press Inc., Totowa, NJ

A contemporary historical histological study demonstrated the presence of PAS-positive material in the arterioles of amputated limb specimens from patients with diabetes *(1)*. Although it was believed for several years that the anatomic changes described were occlusive in nature, in 1984, Logerfo and Coffmann *(2)* recognized that in patients with diabetes, there is no evidence of an occlusive microvascular disease. Subsequent prospective anatomic staining and arterial casting studies have demonstrated the absence of an arteriolar occlusive lesion thus dispelling the hopeless notion of diabetic "occlusive small vessel disease" *(3,4)*.

Although there is no occlusive lesion in the diabetic microcirculation, other structural changes do exist. The thickening of the capillary basement membrane is the dominant structural change in both diabetic retinopathy and neuropathy and is because of an increase in the extracellular matrix. It might represent a response to the metabolic changes related to diabetes and hyperglycemia. However, this alteration does not lead to occlusion of the capillary lumen, and arteriolar blood flow might be normal or even increased despite these changes *(5)*. On the contrary, it might act as a barrier to the exchange of nutrients and/or increase the rigidity of the vessels further limiting their ability to dilate in response to different stimuli *(6)*.

In the kidney, nonenzymatic glycosylation reduces the charge on the basement membrane, which might account for transudation of albumin, an expanded mesangium, and albuminuria *(7)*. Similar increases in vascular permeability occur in the eye and probably contribute to macular exudate formation and retinopathy *(8)*. In simplest terms, microvascular structural alterations in diabetes result in an increased vascular permeability and impaired autoregulation of blood flow and vascular tone.

Many studies have identified a correlation between the development of diabetic chronic complication and metabolic control with perhaps the strongest evidence coming from the Diabetes Control and Complications Trial (DCCT), which enrolled patients with type 1 diabetes, and the United Kingdom Prospective Diabetes Study (UKPDS), which enrolled patients with type 2 diabetes *(9,10)*. The results from both clinical trials clearly showed a delay in the development and progression of retinopathy, nephropathy, and neuropathy with intensive glycemic control, thus supporting the direct causal relationship between hyperglycemia and microcirculation impairment. This was less evident for macrovascular disease, assessed only in the UKPDS.

Although the structural alterations observed in the microcirculation do not affect the basal blood flow, some functional abnormalities of the microvascular circulation that might eventually result in a relative ischemia have been extensively documented. This aspect will be deeply discussed in the "Pathophysiology of microvascular disease and endothelial dysfunction in diabetes" section.

PATHOPHYSIOLOGY OF MICROVASCULAR DISEASE AND ENDOTHELIAL DYSFUNCTION IN DIABETES

Although microvascular diabetic complications have been well-characterized there is still uncertainty regarding the mechanisms that lead to their development. In the past two main pathogenic hypotheses have been proposed: the metabolic hypothesis and the hypoxic hypothesis *(11,12)*. According to the metabolic hypothesis, hyperglycemia is directly responsible of end-organ damage and development of complications through the activation of the polyol pathway. On the other hand, according to the hypoxic hypothesis, the structural alterations detected in kidney, eye, and nerve microvasculature, including basement membrane thickening and endothelial cell proliferation, were considered as the main factor contributing to reduced blood flow and tissue ischemia *(13)*. It is now apparent that both the metabolic and vascular pathways are linked. More specifically, endothelial dysfunction has been suggested as the common denominator between the metabolic and vascular abnormalities detected in diabetes *(14)*. The impaired synthesis and/or degradation of nitric oxide, the main vasodilator released by the endothelium, is believed to determine microvascular insufficiency, tissue hypoxia, and degeneration *(15)*.

Functional Changes

Diabetes mellitus, even in the absence of complications, impairs the vascular reactivity that is the endothelium-dependent and -independent vasodilation in the skin microcirculation *(16)*. Many glucose-related metabolic pathways can determine endothelium dysfunction: increased aldose reductase activity leading to the imbalance in nicotinamide adenine dinucleotide phosphate (NADP)/nicotinamide adenine dinucleotide phosphate reduced form (NADPH); auto-oxidation of glucose leading to the formation of reactive oxygen species; "advanced glycation end products" produced by nonenzymatic glycation of proteins; abnormal n6-fatty acid metabolism and inappropriate activation of protein kinase-C. All these different pathways lead to an increase of oxidative stress which is responsible for a reduced availability of nitric oxide and in turn, for a functional tissue hypoxia and the development of diabetic chronic complications *(17)* (Fig. 1).

Microvascular Dysfunction and Diabetic Neuropathy

Microvascular reactivity is further reduced at the foot level in presence of peripheral diabetic neuropathy. Endothelial nitric oxide synthase (eNOS) is a key regulator of vascular nitric oxide production. Immunostaining of foot skin biopsies in our unit, with antiserum to human eNOS glucose transporter I, which is a functional marker of the endothelium and von Willebrand factor, an anatomical marker, showed no difference among patients with diabetes with or without peripheral neuropathy in the staining of glucose transporter I and von Willebrand factor, whereas the staining for the eNOS was reduced in neuropathic patients (Fig. 2) *(18)*. Another study documented increased levels of iNOS and reduced eNOS levels in skin from the foot of patients with diabetes with severe neuropathy and foot ulceration *(19)*.

It has also been suggested that polymorphism of the *eNOS* gene is implicated in cardiovascular and renal diseases, thus indicating its potential role as a genetic marker of susceptibility to both type 2 diabetes and its renal complications *(20,21)*. However, a relationship between *eNOS* gene polymorphism and diabetic neuropathy has not been clearly demonstrated *(22)*. Nonetheless, all these findings suggest that the reduced eNOS expression/activity might be related to the development of diabetic peripheral neuropathy.

Differences in the microcirculation between the foot and forearm levels have also been investigated, the main hypothesis being that increased hydrostatic pressure in distal

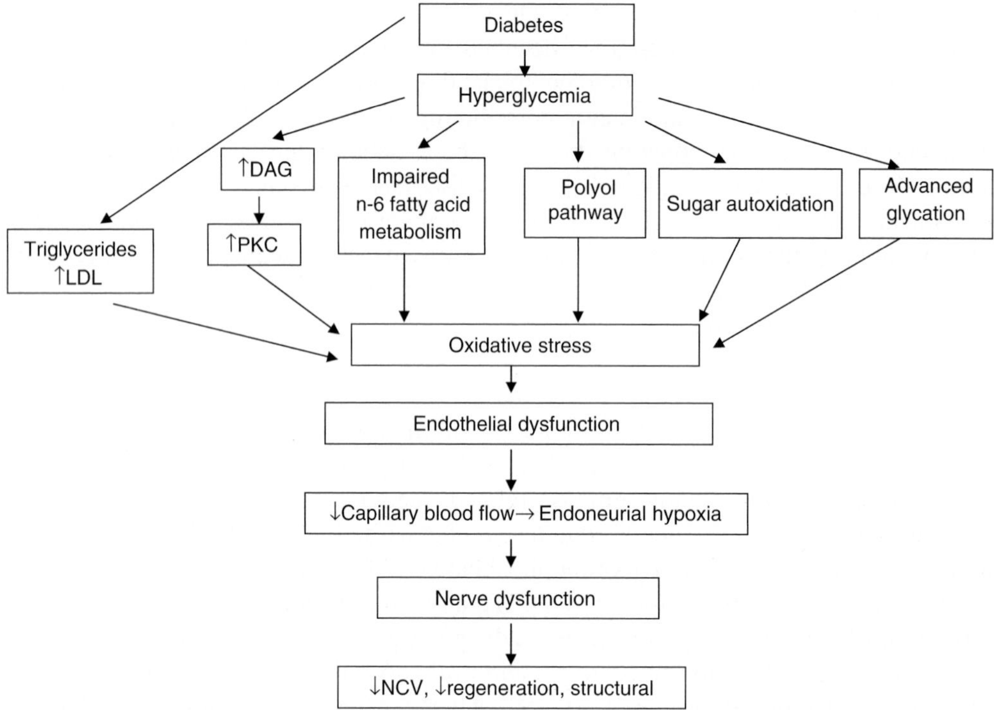

Fig. 1. New concepts in the pathogenesis of diabetic neuropathy.

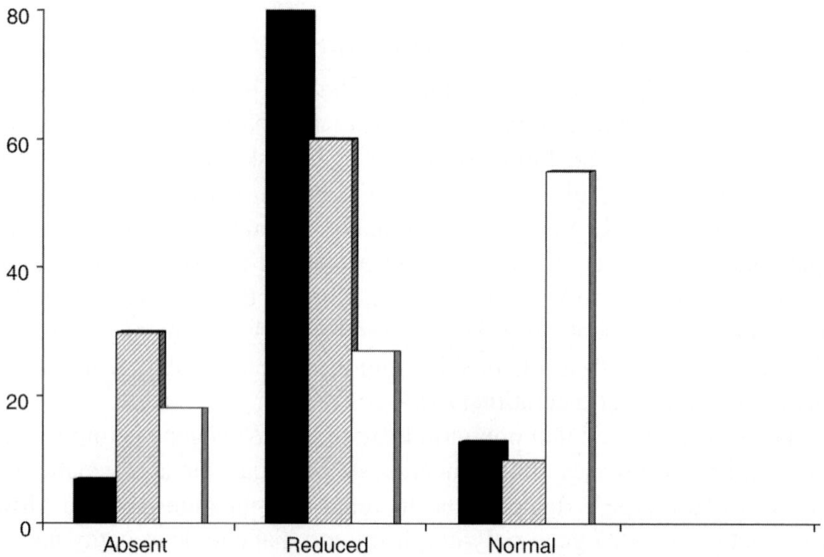

Fig. 2. Expression of eNOS in patients with diabetic neuropathy (black columns), patients with both diabetic neuropathy and peripheral vascular disease (hatched columns) and healthy subjects (white columns). The expression of eNOS was reduced in both the diabetic groups compared with the healthy subjects (data from ref. *18*).

microcirculatory beds, related to the orthostatic posture, affects the foot microcirculation more than at the forearm level. The endothelium dependent and independent vasodilation is in fact lower at the foot level when compared with the forearm in healthy subjects and both nonneuropathic and neuropathic patients with diabetes *(23)*. This forearm-foot gradient exists despite a similar baseline blood flow at the foot and forearm level. Therefore, it is reasonable to believe that erect posture might be a contributing factor for the early development of the nerve damage at the foot, in comparison with the forearm.

Role of Autonomic Neuropathy

Autonomic neuropathy can compromise the diabetic microcirculation because of the development of arterio–venous shunting because of sympathetic denervation. The opening of these shunts might lead to a maldistribution of blood between the nutritional capillaries and subpapillary vessels, and consequent aggravation of microvascular ischemia. Studies using sural nerve photography and fluorescein angiography as well as other elegant techniques seem to support this concept *(24,25)*.

A loss of sympathetic tone is also responsible for an increased capillary permeability in patients with diabetes with neuropathy *(26)*. This might cause endoneurial edema, as demonstrated by using magnetic resonance spectroscopy, which can in turn represent another mechanism leading to a reduction of endoneurial perfusion and a worsening of the nerve damage *(27)*. The increased lower extremity capillary pressure upon assuming the erect posture, because of early loss of postural vasoconstriction (mediated by the sympathetic fibers), might amplify this edematous effect.

Role of Somatic Neuropathy: The Neurovascular Response

Diabetic somatic neuropathy can further affect the skin microcirculation by the impairment of the axon reflex related-vasodilatation (Lewis' flare) *(28)*. Under normal conditions, the stimulus of the *c*-nociceptive nerve fibers not only travels in the normal direction, centrally toward the spinal cord, but also peripherally (antidromic conduction) to local cutaneous blood vessels, causing a vasodilatation by the release of vasoactive substances, such as calcitonin gene-related peptide (CGRP), Neuropeptide Y, substance P, and bradykine by the *c*-fibers and initiates neurogenic inflammation (Fig. 3). This short circuit, or nerve axon reflex, is responsible for the Lewis' triple flare response to injury and plays an important role in increasing local blood flow when it is mostly needed, i.e., in condition of stress.

This neurovascular (N–V) response is significantly reduced at the foot level in patients with diabetes with peripheral somatic neuropathy, autonomic neuropathy, and peripheral artery disease in comparison with patients with diabetes without complications and healthy control subjects (Fig. 4) *(23,29)*. Moreover, local anaesthesia significantly reduces the nerve axon reflex-related vasodilation at the foot of patients without peripheral neuropathy, whereas it has no effect on the amount of the preanesthesia N–V vasodilation—which is already very low—at the foot of neuropathic patients *(30)*. This suggests that the main determinant of the presence of the neurovascular vasodilation is *c*-fiber function and that its measurement could be used as a surrogate measure of the function of these fibers.

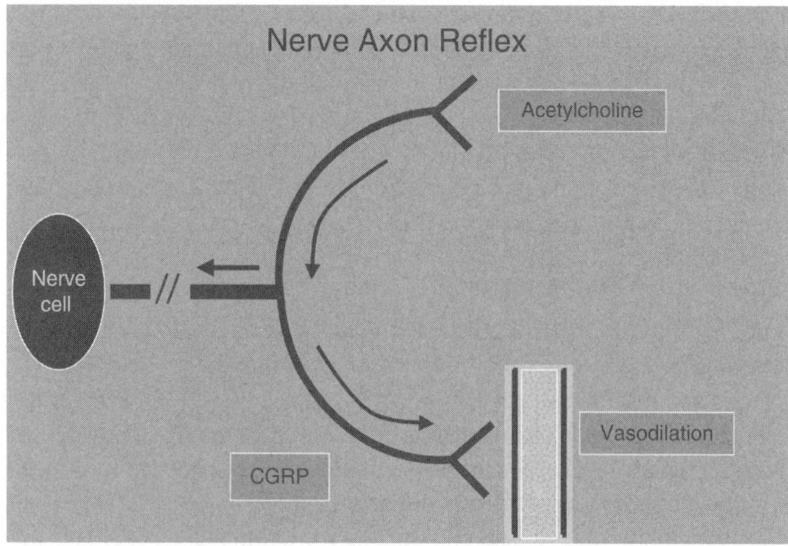

Fig. 3. The nerve axon reflex-related vasodilation or neurovascular response: stimulation of the *c*-nociceptive nerve fibers by acetylcholine or other noxious stimuli leads to antidromic stimulation of the adjacent *c*-fibers, which secrete CGRP that causes vasodilation and increased local blood flow.

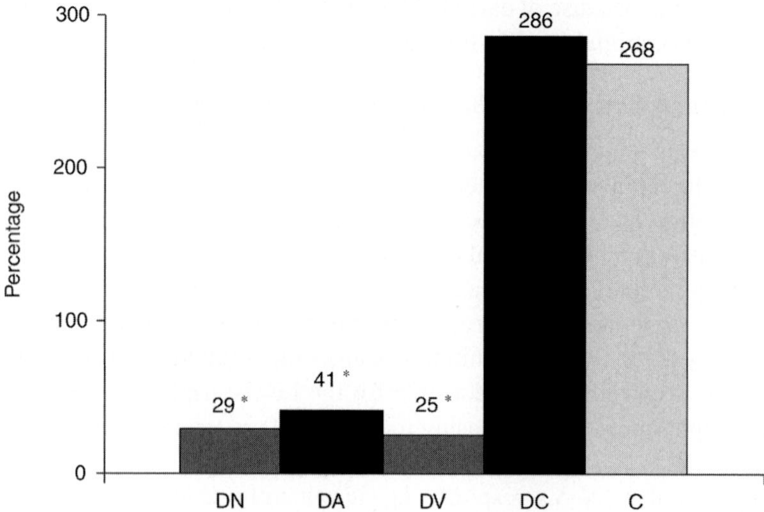

Fig. 4. The neurovascular response (expressed as percentage of blood flow increase over the baseline blood flow) is significantly reduced at the foot level of patients with diabetes with peripheral somatic neuropathy (DN), autonomic neuropathy (DA) and peripheral artery disease (DV) compared with patients with diabetes without complications (DC) and healthy controls (C) $^*p < 0.001$ (data from ref. *29*).

As a matter of fact, it has been shown that the N–V response significantly correlates with different measures of peripheral nerve function *(30,31)*. Studies in our units have shown that a N–V response lower than 50% is highly sensitive (90%) and adequately specific (74%) in identifying patients with diabetes with peripheral neuropathy *(31)*.

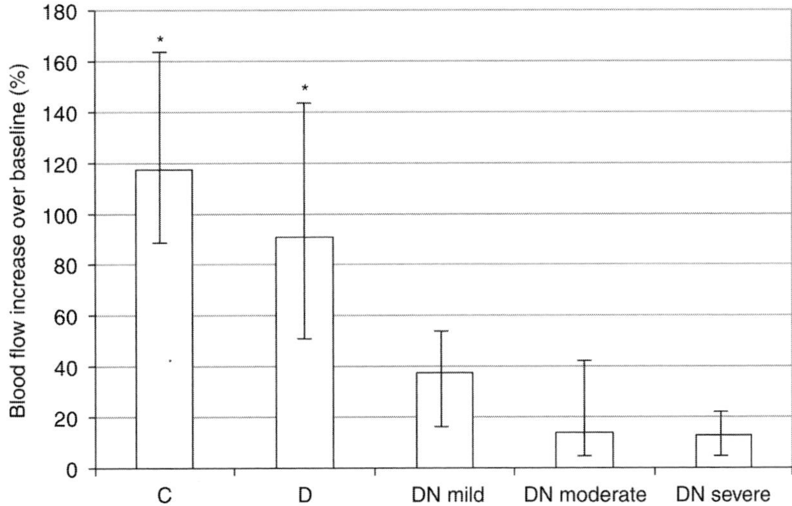

Fig. 5. The nerve axon reflex-related vasodilation at the foot level in a population with diabetes stratified on the basis of the degree of peripheral somatic neuropathy in patients without neuropathy (D), with mild neuropathy (DN mild), with moderate neuropathy (DN moderate) and with severe neuropathy (DN severe) compared with healthy controls (C). Median (25–75 percentile). The nerve axon reflex-related vasodilation is already significantly reduced in the early stages of neuropathy (subclinical neuropathy), supporting the belief that small fiber dysfunction might precede large fiber impairment in the natural history of diabetic nerve damage.

Besides, the finding that this response is significantly reduced even in the early stages of peripheral neuropathy supports the hypothesis that small fiber damage is a precocious event in the clinical history of diabetic neuropathy—even preceding large fibers' impairment (Fig. 5). This leads to impaired vasodilation under conditions of stress, such as injury or inflammation. Therefore, it is possible to speculate that small fiber neuropathy might further contribute to nerve hypoxic damage by the impairment of this hyperemic response, determining a vicious cycle of injury.

The previous conclusions are supported by recent studies in experimental diabetes which have demonstrated that epineurial arterioles of the sciatic nerve are innervated by sensory nerves that contain CGRP and mediate a hyperemic response at this level *(32)*. Furthermore, it has been shown that in long-term diabetic rats the amount of CGRP present in epineurial arterioles is diminished, which could be because of a denervation process *(33)*. Exogenous CGRP-mediated vasodilation of these arterioles is also impaired in experimental diabetes, indicating a reduced CGRP bioactivity *(33)*. All these findings furthermore support a role of small sensory nerve fibers' impairment in the development and progression of diabetic neuropathy.

The impairment of the nerve axon reflex-related vasodilation is not affected by successful bypass surgery in patients with peripheral arterial disease. In addition, the endothelium-dependent and -independent vasodilation that are not related to the nerve axon reflex, remain impaired after successful revascularization. Therefore, despite correction in obstructive lesions and restoration of normal blood flow in the large vessels, the changes in microcirculation continue to be present and cause tissue hypoxia under conditions of stress *(34)*.

Anatomical Changes

Although the structural alterations detected in diabetic capillaries do not cause vessel occlusion, their role in causing a reduction of nerve blood flow supply can not be completely ruled out. According to Pouiselle's law, in fact, the blood flow is proportional to the fourth power of the radius of a vessel. Therefore, the capillary blood flow can be significantly reduced by even slight narrowing of the capillary lumen. Many studies have now confirmed the presence of endoneurial microangiopathy, characterized by basement membrane thickening, endothelial cell hyperplasia and hypertrophy, and pericyte cell degeneration in patients with diabetes with peripheral neuropathy, the degree of which correlates with the severity of the clinical disease *(35,36)*.

In summary, both the functional and structural changes observed in diabetic microcirculation contribute to the shift of blood flow away from the nutritive capillaries to low resistance arterio–venous shunts leading to functional ischemia of tissues including peripheral nerves and, consequently, to the development of diabetic peripheral neuropathy and other diabetic chronic complications.

TECHNIQUES TO ASSESS MICROVASCULAR DYSFUNCTION AND THEIR LIMITATIONS

Endothelial dysfunction, assessed at the macrocirculation, has been proven as an early marker of vascular complications in several diseases, including diabetes, dyslipidemia, and hypertension. The development of techniques capable to measure the skin blood flow has also enabled the study of the vascular reactivity at the microcirculation level. More specifically, the noninvasive measurement of cutaneous blood perfusion can be performed by the laser Doppler.

Currently, laser Doppler flowmetry is the most widely accepted technique for evaluating blood flow in the skin microcirculation. Basically, it measures the capillary flux, which is a combination of the velocity and the number of moving blood cells. This is achieved by using red laser light, which is transmitted to the skin through a fiberoptic cable. The frequency shift of light back-scattered from the moving blood cells beneath the probe tip is computed to give a measure of the superficial microvascular perfusion.

There are mainly two different types of instruments available: the laser Doppler perfusion imager (LDPI) and the laser Doppler blood flow monitor (LDM). The LDPI, or laser scanner, enables the quantification of superficial skin blood perfusion in a multiple number of adjacent sites on the skin and calculates the mean blood perfusion in a particular region (Fig. 6). The LDM, which is characterized for having two single-point laser probes is capable to measure the blood flow changes only in a small skin area (about 2–3 mm diameter)—that corresponds to the area where the probes are placed—and records the blood flow changes in response to the vasodilatory stimulus in a continuous way (Fig. 7).

The LDPI is best-suited for studying the relative changes in flow induced by a variety of physiological manoeuvres or pharmaceutical intervention procedures. The single-point laser probe is used mainly for evaluating the hyperemic response to heat stimulus or for evaluating the nerve-axon related hyperemic response. Both these two laser Doppler instruments have been extensively used to evaluate the skin microcirculatory flow of patients with diabetes in response to the delivery of two vasodilatory substances

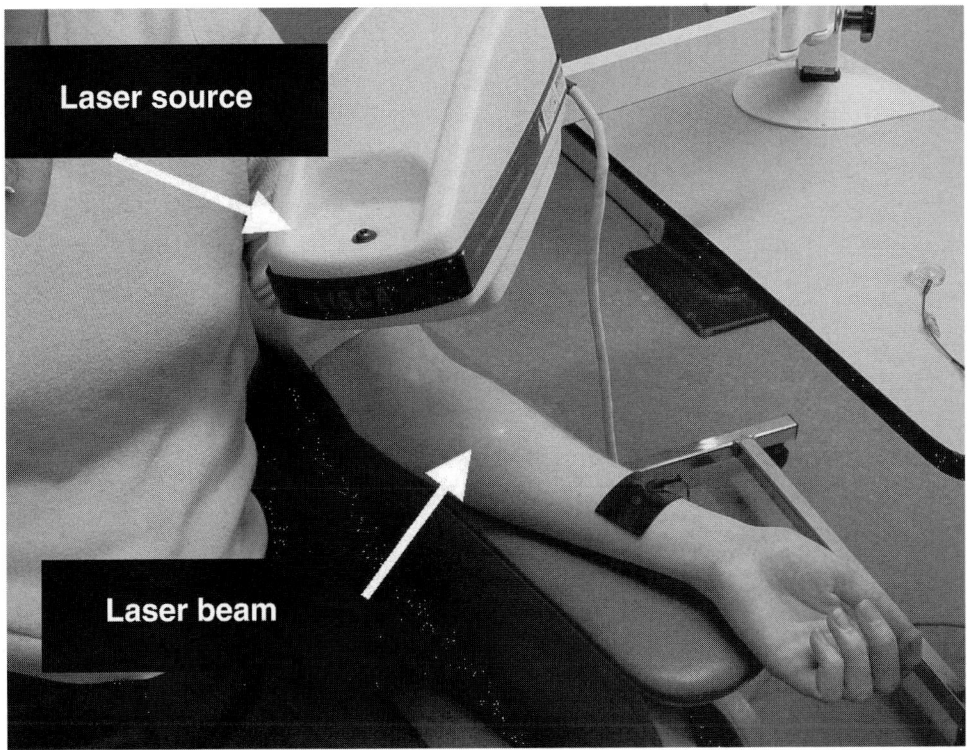

Fig. 6. The LDPI or laser scanner: a helium-neon laser beam is emitted from the laser source to sequentially scan the circular hyperemic area of the skin (surrounding the laser beam) where the hyperemic response is produced by the iontophorized vasoactive substance.

by iontophoresis: a 1% acetylcholine chloride solution (endothelium-dependent vasodilation) and a 1% sodium nitroprusside solution (endothelium-independent vasodilation).

To use these methods for longitudinal analysis, a certain degree of confidence is needed to ensure that the results are not skewed for instrumental inaccuracies or other experimental factors. The main limitation of both techniques is, in fact, the variability, which is higher for the single-point laser Doppler than for the LDPI. The single-point technique has been validated against direct measurements of the capillary blood flow velocity *(37)*. The day-to-day reproducibility of the technique was evaluated in healthy subjects who were repeatedly tested at their foot and arm for 10 consecutive days in our lab. The coefficient of variation for the maximal response to heat was 27.9%, whereas for the maximal hyperemic response after Ach and/or SNP-iontophoresis was 35.2% *(18)*. The variability of this technique is mostly a spatial one, i.e., it is mainly because of the high heterogeneity of the skin microcirculation and not to the technique itself. In fact, the technique reproducibility can be significantly enhanced if one pays attention to place the laser probe approximately at the same skin area for repeated measurements *(38)*.

The laser scanner has a significantly better reproducibility (which is mainly because of the minor spatial variation of blood flow assessment) with the coefficient of variation at the foot and forearms level being between 14 and 19%, and can therefore be used for

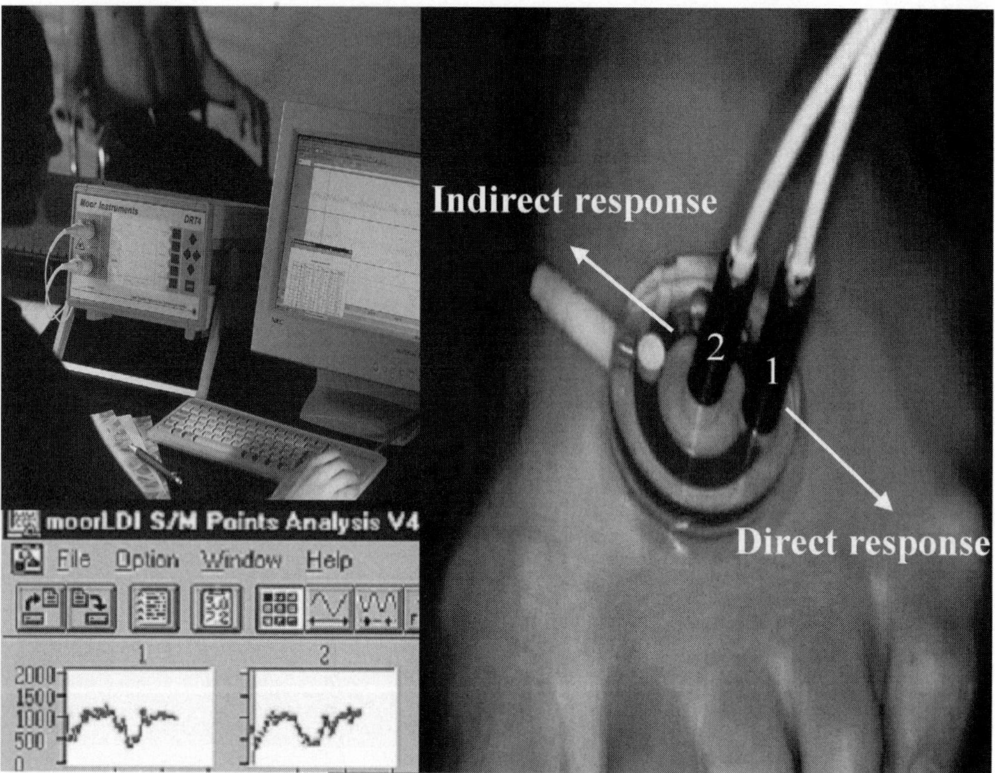

Fig. 7. The LDM or single-point laser doppler: it enables to quantify both the direct and indirect vasodilatory responses to a vasoactive substance. One probe (no. 1) is placed in direct contact to the iontophoresis solution chamber (colored ring) and sequentially measures the blood flow changes in response to the iontophorised solution (direct response). The center probe (no. 2) measures the indirect vasodilatory response which derives from the activation of the nerve axon reflex. Both responses are expressed as percentage of mean blood flow increase over the baseline blood flow.

blood flow assessment in prospective studies *(39,40)*. Nevertheless, some factors, other than the accuracy of the device itself, might also potentially affect the LDPI readings, namely the scanner head height and inclination, tissue heating, prevalence of arm hair, and arm movement.

MACROVASCULAR DISEASE AND DIABETES: AN OVERVIEW

Both type 1 and type 2 diabetes are powerful and independent risk factors for coronary artery disease (CAD), stroke, and peripheral artery disease. More specifically, the Framingham study showed that type 2 diabetes is associated with approximately a twofold increase in CAD in men and a fourfold increase in women *(41)*. It is also known that patients with diabetes have the same risk of acute myocardial infarction than patients without diabetes with a history of previous myocardial infarction, thus all patients with diabetes have to be considered in secondary prevention for CAD *(42)*. Mortality from CAD in individuals with diabetes is also higher than in subjects without diabetes *(43)*.

As opposed to the clear influence of hyperglycemia in the development of microvascular complications in diabetes, hyperglycemia plays a less strong role in the development of macrovascular disease, in particular CAD, as shown by the UKPDS *(10)*. Thus, the risk for macrovascular disease in diabetes seems to rely to a considerable degree on other associated abnormalities, such as hypertension, dyslipidemia, altered fibrinolysis, and obesity, all components of the insulin resistance syndrome *(44)*. Endothelial dysfunction/activation, detected in most of the clinical abnormalities associated to the insulin resistance syndrome, is now considered a precocious event in the clinical history of both micro- and macrovascular complications, contributing to the initiation and progression of the vascular damage in diabetes.

LOWER EXTREMITY ARTERIAL DISEASE AND DIABETES

The concomitant occurrence of atherosclerotic peripheral vascular disease and peripheral neuropathy in patients with diabetes is the main factor in the development of diabetic foot pathology. Although neuropathy has proven the main risk factor for foot ulceration, peripheral arterial disease of the lower extremities is considered the major risk factor for lower-extremity amputation and it is also accompanied by a high likelihood for cardiovascular and cerebrovascular diseases *(45)*. The rate of lower extremity amputation in the population with diabetes is 15 times that seen in the population without diabetes and within 4 years of the first amputation about 50% of contralateral limbs are lost *(46,47)*. Life expectancy is also consistently reduced, as a result *(48)*.

Although the underlying pathogenesis of atherosclerotic disease in diabetics is similar to that noted in nondiabetics, there are significant differences. As previously mentioned, diabetics have a fourfold higher prevalence of atherosclerosis, which progresses at a more rapid rate to occlusion. Patients with diabetes present with the sequelae of atherosclerotic disease at a significantly younger age than their counterparts without diabetes. Occlusive disease in patients with diabetes has a unique distribution, having the propensity to occur in the infrageniculate arteries in the calf. The typically affected arteries are the anterior tibial, posterior tibial, and peroneal. Equally important is the observation that the arteries of the foot, specifically the dorsalis pedis, are often spared of occlusive disease. This provides an excellent option for a distal revascularization target *(49)*.

The clinical presentation of PVD in diabetes is also different because of the coexistence of peripheral neuropathy. In fact, while in patients without diabetes intermittent claudication—defined as pain, cramping or aching in the calves, thighs or buttocks that appears with walking exercise and is relieved by rest—is the initial presenting symptom, followed by rest pain, patients with diabetes might not complain of any ischemic symptom because of the loss of sensitivity or their symptoms can be confused with neuropathic pain. As a consequence, the development of tissue loss (foot ulceration or gangrene) might represent the first sign of lower limb ischemia and because of its limb-threatening potential, it is termed as critical limb ischemia. Therefore, patients with diabetes with a foot ulcer should always be evaluated for ischemia, irrespective of their symptoms, particularly for the increased risk of limb-threatening infection and faulty healing related to PVD *(50)*.

The observations that pedal vessels are often spared from arterial occlusive disease had a crucial impact on the manner in which peripheral vascular disease is approached in the population with diabetes. In the past, based upon the false presumption of small vessel disease, diabetics were not treated as aggressively with revascularization as is now standard. A more aggressive attempt to correct the vascular deficit in diabetic ischemic limbs in addition to more aggressive measures to control local infection has radically altered the prognosis of peripheral vascular disease in the diabetic extremity.

PRINCIPLES OF ARTERIAL RECONSTRUCTION

Patients with diabetes at risk of lower limb amputation because of the presence of a peripheral vascular disease are a growing population because of the higher prevalence of diabetes and to the longer life expectancy of the general population. There is increasing evidence that distal arterial revascularization is effective in preventing major amputations in the population with diabetes *(51)*. The indications for limb revascularization are disabling claudication (not common in patients with diabetes, as previously mentioned) and critical limb ischemia (rest pain or tissue loss), refractive to conservative therapy *(52)*.

Bypass to the tibial or pedal vessels with autogenous veins is the longest experienced technique. In a series of more than 1000 dorsalis pedis bypasses, 5-year secondary potency and limb salvage rates were 62.7 and 78.2%, respectively *(53)*. The increased use of this revascularization option showed to correlate with a decline in the incidence of all levels of amputations. Dorsalis pedis artery bypass can therefore be performed with a high rate of success and low morbidity and mortality, certainly equivalent to that achieved with other lower extremity grafts.

In addition to the traditional approach based on distal bypass surgery, it is gaining importance in terms of feasibility and effectiveness the less invasive approach by percutaneous trasnsluminal angioplasty. This technique allows to dilate also very distal arterial stenosis/obstructions, it can be repeated in case of failure and it allows to spare peripheral veins which might be used in other vascular districts (i.e., the coronary vascular bed) *(54,55)*. In a recently published series of 933 patients with diabetes (mean follow-up 26 ± 15 months) in which this revascularization procedure has been used as a first choice, the 5 years primary patency was 88% *(56)*. Therefore, percutaneous transluminal angioplasty as the first choice revascularisation procedure is feasible, safe, and effective for limb salvage in a high percentage of patients with diabetes.

MACROVASCULAR DISEASE AND DIABETIC NEUROPATHY

Conventional risk factors for macrovascular disease, such as hypertension, raised triglyceride levels, body mass index, and smoking have been shown to be independent predictors of the development of diabetic neuropathy *(57)*. The link between these classical cardiovascular risk factors and diabetic microvascular complications, including neuropathy is not clear, but the development of atherosclerosis of the lower extremities might be one possible explanation. Several of the risk factors associated with neuropathy are also markers of insulin resistance, which is in turn associated with endothelial dysfunction. The latter, as previously discussed, causes tissue functional ischemia and is believed to be a pivotal factor in the development of diabetic neuropathy.

It is clear that impaired blood flow and endoneurial hypoxia are the major pathogenic factors in the development of diabetic peripheral neuropathy. Thus, arterial obstructive lesions, even occurring at the large vessels of the lower extremities might theoretically be responsible for nerve tissue damage by limiting adequate endoneurial oxygenation. This hypothesis was firstly tested by Price more than 100 years ago who detected patchy areas of nerve degeneration in the posterior tibial nerve trunks as a consequence of proximal large vessels atherosclerosis *(58)*. More recent studies in patients without diabetes with peripheral vascular disease confirm the occurrence of significant demyelination and axonal degeneration together with an endoneurial microangiopathy *(59,60)*. Such studies provide support for the role of acute/chronic ischaemic injury resulting in neuronal death.

The most direct evidence of a strict relationship between lower extremity atherosclerosis and diabetic neuropathy is derived from large vessel revascularization studies, which have shown an improvement in nerve conduction velocity in one but not another study *(61,62)*. A longer-term follow-up of the latter study did however show that reversal of hypoxia slows the progression of peroneal nerve conduction velocity deterioration *(63)*. The efficacy of a number of pharmacological treatments that can achieve a similar effect, in improving peripheral nerve function has also been tested. In a double-blind placebo-controlled clinical trial with a vasodilator, Trandalopril, for more than 12 months, peroneal motor nerve conduction velocity, M-wave amplitude F-wave latency, and sural nerve amplitude improved significantly *(64)*. Recently, the appropriate blood pressure control in diabetes trial, aimed to assess the effects of intensive against moderate blood pressure control with either Nisoldipine or enalapril, failed to show any benefit on the progression of diabetic nephropathy, retinopathy, and neuropathy *(65)*.

In summary, despite some evidence that tissue hypoxia related to obstructive atherosclerotic disease can contribute to the development of peripheral neuropathy, the exact mechanisms are not known. Furthermore studies will be required to delineate these mechanisms and the potential of new therapeutic interventions.

CONCLUSION

Changes in the micro- and macrocirculation, both anatomical and functional, contribute to the development of diabetic neuropathy. On the other hand, the development of diabetic neuropathy also affects the vasodilatory capacity of the microcirculation and can interfere with the clinical presentation of peripheral obstructive arterial disease. Thus, the interaction between changes in the vasculature and peripheral nerves is bidirectional and results in changes in both blood flow and neuronal function.

REFERENCES

1. Goldenberg SG, Alex M, Joshi RA, et al. Nonatheromatous peripheral vascular disease of the lower extremity in diabetes mellitus. *Diabetes* 1959;8:261–273.
2. LoGerfo FW, Coffman JD. Current concepts. Vascular and microvascular disease of the foot in diabetes. Implications for foot care. *N Engl J Med* 1984;311:1615–1619.
3. Strandness DE, Priest RE, Gibbons GE. Combined clinical and pathologic study of diabetic and nondiabetic peripheral arterial disease. *Diabetes* 1964;13:366–372.
4. Conrad MC. Large and small artery occlusion in diabetics and nondiabetics with severe vascular disease. *Circulation* 1967;36:83–91.

5. Parving HH, Viberti GC, Keen H, Christiansen JS, Lassen NA. Hemodynamic factors in the genesis of diabetic microangiopathy. *Metabolism* 1983;32:943–949.
6. Flynn MD, Tooke JE. Aetiology of diabetic foot ulceration: A role for the microcirculation? *Diab Med* 1992;8:320–329.
7. Morgensen CE, Schmitz A, Christensen CR. Comparative renal pathophysiology relevant to IDDM and NIDDM patients. *Diab Metab Rev* 1988;4:453–483.
8. Cunha-Vaz JG. Studies on the pathophysiology of diabetic retinopathy. The blood-retinal barrier in diabetes. *Diabetes* 1983;32:20–27.
9. Diabetes Control and Complications Trial Research Group. The effect of intensive treatment of diabetes on the development and progression of long-term complications in insulin-dependent diabetes mellitus. *N Engl J Med* 1993;329:977–986.
10. Intensive blood-glucose control with sulphonylureas or insulin compared with conventional treatment and risk of complications in patients with type 2 diabetes (UKPDS 33). UK Prospective Diabetes Study (UKPDS) Group. *Lancet* 1998;352:837–853.
11. Stevens MJ, Feldman EL, Green DA. The aetiology of diabetic neuropathy: the combined roles of metabolic and vascular defects. *Diab Med* 1995;12:566–579.
12. Feldman EL, Stevens MJ, Green DA. Pathogenesis of diabetic neuropathy. *Clin Neurosci* 1997;4:365–370.
13. Malik RA, Tesfaye S, Thompson SD, et al. Transperineurial capillary abnormalities in the sural nerve of patients with diabetic neuropathy. *Microvasc Res* 1994;48:236–245.
14. Tooke JE. Possible pathophysiological mechanisms for diabetic angiopathy in type 2 diabetes. *J Diab Compl* 2000;14:197–200.
15. Stevens MJ. Nitric oxide as a potential bridge between the metabolic and vascular hypotheses of diabetic neuropathy. *Diab Med* 1995;12:292–295.
16. Morris SJ, Shore AC, Tooke JE. responses of the skin microcirculation to acetylcholine and sodium nitroprusside in patients with NIDDM. *Diabetologia* 1995;38:1337–1344.
17. Cameron NE, Eaton SE, Cotter MA, Tesfaye S. Vascular factors and metabolic interactions in the pathogenesis of diabetic neuropathy. *Diabetologia* 2001;44:1973–1988.
18. Veves A, Akbari CM, Primavera J, et al. Endothelial dysfunction and the expression of endothelial nitric oxide synthetase in diabetic neuropathy, vascular disease, and foot ulceration. *Diabetes* 1998;47:457–463.
19. Jude EB, Boulton AJ, Ferguson MW, Appleton I. The role of nitric oxide synthase isoforms and arginase in the pathogenesis of diabetic foot ulcers: possible modulatory effects by transforming growth beta 1. *Diabetologia* 1999;42:748–757.
20. Monti LD, Barlassina C, Citterio L, et al. Endothelial nitric oxide synthase polymorphisms are associated with type 2 diabetes and the insulin resistance syndrome. *Diabetes* 2003;52: 1270–1275.
21. Noiri E, Satoh H, Taguchi J, et al. Association of eNOS Glu298Asp polymorphism with end-stage renal disease. *Hypertension* 2002;40:535–540.
22. Szabo C, Zanchi A, Komjati K, et al. Poly(ADP-Ribose) polymerase is activated in subjects at risk of developing type 2 diabetes and is associated with impaired vascular reactivity. *Circulation* 2002;106:2680–2686.
23. Arora S, Smakowski P, Frykberg RG, et al. Differences in foot and forearm skin microcirculation in diabetic patients with and without neuropathy. *Diabetes Care* 1998;21:1339–1344.
24. Tesfaye S, Harris N, Jakubowski J, et al. Impaired blood flow and arterio-venous shunting in human diabetic neuropathy: a novel technique of nerve photography and fluorescein angiography. *Diabetologia* 1993;36:1266–1274.
25. Flynn MD, Tooke JE. Diabetic neuropathy and the microcirculation. *Diab Med* 1995;12: 298–301.
26. Lefrandt JD, Bosma E, Oomen PH, et al. Sympathetic mediated vasomotion and skin capillary permeability in diabetic patients with peripheral neuropathy. *Diabetologia* 2003;46:40–47.

27. Eaton RP, Qualls C, Bicknell J, Sibbitt WL, King MK, Griffey RH. Structure-function relationships within peripheral nerves in diabetic neuropathy: the hydration hypothesis. *Diabetologia* 1996;39:439–446.
28. Lewis T. *The blood vessels of the human skin and their responses*. Shaw and Sons, London, 1927.
29. Hamdy O, Abou-Elenin K, LoGerfo FW, Horton ES, Veves A. Contribution of nerve-axon reflex-related vasodilation to the total skin vasodilation in diabetic patients with and without neuropathy. *Diabetes Care* 2001;24:344–349.
30. Caselli A, Rich J, Hanane T, Uccioli L, Veves A. Role of C-nociceptive fibers in the nerve axon reflex-related vasodilation in diabetes. *Neurology* 2003;60:297–300.
31. Caselli A, Spallone V, Marfia G, Battista C, Veves A, Uccioli L. Validation of the nerve axon reflex for the assessment of small nerve fibers' dysfunction. *Diabetologia* 2004; 47:A34.
32. Calcutt NA, Chen P, Hua XY. Effects of diabetes on tissue content and evoked release of calcitonin gene-related peptide-like immunoreactivity from rat sensory nerves. *Neurosci Lett* 1998;254:129–132.
33. Yorek MA, Coppey LJ, Gellett JS, Davidson EP. Sensory nerve innervation of epineurial arterioles of the sciatic nerve containing calcitonin gene-related peptide: effect of streptozotocin-induced diabetes. *Exp Diabesity Res* 2004;5:187–193.
34. Arora S, Pomposelli F, LoGerfo FW, Veves A. Cutaneous microcirculation in the neuropathic diabetic foot improves significantly but not completely after successful lower extremity revascularization. *J Vasc Surg* 2002;35:501–505.
35. Malik RA, Newrick PG, Sharma AK, et al. Microangiopathy in human diabetic neuropathy: relationship between capillary abnormalities and the severity of neuropathy. *Diabetologia* 1989;32:92–102.
36. Britland ST, Young RJ, Sharma AK, Clarke BF. Relationship of endoneurial capillary abnormalities to type and severity of diabetic polyneuropathy. *Diabetes* 1990;39:909–913.
37. Tooke JE, Ostergren J, Fagrell B. Synchronous assessment of human skin microcirculation by laser doppler flowmetry and dynamic capillaroscopy. *Int J Microcirc Clin Exp* 1983; 2:277–284.
38. Vinik AI, Erbas T, Park TS, Pierce KK, Stansberry KB. Methods for evaluation of peripheral neurovascular dysfunction. *Diabete Technol Ther* 2001;3:29–50.
39. Agewall S, Doughty RN, Bagg W, Whalley GA, Braatvedt G, Sharpe N. Comparison of ultrasound assessment of flow-mediated dilatation in the radial and brachial artery with upper and forearm cuff positions. *Clin Physiol* 2001;21(1):9–14.
40. Gaenzer H, Neumayr G, Marschang P, Sturm W, Kirchmair R, Patsch JR. Flow-mediated vasodilation of the femoral and brachial artery induced by exercise in healthy nonsmoking and smoking men. *J Am Coll Cardiol* 2001;38(5):1313–1319.
41. Kannel WB, McGee DL. Diabetes and cardiovascular disease. The Framingham study. *JAMA* 1979;241:2035–2038.
42. Haffner SM, Lehto S, Ronnemaa T, Pyorala K, Laakso M. Mortality from coronary heart disease in subjects with type 2 diabetes and in nondiabetic subjects with and without prior myocardial infarction. *N Engl J Med* 1998;339(4):229–234.
43. Pyorala K, Laakso M, Uusitupa M. Diabetes and atherosclerosis: an epidemiologic view. *Diabete Metab Rev* 1987;3:463–524.
44. Reaven GM, Laws A. Insulin resistance, compensatory hyperinsulinaemia, and coronary heart disease. *Diabetologia* 1994;37:948–952.
45. Reiber GE, Pecoraro RE, Koepsell TD. Risk factors for amputation in patientswith diabetes mellitus. A case-control study. *Ann Intern Med* 1992;117:97–105.
46. Morris AD, McAlpine R, Steinke D, et al. Diabetes and lower-limb amputations in the community. A retrospective cohort study. DARTS/MEMO Collaboration. Diabetes Audit

and Research in Tayside Scotland/Medicines Monitoring Unit. *Diabetes Care* 1998;21: 738–743.

47. Ebskov B, Josephsen P. Incidence of reamputation and death after gangrene of the lower extremity. *Prosthet Orthot Int* 1980;4(2):77–80.
48. Lee JS, Lu M, Lee VS, Russell D, Bahr C, Lee ET. Lower-extremity amputation. Incidence, risk factors, and mortality in the Oklahoma Indian Diabetes Study. *Diabetes* 1993;42(6):876–882.
49. Van Damme H. Crural or pedal artery revascularisation for limb salvage: is it justified? *Acta Chir Belg* 2004;104:148–157.
50. Weitz JI, Byrne J, Clagett GP, et al. Diagnosis and treatment of chronic arterial insufficiency of the lower extremities: a critical review. *Circulation* 1996;94:3026–3049.
51. Holstein P, Ellitsgaard N, Olsen BB, Ellitsgaard V. Decreasing incidence of major amputations in people with diabetes. *Diabetologia* 2000;43:844–847.
52. American Diabetes Association. Peripheral Arterial Disease in people with diabetes. *Diabetes Care* 2003;26:3333–3341.
53. Pomposelli FB, Jr, Kansal N, Hamdan AD, et al. A decade of experience with dorsalis pedis artery bypass: Analysis of outcome in more than 1000 cases. *J Vasc Surg* 2003;37: 307–315.
54. Kumpe DA, Rutherford RB. Percutaneous transluminal angioplasty for lower extremity ischemia, in *Vascular Surgery* (Rutherford RB, ed.), 3rd ed., WB Saunders, Philadelphia PA, 1992, pp. 759–761.
55. London NJ, Varty K, Sayers RD, Thompson MM, Bell PR, Bolia A. Percutaneous transluminal angioplasty for lower-limb critical ischaemia. *Br J Surg* 1995;82(9):1232–1235.
56. Faglia E, Dalla Paola L, Clerici G, et al. Peripheral angioplasty as the first-choice revascularization procedure in diabetic patients with critical limb ischemia: prospective study of 993 consecutive patients hospitalized and followed between 1999 and 2003. *Eur J Vasc Endovasc Surg* 2005;29(6):620–627.
57. Tesfaye S, Chaturvedi N, Eaton SE, et al. Vascular risk factors and diabetic neuropathy. *N Engl J Med* 2005;352(4):341–350.
58. Pryce TD. On diabetic neuritis, with a clinical and pathological description of three cases of diabetic pseudo-tabes. *Brain* 1893;16:416.
59. Nukada H, van Rij AM, Packer SG, McMorran PD. Pathology of acute and chronic ischaemic neuropathy in atherosclerotic peripheral vascular disease. *Brain* 1996;119: 1449–1460.
60. McKenzie D, Nukada H, van Rij AM, McMorran PD. Endoneurial microvascular abnormalities of sural nerve in non-diabetic chronic atherosclerotic occlusive disease. *J Neurol Sci* 1999;162:84–88.
61. Young MJ, Veves A, Walker MG, Boulton AJ. Correlations between nerve function and tissue oxygenation in diabetic patients: further clues to the aetiology of diabetic neuropathy? *Diabetologia* 1992;35:1146–1150.
62. Veves A, Donaghue VM, Sarnow MR, Giurini JM, Campbell DR, LoGerfo FW. The impact of reversal of hypoxia by revascularization on the peripheral nerve function of diabetic patients. *Diabetologia* 1996;39:344–348.
63. Akbari CM, Gibbons GW, Habershaw GM, LoGerfo FW, Veves A. The effect of arterial reconstruction on the natural history of diabetic neuropathy. *Arch-Surg* 1997;132:148–152.
64. Malik RA, Williamson S, Abbott CA, et al. Effect of angiotensin-converting enzyme (ACE) inhibitor trandalopril on human diabetic neuropathy: randomised double-blind controlled trial. *Lancet* 1998;352:1978–1981.
65. Estacio RO, Jeffers BW, Gifford N, Schrier RW. Effect of blood pressure control on diabetic microvascular complications in patients with hypertension and type 2 diabetes. *Diabetes Care* 2000;23:B54–B64.

16

Clinical Diagnosis of Diabetic Neuropathy

Vladimir Skljarevski and Rayaz A. Malik

SUMMARY

Diabetic neuropathies are among most common long-term complications of diabetes. Clinical assessment of diabetic neuropathies typically involves evaluation of subjective symptoms and neurological deficits since an alteration in the former does not necessarily reflect an improvement in nerve function. A number of clinical symptom and/or deficit scales have been developed for either mass screening or focused research purposes. The assessment may additionally be quantified using more or less sophisticated tools. The Semmes-Weinstein monofilaments and graduated tuning fork can detect patients with advanced neuropathy, while quantitative sensory testing and nerve conduction studies are much more sensitive to subtle changes in nerve function. Sophisticated techniques like axon reflex, magnetic resonance imaging and corneal confocal microscopy are rarely used outside research environment. Recent years have brought a significant progress in symptomatic treatment of painful diabetic neuropathies. However, an effective treatment of the underlying pathology is still lacking.

Key Words: Clinical assessment; diabetic neuropathies; clinical trials; symptoms; deficits; screening tools.

INTRODUCTION

The neuropathies are among the most common of the long-term complications of diabetes, affecting up to 50–60% of patients. Progressive loss of nerve fibres might affect both somatic and autonomic divisions, producing a wide range of symptoms and signs, which can be assessed using an array of measures, that differ when used for screening as opposed to detailed quantification for research or when assessing the benefits of therapeutic intervention. For the latter, two major types of end point are utilized: (1) those which assess symptoms for defining efficacy in painful diabetic neuropathy and (2) those which assess neurological deficits. An alteration in symptoms does not necessarily reflect an improvement in nerve function. Furthermore, tests which might accurately detect structural repair on repeat nerve or skin biopsy might not necessarily translate to improved neuronal function and vice versa. Thus, although there is considerable enthusiasm to develop new therapies for both symptoms and deficits, the criteria used to determine therapeutic efficacy are varied and lacking consensus.

From: *Contemporary Diabetes: Diabetic Neuropathy: Clinical Management, Second Edition*
Edited by: A. Veves and R. Malik © Humana Press Inc., Totowa, NJ

CLINICAL SYMPTOMS

Symptomatic diabetic neuropathy might affect 30–40% of diabetic patients with neuropathy. The most commonly reported symptom is pain in the distal extremities, in the legs more than in the arms with nocturnal exacerbation. Patients report deep aching pain, a burning feeling, sharp "shock-like" pain, or a more constant squeezing sensation (pressure myalgia). These symptoms are called positive sensory symptoms because of apparent "hyperactivity" of nerves and perceived as a presence of something that is normally absent. Negative sensory symptoms include "numbness," "wooden, rubber, or dead feet" feeling and commonly used descriptors are "a wrapped feeling," "retained sock feeling," "cotton wool under soles," and so on. Hyperalgesia and allodynia are also prominent elements of the neuropathic sensory symptom complex and are defined as hypersensitivity to a normally mild painful stimulus and painful sensation evoked by a normally nonpainful stimulus, respectively. In the vast majority of patients both positive and negative sensory symptoms coexist but they are typically picked up only by systematic questioning, as spontaneous reporting tends to favor the positive symptoms.

Because current treatments of painful diabetic neuropathy display limited efficacy and a troublesome side effect profile it forms a major target for clinical trials of patients with diabetic neuropathy *(1)*. However, many patients have difficulty in describing their symptoms accurately and consistently, and many of the symptom questionnaires do not necessarily capture all of the many attributes of symptomatic diabetic neuropathy. Thus, a range of symptom questionnaires are available to record symptom quality and severity, many of which have been imported from pain states in general, and are therefore not specific to diabetic neuropathy. Although the most common outcome measure of pain response is the 11-point Likert scale, many other measures are used and there is no gold standard (Table 1) *(2–14)*.

Moreover, there is no accepted cutoff for a level of pain response, which might be deemed clinically significant, with most studies accepting responses ranging from 30 to 50%, knowing that there is about 20–30% placebo response. To assess and compare therapeutic response between different drugs, responder rates should be considered across a range of responses from 30 to 90%. Limited head-to-head studies make comparison of relative efficacy between different therapies impossible. This compels us to develop a uniform, validated, and internationally accepted tool to quantify painful diabetic neuropathy.

Many of the drugs for painful diabetic neuropathy can result in significant side effects, particularly at higher doses. Therefore, in any clinical trial, adverse effects, maximal tolerated doses, mood, and quality of life should be evaluated as secondary outcome measures. This is particularly important in a "real world" scenario as opposed to a clinical trial in which treatment is often stopped by the patient or switched by the physician as a result of adverse effects.

To try and standardize and compare treatment efficacy with safety, the number-needed-to-treat (NNT) (reciprocal of the absolute risk reduction) for one patient to achieve at least 50% pain relief should be calculated in addition to the relative risk (RR) and number-needed-to-harm for adverse effects and drug-related study withdrawal. Eventhough the proposed approach is more systematic it is not without its problems particularly when combining different studies. Variable durations and numbers of patients in different clinical trials limit the usefulness of a summated analysis and extrapolation

Table 1
Variety of Outcome Measures Used in Epidemiological and Interventional Studies of Painful Diabetic Neuropathy

Outcome measure	Study
Neuropathy symptom score	*2,3*
Simple visual analog or verbal descriptive scales	*4,5*
Brief pain inventory	*6*
Mean daily pain intensity	*7*
Short-form McGill Pain Questionnaire	
Weekly mean pain scores	*8*
Sleep interference scores	
Visual analog pain intensity	*9*
Visual analog pain relief	
Clinical global impression-severity of illness	*9*
Clinical global impression-improvement	
Patient global rating of pain relief	
NeuroQoL	*10*
0–100 mm visual analog scale and a 0–10 Likert scale	*11*
50% reduction in the 24-h average pain score	*12*
Mean pain score, sleep interference, past week and present pain intensity, sensory and affective pain scores, and bodily pain	*13*
Total symptom score	*14*

to an “average” duration or population size. There are also basic mathematical constraints, i.e., it is not appropriate to calculate confidence intervals in crossover studies, and the mean NNT for several studies is actually the reciprocal of the arithmetic mean of the individual weighted absolute risk reductions and not the average of all weighted NNT’s. If the end points move in the same direction for both placebo and drug, NNT’s might be overestimated. Finally, the validity of meta-analyses should be questioned if the reduction in RR exceeds 20% between studies.

Use of the aforementioned methods with an awareness of their caveats might ensure that treatment on a robust evidence base is advocated as opposed to the current situation, where a number of national and international guidelines still recommend tricyclic antidepressants as first line treatment for painful diabetic neuropathy. This is despite the fact that studies assessing the efficacy of amitriptyline are limited to five small clinical trials with heterogeneous patient groups, end points and analyses, which have never enabled it to secure an indication for diabetic neuropathy *(1)*.

CLINICAL DEFICITS

A number of scoring systems have been proposed to quantify clinically neurological deficits and hence, define the presence and severity of neuropathy. This approach was originally pioneered by Dyck et al. *(15)* in the Mayo Clinic who described the neuropathy disability score (Mayo NDS). A comprehensive evaluation of muscular strength in the face, torso and extremities, reflexes of the upper and lower extremities and sensation to pain, vibration, and joint position at the index finger and great toe scored on a scale of

Table 2
Modified Neuropathy Disability Score

Neuropathy disability score		Right	Left
Vibration perception threshold			
128-Hz tuning fork; apex of big toe: normal = can distinguish vibrating/not vibrating	Normal = 0 Abnormal = 1		
Temperature perception on dorsum of the foot			
Use tuning fork with beaker of ice/warm water			
Pin-prick			
Apply pin proximal to big toe nail just enough to deform the skin; trial pair = sharp, blunt; normal = can distinguish sharp/not sharp			
Achilles reflex	Present = 0 Present with reinforcement = 1 Absent = 2		
	NDS Total out of 10		

0–4 produces an accurate and reproducible measure of the severity of diabetic neuropathy *(16)*. However, because it should be performed by well-trained neurologist who can accurately evaluate muscle strength and grade the severity of sensory deficits, it renders it a useful research tool but limits its role in daily clinical practice. A modified NDS first described by Young et al. *(17)* can be performed by a nonspecialist and provides a sum of the sensory and reflex deficits totalling 28. The sensory score is derived from an evaluation of pain (pin prick), touch (cotton wool), cold (tuning fork immersed in icy water), and vibration (128 Hz tuning fork), graded according to the anatomical level at which sensation is impaired (no abnormality [0], base of toes [1], midfoot [2], ankle [3], midleg [4], knee [5]). The average of both feet for each modality is calculated and the sum of all four deficits represents the sensory score. The reflex score is derived from the knee and ankle reflexes (normal 0, elicited with reinforcement 1 and absent 2). A score from 1 to 5 represents mild, 6–16 moderate, and 17–28 severe neuropathy. A furthermore simplification of the NDS is provided by a tool which takes only a minute or so to complete and ranges from zero (normal) to 10 (maximum deficit score) indicating a complete loss of sensation to all sensory modalities and absent reflexes *(18)* (Table 2). Of direct clinical relevance a NDS score of more than 6/10 predicts the risk of foot ulceration better than the monofilament and was found to be second only to past or present history of ulceration *(19)*. Alternative methods to diagnose and stage diabetic neuropathy on an out-patient basis include the Michigan Neuropathy Screening Instrument, which consists of 15 "yes or no" questions for symptoms related to sensation, general asthenia, and peripheral vascular disease in addition to inspection of the foot, assessment of vibration sensation, and ankle reflexes *(20)*. Those with an abnormal Michigan Neuropathy Screening Instrument score undergo a more detailed evaluation, the Michigan Diabetic Neuropathy Score, which involves assessment of vibration perception thresholds, pain,

Table 3
Toronto Clinical Neuropathy Scoring System

Symptom scores	Reflex scores	Sensory test scores
Foot	Knee reflexes	Pinprick
Pain	Ankle reflexes	Temperature
Numbness		Light touch
Tingling		Vibration
Weakness		Position
Ataxia		
Upper-limb symptoms		

Symptom scores: present, 1; absent, 0.
Reflex scores: absent, 2; reduced, 1, normal, 0.
Sensory test score: abnormal, 1; normal, 0.
Total scores range from normal 0 to Maximum of 19.

light touch, 10 g monofilament, and nerve electrophysiology that are scored and graded into normal, mild, moderate, or severe neuropathy. More recently the Toronto clinical scoring system (Table 3) has been validated against neurophysiological and pathological deficits obtained on sural nerve biopsy *(21)*. It is weighted to emphasize sensory symptoms and deficits as opposed to motor deficits, which is a criticism of the original NDS *(15)*. Thus, patients are questioned as to the presence or absence and characteristics (burning, stabbing, or shock-like) of neuropathic pain, numbness, tingling, and weakness in the feet; the presence or absence of similar upper-limb symptoms; and the presence or absence of unsteadiness on ambulation. Sensory testing is performed on the first toe and rated as normal or abnormal while knee and ankle reflexes are graded as normal, reduced, or absent.

Clinical Screening Devices

The Semmes–Weinstein monofilament, graduated Rydel–Seiffer tuning fork, tactile circumferential discriminator, and Neuropen (Fig. 1) can detect those at risk of ulceration *(18)*. However, their ability to detect mild neuropathy and minimal change is limited and therefore, they should not be used in clinical trials to determine treatment efficacy.

Quantitative Sensory Testing

Formal quantitative sensory testing (QST), where the intensity and characteristics of the stimuli are well-controlled, and where the detection threshold is determined in parametric units that can be compared with established "normal" values is essential for accurate quantification of neuropathy. It allows:

1. Serial standardized evaluations at multiple body sites;
2. Accurate control of stimulus characteristics in a wide dynamic range;
3. Assessment of multiple sensory modalities; and
4. Comparison of individual test results with normative databases, and is noninvasive.

The main disadvantages are: (1) lack of objectivity and (2) the examinee's response, which depends on their cooperation and concentration as well as expectations *(18)*. QST measures of vibration using the Biothesiometer or Neurothesiometer

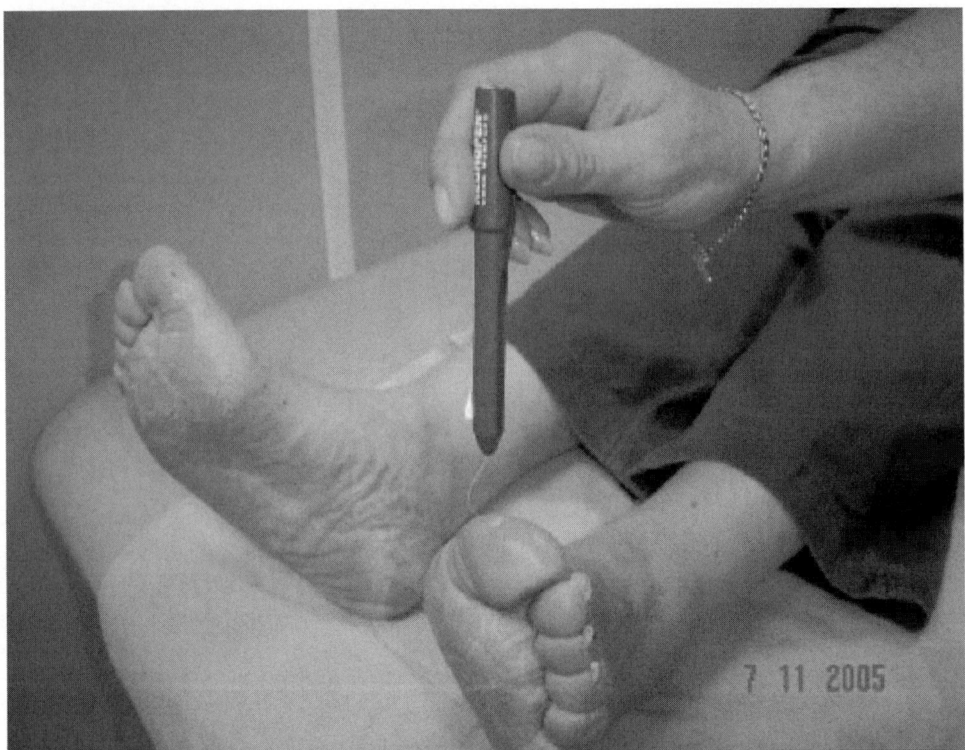

Fig. 1. Using the Neuropen to establish risk of foot ulceration.

(Fig. 2), thermal and pain thresholds, have proven valuable to identify diabetic patients with subclinical neuropathy *(18)*, track progression *(22)*, and predict those "at risk" for foot ulceration *(23)*. Thus, a consensus subcommittee of the American Academy of Neurology have stated that "QST testing for vibratory and cooling thresholds receives a Class II rating as a diagnostic test. Further, QST is designated as safe, effective, and established, with a type B strength of recommendation. Thus, QST is accepted and has been used as a primary end point in several recent clinical trials of diabetic neuropathy *(25,26)*; however, QST is unacceptable as the sole criteria to define diabetic neuropathy" *(24)*.

Electrophysiology

Attributes of nerve conduction are reliable, reproducible, and form objective primary outcome measures in trials evaluating pharmaceutical treatment of diabetic peripheral neuropathy. However, they must be performed in triplicate samples and by trained individuals, as a recent study has demonstrated a sixfold difference in the ability to detect polyneuropathy (11.9% by neurologists to 2.4% by podiatrists) *(27)*. Furthermore, maximal nerve conduction velocity (NCV) only reflects a limited aspect of neural activity of a small subset of large diameter and heavily myelinated axons and is insensitive to early functional alterations such as a reduction in Na^+/K^+ ATPase activity *(28)*. Despite these obvious limitations multiple consensus panels have recommended the inclusion of whole nerve electrophysiology (e.g., NCV, F-waves, sensory,

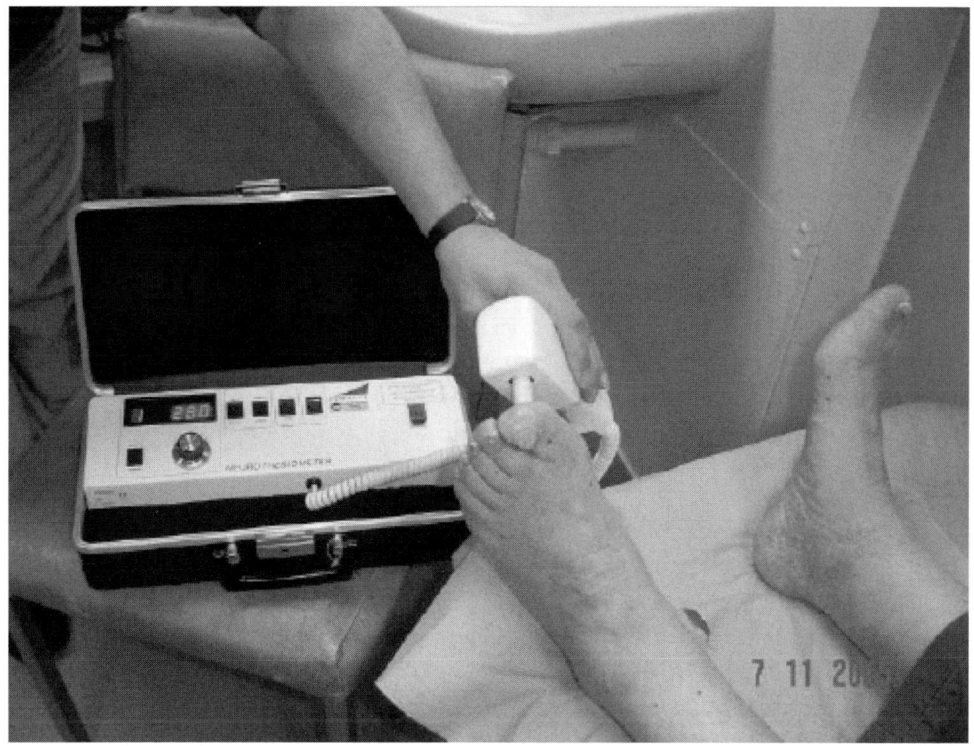

Fig. 2. Using the Neurothesiometer to establish the vibration perception threshold in a diabetic patient with established neuropathy.

and/or motor amplitudes) as surrogate measures in multicentre clinical trials of human diabetic neuropathy *(29)*.

NCV

The principal factors deemed to influence NCV are: the integrity and degree of myelination of the largest diameter fibres; the mean axonal cross-sectional diameter; the representative internodal distance, and the distribution of nodal ion channels. Although demyelination can produce a profound deficit in NCV, it has been proposed to play only a minor role in slowing of NCV in diabetic peripheral neuropathy (DPN) *(30)*. It has been suggested that the initial structural deficit responsible for NCV slowing is likely a diminished "length constant" of large diameter axons because of axonal atrophy. However, in a recent study of 57 patients with diabetes an amplitude-independent slowing of NCV supported the occurrence of demyelination *(31)*. Furthermore, our recent study in patients with diabetes with early neuropathy demonstrated significant paranodal demyelination and remyelination with no evidence of axonal atrophy *(32)*.

To establish a perspective on the expected rate of decline in NCV and the factors which might influence it, it is important to analyze in detail the results from several published studies. In the Diabetic Control and Complications Trial (type 1 diabetes) the sural and peroneal nerve velocities in the conventionally treated group diminished by 0.56 and 0.54 m per second per year, respectively, for 5 years *(33)*. In a prospective 8 year study of 45 type 1 diabetic patients a 1% rise in HbA1c was associated with a

1.3 m per second decrease in maximal nerve conduction velocity *(34)*. In patients with type 2 diabetes a lower rate of decline was observed in a 10-year natural history study of 133 patients with newly diagnosed type 2 diabetes in which NCV deteriorated by 0.39 m per second per year in the sural and 0.3 m per second per year in the peroneal nerves *(35)*. Recently, some composite scores of nerve conduction and selected individual attributes of nerve conduction have been shown to be superior to symptoms or quantitative sensation when assessing a worsening of early neuropathy *(36)*. A part of the alteration in NCV might well depend on nodal ion channel function as opposed to frank structural alterations such as demyelination and axonal atrophy. Recently, the relatively new technique of threshold tracking which measures nodal ion channel function has shown that reduced nodal/paranodal potassium currents are related to glycemic control *(37)*. This technique might well be used in the future together with standard NCV assessment to define therapeutic responses.

Amplitude

Peak amplitude of either the sensory response sensory nerve action potential (SNAP) or the compound muscle action potential (CMAP) reflects the number of responding fibres and the synchrony of their activity. A strong correlation ($r = 0.74$; $p < 0.001$) between myelinated fibre density and whole nerve sural amplitude in DPN *(38)* has been previously demonstrated. Others have shown that a change of 1 μV in sural nerve SNAP is associated with a decrease of approximately 150 fibers/mm^2 and a loss of 200 fibres/mm^2 is associated with an approximate 1 mV reduction in the mean amplitude of the ulnar, peroneal, and tibial nerves CMAP *(39)*. In a longitudinal study of patients with type 2 diabetes an approximate 5% per year loss of SNAP has been demonstrated *(35)*.

F-Waves

F-Waves detect any abnormality in the antidromic conduction of the compound neural volley to the ventral spinal cord, the activation of a subpopulation of spinal motor neurons, the orthodromic conduction of the newly established volley, and the postsynaptic activation of muscle fibres in the innervated muscle. The “long-loop” nature, of this measure increases the sensitivity to detect factors that alter the speed of conduction, which might be widely distributed along a nerve. Thus, a subtle change affecting each node might not be detected in measures focused on an isolated distal segment, but might accumulate and become evident in the long latency F-wave response. F-wave latency has been shown to be the most reproducible measure in nerve conduction studies of diabetic polyneuropathy *(40)*. Although minimal latency is the most frequent measures of F-wave activity, the addition of chronodispersion, duration, persistence, and amplitude might add sensitivity to detect an abnormality in slower conducting axons *(41)*.

Distribution of Velocities

The fusion of a collision technique with an analysis of the distribution of conduction velocities has proven to be valuable in exploring the effects of DPN on slower fibres *(42)*. Using a computer-assisted collision procedure with an assessment of velocities in slower conducting fibres, subclinical neuropathy was detected in 58% of subjects compared with only 11% of subjects using standard electrophysiology *(42)*.

Table 4
Frequency of Detection and Sensitivity and Specificity for Detection of Diabetic Polyneuropathy

	Frequency of diabetic polyneuropathy	Sensitivity	Specificity
NIS (LL) + seven tests	58/195 = 29.5%	58/58 = 100%	137/137 = 100%
NIS (LL)	58/195 = 29.5%	40/58 = 69%	119/137 = 86.9%
Abnormal ankle reflex	48/195 = 24.6%	35/58 = 60.3%	124/137 = 90.5%
Abnormal vibration sensation (tuning fork)	15/195 = 7.7%	10/58 = 17.2%	132/137 = 96.4%
VPT	15/195 = 7.7%	15/54 = 27.8%	141/141 = 100%
More than two abnormal tests	73/195 = 37.4%	51/58 = 87.9%	115/137 = 83.9%
More than two abnormal tests and NC abnormal	112/195 = 57.4%	54/58 = 93.1%	79/137 = 57.7%
More than two nerves with NC abnormal	59/195 = 30.3%	47/58 = 81%	125/137 = 91.2%
More than one nerve with NC abnormal	112/195 = 57.4%	54/58 = 93.1%	79/137 = 57.7%
NIS (LL) + VDT (abnormal at 99th percentile)	28/195 = 14.4%	27/54 = 50%	140/141 = 99.3%

COMPOSITE SCORES

The reproducibility of the different measures of neuropathy and interobserver agreement varies markedly between tests. This leads to the situation where the analysis for a clinical trial produces some results which are found to be significant whereas others are not, yet they might be assessing the same modality. To overcome this, Dyck and coworkers *(43)* pioneered composite scores such as the NDS and later the neuropathy impairment score (NIS). This allows an assessment of an alteration in function of several classes of nerve fibres, all of which are likely to be affected by diabetes. In the Rochester longitudinal study the NIS [LL] + 7 (vibration perception threshold [VPT] great toe, R–R variation to deep breathing, peroneal motor nerve conduction velocity, CMAP, and motor nerve distal latency, tibial motor nerve distal latency, and sural SNAP) have been shown to be 100% sensitive and specific in comparison with an abnormal VPT, which had a sensitivity of 27.8% (Table 4). Based on the findings of the Rochester study *(43)*, a treatment effect of two points in NIS is deemed clinically meaningful. Therefore, to achieve a power of 0.90, about 140 patients need to be randomized to active and placebo arms for at least 2 years to detect a statistically significant difference at $p = 0.05$. However, if the primary end point is prevention of progression then the duration of the trial needs to be extended to about 4 years. A significant shortcoming of such composite scores arises when assessing the therapeutic benefits of agents which target a subclass of nerve fibres, e.g., NGF and C-fibres, where ideally one should focus on a small fibre abnormality *(44)*.

OTHER METHODS OF ASSESSMENT

Axon Reflex

Capillary dilatation because of an injury response (caused by histamine and other mediators of vasodilatation released from damaged tissues) can be captured as a red flare as a result of arteriolar dilatation through a local axon reflex. The axon reflex might be elicited by stimulation of pain nerve fibers *(45)* or through iontophoresis of acetylcholine, which mediates the release of nitric oxide through the axon reflex *(46)*. A recent study has used heating the skin to 44°C to evoke the flare *(LDIflare)* and assessed it using a laser Doppler imager to show that it demonstrates C-fibre dysfunction before it can be detected by CASE IV *(47)*.

Nerve Biopsy

Nerve biopsy, typically of the sural nerve has been used for many years in the study of peripheral neuropathy, particularly when the etiology is unclear or in patients with diabetes with atypical neuropathies *(48)*. However, this is an invasive procedure with recognized sequelae, which might include postoperative pain at the site of biopsy, sensory deficits in the nerve distribution and allodynia, particularly in diabetic patients *(49)*. A number of morphological parameters including myelinated fibre density, regenerative cluster density, axonal atrophy, and axo-glial dysjunction have been used as morphological end points to determine treatment efficacy *(50,51)*. However, the need to repeat contra-lateral nerve biopsy and questions on the utility and reliability of the methods used to evaluate axo-glial dysjunction and axonal atrophy has posed serious questions regarding its use as an end point in any future trials of human diabetic neuropathy.

Skin Biopsy

An alternative less invasive technique of a 3-mm skin biopsy enables a direct study of small nerve fibres and has been proposed for use in clinical trials *(52)*. Although a number of neuronal markers including neurone-specific enolase and somatostatin have been used to immunostain skin nerves, protein gene product-9.5 has proven to be the best cytoplasmic axonal marker. To define alterations in the most distal nerves and hence those likely to sustain the earliest damage, 50 μm formalin-fixed frozen sections have been used to visualize and quantify intraepidermal nerve fibres (IENF) density, as number/length of epidermis in idiopathic sensory neuropathy and in patients with impaired glucose tolerance *(53,54)*. A recent study used a new morphometric modification to assess nerves per epidermal area, which correlated highly ($r = 0.945$) with the accepted gold standard assessment of nerves per epidermal length *(55)*. This method appears reproducible, diagnostically sensitive, less time-consuming than IENF-counting, and might be adopted in any laboratory familiar with basic immunohistochemical methodology for protein gene product-9.5 staining *(55)*. It has been proposed that the rate of epidermal nerve fibre regeneration before and after intervention could be utilized as an end point in clinical trials *(56)*.

Magnetic Resonance Imaging

Magnetic resonance imaging has been used to demonstrate that patients with DPN have a lower cross-sectional spinal cord area than healthy controls in the cervical and thoracic regions *(57)*. However, progression or regression of this abnormality has not been evaluated in prospective studies, and therefore, the potential for its use as an end point in clinical trials of human diabetic neuropathy remains to be established.

Corneal Confocal Microscopy

The cornea is the most densely innervated part of the human body containing Aδ and unmyelinated C-fibres and derives its innervation from the ophthalmic division of the trigeminal nerve. Corneal confocal microscopy (CCM) permits sequential observations of the corneal subbasal nerve plexus comparable or even superior to that obtained with histopathological examination *(58)*. CCM detects significant alterations in corneal nerve fibre density, branching, and tortuosity in patients with mild diabetic neuropathy and these alterations relate to the severity of somatic neuropathy *(59,60)* (Fig. 1). Furthermore, in a recent prospective study corneal nerve fibre density has been shown to improve with improved glycemic control *(61)*. Therefore, the ability of CCM to define the extent of nerve damage and repair cross-sectionally but also longitudinally in patients with diabetes appears significant. In particular the noninvasive and hence, reiterative facility of CCM provides a means of expediting drug development programmes of therapies deemed to be beneficial in the treatment of diabetic peripheral neuropathy (Fig. 3).

Assessing Risk of Ulceration

At present there is no effective treatment for neuropathy therefore, the focus of defining those with neuropathy should be on those who have a significant risk of foot ulceration. The methods used for this purpose must be rapid, simple, and predict ulceration. In a recent study of 2022 diabetic subjects and 175 nondiabetic control subjects, "peripheral polyneuropathy" was diagnosed by assessing VPT at the tip of both great toes using a Rydel–Seiffer 128-Hz tuning fork and a neurothesiometer, abnormal 10-g monofilament test, and the presence of neuropathic symptoms. 5.2% of patients with diabetes had an abnormal vibration test, of whom 66.7% had an abnormal monofilament response and 68.6% had a missing Achilles' tendon reflex. But those with an abnormal tuning fork test had a significantly higher vibration perception threshold (32 +/– 9.8 vs 12.5 +/– 6.4 V), which would be consistent with defining those at risk of ulceration. Thus, it would appear that the simple tuning fork was a useful screening test for those at risk of ulceration rather than diabetic neuropathy as concluded by the authors *(62)*. The predictive value of defining vibration perception threshold was established more than 10 years ago in a large prospective study, which showed that a VPT >25 effectively predicted the risk of foot ulceration in diabetes *(63)*. In a multicenter prospective follow-up study to determine which risk factors in foot screening have a high association with the development of foot ulceration, 248 patients underwent an assessment of the neuropathy symptom score, NDS, VPT, Semmes–Weinstein monofilaments, joint mobility, peak plantar foot pressures, and vascular status at baseline and every 6 months for a mean period of 30 months (range 6–40) *(64)*. Foot ulcers developed in a high proportion (29%) of patients suggesting they were all extremely at high risk. They were more frequently men, had a longer duration of diabetes, nonpalpable pedal pulses, reduced joint mobility, higher NDS, higher VPT, and an inability to feel a 5.07 monofilament. The NDS alone had the best sensitivity, whereas the combination of the NDS and the inability to feel a 5.07 monofilament reached a sensitivity of 99% *(64)*.

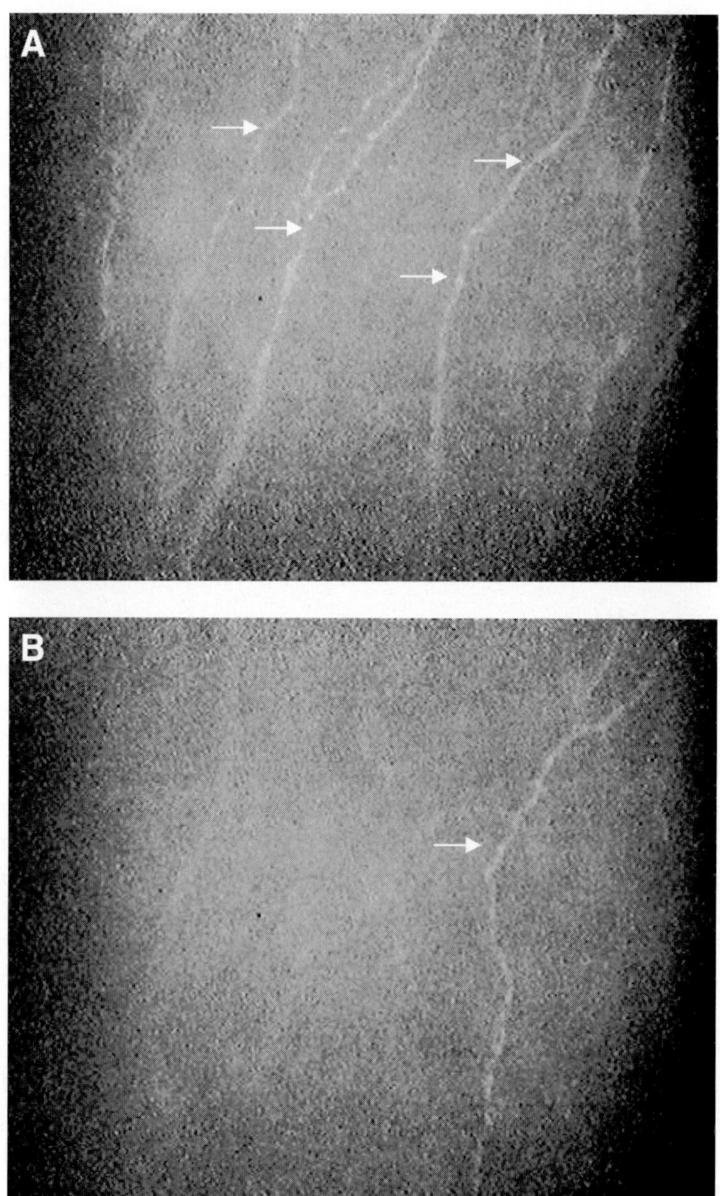

Fig. 3. Corneal confocal images showing loss of corneal never fibres in diabetic neuropathy. **(A)** Confocal image of a control subject with many corneal nerves (→). **(B)** Diabetic patient with neuropathy and only one corneal nerve fibre (→).

To determine the incidence of, and clinically relevant risk factors for new foot ulceration in a large cohort of patients with diabetes in the community healthcare setting, 9710 patients with diabetes underwent an assessment of the neuropathy symptom score, NDS, sensitivity to the 10 g monofilament, foot deformities, and peripheral pulses at baseline for 2 years in six districts of North-West England *(19)*. The annual incidence of new foot ulcers was 2.2% and the following factors independently predicted new foot ulcer risk: ulcer present at baseline (RR [95% confidence interval]) 5.32 (3.71–7.64), past history of ulcer 3.05 (2.16–4.31), abnormal NDS (≥6/10) 2.32 (1.61–3.35), any previous podiatry attendance 2.19 (1.50–3.20), insensitivity to the 10 g monofilament 1.80 (1.36–2.39), reduced pulses 1.80 (1.40–2.32), foot deformities 1.57 (1.22–2.02), abnormal ankle reflexes 1.55 (1.01–2.36), and age 0.99 (0.98–1). Thus, the study recommended that the NDS, 10 g monofilament and palpation of foot pulses be used as screening tools in general practice *(19)*.

Best Methods for Clinical Trials

Methodological issues of paramount importance for success of any DPN trial are: (1) population selection, (2) end points, (3) study duration, and (4) confounding factors.

Population Selection

Because DPN is a complex disease of multifactorial etiology, a randomly chosen population of patients with this condition are likely to be heterogenous not only with respect to the form and severity of neuropathy but also with respect to the type of diabetes and other risk factors for neuropathy *(22)*. Therefore, to detect a significant drug effect in such a population large numbers of patients and/or impractically long study durations are required. Additionally, DPN evolves from a stage of subclinical alteration with early neurophysiological dysfunction *(36)* to eventual significant clinical and pathological deficits *(43)*. It is reasonable to assume that any therapeutic intervention is likely to be more beneficial earlier in the course of the disease. For the purpose of a clinical trial, patients with clinical stage 1 or 2a should be targeted. Those with more advanced disease—stage 2b and, especially, stage 3, are less likely to respond to any given therapeutic intervention. Furthermore to limit variability in the assessment of neuropathy because of the involvement of multiple examiners participating in a multicenter trial, it is desirable to establish entry criteria, such as nerve conduction attributes or quantitative sensory tests to optimize homogeneity. To eliminate the possible effects of glycemic control over the duration of the trial it is important to have a run-in period reserved for optimizing glycemic control and eliminating those who are unable to achieve acceptable levels of HbA1C (i.e., 9%). Because patients with type 1 and type 2 diabetes differ considerably in demographic characteristics, comorbidities, concomitant medication, and incidence of neuropathy, proper stratification techniques, and/or study analysis methods are necessary. Regarding neuropathy itself, patients not experiencing steady levels of symptoms and signs for at least 6–12 months should be excluded and the adjustment should be done for the duration of both diabetes and neuropathy. This approach is desirable but might limit recruitment. An effective compound will only succeed if a fair balance is established for study entry criteria that reflect the population with diabetic neuropathy in general.

End Points

Ideally, the end points should be clinically relevant, such as the development of clinically manifest neuropathy or progression of existing neuropathy to the point of an insensate foot or foot ulceration. However, because of the natural history of the disease, use of such endpoints makes studies prohibitively long, expensive, and potentially obsolete.

Thus, one has to rely on surrogate end points, which by definition exhibit a causal relationship with the clinical outcome and are laboratory measurements or physical signs which can be measured rapidly with good sensitivity and specificity.

Study Duration

The duration of the trial needed to demonstrate a difference in outcomes between active and placebo groups is directly dependent on the desired statistical power of the study and relative success rates observed in both groups. This success rate will depend on the severity and evolution of change in the chosen end point and the duration of treatment. In patients with mild neuropathy, using outcome measures such as nerve conduction studies (NCS) and QST, it might take 3–5 years to demonstrate a clinically meaningful difference. If clinical signs of neuropathy or composite scores consisting of signs, NCS and QST are being used, it has been postulated that the trial should recruit at least 68 patients per treatment arm and should last 3.7 years *(43)*. If however, one chooses a hard end point like the annual incidence of foot ulceration then approximately 3000 patients are required in 5 years *(65)*.

Confounding Factors

First, the phenomenon of "regression to the mean" is particularly relevant to trials of symptomatic human diabetic neuropathy. Thus, patients who enroll in a trial might do so when their symptoms are at their peak. Because the natural history of painful diabetic neuropathy is one of spontaneous improvement then the next assessment after being randomized, irrespective of treatment benefit is biased toward an improvement. Second, the placebo effect might play a significant role, especially as this might be higher than the conventionally quoted 20–30% particularly in painful diabetic neuropathy.

CONCLUSION

Progress has been made in the development of more effective treatments for painful diabetic neuropathy in the last 5 years. The improved clinical trial design, use of clinically relevant end points with drugs that have plausible pharmacological mechanisms and hence greater efficacy with lesser side effects, has led the FDA to approve pregabalin and duloxetine for painful diabetic neuropathy in 2005. Positive data have also been published for acetyl-L-carnitine *(51)*, α-lipoic acid *(14)*, and C-peptide *(66)* for symptoms and some deficits in patients with diabetic neuropathy. Long-term data for the benefits of α-lipoic acid in relation to nerve function should be available by 2006/2007. Although two recent phase-3 clinical trials with the protein kinase-C β-inhibitor, ruboxistaurin, have failed to improve neuropathic symptoms the Phase-3 trial to define the effects on nerve function continues and is because of report in 2008. A number of phase-2 and -3 studies are planned or are underway with new agents both for symptomatic neuropathy (NMDA receptor antagonists) and to improve deficits (aldose reductase inhibitor's).

REFERENCES

1. Malik RA. Current and future strategies for the management of diabetic neuropathy. *Treat Endocrinol* 2003;2:389–400.
2. Young MJ, Boulton AJ, McLeod AF, Williams DR, Sonksen PH. A multicentre study of the prevalence of diabetic peripheral neuropathy in the UK hospital clinic population. *Diabetologia* 1993;36:150–156.

3. Cabezas-Cerrato J. The prevalence of diabetic neuropathy in Spain: a study in primary care and hospital clinic groups. *Diabetologia* 1998;41:1263–1269.
4. Scott J, Huskisson EC. Graphic representation of pain. *Pain* 1976;2:175–186.
5. Meijer JW, Smit AJ, Sondersen EV, Groothoff JW, Eisma WH, Links TP. Symptom scoring systems to diagnose distal polyneuropathy in diabetes; the Diabetic Neuropathy Symptom Score. *Diabetic Med* 2002;19:962–965.
6. Zelman DC, Gore M, Dukes E, Tai KS, Brandenburg N. Validation of a modified version of the brief pain inventory for painful diabetic peripheral neuropathy. *J Pain Symptom Manage* 2005;29:401–410.
7. Gilron I, Bailey JM, Tu D, Holden RR, Weaver DF, Houlden RL. Morphine, gabapentin, or their combination for neuropathic pain. *N Engl J Med* 2005;352:1324–1334.
8. Frampton JE, Scott LJ. Pregabalin: in the treatment of painful diabetic peripheral neuropathy. *Drugs* 2004;64:2813–2820.
9. Rowbotham MC, Goli V, Kunz NR, Lei D. Venlafaxine extended release in the treatment of painful diabetic neuropathy: a double-blind, placebo-controlled study. *Pain* 2004; 110:697–706.
10. Vileikyte L, Peyrot M, Bundy C, et al. The development and validation of a neuropathy- and foot ulcer-specific quality of life instrument. *Diabetes Care* 2003;26:2549–2555.
11. Atli A, Dogra S. Zonisamide in the treatment of painful diabetic neuropathy: a randomized, double-blind, placebo-controlled pilot study. *Pain Med* 2005;6:225–234.
12. Goldstein DJ, Lu Y, Detke MJ, Lee TC, Iyengar S. Duloxetine vs. placebo in patients with painful diabetic neuropathy. *Pain* 2005;116:109–118.
13. Richter RW, Portenoy R, Sharma U, Lamoreaux L, Bockbrader H, Knapp LE. Relief of painful diabetic peripheral neuropathy with pregabalin: a randomized, placebo-controlled trial. *J Pain* 2005;6:253–260.
14. Ziegler D, Nowak H, Kempler P, Vargha P, Low PA. Treatment of symptomatic diabetic polyneuropathy with the antioxidant alpha-lipoic acid: a meta-analysis. *Diabet Med* 2004;21:114–121.
15. Dyck PJ, Karnes J, O'Brien PC, Swanson CJ. Neuropathy symptom profile in health, motor neuron disease, diabetic neuropathy, and amyloidosis. *Neurology* 1986;36:1300–1308.
16. Dyck PJ, Kratz KM, Lehman KA, et al. The Rochester diabetic neuropathy study: Design, criteria for types of neuropathy, selection bias, and reproducibility of neuropathic tests. *Neurology* 1991;41:799–807.
17. Young RJ, Zhou YQ, Rodriguez E, Prescott RJ, Ewing DJ, Clarke BF. Variable relationship between peripheral somatic and autonomic neuropathy in patients with different syndromes of diabetic polyneuropathy. *Diabetes* 1986;35:192–197.
18. Boulton AJ, Malik RA, Arezzo JC, Sosenko JM. Diabetic somatic neuropathies. *Diabetes Care* 2004;27:1458–1486.
19. Abbott CA, Carrington AL, Ashe H, et al. North-West Diabetes Foot Care Study. The North-West Diabetes Foot Care Study: incidence of, and risk factors for, new diabetic foot ulceration in a community-based patient cohort. *Diabet Med* 2002;19:377–384.
20. Feldman EL, Stevens MJ, Thomas PK, Brown MB, Canal N, Greene DA. A practical two-step quantitative clinical and electrophysiological assessment for the diagnosis and staging of diabetic neuropathy. *Diabetes Care* 1994;17:1281–1289.
21. Bril V, Perkins BA. Validation of the Toronto Clinical Scoring System for diabetic polyneuropathy. *Diabetes Care* 2002;25:2048–2052.
22. Dyck PJ, Dyck PJ, Velosa JA, Larson TS, O'Brien PC. The Nerve Growth Factors Study Group. Patterns of quantitative sensation testing of hypoesthesia and hyperalgesia are predictive of diabetic polyneuropathy. A study of three cohorts. *Diabetes Care* 2000;23:510.
23. Sosenko JM, Kato M, Soto R, Bild DE. Comparison of quantitative sensory-threshold measures for their association with foot ulceration in diabetic patients. *Diabetes Care* 1990;13:1057–1061.

24. Shy ME, Frohman EM, So YT, Arezzo JC, Cornblath DC, Giuliani MJ. Quantitative sensory testing: report of the Therapeutics and Technology Assessment the Subcommittee of the American Academy of Neurology. *Neurology* 2003;602:898–906.
25. Apfel SC, Schwartz S, Adornato BT, et al. Efficacy and safety of recombinant human nerve growth factor in patients with diabetic polyneuropathy: A randomized controlled trial. *JAMA* 2000;284:2215–2221.
26. Ekberg K, Brismar T, Johansson BL, Jonsson B, Lindstrom P, Wahren J. Amelioration of sensory nerve dysfunction by C-Peptide in patients with type 1 diabetes. *Diabetes* 2003;52:536–541.
27. Dillingham TR, Pezzin LE. Under-recognition of polyneuropathy in persons with diabetes by non-physician electrodiagnostic services providers. *Am J Phys Med Rehabil* 2005;84:399–406.
28. Hohman TC, Cotter MA, Cameron NE. ATP-sensitive K (+) channel effects on nerve function, Na (+), K (+) ATPase, and glutathione in diabetic rats. *Eur J Pharmacol* 2000;3(397):335–341.
29. Peripheral Nerve Society: Diabetic polyneuropathy in controlled clinical trials: consensus report of the peripheral nerve society. *Am Neurol* 1995;38:478–482.
30. Valk GD, Grootenhuis PA, van Eijk JT, Bouter LM, Bertelsmann FW. Methods for assessing diabetic polyneuropathy: validity and reproducibility of the measurement of sensory symptom severity and nerve function tests. *Diabetes Res Clin Pract* 2000;47:87–95.
31. Herrmann DN, Ferguson ML, Logigian EL. Conduction slowing in diabetic distal polyneuropathy. *Muscle Nerve* 2002;26:232–237.
32. Malik RA, Tesfaye S, Newrick PG, et al. Sural nerve pathology in diabetic patients with minimal but progressive neuropathy. *Diabetologia* 2005;48:578–585.
33. DCCT research group. The effect of intensive diabetes therapy on the development and progression of neuropathy. *Ann Int Med* 1995;122:561–568.
34. Amthor KF, Dahl-Jorgensen K, Berg TJ, et al. The effect of 8 years of strict glycaemia control on peripheral nerve function in IDDM patients: the Oslo Study. *Diabetologia* 1994; 37:579–784.
35. Partanen J, Niskanen L, Lehtinen J, Mervaala E, Siitonen O, Uusitupa M. Natural history of peripheral neuropathy in patients with non-insulin dependent diabetes. *NEJM* 1995;333: 39–84.
36. Dyck PJ, O'Brien PC, Litchy WJ, Harper CM, Klein CJ, Dyck PJ. Monotonicity of nerve tests in diabetes: subclinical nerve dysfunction precedes diagnosis of polyneuropathy. *Diabetes Care* 2005;28:2192–2200.
37. Misawa S, Kuwabara S, Kanai K, et al. Axonal potassium conductance and glycemic control in human diabetic nerves. *Clin Neurophysiol* 2005;116:1181–1187.
38. Veves A, Malik RA, Lye RH, et al. The relationship between sural nerve morphometric findings and measures of peripheral nerve function in mild diabetic neuropathy. *Diabetic Med* 1991;8:917–921.
39. Russell JW, Karnes JL, Dyck PJ. Sural nerve myelinated fibre density differences associated with meaningful changes in clinical and electrophysiologic measurements. *J Neurol Sci* 1996;135:114–117.
40. Kohara N, Kimura J, Kaji R, et al. F-wave latency serves as the most reproducible measure in nerve conduction studies of diabetic polyneuropathy: multicentre analysis in healthy subjects and patients with diabetic polyneuropathy. *Diabetologia* 2000;43:915–921.
41. Caccia MR, Salvaggi A, Dezuanni E. An electrophysiological method to assess the distribution of the sensory propagation velocity of the digital nerve in normal and diabetic subjects. *Electroencephal Clin Neurophysiol* 1993;89:88–94.
42. Bertora P, Valla P, Dezuanni E. Prevalence of subclinical neuropathy in diabetic patients: assessment by study of conduction velocity distribution within motor and sensory nerve fibres. *J Neurol* 1998;245:81–86.

43. Dyck PJ, Davies JL, Litchy WJ, O'Brien PC. Longitudinal assessment of diabetic polyneuropathy using a composite score in the Rochester Diabetic Neuropathy Study cohort. *Neurology* 1997;49:229–239.
44. Apfel SC, Schwartz S, Adornato BT, et al. Efficacy and safety of recombinant human nerve growth factor in patients with diabetic polyneuropathy: A randomized controlled trial. *JAMA* 2000;284:2215–2221.
45. Magerl W, Treede RD. Heat-evoked vasodilatation in human hairy skin: axon reflexes due to low-level activity of nociceptive afferents. *J Physiol* 1996;15:837–848.
46. Hamdy O, Abou-Elenin K, LoGerfo FW, Horton ES, Veves A. Contribution of nerve-axon reflex-related vasodilation to the total skin vasodilation in diabetic patients with and without neuropathy. *Diabetes Care* 2001;24:344–349.
47. Krishnan ST, Rayman G. The LDIflare: a novel test of C-fibre function demonstrates early neuropathy in type 2 diabetes. *Diabetes Care* 2004;27:2930–2935.
48. Thomas PK. Nerve biopsy. *Diabetic Med* 1997;16:351–352.
49. Dahlin LB, Erikson KF, Sundkvist G. Persistent postoperative complaints after whole nerve sural nerve biopsies in diabetic and non-diabetic subjects. *Diabetic Med* 1997;14:353–356.
50. Greene DA, Arezzo JC, Brown MB. Effect of aldose reductase inhibition on nerve conduction and morphometry in diabetic neuropathy. Zenarestat Study Group. *Neurology* 1999;53:580–591.
51. Sima AA, Calvani M, Mehra M, Amato A. Acetyl-L-Carnitine Study Group. Acetyl-L-carnitine improves pain, nerve regeneration, and vibratory perception in patients with chronic diabetic neuropathy: an analysis of two randomized placebo-controlled trials. *Diabetes Care* 2005;28:89–94.
52. McCarthy BG, Hsieh ST, Stocks A, et al. Cutaneous innervation in sensory neuropathies: evaluation by skin biopsy. *Neurology* 1995;45:1848–1855.
53. Holland NR, Crawford TO, Hauer P, Cornblath DR, Griffin JW, McArthur JC. Small-fiber sensory neuropathies: clinical course and neuropathology of idiopathic cases. *Ann Neurol* 1998;44:47–59.
54. Polydefkis M, Griffin W, McArthur J. New insights into diabetic polyneuropathy. *JAMA* 2003;371–1376.
55. Koskinen M, Hietaharju A, Kylaniemi M, et al. A quantitative method for the assessment of intraepidermal nerve fibres in small-fibre neuropathy. *J Neurol* 2005;252:789–794.
56. Yaneda H, Tereda M, Maeda K, et al. Diabetic neuropathy and nerve regeneration. *Prog Neurobiol* 2003;69:229–285.
57. Eaton SE, Harris ND, Rajbhandari SM, et al. Spinal-cord involvement in diabetic peripheral neuropathy. *Lancet* 2001;358:35–36.
58. Oliviera-soto L, Efron N. Morphology of corneal nerves using confocal microscopy. *Cornea* 2001;21:246–248.
59. Malik RA, Kallinikos P, Abbott CA, et al. Corneal confocal microscopy: a non-invasive surrogate of nerve fibre damage and repair in diabetic patients. *Diabetologia* 2003;46: 683–688.
60. Kallinikos P, Berhanu M, O'Donnell C, et al. Corneal nerve tortuosity in diabetic patients with neuropathy. *Invest Ophthalmol Vis Sci* 2004;45:418–422.
61. Iqbal I, Kallinikos P, Boulton AJ, Efron N, Malik RA. Corneal nerve morphology: A surrogate marker for human diabetic neuropathy improves with improved glycaemic control. *Diabetes* 2005;54:871.
62. Kastenbauer T, Sauseng S, Brath H, Abrahamian H, Irsigler K. The value of the Rydel-Seiffer tuning fork as a predictor of diabetic polyneuropathy compared with a neurothesiometer. *Diabet Med* 2004;21:563–567.
63. Young MJ, Breddy JL, Veves A, Boulton AJM. The prediction of diabetic foot ulceration using vibration thresholds: A prospective study. *Diabetes Care* 1994;17:557–560.

64. Pham H, Armstrong DG, Harvey C, Harkless LB, Giurini JM, Veves A. Screening techniques to identify people at high risk for diabetic foot ulceration: a prospective multicenter trial. *Diabetes Care* 2000;23:606–611.
65. Nicolucci A, Carnici F, Cavaliere D, et al. On behalf of the Italian study group for the implementation of the St. Vincent Declaration. A meta-analysis of trials on aldose reductase inhibitors in diabetic peripheral neuropathy. *Diabet Med* 1996;13: 1017–1026.
66. Ekberg K, Brismar T, Johansson BL, Jonsson B, Lindstrom P, Wahren J. Amelioration of sensory nerve dysfunction by C-Peptide in patients with type 1 diabetes. *Diabetes* 2003;52: 536–541.

17
Punch Skin Biopsy in Diabetic Neuropathy

Michael Polydefkis, MD

SUMMARY

Measurement of unmyelinated C and A delta nociceptors through punch skin biopsy has been an important development in diabetic peripheral neuropathy over the past decade. The technique provides an objective pathological window into a population of fibers that is invisible to standard electrophysiological techniques and as a result has been difficult to investigate. Clinically, the punch biopsy technique is most often used to define a length-dependent peripheral neuropathy, but can also be used to follow patients longitudinally over time. Epidermal nerve fibers are often lost early in diabetes or impaired glucose tolerance and can be the only objective measure of neuropathy in these patients. The accessibility of cutaneous nerve fibers has also given rise to several nerve injury paradigms from which regeneration can be efficiently measured. The chapter will review the skin biopsy technique and recent findings with respect to diabetes.

Key Words: Epidermal nerve fiber; nociceptor; skin biopsy; regeneration.

INTRODUCTION

This chapter describes the skin biopsy and skin blister technique and their role in the evaluation of unmyelinated nerve fibers in skin biopsies from patients with diabetes and impaired glucose tolerance. These techniques are a reliable and reproducible means of assessing C-fiber nociceptors. Historically, pathological examination of these fibers has been limited to nerve biopsies, primarily of the sural nerve. The invasive nature of these biopsies, the insensitivity to detect small degrees of unmyelinated nerve fiber loss, and the wide range of normal values all limited assessment of this population of fibers. Further complicating interpretation of nerve biopsies is the difficulty to discern differences between somatic and autonomic small caliber unmyelinated nerve fibers. Clinically, these fibers are "invisible" because nerve conduction testing assesses only myelinated large sensory and motor fibers. These limitations and the observations that individuals with sensory neuropathies have spontaneous acral neuropathic pain with allodynia led investigators to seek alternative means to assess this population of nerve fibers, and skin biopsy/blister has emerged as a result.

Early studies of epidermal innervation focused on the density and distribution of Meissner's corpuscles *(1,2)*. The availability of antibody to protein gene product (PGP) 9.5, a neuronal ubiquitin hydrolase, rapidly led to sensitive immunohistochemical techniques to visualize nerve fibers in the skin *(3)*. Epidermal innervation has received the most attention although myelinated fibers and autonomic fibers innervating sweat

From: *Contemporary Diabetes: Diabetic Neuropathy: Clinical Management, Second Edition*
Edited by: A. Veves and R. Malik © Humana Press Inc., Totowa, NJ

glands or arrector pili muscles in the deep dermis can also be assessed *(4–6)*. Epidermal fibers represent nociceptors and include both C and Aδ fibers. Robust normative data have been developed *(7,8)* and a distal predominant pattern of nerve fiber loss has been demonstrated in several conditions including diabetes, HIV, and idiopathic small fiber neuropathies *(9)*. Less marked reductions in epidermal nerve fiber density as well as morphological changes such as prominent nerve fiber swelling are often present at more proximal and even asymptomatic sites *(9)*.

The association between neuropathic pain and epidermal nerve fiber loss is counterintuitive as nerve fiber loss is generally associated with the absence of sensation. Neuropathic pain has been correlated with epidermal nerve fiber loss in small fiber sensory neuropathy, post herpetic neuralgia (PHN), HIV-SN, and diabetes *(9–12)*. There are several explanations for this apparent paradox. The distal ends of nerve fibers that have withdrawn from the epidermis may act as sensitized nociceptors with reduced thresholds to noxious stimuli (hyperalgesia). Alternatively, spontaneous pain may result from ectopic discharges in peripheral nociceptors. Finally, central changes such as sprouting of injured Aδ fibers from deep dorsal horn lamina into superficial lamina or changes in descending modulatory pathways may result in innocuous peripheral stimulation being misinterpreted as painful.

Nerves innervating the skin arise within the dorsal root and sympathetic ganglia. As they project toward the skin surface, myelinated fibers branch off to innervate sweat glands, Meisner's corpuscles, and Merkel complexes. Similarly, autonomic fibers envelope sweat glands in a dense matrix of fibers, whereas arrector pili are innervated in a characteristic striated pattern (Fig. 1). Hair follicles are innervated by both myelinated and unmyelinated fibers with specialized nerve endings at the base of the hair shaft. Unmyelinated sensory fibers consist the majority of dermal fibers and project vertically to the subepidermal dermis where they form a horizontally oriented nerve fiber plexus. From this plexus, branches project toward the skin surface penetrating the dermal-epidermal junction. The fibers lose their Schwann cell ensheathment as they enter the epidermis and extend between keratinocytes and Langerhans cells and project toward the stratum corneum as free nerve endings. During embryogenesis, nerve growth factor (NGF) expression within the epidermis is responsible for neuronal survival and targeted growth into the skin *(13)*. Later in development, roughly half of these fibers lose their responseiveness to NGF, becoming dependent on glial derived neurotrophic factor (GDNF). NGF-dependent cutaneous nerve fibers respond to noxious stimuli and express neuropeptides including calcitonin gene related product (CGRP) and SP, whereas GDNF dependent fibers bind the Griffonia lectin IB4 and express thimidine monophosphate and P2X3 but generally not CGRP or SP. Axons from NGF responsive neurons express the high-affinity NGF receptor TrkA as well as the low-affinity receptor p75. GDNF responsive neurons express c-Ret as well as other markers. Abnormalities in both NGF and GDNF have been implicated in the pathogenesis of diabetic neuropathy.

SELECTION OF BIOPSY SITE AND PROCESSING TECHNIQUE

Generally, skin biopsies are very well tolerated and result in negligible scarring in individuals without a predilection to keloid formation. Discoloration at the biopsy site tends to be more prominent among darker pigmented individuals. The rate of infection even among neuropathic populations is small, approximately 1:500. Biopsy sites

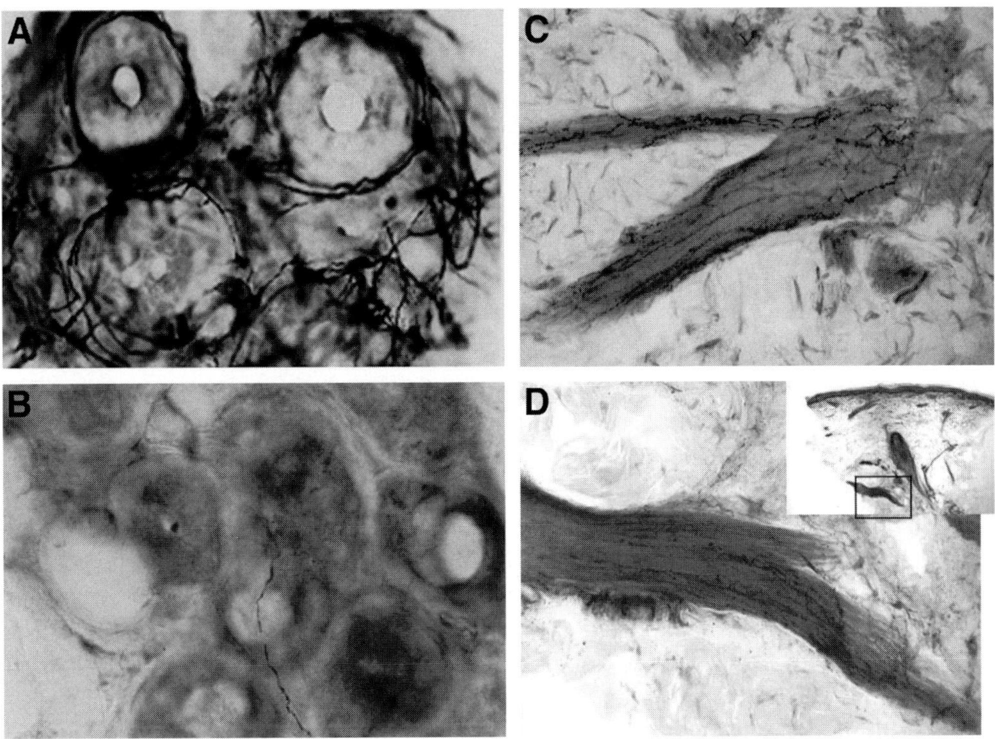

Fig. 1. Example of innervation of dermal appendages. Examples of dermal appendages stained with PGP 9.5. **(A)** Sweat gland from a normal control that is robustly innervated. **(B)** Denervated sweat gland, as evidenced by the relative paucity of PGP 9.5 staining. **(C)** Example of a normally innervated arrector pili muscle. **(D)** Example of a denervated arrector pili muscle from a distal leg biopsy in a patient with small fiber neuropathy. From ref. *43*.

generally heal through a process of granulation without a need for cautery of suturing. Selection of the biopsy site depends on the clinician's intent. If the intent is to diagnose small fiber neuropathy, the availability of normative data is important. These data are available for several locations in the lower extremity by different processing techniques and to a lesser extent in the arm *(7,8)*. Areas of trauma or where scar formation is present should be avoided as these can artificially lower epidermal nerve fiber densities. In general, a distal location where there are abnormalities on examination, particularly decreased sensibility to pin prick or thermal sensation, or where the patient has symptoms is best. Biopsies from the dorsum of the foot, distal, or proximal calf often have reduced nerve fiber densities or are denervated altogether in patients with neuropathy. In our experience, sites within the foot are prone to trauma and this can limit interpretation of the biopsy. In addition, sites within the foot are more prone to infection and for these reasons the distal leg for a caudal biopsy site is prefered. Additional biopsies from more proximal locations can provide additional information allowing the severity of the nerve fiber loss to be assessed as well as providing an internal control. If the intent of the biopsy is to follow a patient longitudinally for neuropathy progression or to monitor a treatment effect, the site chosen should have proximity to the symptomatic area, but should retain enough innervation to provide a substrate for nerve regeneration or

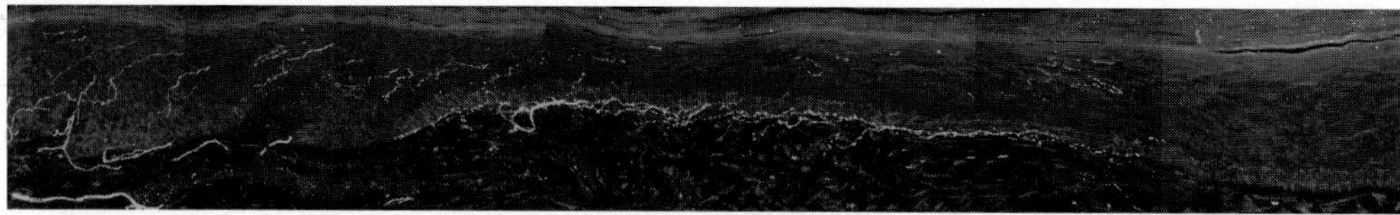

Fig. 2. Example of crush. **Panel C** shows an entire skin section at low magnification. The crushed region appears pale and has reduced PGP 9.5 staining. **Panels A** and **B** show region without **(A)** and with **(B)** crush artifact. Arrows indicate epidermal nerve fibers.

allow documentation of further degeneration. Future biopsies should be performed adjacent to the original biopsy at a distance of 5–10 mm. One distinct advantage of the technique is that nearly any site can be assessed in contrast to electrophysiology where testing is limited to specific nerves at specified sites. In patients being evaluated for asymmetric, focal symptoms in sites where normative data are not available, biopsies can be performed bilaterally using the asymptomatic site as an internal control.

Two biopsy techniques have been described: punch skin biopsy and skin blister formation *(14)*. Punch biopsy is the most widely used and is performed with a 3-mm diameter circular biopsy instrument. Generally biopsies are performed to a depth of 2–3 mm. This facilitates the removal of the tissue plug and allows innervation of dermal appendages to be assessed. If one is interested only in epidermal innervation it is possible to perform a shallower biopsy. It is crucial to avoid crushing or pinching the biopsy tissue, which can produce artifact resembling denervation (Fig. 2). An alternative biopsy procedure is achieved by application of 300 mmHg negative pressure to a 3 mm blister capsule. This approach has the advantage of being less invasive though blister formation is dependent on maintenance of a tight seal for 20–40 minutes. Application of a heating pad can reduce the time needed and is necessary to achieve blister formation in younger subjects. Blisters are removed with microscissors or superficial skin punches and processed as whole mounts. Both forms of biopsy tissue are immediately placed into refrigerated fixative solution for 12–18 hours at 4°C. Zamboni (2% paraformaldehyde, picric acid), Lana (4% formaldehyde, picric acid), and PLP (paraformaldehyde, lysine, periodate) fixatives all preserve antigenic integrity and are routinely used. If these fixatives are not available, an acceptable alternative is 10% formalin; however this produces a more fragmented appearance of the epidermal nerves and is suboptimal. Glutaraldehyde destroys the antigens and should not be used. Following fixation, the biopsy tissue is transferred to 20% sucrose in phosphate buffered saline cryoprotectant where it can remain for up to 1 month at 4°C or frozen for longer periods. In multicenter trials, or in instances where biopsies need to be sent to a processing center, they should be shipped after fixation and in cryoprotectant overnight on wet ice.

Two similar protocols for processing and imaging fixed biopsy tissue have emerged *(15,16)*. Frozen 50–100 μ*M* skin sections are cut perpendicular to the skin surface. Sections are immunohistochemically stained as free floating sections in reagents containing the detergent Triton-X-100. The free floating technique and use of a detergent are critical to achieve antibody penetration into the thick sections. After blocking, sections are incubated with a primary anti-PGP 9.5 antibody overnight. After washing, sections are incubated with a secondary antibody directed against the Fc region of the primary

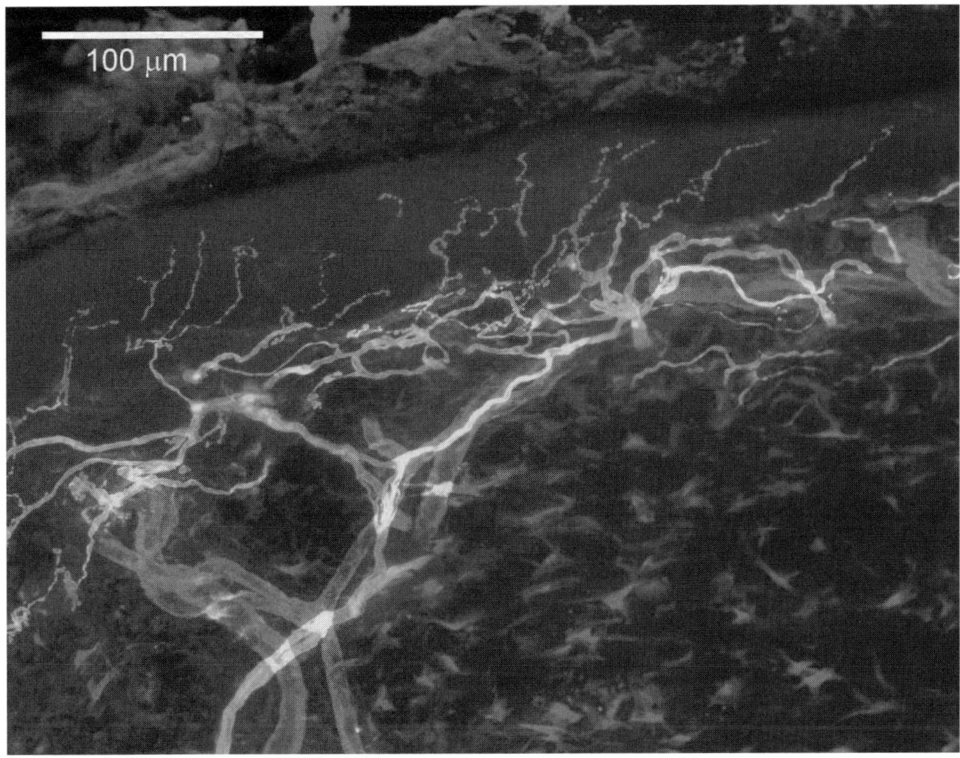

Fig. 3. Normal human epidermal and dermal innervation visualized with confocal microscopy. Nerves are localized with antibody to PGP 9.5 and basement membrane is demarcated with antibody to type IV collagen. Vasculature is labeled with Ulex europaeus agglutinin type I. Epidermal nerve fibers appear aqua and lie within the blue epidermis. The subepidermal neural plexus appears green or yellow. The dermal epidermal junction appears as a red ribbon. Capillaries appear magenta. Nerve fibers (green and aqua) course in bundles through the dermis and branch in the papillary dermis to form the subepidermal neural plexus. Fibers arise from this plexus and penetrate the epidermal basement membrane to enter the epidermis. Some non-neuronal fibroblasts appear green as a result of nonspecific PGP9.5 binding. Figure courtesy of William Kennedy and Gwen Wendelschafer-Crabb.

antibody species (e.g., goat antirabbit secondary with rabbit anti-PGP 9.5 primary antibody). If the sections are imaged using confocal microscopy, the secondary antibody must be labeled with a stable fluorescent marker, whereas imaging by light microscopy uses a peroxidase labeled secondary. Multiple individual sections from each biopsy should be stained in order to address concerns of sampling error. Confocal imaging has the advantage that multiple targets can be visualized simultaneously provided secondary antibodies with different fluorochromes are used. Different imaging planes or stacks can be compressed allowing innervation occurring within three dimensions to be viewed in two dimensions. These images are particularly convenient for publication and can facilitate quantification of epidermal nerves though it is possible that overlapping nerve fibers at different depths will be mistakenly viewed as a single fiber once the perspective of the tissue depth is removed (*see* Fig. 3). The time and expense required to produce such images make such an approach less practical in the setting of clinical trials or longitudinal studies, where large numbers of samples need to be processed quickly. Light microscopy-based techniques are better suited toward such applications where the focus is on determining epidermal nerve fiber densities for which only a signal antigenic determinant is stained (Fig. 4). Recently developed software programs such as Helicon Focus allow multiple light microscopy focal planes to be compressed into a single image—in effect producing a "poor man's" compressed confocal z series.

Most attention has been directed toward staining nerve fibers with antibody directed against PGP 9.5 though other markers have been identified that stain all epidermal nerve fibers such as TuJ1 *(17)*, Gα0 *(18)*, and TRPV1 *(19)*. Specialized stains have also demonstrated IgM deposits in dermal nerve fibers from glabrous skin biopsies in patients with anti-myelin associated glycoprotein (MAG) neuropathy. This suggests that skin biopsies may also be used to assess demyelinating conditions. Interestingly, the deposits of IgM were greatest in the most distal skin biopsies correlating with the electrophysiological hallmark of prolongation of distal motor latencies in anti-MAG neuropathy. Analysis of skin biopsy samples from patients with inherited demyelinating conditions also reproduced the observations from sural nerve biopsies suggesting that skin biopsies will be helpful in the study of these patients as well. Myelinated nerve fibers from skin biopsies have not yet been studied systematically in patients with diabetes.

CORRELATION BETWEEN EPIDERMAL NERVE AND SURAL NERVE

Twenty six patients with neuropathic complaints had sural nerve morphometry and determination of epidermal nerve fiber density at the distal part of the leg *(20)*. The intraepidermal nerve fiber (IENF) density correlated with the densities of total myelinated fibers within the sural nerve ($r = 0.57$, $p = 0.0011$), small myelinated ($r = 0.53$, $p = 0.029$), and large myelinated fibers ($r = 0.49$, $p = 0.0054$). There was a trend toward an association between intraepidermal nerve fiber density and sural nerve unmyelinated nerve fiber densities ($r = 0.32$, $p = 0.054$). Sensory nerve action potential amplitudes and large myelinated nerve fiber densities were highly correlated ($r = 0.87$, $p < 0.0001$). Intraepidermal nerve fiber density and sural nerve small fiber measures were concordant in 73% of patients. In 23% of cases, reduced intraepidermal nerve fiber density was the only indicator of small fiber depletion. An editorial in Neurology suggested that determination of distal leg intraepidermal nerve fiber density may be more sensitive than sural nerve biopsy in identifying small fiber sensory neuropathies *(21)*.

Measurement of cutaneous innervation has proven to be particularly useful in the study of diabetic neuropathy. Abnormalities in epidermal innervation have been demonstrated to be more sensitive for the diagnosis of diabetic neuropathy than clinical or electrophysiological methods. Several investigators have demonstrated that dermal PGP immunoreactivity was reduced in subjects with diabetes testing normal on clinical examination, electrophysiology, and quantitative sensory testing (QST) when compared with healthy control subjects *(22)*. This likely reflects the observation that small unmyelinated nerve fibers are vulnerable early in diabetes *(23)*. Evaluation of epidermal nerve fibers (ENFs) appear to be even more sensitive, perhaps because of their further distance from the cell body, absence of a Schwann cell or collagen covering sheath, and the avascular nature of the epidermis that increase their susceptibility to disease. Kennedy demonstrated that subjects with diabetes had reduced innervation densities and nerve fiber lengths with many

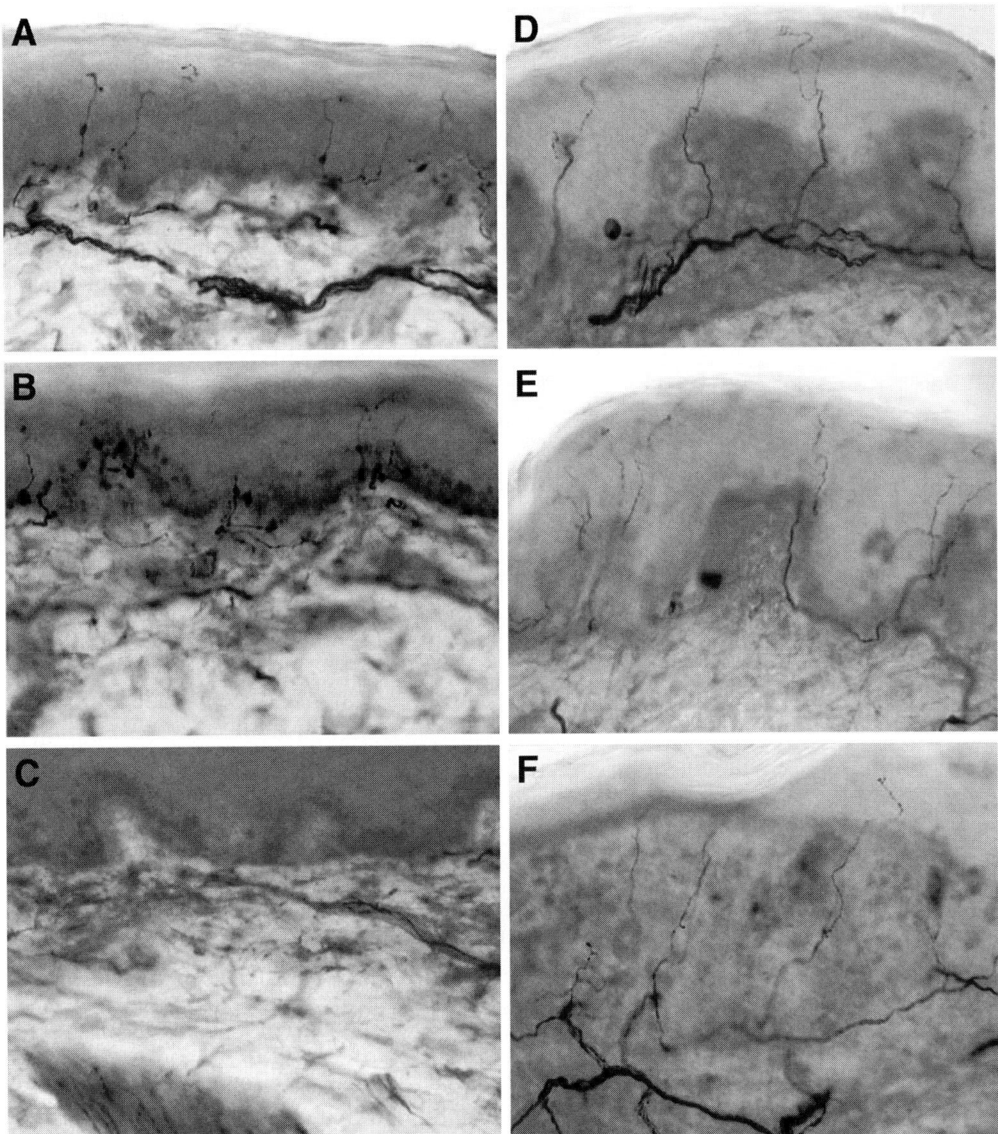

Fig. 4. Example of neuropathy diagnosis by skin biopsy. Representative skin biopsy sections from a diabetic individual with small fiber sensory neuropathy (**panels A–C**) and comparable biopsy sections from a normal control subject (**panels D–F**). **Panels A** and **D** are skin sections from the proximal thigh; B and E from the distal thigh; C and F from the distal leg. The epidermal nerve fiber densities from both proximal thigh sites are within a normal range, although the section from the diabetic patient (**panel A**) contains several small swellings. At the distal thigh site (**panels B** and **E**), the ENF densities are again within a normal range, though the morphological abnormalities such as nerve fiber swellings are more prominent in the **panel B**. In **panel C**, the epidermis is completely denervated, while the skin section form the normal control subject (**panel F**) has a normal ENF density. The bottom of **panel C** contains an arrector pili muscle fragment that is well innervated which may suggest a relative sparing of large fiber function. From ref. *43*.

subjects being completely denervated *(12)*. Changes in fiber morphology such as increased branching patterns or the presence of swellings are also noted to be present in subjects with diabetes and may represent degenerative changes *(24,25)*. Increased numbers of large axonal swellings predict the degeneration of epidermal nerve fibers and progression of neuropathy in diabetes as well as other forms of neuropathy *(26)*. Nerve fiber swellings stained positively for PGP and tubulin and less prominently for neurofilament markers, suggesting that tubules are the main component of epidermal nerve fiber (ENF) cytoskeleton and that they accumulate with ubiquitin-associated proteins within swellings *(26)*. IENF density has been shown to be inversely related to diabetes duration in people with type 2 diabetes, but not to HbA1C levels *(27)*. The latter might represent an effect of historical glycemic control or "metabolic memory" as has been demonstrated for other diabetes end organ complications *(28)*.

Many patients with idiopathic small fiber predominant neuropathy symptoms have been found to have either occult diabetes or impaired glucose tolerance after rigorous assessment with an oral glucose tolerance test *(29,30)*. The diagnosis of diabetes was missed in these patients because of the inappropriate use of glycated hemoglobin as a screening test for diabetes. Using fasting 75 g oral glucose tolerance testing (OGTT), nearly 60% of patients were found to have diabetes or impaired glucose tolerance (IGT) *(31)*. It is possible, but unlikely that the association between neuropathy and abnormalities on OGTT represents a spurious overlap of two common conditions, as the prevalence of IGT in the neuropathy populations was two- to threefold more than what would have been predicted by the National Health and Nutrition Examination Study (NHANES) study. Furthermore, there was a dose response relationship between the pathological and electrophysiological severity of neuropathy and the degree of hyperglycemia *(31)*. In this study, the IENF density was the most sensitive measure of neuropathy and was abnormally low compared with control subjects in both subjects with diabetes and IGT. This observation is consistent with the clinical impression that patients with idiopathic small fiber neuropathy are indistinguishable to those with early diabetic neuropathy. Longitudinal follow-up of subjects with IGT-associated or de-novo diabetes associated neuropathy suggest that the rate of neuropathy progression is slower in those with IGT-associated neuropathy compared with *de novo* diabetes (Mammen, Polydefkis, unpublished).

A subsequent study that investigated factors associated with neuropathy among 50 idiopathic neuropathy patients and controls concluded that triglyceride levels and not hyperglycemia was the strongest predictor of neuropathy irrespective of pain *(32)*. Together, these results suggest that it may be a combination of diabetic risk factors, perhaps even the metabolic syndrome that are responsible for neuropathy in these patients *(33)*. Impaired glucose tolerance is a potentially reversible entity with diet and exercise having been demonstrated to slow or prevent progression to diabetes *(34)*. Based on these studies, patients with IGT-associated neuropathy are routinely advised to adopt a diet and exercise regimen. Many patients who have succeeded in doing so have also reported improvements in their neuropathic pain. Weight loss and exercise can have dramatic effects on an individual's sense of well-being and pain perception. It remains unclear whether these patients' reductions in neuropathic pain are related to improvements in nerve function or the constitutional effects of exercise and weight loss.

EPIDERMAL INNERVATION IN CLINICAL TRIALS

Skin biopsy with determination of epidermal nerve fiber density lends itself to application as an outcome measure in regenerative and longitudinal studies. The technique offers the advantage over NCVs that it focuses on a larger subset of nerve fibers than nerve conduction testing and unmyelinated nerve fibers appear to be a more sensitive measure of neuropathy than large myelinated nerve fibers. Several small studies have used serial skin biopsies as an outcome measure. In a trial of recombinant human nerve growth factor (NFG) in HIV-sensory neuropathy, 62 of 270 patients who participated in the trial were included in a substudy examining the density of intraepidermal nerve fibers. Fiber density was inversely correlated with neuropathic pain as measured both by patient and physician global pain assessments *(10)*. The intrasubject reproducibility of the technique, as assessed from correlation between baseline and the week 18 densities was 81% in the distal part of the leg, and 77% in the upper thigh. Although decreased intraepidermal nerve fiber density at the distal leg was associated with lower CD4 counts and higher plasma HIV RNA levels, there was no treatment effect in the relatively short period of 18 weeks *(35)*. The reproducibility of the technique was good in this study and suggests that it could be incorporated in future trials of regenerative agents for sensory neuropathies. An open-label pilot study of acetyl-L-carnitine in patients with antiretroviral toxic neuropathy associated with HIV treatment demonstrated a significant increase in immunoreactivity for PGP9.5 as well as other specific fiber type neurotransmitters. This provocative study used unconventional measures of epidermal innervation and a larger controlled study is currently underway *(36)*. In a small, 18 week open label trial of topiramate in people with moderate diabetic neuropathy, Vinik et al. reported that treatment was associated with improvements in epidermal nerve fiber density and length *(37)*. Enhanced nerve fiber length was observed at all tested sites including the forearm although increases in ENF density were seen only at the proximal leg site. Although further analyses need to be performed, this finding suggests that nerve fiber length may be a useful adjunct measure. There is relatively little longitudinal data using skin biopsy in people with diabetes. Several small series suggest that at the distal thigh, the ENF density declines at a rate of about 1 fiber/mm per year. This combined with the observation that ENF density is correlated with heat pain threshold after adjusting for diabetes duration, age, and gender *(27)* suggest that a change of 2–3 fibers/mm may represent a clinically meaningful change.

Epidermal nerve fibers offer an additional advantage that they can be easily and repeatedly sampled over time. Their superficial nature also allows them to be injured in a standardized fashion and recovery from such nerve injuries have been used as a measure of nerve fiber regeneration. Several models based on such an approach have been developed to measure collateral *(38)* and regenerative *(18)* sprouting in human subjects. Reinnervation of the epidermis following removal of a 3 mm diameter cylindrical tissue plug allows collateral sprouting to be efficiently measured. Following removal of a conventional 3 mm skin biopsy, the site heals by a process of granulation and eventually becomes re-epithelialized. The collagen plug within the dermis of the healing biopsy site acts as a barrier to the distal ends of the transected nerves. Therefore, reinnervation of the epidermis within the original 3 mm biopsy site can only occur through sprouting of uninjured fibers peripheral to the incision line (Figs. 5 and 6). The degree of collateral

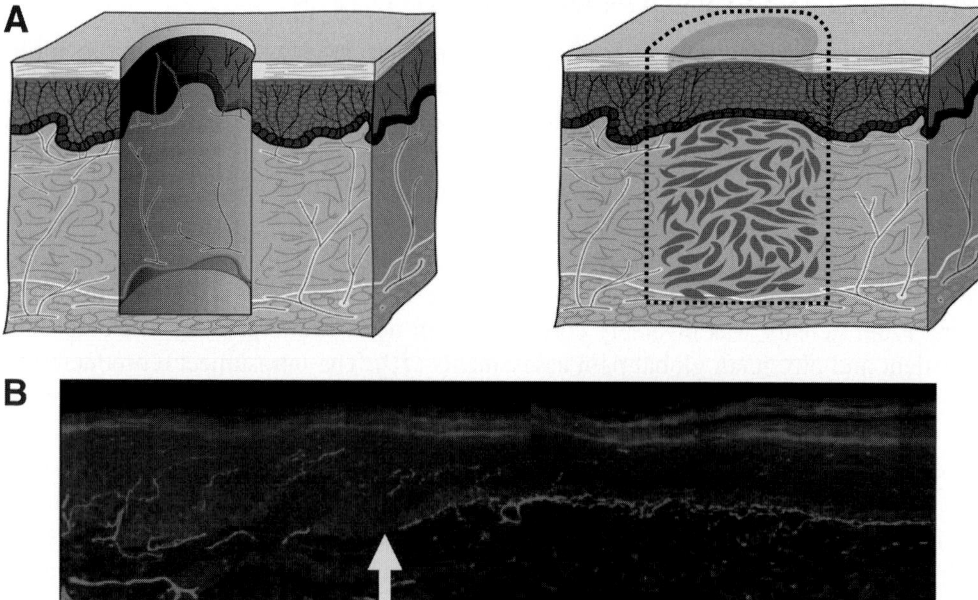

Fig. 5. (A) Method to measure collateral sprouting of human epidermal nerve fibers. Following removal of a standard 3 mm biopsy tissue plug (left frame), the site heals by a process of granulation (right frame). Nerve fibers within the dermis are not able to penetrate the collagen scar that forms in the healed biopsy site. The only mechanism for the re-epithelialized epidermis to become reinnervated is for fibers to sprout from the epidermis peripheral to the healed 3 mm incision line into denervated central zone. This collateral sprouting can be assessed by taking a larger concentric biopsy centered on the healed, original 3 mm biopsy site (dotted line, right panel). **(B)** Example of collateral sprouting. The yellow arrow indicated the location of the original 3 mm biopsy incision. Epidermal nerve fibers peripheral to the incision line grow into the central denervated epidermis by a process of collateral sprouting. These sprouts frequently grow along the epidermal side of the dermal-epidermal junction adjacent to the basal keratinocytes which are known to be a source of neurotrophin production. Adapted from ref. *38*.

sprouting can be measured by a concentric 4 or 5 mm biopsy centered on the healed 3 mm biopsy site (Fig. 5). Although detailed time course experiments have not been published in people with diabetes, preliminary evidence suggests that collateral sprouting is reduced in neuropathic states such as diabetes and HIV infection *(39)*.

Regenerative sprouting has been systematically measured following a "chemical axotomy" produced by topical capsaicin *(18)*. Application of capsaicin either topically as a cream or injected into the epidermis has been shown to produce a superficial denervation of the skin *(40,41)*. When applied topically in an occlusive bandage, capsaicin produces a standardized injury that is reproducible and well-tolerated (Fig. 6) *(18)*. Studies in healthy control subjects and people with diabetes have demonstrated that functional abnormalities in regenerative sprouting are present among subjects with diabetes with no signs or symptoms of neuropathy (Fig. 7). This observation suggests that nerve is affected early in the course of diabetes and that regenerative abnormalities may be the earliest sign of nerve dysfunction. It could be speculated that an abnormality in nerve

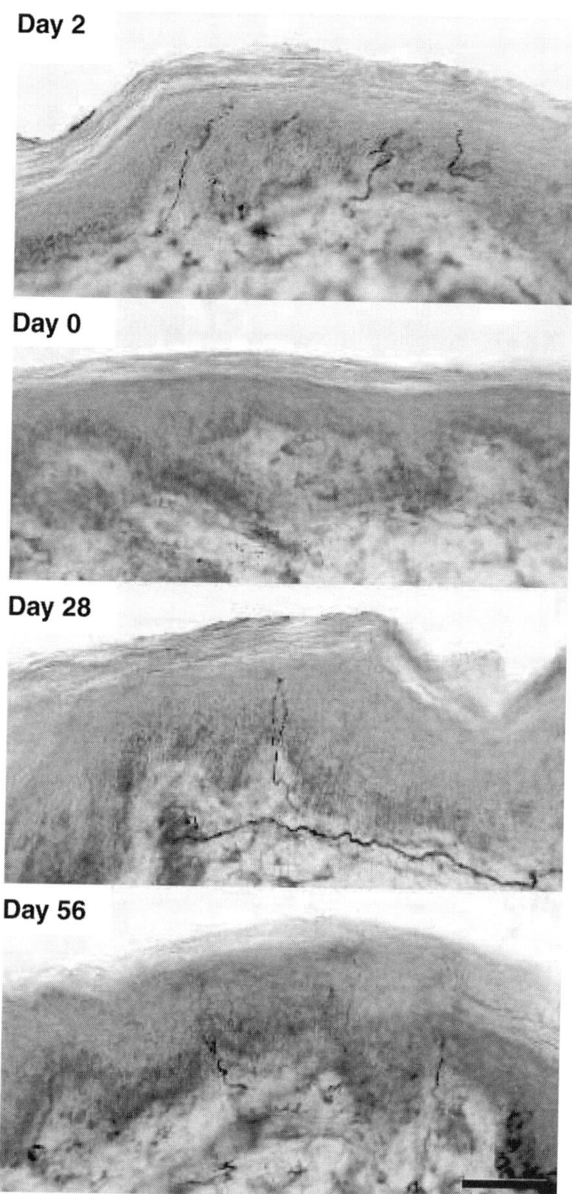

Fig. 6. Representative skin biopsy sections demonstrating that topical capsaicin application produces a superficial denervation. The epidermis becomes reinnervated over several months. The day -2 biopsy depicts normal epidermal innervation at baseline. Following capsaicin treatment (day 0), there is complete denervation of the epidermis and subepidermal dermis. Biopsies at 28 and 56 days demonstrate reinnervation of the epidermis. Recovery of ENF density has been correlated with heat pain. From ref. *44*.

regeneration is followed by development of swellings that are in turn followed by development of neuropathy. Correction of subclinical abnormalities in regeneration as an outcome measure has several attractive features. First, it would allow recruitment of a non-neuropathic population of people with diabetes. This will simplify trial designs and

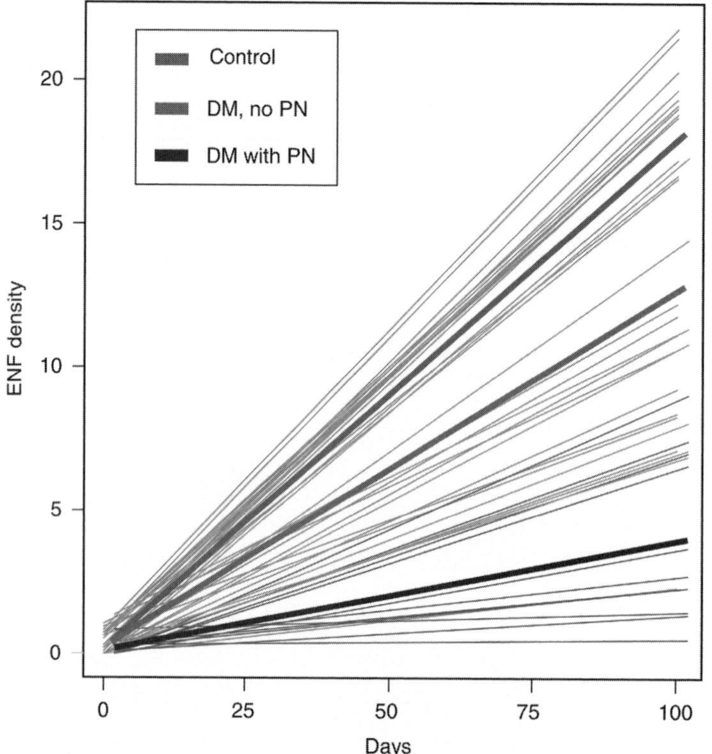

Fig. 7. For each subject, a regression line from postcapsaicin time-points is generated and the slope of this line is used as the rate of regeneration. The mean line for each group is shown as a thick solid line. The rate of regeneration following denervation is 0.177 ± 0.075 fibers per mm/day for control subjects (red), 0.10 ± 0.07 fibers per mm/day ($p = 0.03$) for subjects with diabetes but no neuropathy (green), and 0.04 ± 0.03 fibers per mm/day ($p = 0.03$) for subjects with diabetes and neuropathy (blue).

facilitate the recruitment of homogeneous study subject populations. Second, correction or partial correction of abnormalities in regeneration is a concrete target with a clear clinical interpretation. Furthermore, an improvement in the regeneration rate will precede an improvement in nerve fiber density and is likely to be a more sensitive measure. Finally, such a study designed to detect a 50% normalization of regeneration with 80% power in nonneuropathic subjects with diabetes would require about 65 subjects per treatment arm. A recent trial of Timcodar dimesylate in healthy control subjects used such measures of collateral and regenerative sprouting as outcome measures. Although the compound did not accelerate regeneration by either measure, the trial did demonstrate that such an approach was feasible and the measures were reproducible and robust *(42)*.

In conclusion, skin biopsy with determination of epidermal nerve fiber density is a powerful tool that provides investigators insight into a population of nerve fibers that is prominently affected in diabetes and yet has been relatively under investigated. The superficial nature of epidermal nerve fibers allows repeated sampling of these nerves in a relatively non invasive fashion, and in sites that cannot be assessed through conventional electrodiagnostical techniques. These features have allowed investigators to diagnose neuropathy earlier and to define an association between neuropathy and impaired glucose tolerance. Finally, the ability to injure these fibers in a standardized fashion has led to novel measures of human axonal regeneration that may provide a more sensitive scale by which to assess promising regenerative compounds.

REFERENCES

1. Bolton CF, Winkelmann RK, Dyck PJ. A quantitative study of Meissner's corpuscles in man. *Neurology* 1966;16(1):1–9.
2. Dyck PJ, Winkelmann RK, Bolton CF. Quantitation of Meissner's corpuscles in hereditary neurologic disorders. Charcot-Marie-Tooth disease, Roussy-Levy syndrome, Dejerine-Sottas disease, hereditary sensory neuropathy, spinocerebellar degenerations, and hereditary spastic paraplegia. *Neurology* 1966;16(1):7–10.
3. Dalsgaard CJ, Rydh M, Haegerstrand A. Cutaneous innervation in man visualized with protein gene product 9.5 (PGP 9.5) antibodies. *Histochemistry* 1989;92(5):385–390.
4. Kennedy WR, Wendelschafer-Crabb G, Brelje TC. Innervation and vasculature of human sweat glands: an immunohistochemistry-laser scanning confocal fluorescence microscopy study. *J Neurosci* 1994;14(11 Pt 2):6825–6833.
5. Nolano M, Provitera V, Crisci C, et al. Quantification of myelinated endings and mechanoreceptors in human digital skin. *Ann Neurol* 2003;54(2):197–205.
6. Lombardi R, Erne B, Lauria G, et al. IgM deposits on skin nerves in anti-myelin-associated glycoprotein neuropathy. *Ann Neurol* 2005;57(2):180–187.
7. McArthur JC, Stocks EA, Hauer P, Cornblath DR, Griffin JW. Epidermal nerve fiber density:normative reference range and diagnostic efficiency. *Arch Neurol* 1998;55(12): 1513–1520.
8. Kennedy WR, Wendelschafer-Crabb G, Polydefkis M, McArthur JC. Pathology and quantitation of cutaneous innervation, in *Peripheral Neuropathy.* (Dyck PJ, Thomas PK, eds.) Elsevier Saunders, Philadelphia, 2005, pp. 869–897.
9. Holland NR, Stocks A, Hauer P, Cornblath DR, Griffin JW, McArthur JC. Intraepidermal nerve fiber density in patients with painful sensory neuropathy. *Neurology* 1997;48(3):708–711.
10. Polydefkis M, Yiannoutsos C, Cohen B, et al. Reduced intraepidermal nerve fiber density in HIV-associated sensory neuropathy. *Neurology* 2002; in press.
11. Rowbotham MC, Yosipovitch G, Connolly MK, Finlay D, Forde G, Fields HL. Cutaneous innervation density in the allodynic form of postherpetic neuralgia. *Neurobiol Dis* 1996;3(3):205–214.
12. Kennedy WR, Wendelschafer-Crabb G, Johnson T. Quantitation of epidermal nerves in diabetic neuropathy. *Neurology* 1996;47(4):1042–1048.
13. Silos-Santiago I, Molliver DC, Ozaki S, et al. Non-TrkA-expressing small DRG neurons are lost in TrkA deficient mice. *J Neurosci* 1995;15(9):5929–5942.
14. Kennedy WR, Nolano M, Wendelschafer-Crabb G, Johnson TL, Tamura E. A skin blister method to study epidermal nerves in peripheral nerve disease. *Muscle Nerve* 1999;22(3):360–371.
15. Kennedy WR, Wendelschafer-Crabb G. The innervation of human epidermis. *J Neurol Sci* 1993;115(2):184–190.
16. McCarthy BG, Hsieh ST, Stocks A, et al. Cutaneous innervation in sensory neuropathies: evaluation by skin biopsy. *Neurology* 1995;45(10):1848–1855.
17. Lauria G, Borgna M, Morbin M, et al. Tubule and neurofilament immunoreactivity in human hairy skin: markers for intraepidermal nerve fibers. *Muscle Nerve* 2004;30(3): 310–316.

18. Polydefkis M, Hauer P, Sheth S, Sirdofsky M, Griffin JW, McArthur JC. The time course of epidermal nerve fibre regeneration: studies in normal controls and in people with diabetes, with and without neuropathy. *Brain* 2004;127(Pt 7):1606–1615.
19. Lauria G, Morbin M, Borgna M, et al. Vanilloid receptor (VR1) expression in human peripheral nervous system. *J Periph Nerv Sys* 2003;8(S1):1–78.
20. Herrmann DN, Griffin JW, Hauer P, Cornblath DR, McArthur JC. Epidermal nerve fiber density and sural nerve morphometry in peripheral neuropathies. *Neurology* 1999;53(8): 1634–1640.
21. Kennedy WR, Said G. Sensory nerves in skin: answers about painful feet? *Neurology* 1999;53(8):1614–1615.
22. Levy DM, Terenghi G, Gu XH, Abraham RR, Springall DR, Polak JM. Immunohistochemical measurements of nerves and neuropeptides in diabetic skin: relationship to tests of neurological function. *Diabetologia* 1992;35(9):889–897.
23. Brown MJ, Martin JR, Asbury AK. Painful diabetic neuropathy. A morphometric study. *Arch Neurol* 1976;33(3):164–171.
24. Hsieh ST, Chiang HY, Lin WM. Pathology of nerve terminal degeneration in the skin. *J Neuropathol Exp Neurol* 2000;59(4):297–307.
25. Pan CL, Tseng TJ, Lin YH, Chiang MC, Lin WM, Hsieh ST. Cutaneous innervation in Guillain-Barre syndrome: pathology and clinical correlations. *Brain* 2003;126(Pt 2): 386–397.
26. Lauria G, Morbin M, Lombardi R, et al. Axonal swellings predict the degeneration of epidermal nerve fibers in painful neuropathies. *Neurology* 2003;61(5):631–636.
27. Shun CT, Chang YC, Wu HP, et al. Skin denervation in type 2 diabetes: correlations with diabetic duration and functional impairments. *Brain* 2004;127(Pt 7):1593–1605.
28. Sustained effect of intensive treatment of type 1 diabetes mellitus on development and progression of diabetic nephropathy:the Epidemiology of Diabetes Interventions and Complications (EDIC) study. *Jama* 2003;290(16):2159–2167.
29. Singleton JR, Smith AG, Bromberg MB. Increased prevalence of impaired glucose tolerance in patients with painful sensory neuropathy. *Diabetes Care* 2001;24(8): 1448–1453.
30. Singleton JR, Smith AG, Bromberg MB. Painful sensory polyneuropathy associated with impaired glucose tolerance. *Muscle Nerve* 2001;24(9):1225–1228.
31. Sumner CJ, Sheth S, Griffin JW, Cornblath DR, Polydefkis M. The spectrum of neuropathy in diabetes and impaired glucose tolerance. *Neurology* 2003;60(1):108–111.
32. Hughes RA, Umapathi T, Gray IA, et al. A controlled investigation of the cause of chronic idiopathic axonal polyneuropathy. *Brain* 2004;127(Pt 8):1723–1730.
33. Smith AG, Singleton JR. Peripheral neuropathy and the metabolic syndrome. *Annals of Neurology* 2005;58(S9):S31.
34. Knowler WC, Barrett-Connor E, Fowler SE, et al. Reduction in the incidence of type 2 diabetes with lifestyle intervention or metformin. *N Engl J Med* 2002;346(6):393–403.
35. McArthur JC, Yiannoutsos C, Simpson DM, et al. A phase II trial of nerve growth factor for sensory neuropathy associated with HIV infection. AIDS Clinical Trials Group Team 291. *Neurology* 2000;54(5):1080–1088.
36. Hart AM, Wilson AD, Montovani C, et al. Acetyl-l-carnitine: a pathogenesis based treatment for HIV-associated antiretroviral toxic neuropathy. *Aids* 2004;18(11):1549-1560.
37. Pittenger GL, Simmons K, Anandacoomaraswamy D, Rice A, Barlow P, Vinik A. Topiramate improves intraepidermal nerve fiber morphology and quantitative measures in diabetic neuropathy patients. *J Periph Nerv Sys* 2005;10(S1):73.
38. Rajan B, Polydefkis M, Hauer P, Griffin JW, McArthur JC. Epidermal reinnervation after intracutaneous axotomy in man. *J Comp Neurol* 2003;457(1):24–36.

39. Hahn K, Brown A, Hauer P, McArthur J, Polydefkis M. Epidermal reinnervation after mechanical intracutanous axotomy in skin biopsies in normal controls and in people with HIV. *Neurology* 2005;64(6 S1):A245–A246.
40. Simone DA, Nolano M, Johnson T, Wendelschafer-Crabb G, Kennedy WR. Intradermal injection of capsaicin in humans produces degeneration and subsequent reinnervation of epidermal nerve fibers: correlation with sensory function. *J Neurosci* 1998;18(21): 8947–8959.
41. Nolano M, Simone DA, Wendelschafer-Crabb G, Johnson T, Hazen E, Kennedy WR. Topical capsaicin in humans: parallel loss of epidermal nerve fibers and pain sensation. *Pain* 1999;81(1–2):135–145.
42. Polydefkis M, Sirdofsky M, Hauer P, Petty BG, Murinson BB, McArthur JC. Factors influencing nerve regeneration in a trial of Timcodar dimesylate. *Neurology* 2006; 66(2):259–261.
43. Polydefkis M, Hauer P, Griffin JW, McArthur JC. Skin biopsy as a tool to assess distal small fiber innervation in diabetic neuropathy. *Diabetes Technol Ther* 2001;3:23–28.
44. Polydefkis M, Griffin JW, McArthur J. New insights into diabetic polyneuropathy. *JAMA* 2003;290:1371–1376.

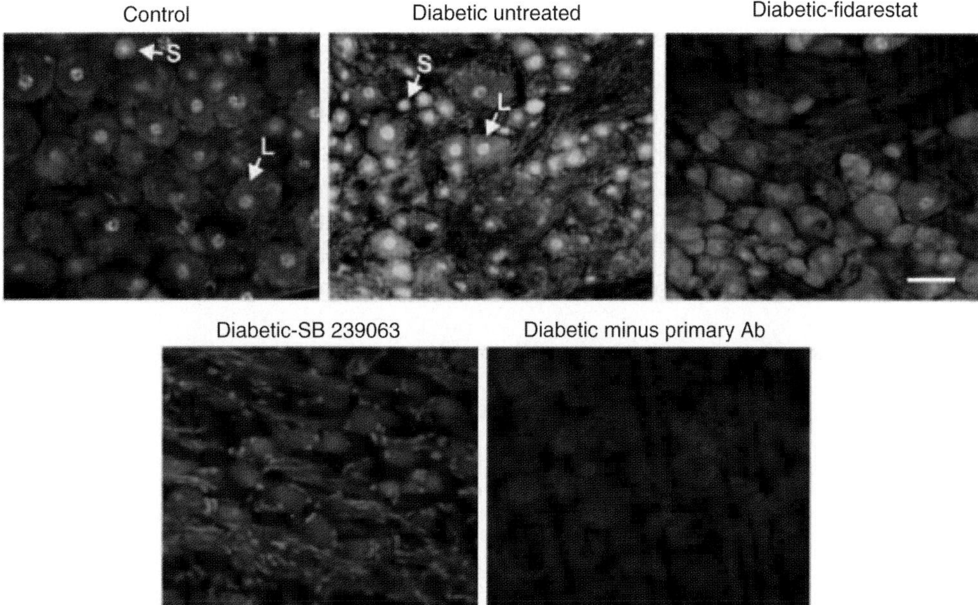

Color Plate 1. Bar charts and Western blots showing the effects of insulin, fidarestat and the p38 mitogen-activated protein kinases inhibitor, SB239063. (Fig. 5, Chapter 6; *see* complete caption on p. 103.)

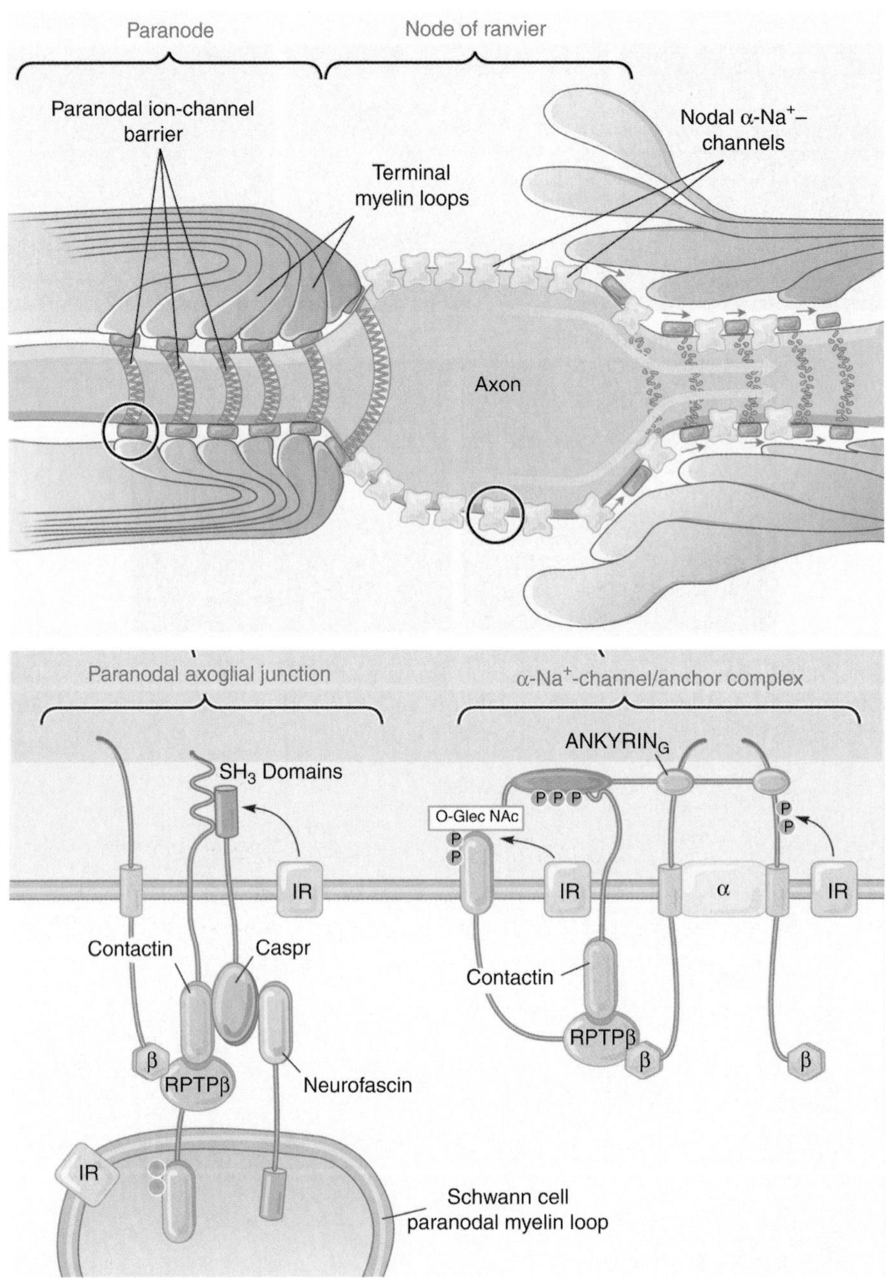

Color Plate 2. Axoglial dysjunction is a characteristic degenerative change of type 1 DPN. (Fig. 5, Chapter 8; *see* complete caption on p. 142.)

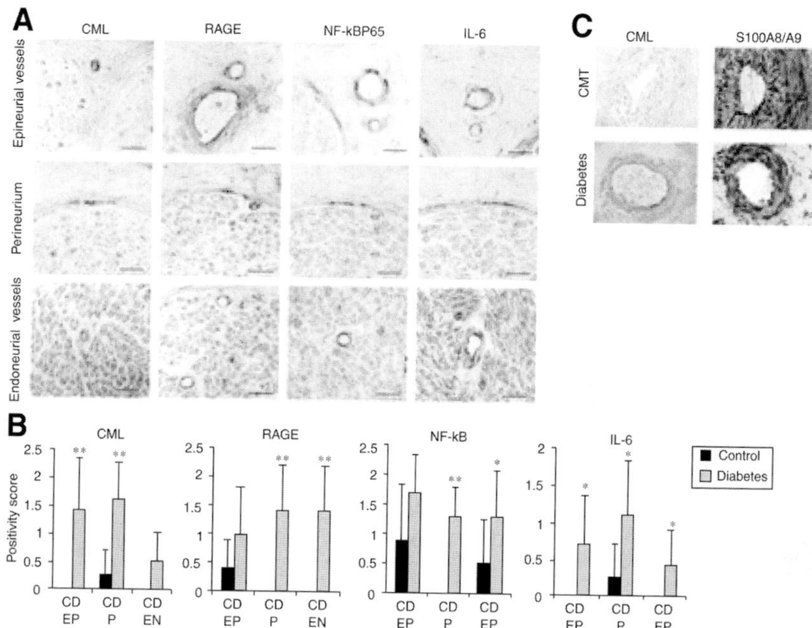

Color Plate 3. **(A)** Localization of CML. **(B)** Quantification of staining intensities of epineurial vessels, perineurium, and endoneurial vessels. **(C)** Comparison of the staining intensity for CML and the receptor for advanced glycation end products. (Fig. 2, Chapter 13; *see* complete caption on p. 234.)

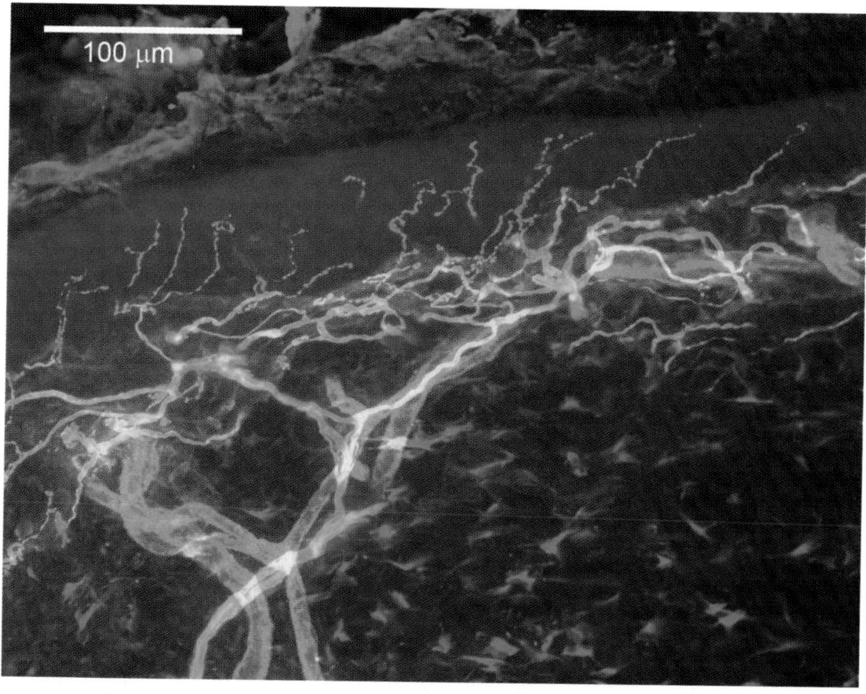

Color Plate 4. Normal human epidermal and dermal innervation visualized with confocal microscopy. (Fig. 3, Chapter 17; *see* complete caption on p. 297.)

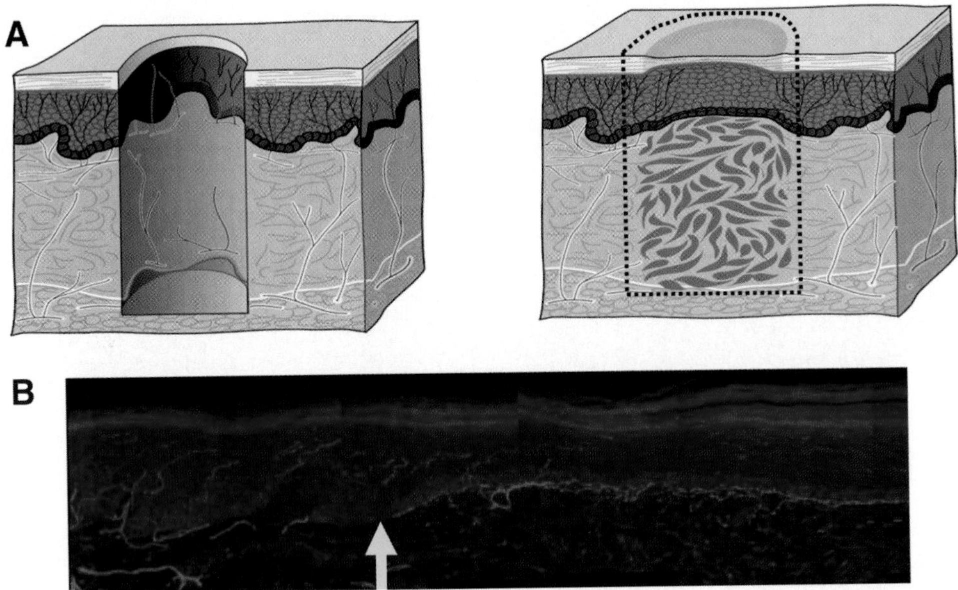

Color Plate 5. (A) Method to measure collateral sprouting of human epidermal nerve fibers. **(B)** Example of collateral sprouting. (Fig. 5, Chapter 17; *see* complete caption on p. 302.)

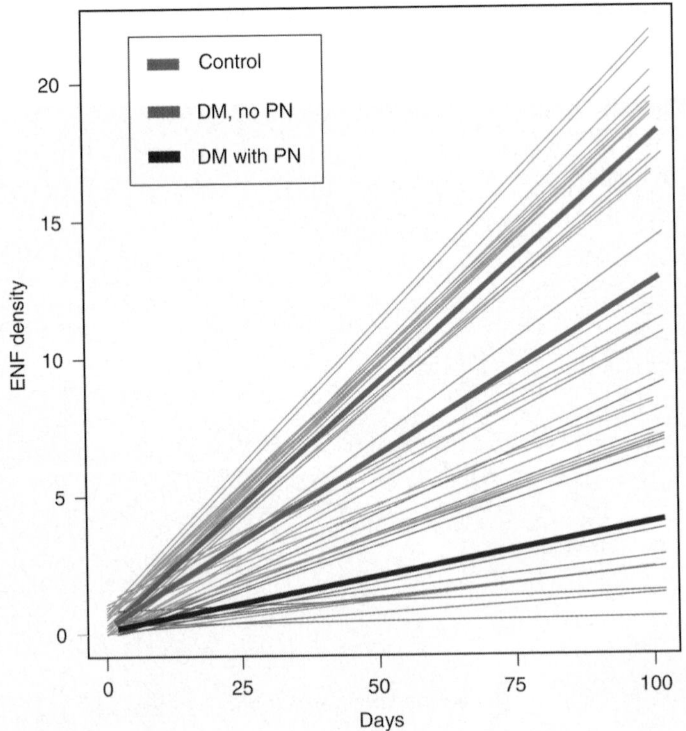

Color Plate 6. For each subject, a regression line from postcapsaicin time-points is generated and the slope of this line is used as the rate of regeneration. (Fig. 7, Chapter 17; *see* complete caption on p. 304.)

18
Aldose Reductase Inhibitors for the Treatment of Diabetic Neuropathy

Aristidis Veves, MD, DSc

SUMMARY

It has been more than 30 years since the first aldose reductase inhibitor (ARI) was tested in diabetic and galactosemic rats and found to control the polyol accumulation. Since then, a considerable number of ARIs have been tested in experimental and human diabetes. Despite the initial encouraging results from tests that were conducted for the past 20 years, ARIs have not been established for the treatment of diabetic neuropathy yet. The main reasons for this are inconsistent results and the unacceptable high rate of side-effects associated with the initially tested compounds. The lack of well-defined end points and the inability to produce an inhibitor that achieves satisfactory tissue penetration and enzyme inhibition are other major contributing factors for this failure. This chapter focuses on the clinical trials that have examined the effect of all tested ARIs on human diabetic neuropathy.

Key Words: Aldose reductase inhibitors; clinical trials; human diabetic neuropathy; efficacy; side effects; clinical use.

INTRODUCTION

It has been more than 30 years since the first aldose reductase inhibitor (ARI) was tested in diabetic and galactosemic rats and found to control the polyol accumulation *(1)*. Since then, a considerable number of ARIs have been tested in experimental and human diabetes. However, very few new information have become available since the last edition of this book, probably an indication that either interest in these compounds is waning down in the scientific community or that despite all the intensive efforts, the ideal compound that will offer satisfactory enzyme inhibition with minimal side-effect has not been discovered as yet. A thorough review of work on experimental diabetes would be out of the spirit of this chapter; however, more information is provided in chapters of this edition. The following chapter will focus on the results from clinical trials in diabetic neuropathy *(2)*.

END POINTS FOR CLINICAL TRIALS IN DIABETIC NEUROPATHY

Painful symptoms and foot ulceration are the two most important clinical problems related to peripheral somatic diabetic neuropathy. The conduction of clinical trials, which test the efficacy of new therapies for painful neuropathy is straight forward:

From: *Contemporary Diabetes: Diabetic Neuropathy: Clinical Management, Second Edition*
Edited by: A. Veves and R. Malik © Humana Press Inc., Totowa, NJ

patients with this condition are provided trial medication and the primary end point is the reduction of the symptoms, which is expected to occur during a reasonable period after the treatment has been initiated. In contrast, foot ulcers develop long after the initiation of events which lead to nerve damage and, by this time, the possibility of restoring the nerve lesions, or halting their progression, is close to nonexisting. Therefore, if a study was to be conducted having as primary end point the prevention of foot ulceration it should involve patients who have diabetic neuropathy in the early stages and follow them until they reach the very late stages of the disease. This would mean that a large number of patients should be followed for prolonged periods of time, even decades, before any conclusion would be reached.

It is obvious from the aforementioned that more practical end points should be used in order to conduct clinical therapeutic trials, which will be financially supported by the pharmaceutical industry where efficient development of new medications are of paramount importance. In addition, these end points should give an accurate and more detailed picture about the effects of the treatment on the progression of the disease, mainly to what extent it can restore the already established lesions.

Sural nerve biopsies were initially considered to be the best method for evaluating new medications. However, the interpretation of the biopsy results was found to be more difficult than was originally believed and as a result, nerve biopsies fall out of favor. Most recent studies have used surrogate measurements, mainly nerve electrophysiological measurements and quantitative sensory testing. Regarding the electrophysiological measurements, Dyck and O'Brian, based on epidemiological data, initially suggested that a mean change of 2.9 m per second in the combined conduction velocities of the ulnar, median, and peroneal nerves, or a change of 2.2 m per second in the peroneal nerve alone should be achieved in order that the results can have a meaningful clinical significance *(4)*. However, it should be emphasized that the selection of end points is not the only issue with the design of new clinical trials. Thus, the current prevailing opinion is that future studies will have to include large number of patients and be of long enough duration (probably around 18–24 months), pay particular attention to the variability of the end point measurements, and have rigorous quality control in order to allow the drawing of definite conclusions regarding the efficacy of ARIs in treating diabetic neuropathy.

CLINICAL TRIALS WITH ARIS

Alrestatin

Alrestatin was the first ARI to be tried in human diabetic neuropathy. In the first, uncontrolled study conducted in 1981, 10 patients with symptomatic neuropathy were treated with intravenous infusions of alrestatin for 5 days *(5)*. Although, symptomatic improvement was noticed in seven patients, objective measurements failed to improve. Therefore, as the trial was not controlled, a placebo effect accounting for the symptomatic improvement cannot be excluded. No adverse effects of alrestatin were noticed in this trial (Table 1).

The next trial included nine patients with diabetes with severe symptomatic neuropathy, which had necessitated at least one hospital admission before the study *(6)*. The trial was a single-blind, nonrandomized, placebo-crossover, which lasted for 4 months. Each patient received the maximum tolerated oral dose for 2 months and was on placebo for the other two. Subjective improvement was noted by most of the patients

Table 1
ARIs Trials in Human Neuropathy

Authors	Design	Duration of active treatment	Results
Alrestatin			
Culebras (1981)	Uncntr	5 days	Symptomatic improvement
Handelsman (1981)	sb, nonrmd, co	4 months	Symptomatic improvement
Fagious (1981)	db, rmd	12 weeks	Improvement of symptoms, VPT and ulnar mcv
Sorbinil			
Judzewitsch (1983)	db, rmd	9 weeks	Improvement of peroneal mcv and median mcv and scv
Jaspan (1983)	sb	3–5 weeks	Symptomatic improvement
Young (1983)	db, rmd, co	4 weeks	Improvement of symptoms and sural sap
Lewin (1984)	db, rmd, co	4 weeks	No improvement
Fagious (1985)	db, rmd	6 months	Improvement of posterior tibial mcv and ulnar nevre F wl and dsl
O'Hare (1988)	db, rmd	12 months	No benefit
Guy (1988)	db, rmd	12 months	No benefit
Sima (1988)	db, rmd	12 months	Improvement of symptoms, sural sap and mfd
Ponalrestat			
Ziegler (1991)	db, rmd	12 months	No benefit
Krentz (1992)	db, rmd	12 months	No benefit
Tolrestat			
Ryder (1986)	db, rmd	8 weeks	Improvement of median mcv
Boulton (1990)	db, rmd	12 months	Improvement of paraesthetic symptoms and peroneal mcv
Macleod (1992)	db, rmd	6 months	Improvement of VPT, median and ulnar mcv
Boulton (1992)	db, rmd, withdrawal	12 months	Improvement of symptoms, median and peroneal mcv
Giugliano (1993)	db, rmd	12 months	Improvement of autonomic measurements and VPT
Giugliano (1995)	db, rmd	12 months	Improvement of autonomic measurements and VPT
Didangelos (1999)	db, rmd	24 months	Improvement of autonomic measurements
Greene (1999)	db, rmd	12 months	Increase in small diameter myelinated fibers
Hotta (2001)	db, rmd	12 months	Improvement of symptoms, median fcv and median F-wave latency
Johnson (2004)	db, rmd	12 months	Exercise LVEF and cardiac stroke volume

sb, single blind; db, double-blind; Uncntr, uncontrolled; nonrmd, nonrandomized; rmd, randomized; co, crossover; mcv, motor nerve conduction velocity; scv, sensory nerve conduction velocity; sap, sensory action potential; wl, wave latency; dsl, distal sensory latency; VPT, vibration perception threshold; mfd, myelinated fibre density.

(eight out of nine), but electrophysiological measurements remained virtually unchanged. The most notable side-effects were nausea, and photosensitivity, which was severe in two cases.

Around the same time, the most comprehensive trial of alrestatin was conducted. Thirty patients with long-standing diabetes and mild to moderate neuropathy were studied in a double-blind, randomized, placebo-controlled trial, which lasted 12 weeks *(7)*. Symptomatic improvement, reduction of the sensory impairment score, and improvement of vibration perception threshold and ulnar nerve conduction velocity were noticed, but the rest of the electrophysiological measurements in the median, peroneal, and sural nerves did not show any significant difference.

The earlier-mentioned studies indicated that treatment with ARIs might be helpful in treating diabetic neuropathy and also highlighted the need for well-conducted long-term trials in order to fully explore the potential of this new therapeutic approach. On the down side, the high incidence of side-effects of alrestatin prohibited its further development. This led the way for using some newly discovered compounds such as sorbinil and tolrestat.

Sorbinil

Sorbinil was the second ARI to be tested in human diabetic neuropathy and a considerable number of studies were conducted during the last decade using this drug. An early study using sorbinil for the treatment of neuropathy was published in 1983 and included 39 patients with stable diabetes and no clinical symptoms of neuropathy *(8)*. The design of the study was randomized, double-blind, crossover and each patient received active treatment for 9 weeks. The results showed a small but statistically significant increase of the conduction velocity of the peroneal motor nerve (0.70 m per second), the median motor nerve (0.66 m per second), and the median sensory nerve (1.16 m per second) during the treatment with the active drug. Another important finding was that the increase declined rapidly after cessation of the treatment so that the nerve conduction velocity was similar to pretreatment levels 3 weeks later. Five patients were withdrawn from the study because of fever and rash, which were attributed to sorbinil.

In contrast with the previous trial, the ones which followed included mainly patients with diabetes with symptomatic neuropathy. The first one studied 11 patients with severely painful neuropathy who failed to respond to conventional treatment with analgesics or tricyclic antidepressants *(10)*. In a single blind design the patients were treated with sorbinil for 3–5 weeks and the pain relief was measured using a graphic scale. Marked to moderate pain relief was noted in eight patients usually 3–4 days after being on treatment, whereas the pain returned to pretreatment levels in seven of the responders when they stopped taking the drug. The motor and sensory conduction velocities of the median nerve improved in four patients, whereas the peroneal motor conduction velocity improved in two patients. It is of interest however, that in four patients who responded to the treatment the pain was related to proximal motor neuropathy, a condition, which is thought to be caused by mechanisms not related to polyol accumulation. No significant side-effects were noted in the 11 patients who finished the study whereas 12th patient who started the study was withdrawn because of rash.

The next study had a double-blind, randomized, placebo-controlled crossover design, and included 15 patients with painful symptoms, which were present for more than 1 year *(10)*. The patients were observed for 16 weeks but they were on active treatment for only 4 weeks, either from week 5 to 8 or from 9 to 12. Painful symptoms were assessed using a standardized symptom score, whereas other measurements included neurological findings on clinical examination, vibration perception threshold, motor and sensory nerve conduction velocities, and autonomic system function tests. A significant number of patients reported improvement of painful symptoms while on the active treatment, but when the pain score was calculated using their diaries no difference was found between sorbinil and placebo treatment. Significant improvement was also noticed in the sural sensory potential action, whereas the rest of the electrophysiological measurements remained unchanged. The number of patients who withdrew because of side-effects (mainly rash and fever) had increased in comparison with the previous study; four patients in total had an idiosyncratic reaction which resolved rapidly after the discontinuation of the drug.

The next trial used the same layout, i.e., double-blind, placebo-controlled crossover, and included 13 patients with diabetes with chronic symptomatic neuropathy (mean duration of symptoms 6 years) *(11)*. The duration of treatment with sorbinil was the same as in the previous trial, 4 weeks out of a total study period of 16 weeks. The pain intensity was measured using a 100-mm visual analog scale whereas other measurements included vibration perception threshold, motor and sensory conduction velocities, autonomic function tests, and duration of sleep. In contrast to the previous study, no difference was found in any parameter, including the severity of neuropathic symptoms and the objective measurements of peripheral nerve function. Side-effects were present only in one patient who took sorbinil in the form of a febrile rash necessitating his withdrawal from the study.

The aforementioned short-term trials were followed by long-term ones, which examined the effects of aldose reductase inhibition for periods of 6–12 months. The first long-term study studied 55 male patients with diabetes with symptomatic neuropathy for 6 months in a double-blind placebo-controlled parallel group design *(12)*. To avoid a possible long-term effect of the drug, the authors elected to randomize their patients to active- and placebo-treatment and to avoid the crossover design. Patients assessment included clinical examination, neurophysiological measurements, thermal and vibration perception thresholds, and autonomic system function tests.

No significant improvement was found in the sorbinil-treated group when it was compared with the placebo group, although three sorbinil-treated patients reported a marked overall improvement compared with none from the placebo group. When these three patients were compared with the whole sorbinil-treated group their age was lower than the mean group age and the neuropathy assessed by electrophysiology was less severe. All three patients worsened to pretreatment levels when sorbinil was discontinued. No significant changes were found in the vibration and thermal discrimination threshold. From the electrophysiological measurements improvement was noticed in the motor posterior tibial nerve conduction velocity (approximately 1.5 m per second), F-wave latency of the ulnar nerve, and the distal sensory latency of the ulnar nerve. From the autonomic tests, a significant improvement in the R–R interval variation during deep breathing was found in the sorbinil-treated group. The number of patients with serious side-effects was smaller in this study; only two patients had to be withdrawn from the study because of rash and lymphadenopathy.

The next long-term study included 31 patients with mild to moderate neuropathy and lasted for 14 months (including a 2-month run-in period) *(13)*. The study was designed as double-blind, randomized, placebo-controlled, and two-third of patients were treated with sorbinil whereas one-third received placebo. Assessments of the patients response were performed every 3 months and included the measurement of symptoms such as pain, tingling, and temperature insensitivity using a 100 mm visual analog scale, clinical examination, vibration perception thresholds, electrophysiology, and autonomic function tests. The results indicated no benefit for the sorbinil-treated patients in any of the measured parameters. In addition, as similar doses of the drug were used in this trial and the previous ones, and was accompanied by serum sorbinil levels measurements, inadequate drug dosage or poor patient compliance could not be held responsible for the observed discrepancies. Hypersensitivity reactions with fever, rash, and myalgia occurred in two patients who recovered completely after the drug was discontinued.

No improvement was also found in another double-blind, randomized trial, which lasted for 12 months and included patients with severe neuropathy with or without symptoms *(14)*. Thirty nine patients took part in this study and the severity of neuropathy is indicated by the fact that a history of foot ulceration was present in 21 patients. Efficacy assessments included clinical evaluation, vibration and thermal perception thresholds, nerve conduction velocities in 12 nerves, and somatosensory-evoked potentials. The results showed no difference in any of the above measurements between sorbinil and placebo-treated patients, both for the lower and upper extremities, despite the fact that the arms were less severely affected.

As it can be seen from the aforementioned studies, the beneficial results, which were initially reported failed to be confirmed in subsequent, better designed, long-term trials. In an effort to clear the confusion, the next trial used sural nerve biopsies, which allow more precise evaluation of the therapeutic efficacy *(15)*. This trial included 16 patients with established peripheral neuropathy and involved subjects undergoing fascicular sural nerve biopsies of the same limb at the beginning and the end of the study *(16)*. The design of the trial was double-blind, randomized, placebo-controlled, and lasted 12 months. Additional investigations included clinical neurological assessments, thermal perception thresholds, and electrophysiological measurements. Although both actively- and placebo-treated groups showed some clinical improvement at the end of the study this was more pronounced in the sorbinil-treated group. The nonbiopsised sural nerve of the sorbinil group showed an improvement of 1 μV in the action-potential amplitude and of 2 m per second in the sensory conduction velocity (2 m per second), results that were not found in the placebo group.

The analysis of the sural nerve biopsies showed that the sorbitol levels in the sorbinil group were reduced, indicating a successful aldose reductase inhibition in the nerve tissue. The myelinated fibers density, the best single histopathological criterion to quantify neuropathy, was similarly reduced at baseline by 50% in both the sorbinil and placebo groups when they were compared with age-matched nondiabetic subjects. After 12 months of treatment, a significant increase of 33% was found in the sorbinil group, whereas no difference was noted in the placebo group. The regeneration and remyelination activity in the sorbinil group was also increased, whereas no change was noticed in the placebo group. Important changes were also noticed in the degree of paranodal demyelination, segmental demyelination, and myelin wrinkling. The main importance of this study lies in the fact that it was the first to demonstrate morphological improvements in nerve biopsies after long-term aldose reductase inhibition in humans and suggested that long-term treatment in properly selected patients might be the most beneficial.

A second clinical trial, which used repeated sural nerve biopsies, assessed the changes in nerve concentrations of alcohol sugars after a 12-month period with sorbinil treatment *(17)*. Six patients took part in this study and histochemical measurements showed a significant decrease in nerve sorbitol and fructose levels in the follow-up visit compared with baseline, whereas the levels of glucose and myo-inositol remained unchanged. The earlier findings were interpreted by the investigators as indicating that sorbinil is an effective inhibitor of aldose reductase, but raised doubts about the role of myo-inositol in the pathogenesis of diabetic neuropathy.

A common factor, present in virtually all the earlier studies which used sorbinil was the relatively high rate of side-effects. The main adverse reactions were rash, fever, and lymphadenopathy, which subsided when the drug was discontinued. Nevertheless, these adverse reactions would make the use of sorbinil for prolonged period of time in relatively asymptomatic patients unacceptable, and therefore, the compound was withdrawn.

Ponalrestat

The main characteristic of ponalrestat compared with the previous two drugs was its safety profile: very few adverse reaction were reported during the preliminary safety trials, making it ideal for long-term usage. These early expectations were soon dashed as it became apparent that the nerve-tissue concentration levels were probably insufficient to inhibit aldose reductase. Therefore, it is hardly surprising that the few properly conducted trials with this compound reported negative results, despite some modest improvements, which were reported in short, preliminary trials *(18,19)*.

An example of a published paper with ponalrestat was that by Ziegler et al. *(20)*, who reported a randomized, double-blind, placebo-controlled trial of 60 patients with chronic symptomatic peripheral diabetic neuropathy for 12 months. No difference in any peripheral nerve function measurements, including electrophysiology, were documented at the end of the study. As was expected, the drug was well tolerated and no significant side-effects were present during the study. Similar results were subsequently reported by Krentz et al. *(21)* in a study with almost identical design.

Tolrestat

Tolrestat was the first ARI to be licensed for the treatment of diabetic neuropathy in certain countries all over the world including Italy, Mexico, and Ireland. Given orally, tolrestat is rapidly absorbed at a rate of 60–70%. Its plasma half-life is 10 hours and in clinical practice a dose of 200 mg per day is sufficient to provide satisfactory inhibition of the aldose reductase for 24 hours. Excretion is mainly through kidneys (70%), whereas a further 25% of the dose is excreted in the feces.

In a multicenter, double-blind, randomized, placebo-controlled trial, which lasted for 12 months the efficacy of tolrestat on symptomatic neuropathy was studied in 556 patients with either type 1 or type 2 diabetes *(22)*. Inclusion criteria were stable or increasing severity of neuropathic symptoms, and abnormal motor or sensory nerve electrophysiological measurements in at least three of six tested nerves. Patients were randomized to doses from 50 to 200 mg daily and efficacy assessments included the response of the painful and paraesthetic symptoms and electrophysiological measurements.

The painful symptoms improved in both the tolrestat- and placebo-treated patients but the paraesthetic symptoms improved significantly in patients treated with 200 mg tolrestat daily over placebo. From the objective measurements, a significant improvement (up to 2 m per second) was noticed for the tibial and peroneal nerve conduction velocities when they were compared both with the baseline measurements and with the placebo-treated group. Improvement in both symptoms and electrophysiological measurements was found in 28% of tolrestat-treated patients, significantly higher when compared with the 5% of the placebo-treated patients who had a similar response. The adverse reaction profile of the tolrestat was also satisfactory. The only symptom which occurred more frequently in the tolrestat group was dizziness. Elevation of transaminases was found in 13 (2.9%) patients with diabetes treated with tolrestat on any dose, but the transaminases returned to normal levels within 8–16 weeks after the drug was discontinued. There was no evidence of severe liver dysfunction in any of the patients. A small but significant drop of the blood pressure, up to 7 mmHg in the systolic and 3.4 mm in the diastolic was also noticed without any consequences. No hypersensitivity reactions similar to the ones which were present with other ARIs were noticed.

The same design with the previous study was adopted by a multicentre European study, which enrolled 190 patients with symptomatic diabetic neuropathy *(23)*. The study lasted for 6 months and patients were randomized to take either placebo or tolrestat 200 mg per day. The efficacy analysis included measurements of painful and paraesthetic symptoms, vibration perception threshold in three sites, and nerve conduction velocities of four motor and two sensory nerves. No difference in the painful symptoms was found between the placebo and tolrestat group at the end of the study, although both groups improved in comparison with baseline measurements. In contrast, a significant improvement of paraesthetic symptoms was noticed in the placebo group compared both with tolrestat group and with baseline measurements. Regarding the vibration perception threshold measurements, a significant change in favor of tolrestat-treated patients was found in one of the three sites it was measured (carpal site, which was located at the dorsum of the second metacarpal bone).

Significant increases in the motor conduction velocities in tolrestat-treated patients were recorded at the median nerve compared both with baseline (2 m per second) and with the placebo group, and in the ulnar nerve compared with baseline. When the changes of all motor conduction velocities were combined together, a significant improvement was found at the end of the study, compared with baseline measurements and with the placebo group. All the above changes were present only at the end of the study, after 24 weeks of treatment. At the same time, 48% of the tolrestat-treated patients showed an improvement in three of the four motor nerve conduction velocities, whereas in the placebo-treated patients similar response was noticed in 28%. No changes in the two sensory nerve function measurements were present at the end of the study, although the heart rate in the tolrestat group was slower compared with baseline measurements of the same group and with the placebo group. Six tolrestat-treated and two placebo-treated patients were discontinued from the study because of elevated liver enzymes.

A considerable number of patients who took part in the aforementioned studies continued to take the drug for several years after the studies were completed and were the cohort of the subsequent trial, which was designed as a randomized, double-blind, placebo-controlled withdrawal study *(24)*. Thus, 372 patients who had already received tolrestat for a mean period of 4.2 years were randomly selected either to continue receiving tolrestat at a dose of 200 or 400 mg or to switch to placebo for 1 year. Another interesting feature of the design of this trial was the fact that patients were given the option to change treatment on one occasion after the first three months of the study without breaking the code and therefore, maintaining the double-blind design of the trial. The symptom score and the motor conduction velocities of four nerves were used as end points.

A significant deterioration of the symptom score was noticed at the 24th and 36th weeks in the placebo group compared with the tolrestat group. However, at the end of the study, although a small difference still existed between the two groups, it failed to reach statistical significance. The conduction velocities of three out of the four motor nerves also deteriorated considerably in the patients who switched to placebo, whereas no change was noticed in the patients who continued on tolrestat. Thus, in the median nerve there was a drop of 0.9 m per second, in the ulnar 1.3 m per second, and in the peroneal 0.8 m per second, whereas the mean reduction of both nerves was 0.9 m per second. In addition, in patients who switched from tolrestat to placebo during the study there was a mean drop of 1.3 m per second for all four nerves, whereas in the patients who switched from placebo to tolrestat an improvement of 1 m per second was recorded. Therefore, a small but significant benefit of long-term treatment with tolrestat which can disappear when the treatment is discontinued was the main finding of the aforementioned study.

In a parallel study, sural nerve biopsies were obtained at the end of the earlier-mentioned trial from 13 patients who continued to receive tolrestat and 14 patients who received placebo *(25)*. Morphometric analysis showed no difference between the above two groups, but when compared with nerve biopsies from untreated neuropathic patients both groups showed increased nerve fiber regeneration. In addition, treatment with tolrestat was found to ameliorate the increase in the sorbitol and fructose levels in the nerve tissue indicating that tolrestat can achieve satisfactory concentration levels in the peripheral nerves.

The following two trials with tolrestat were performed at the University of Naples and were both randomized, placebo-controlled, double-blind, parallel trials of 52 weeks duration. The first one examined the effect of 200 mg daily tolrestat on patients with asymptomatic autonomic diabetic neuropathy, defined as at least one abnormal cardiovascular reflex *(26)*. At end of the study, improvement in the tolrestat-treated group was found in all autonomic tests, which included deep breathing (E/I ratio), lying to standing (30/15) ratio, Valsalva (L/S ratio), and postural hypertension. In contrast to this improvement, a worsening in all the above parameters except the orthostatic hypotension was observed in the placebo-treated group. Similar results, namely an improvement in the tolrestat group and a worsening in the placebo group, were found in vibration perception threshold measurements, the only reported assessment of the peripheral somatic nerve function. Similar results were reported in the second study, which included patients with subclinical neuropathy, defined as abnormality in only one autonomic test, the squatting test *(27)*. Improvement was found in all the autonomic tests and the vibration perception thresholds in the tolrestat group, whereas deterioration was observed in the placebo group in all but the orthostatic hypotension tests.

In one of the last studies that were conducted with tolrestat, patients with diabetes with clinical autonomic neuropathy were randomized to either tolrestat (200 mg daily) or placebo for a period of 2 years. As with the earlier studies, treatment with tolrestat resulted in improvement of most standard cardiovascular reflex test, in comparison with both the baseline measurements and also to the changes that were observed in the placebo group *(28)*. Despite the initially promising results, tolrestat was subsequently withdrawn from clinical use as it was associated to serious side-effects, mainly related to liver failure.

Zenarestat

Zenarestat was an ARI that was shown to achieve very good penetration in the nerve tissue. Initial studies indicated that in patients who achieved more than 80% sorbitol suppression in sural nerve biopsies after a 52-week treatment with agent, there was a significant increase in the density of small diameter sural nerve myelinated fibers *(29)*. However, an unfavorable risk/benefit ratio, mainly related to kidney problems, prohibited the conduction of large pivotal studies, and zenarestat was withdrawn.

Fidarestat

In animal models, Fidarestat was shown to be one of the most potent AR inhibitors. As a result, a large multicenter placebo-controlled randomized study that used 1 mg of Fidarestat once a day and lasted for 52 weeks was conducted *(30)*. A total of 279 patients with mild diabetic neuropathy were included. Fidarestat-treated patients showed an improvement in two out of eight nerve electrophysiological measures (median nerve FCV and F-wave latency) that were recorded and in subjective symptoms.

Zopolrestat

Zopolrestat is an interesting ARI as there are no published clinical trials indicating favorable effects on diabetic neuropathy. However, a recently published randomized, placebo-controlled, double-blind, parallel trial of 52 weeks duration examined the efficacy of 500 or 1000 mg daily in patients with low diastolic peak filling rate or impaired augmentation of left ventricular ejection fraction (LVEF) and absence of coronary artery disease, left ventricular hypertrophy, and valvular heart disease *(30)*. Treatment with either dose of zopolrestat resulted in a small improvement of the exercise LVEF and stroke volume when compared with the placebo-treated patients. Although, the clinical significance of these results is small, they do indicate that diabetic cardiomyopathy may not be exclusively related to coronary artery disease, but it might also be associated to activation of the polyol pathway in the cardiac myocytes. It is also of interest that no improvement was noticed in the peripheral somatic or autonomic neuropathy in the patients who participated in the aforementioned study.

CONCLUSION

Despite the initial encouraging results from trials that were conducted during the last 20 years, ARIs have not been established for the treatment of diabetic neuropathy yet. The main reasons for this are inconsistent results in subsequent trials and the unacceptable high rate of side-effects associated with the initially tested compounds. The lack of well-defined end points and the conduction of numerous small trials, instead of focussing on the most promising agents and conducting large pivotal trials is one of the reasons that are related to this outcome. In addition, the inability to produce an inhibitor that achieves satisfactory tissue penetration and enzyme inhibition, whereas at the same time is devoid of serious side-effects have also played a significant role. Currently, it seems that the interest in ARIs is significantly reduced and is doubtful if new ARIs will be tested clinically in the near future.

REFERENCES

1. Dvornik D, Simard-Duquesne N, Krami M, et al. Polyol accumulation in galactosemic and diabetic rats: control by an aldose reductase inhibitor. *Science* 1973;182:1146–1148.
2. Tomlinson DR, Willars GB, Carrington AL. Aldose reductase inhibitors and diabetic complications. *Pharmacol Ther* 1992;54:151–194.
3. Pfeifer MA, Schumer MP, Gelber DA. Aldose reductase inhibitors: the end of an era or the need for different trial designs? *Diabetes* 1997;46(Suppl 2):S82–S89.
4. Dyck PJ, O'Brian PC. Meaningful degrees of prevention or improvement of nerve conduction in controlled clinical trials of diabetic neuropathy. *Diabetes Care* 1989;12: 649–652.
5. Culebras A, Alio J, Herrera JL, Lopez-Fraile IP. Effect of an aldose reductase inhibitor on diabetic peripheral neuropathy. *Arch Neurol* 1981;38:133–134.
6. Handelsman DJ, Turtle JR. Clinical trial of an aldose reductase inhibitor in diabetic neuropathy. *Diabetes* 1981;30:459–464.
7. Fagius J, Jameson S. Effects of aldose reductase inhibitor treatment in diabetic polyneuropathy—a clinical and neurophysiological study. *J Neurol Neurosurg Psychiatr* 1981;44: 991–1001.
8. Judzewitsch RG, Jaspan JB, Polonsky KS, et al. Aldose reductase inhibition improves nerve conduction velocity in diabetic patients. *N Engl J Med* 1983;308:119–125.
9. Jaspan J, Maselli R, Herold K, Bartkus C. Treatment of severely painful diabetic neuropathy with an aldose reductase inhibitor: relief of pain and improved somatic and autonomic nerve function. *Lancet* 1983;ii:758–762.
10. Young RJ, Ewing DJ, Clarke BF. A controlled trial of sorbinil, an aldose reductase inhibitor, in chronic painful diabetic neuropathy. *Diabetes* 1983;32:938–942.
11. Lewin IG, O'Brien AD, Morgan MH, Corrall RJM. Clinical and neurophysiological studies with the aldose reductase inhibitor, sorbinil, in symptomatic diabetic neuropathy. *Diabetologia* 1984;26:445–448.
12. Fagius J, Brattberg A, Jameson S, Berne C. Limited benefit of treatment of diabetic neuropathy with an aldose reductase inhibitor: a 24-week controlled trial. *Diabetologia* 1985;28:323–329.
13. O'Hare JP, Morgan MH, Alden P, Chissel S, O'Brien AD, Corrall RJM. Aldose reductase inhibition in diabetic neuropathy: Clinical and neurophysiological studies of one year's treatment with sorbinil. *Diabet Med* 1988;5:537–542.
14. Guy RJC, Gilbey SG, Sheehy M, Asselman P, Watkins P. Diabetic neuropathy in the upper limb and the effect of twelve months sorbinil treatment. *Diabetologia* 1988;31: 214–220.

15. Consensus Statement. Report and Recommendations of the San Antonio Conference on Diabetic Neuropathy. *Diabetes* 1988;37:1000–1004.
16. Sima AAF, Brill V, Nathaniel T, et al. Regeneration and repair of myelinated fibres in sural nerve biopsy specimens from patients with diabetic neuropathy treated with sorbinil. *N Engl J Med* 1988;319:548–555.
17. Dyck PJ, Zimmerman BR, Vilen TH, et al. Nerve glucose, fructose, sorbitol, myo-inositol, and fiber degeneration and regeneration in diabetic neuropathy. *N Engl J Med* 1988;319: 542–548.
18. Gill JS, Williams G, Ghatei MA, Hetreed AH, Mather HM, Bloom SR. Effect of the aldose reductase inhibitor, ponalrestat, on diabetic neuropathy. *Diabete Metab* 1990;16:296–302.
19. Price DE, Alani SM, Wales JK. Effect of aldose reductase inhibition on resistance to ischemic conduction block in diabetic subjects. *Diabetes Care* 1991;14:411–413.
20. Ziegler D, Mayer P, Rathmann W, Gries FA. One-year treatment with the aldose reductase inhibitor, ponalrestat, in diabetic neuropathy. *Diabetes Res Clin Pract* 1991;14:63–73.
21. Krentz AJ, Honigsberger L, Ellis SH, Hardman M, Nattrass M. A 12-month randomized controlled study of the aldose reductase inhibitor ponalrestat in patients with chronic symptomatic diabetic neuropathy. *Diabet Med* 1992;9:463–468.
22. Boulton AJM, Levin S, Comstock J. A multicentre trial of the aldose reductase inhibitor, tolrestat, in patients with symptomatic diabetic neuropathy. *Diabetologia* 1990;33: 431–437.
23. Macleod AF, Boulton AJM, Owens DR, et al. A multicentre trial of the aldose reductase inhibitor tolrestat in patients with symptomatic diabetic peripheral neuropathy. *Diabete Metab* 1992;18:14–20.
24. Santiago JV, Sonksen PH, Boulton AJM, et al. Withdrawal of the aldose reductase inhibitor tolrestat in patients with diabetic neuropathy: Effect on nerve function. *J Diab Comp* 1993;7:170–178.
25. Sima AAF, Greene DA, Brown MB, et al. Effect of hyperglycemia and the aldose inhibitor tolrestat on sural nerve biochemistry and morphometry in advanced diabetic peripheral polyneuropathy. *J Diab Comp* 1993;7:157–169.
26. Giugliano D, Marfella R, Quatraro A, et al. Tolrestat for mild diabetic neuropathy. A 52-week, randomized, placebo controlled trial. *Ann Int Med* 1993;118:7–11.
27. Giugliano D, Acampora R, Marfella R, et al. Tolrestat in the primary prevention of diabetic neuropathy. *Diabetes Care* 1995;18:536–541.
28. Didangelos TP, Karamitsos DT, Athyros VG, Kourtoglou GI. Effect of aldose reductase inhibition on cardiovascular reflex tests in patients with definite diabetic autonomic neuropathy over a period of 2 years. *J Diab Comp* 1998;12:201–207.
29. Greene DA, Arezzo J, Brown M. Effects of aldose reductase inhibition on nerve conduction and morphometry in diabetic neuropathy. *Neurology* 1999;53:580–591.
30. Hotta N, Toyota T, Matsuoka K, et al. Clinical efficacy of fidarestat, a novel aldose reductase inhibitor, for diabetic peripheral neuropathy: a 52-week multicenter placebo-controlled double-blind parallel group study. *Diabetes Care* 2001;24:1776–1782.
31. Johnson BF, Nesto RW, Pfeifer MA, et al. Cardiac abnormalities in diabetic patients with neuropathy: effects of aldose reductase inhibitor administration. *Diabetes Care* 2004;27: 448–454.

19

Other Therapeutic Agents for the Treatment of Diabetic Neuropathy

Gary L. Pittenger PhD, **Henri Pharson** PhD, **Jagdeesh Ullal** MD, **and Aaron I. Vinik** MD, PhD

SUMMARY

The pathogenesis of diabetic neuropathy is complex and it is important to understand the underlying pathology leading to the complication in order to best tailor treatment for each individual patient. It is unlikely that reversing any single mechanism will prove sufficient for reversing nerve damage. Several drugs, such as antioxidant, PKC inhibitors and nerve growth factors can have effects on multiple systems that are compromised in diabetic neuropathy, yet even those may not be enough in and of themselves to completely restore neurological function. Combination therapy may prove to be the best long term approach, and studies of those combinations should prove revealing as to the relative roles of metabolic dysfunction, microvascular insufficiency and autoimmunity in the diabetic neuropathy patient population.

Key Words: Antioxidant; PKC inhibitors and nerve growth factors; VEGF.

INTRODUCTION

Neuropathy is one of the most common complication of diabetes with a heterogeneous clinical presentation and a wide range of abnormalities. As a result, there is still not a single therapeutic agent for diabetic neuropathy that consistently gives more than mild relief. There is a plethora of studies in the literature indicating that metabolic, microvascular, and autoimmune dysfunction all play a role in the progression of diabetic neuropathy. Given the potential significance of each of these different systems in diabetes, it is not surprising that treatments targeted to specific pathways in these systems have commonly proven disappointing in their efficacy. Our "simple" concept of the various functional changes leading to peripheral nerve disease in diabetes is presented in (Fig. 1) *(1)*. Thus, although clinical studies with thousands of patients have shown that hyperglycemia is at the center of diabetic neuropathy *(2,3)*, finding specific biochemical pathways to manipulate for therapy has proven difficult.

From: *Contemporary Diabetes: Diabetic Neuropathy: Clinical Management, Second Edition*
Edited by: A. Veves and R. Malik © Humana Press Inc., Totowa, NJ

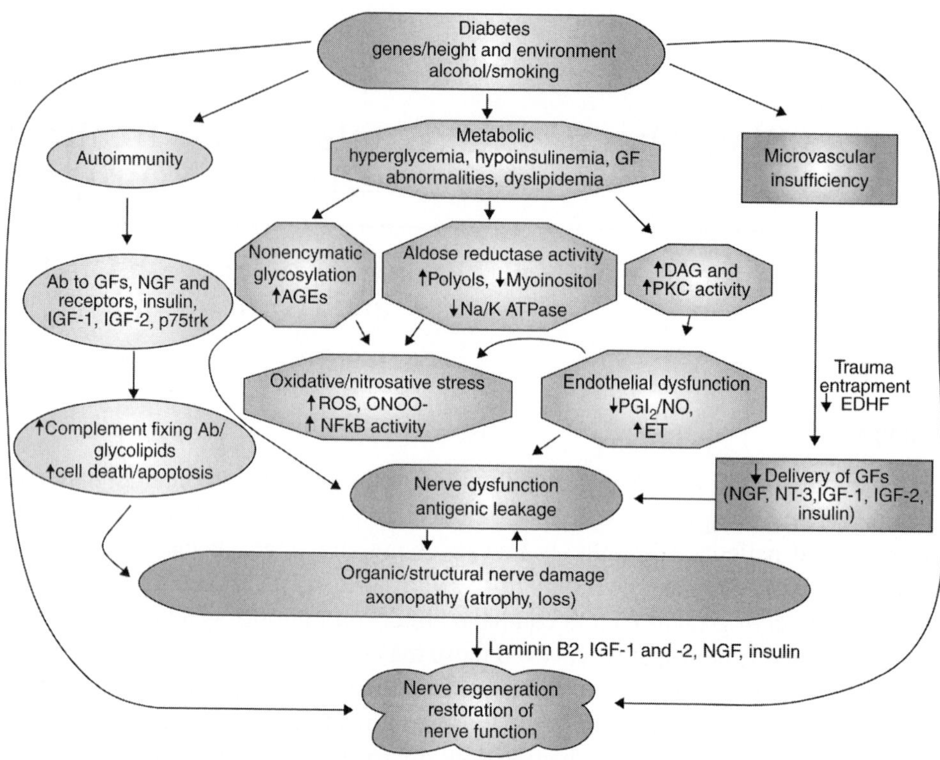

Fig. 1. Diagram of the pathologies underlying the development of diabetic neuropathy, beginning with hyperglycemia, possibly exacerbated by alcohol or smoking Adapted from ref. *1*.

END POINTS FOR CLINICAL TRIALS IN DIABETIC NEUROPATHY

Among the challenges for studies of diabetic neuropathy is the selection of the measures that can be used to determine the efficacy of the agents. Common end points include:

1. Subjective measures of symptoms (e.g., nerve symptom scores).
2. Questionnaires that allow for quantification of any changes in the symptoms of diabetic neuropathy, or the quality of life of the patient (e.g., neuropathy symptom scores, total neuropathy scores).
3. Objective neurological examinations focussing on distal sensorimotor function, including combinations giving a single score (e.g., NTSS-6, a combination of numbness, prickling sensation, aching pain, burning pain, lancinating pain, and allodynia scores).
4. Electrophysiology (nerve conduction velocity, amplitudes [especially sural nerve amplitude], F-wave latencies).
5. Quantitative tests of sensory and motor modalities that allow more precise measures of nerve function.
6. Autonomic measures (e.g., cardiac function or neurovascular measures).
7. Skin biopsy, which allows direct observation of the morphology of sensory nerve fibers.
8. Instruments that entail various combinations of the above.

The following summarizes the view of prospective end points in diabetic neuropathy trials:

Table 1
Mechanisms for Pathogenesis of Diabetic Neuropathy and Therapies That Have Been Tested Addressing Them

Metabolic dysfunction	Microvascular insufficiency	Autoimmunity	Nerve regeneration
ARIs	PKC-β Inhibitor	Steroidal anti-inflammatories	Neurotrophins
Antioxidants	Vasodilators	IVIg	Topiramate
Inhibitors of glycation	Antioxidants	Plasmaphoresis	–

1. Symptoms (forms and questionnaires)—*subjective.*
2. Quality of life (questionnaire)—*subjective.*
3. Quantitative neurological examination focussing on distal sensorimotor function (sensation, strength, and reflexes)—*semiobjective.*
4. Neurophysiology (nerve conduction velocity, amplitudes, F-wave latencies; multiple nerves, both sensory and motor)—*objective.*
5. Quantitative sensory testing (vibration, thermal, pain, and NTSS-6)—*semiobjective* 6. Autonomic testing (microvascular, cardiac measures)—*objective.*
7. Morphology—(skin biopsy—nerve density and length, branching pattern)—*objective.*
8. Combinations (e.g., NIS-LL + 7 = objective neurological examination of the lower limbs + 4 measures of nerve electrophysiology + QAFT + QST).

Unfortunately, subjective measures may not be sensitive enough to discern small changes in nerve fiber functions in a small test group during a short period of time. Unless a study includes a large number of subjects and a sufficient period of time significant changes may not be detectable, particularly in the short time periods that most efficacy trials are designed for. Thus, objective tests may be more useful for studies of shorter duration.

TREATMENTS

Therapies for diabetic neuropathy are generally directed at the 3 primary mechanisms shown in Fig. 1: metabolic dysfunction, autoimmunity, or microvascular insufficiency. Several of these agents, for example, antioxidants or neurotrophins (NTs), can affect more than one of the pathogenetic mechanisms, as shown in Table 1.

THERAPIES TARGETED TO METABOLIC PATHWAYS

Note: The aldose reductase inhibitors are discussed elsewhere (*see* Chapter 18).

Antioxidants

Hyperglycemia has been shown in a number of studies to cause oxidative stress in tissues that are susceptible to the complications of diabetes, including peripheral nerves. In turn, the oxidative stress leads to the generation of free radicals that can attack the lipids, proteins, and nucleic acids of the affected tissues directly, compromising physiological function. The end result is the loss of axons and disruption of the microvasculature in the peripheral nervous system (Fig. 2). It has been shown that there is an increased presence of markers of oxidative stress, such as superoxide and peroxynitrite ions, and that antioxidant moieties were reduced in patients with diabetic peripheral

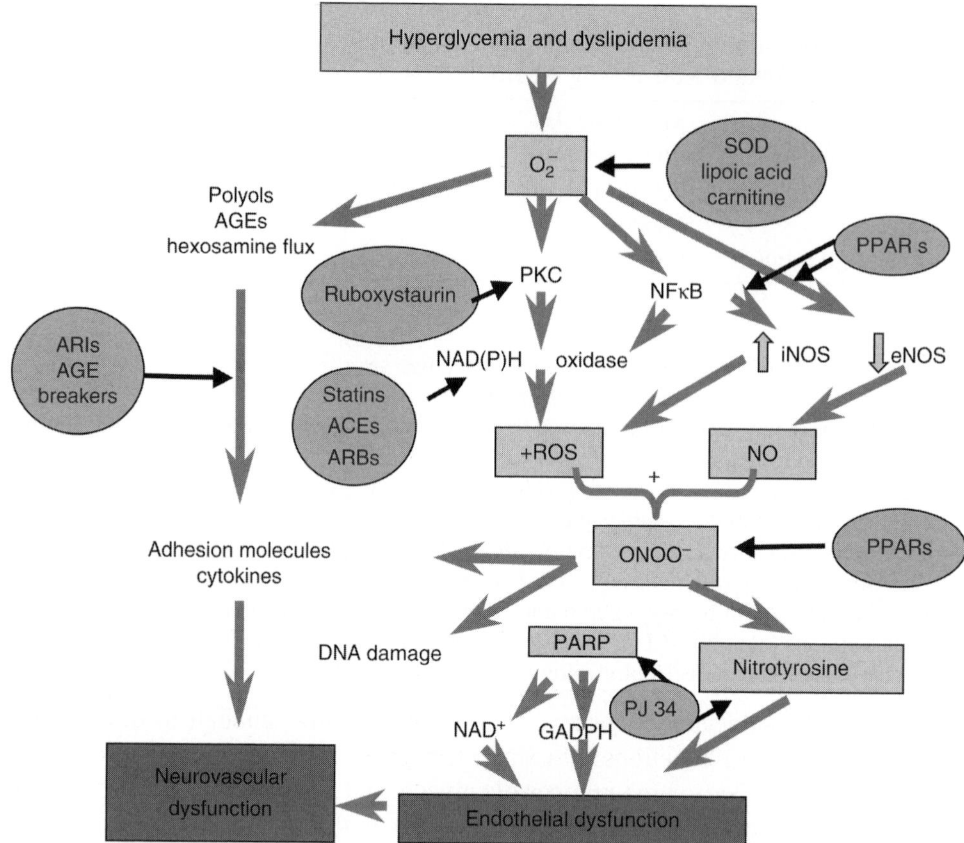

Fig. 2. The interactions of pathways leading to neurovascular and endothelial dysfunction and the actions of drugs that alter those mechanisms and are being tested in models of neuropathy.

neuropathy *(4)*. Therefore, it is reasonable to use therapies that are known to reduce oxidative stress in tissues, and antioxidants. Although a host of antioxidants have been tested in animal models (for review *see* ref. *5*), those that have been tested in human studies will be addressed.

α-Lipoic Acid

α-lipoic acid is the best studied antioxidant therapy used in diabetic neuropathy. Lipoic acid (1,2-dithiolane-3-pentanoic acid), a derivative of octanoic acid, is present in food and is also synthesized by the liver. It is a natural cofactor in the pyruvate dehydrogenase complex where it binds acyl groups and transfers them from one part of the complex to another. α-lipoic acid, also known as thioctic acid, has generated considerable interest as a thiol replenishing and redox modulating agent. In streptozotocin (STZ)-diabetic rats α-lipoic acid has been shown to prevent slowing of peripheral nerve conduction velocity and to maintain peripheral nerve blood flow *(6–8)*. It has also been shown to be effective in ameliorating both the somatic and autonomic neuropathies in diabetes *(9–11)*. It is not clear that the positive effects are limited to the antioxidant properties of α-lipoic acid, and studies are ongoing to determine its range of effects. α-lipoic acid is licensed for use in diabetes in Germany and it is currently undergoing extensive trials in the US as both an antidiabetic agent and for the treatment of diabetic neuropathy.

γ-Linolenic Acid

Linoleic acid is an essential fatty acid that is metabolized to di-homo-γ-linolenic acid (GLA), which in turn serves as an important constituent of neuronal membrane phospholipids. In addition it can serve as a substrate for prostaglandin E synthesis, which may be important for preservation of nerve blood flow. In diabetes, conversion of linoleic acid to GLA and subsequent metabolites is impaired, possibly contributing to the pathogenesis of diabetic neuropathy *(12,13)*. A multicenter, double-blind placebo-controlled trial using GLA for 1 year demonstrated significant improvements in both clinical measures and electrophysiological testing *(14)*.

Tocopherol (Vitamin E)

The tocopherols, especially the α-tocopherol isoform, have been promoted as effective antioxidant therapy for a number of neurological diseases, including Alzheimer's disease, epilepsy, cerebellar ataxia, and diabetic neuropathy. In studies of patients with diabetes vitamin E has been shown to decrease 8-isoprostane F2α *(15)*, decrease low density lipoprotein-C oxidation at high doses *(16)*, and increase skin blood flow and reduce free radicals in skin with topical application *(17)*. Human studies of vitamin E using combined oral therapy with vitamin C, another well-established antioxidant have shown improved vascular function, but only in type 1 patients *(18)*. Thus, vitamin E appears to exert antioxidant protective effects on neurons in diabetes although efficacy has not yet been demonstrated.

INHIBITORS OF GLYCATION

It is apparent that advanced glycosylation end products (AGEs) contribute to nerve damage either by direct action on neurons and myelin or by enhancing oxidative stress under hyperglycemic conditions. Thus, there is a great deal of interest in agents that either prevent the formation of AGEs or agents that reverse the nonenzymatic glycation of proteins.

Aminoguanidine

Animal studies using aminoguanidine, an inhibitor of the formation of AGEs, showed improvement in nerve conduction velocity in rats with STZ-induced diabetic neuropathy. However, controlled clinical trials to determine its efficacy in humans have been discontinued because of toxicity *(19,20)*. However, there are compounds related to aminoguanidine that reduced AGE formation and hold promise for this approach, although these have not been systematically studied in humans *(21–24)*.

THERAPIES FOR MICROVASCULAR INSUFFICIENCY

Although it is clear that there are significant alterations of blood vessels in diabetes, data thus far has been conflicting whether neuropathy promotes the changes in the microvasculature or whether it is the changes in the microvessels of the nerves that lead to neuropathy. Whatever the case, evidence is growing that re-establishing more normal patterns of blood flow to the nerves results in improved neurological function.

Protein Kinase C Inhibitors

Protein kinase C (PKC) and diacylglycerol (DAG) are intracellular signaling molecules that regulate vasculature by endothelial permeability and vasodilation. The PKC isozymes are a family of 12 related serine/threonine kinases *(25)* whose normal function is the activation of essential proteins and lipids in cells essential for cell survival. PKC-β is expressed in the vasculature *(26,27)* and belived to be involved in cell proliferation, differentiation, and apoptosis. PKC is activated by oxidative and osmolar stress, both of which are a consequence of the dysmetabolism of diabetes. Increased polyol pathway activity and pro-oxidants bind to the catalytic domain of PKC and it is disinhibited. PKC-β overactivation is induced by hyperglycemia or fatty acids through receptor-mediated activation by phospholipase C. It is hypothesized that AGEs and oxidants produced by nonenzymatic glycation and the polyol pathway, respectively, increase the production of DAG *(28)*. Increased DAG and calcium promotes the overactivation of PKC-β *(29)*. Activation of PKC-β activates MAP kinase and, subsequently, phosphorylation of transcription factors that are involved in angiogenesis, increased stress-related genes, *c-Jun* kinases and heat shock proteins, all of which can damage cells and vascular endothelial growth factor (VEGF) *(30)*, which is known to play a critical role in nerve development *(31)*. Diabetic animal models have shown high levels of PKC-β in a number of tissues *(28)*, including nerves and endothelium *(32)*. Activation of PKC-β causes vasoconstriction and tissue ischemia, whereas high levels may impair neurochemical regulation. PKC-β hyperactivity leads to increased vascular permeability, nitric oxide dysregulation *(33)*, increased leukocyte adhesion *(34)*, and altered blood flow *(35)*. Furthermore, PKC-β hyperactivity in the neural microvessels causes vasoconstriction, which might lead to decreased blood flow, resulting in nerve dysfunction and hypoxia *(35)*. Nerve hypoxia, oxidative nitrosative stress, and an increase in NFκB causes endothelial damage, leading to depletion of nerve growth factors, VEGF, and TGF-α autoimmunity and may further accelerate the loss of nerve conduction *(31)*. Both animal models and human clinical trials investigating complications of diabetes have shown that blockade of PKC-β slows the progression of complications *(33,36–47)*.

Multiple studies using a specific PKC-β inhibitor, ruboxistaurin mesylate (LY333531), have shown improvements in diabetic neuropathy. One study in obese rats observed that ruboxistaurin increased resting nitric oxide concentration, and reduced nitric oxide by 15%, indicating that this action is a PKC-β dependent phenomenon *(33)*. Ruboxistaurin has been shown to improve nitric oxide-dependent vascular and autonomic nerve dysfunction in diabetic mice *(46)*. In addition to improving nitric oxide levels, ruboxistaurin improves nerve function and blood flow. Ruboxistaurin corrected the diabetic reduction in sciatic endoneurial blood flow, sciatic motor, and saphenous sensory nerve conduction velocity in diabetic rats *(40,43)*. In another study, the investigators measured sciatic nerve, superior cervical ganglion blood flow, and nerve conduction velocity in STZ treated rats. After 8 weeks, the authors observed that diabetes reduced sciatic nerve and superior cervical ganglion blood flow by 50% and produced deficits in saphenous nerve sensory conduction velocity *(48)*. After 2 weeks of treatment with ruboxistaurin, the sciatic nerve, and ganglion blood flow were improved. Additionally, nerve dysfunction is commonly attributed to alterations of the nerve transporters. Other studies demonstrated that a specific inhibitor of the PKC-β, (ruboxistaurin), prevents PMA-dependent activation of Na^+, K^+-ATPase in rats *(44,45)*. In addition to improvements with blood flow nerve function and ion transport, ruboxistaurin corrected thermal hyperalgesia *(48,49)*.

These observations have been supported in preliminary clinical studies. In healthy humans, ruboxistaurin blocked the reduction in endothelium-dependent vasodilation induced by acute hyperglycemia *(47)*, suggesting that the hyperglycemic effects on vasodilation are mediated through PKC-β. More recently, a 1-year double-blind, parallel clinical trial with 205 patients with type 1 or 2 diabetes and DPN was performed to assess the impact of ruboxistaurin on vibration perception in patients with DPN compared with placebo. In patients with DPN, ruboxistaurin treatment improved symptoms and vibratory sensation with a significant correlation between the two compared with placebo group *(50)*. Another recent report indicates that ruboxistaurin is particularly effective in neuropathy patients with intact sural nerve amplitudes *(51)*. A phase II study using NTSS-6 to assess the intensity and frequency of sensory neuropathy symptoms further suggested that ruboxistaurin slows the progression of hyperglycemia-induced microvascular damage *(52)*. Together, these studies support the belief underlying a role for PKC-β in the etiology of diabetes-induced neuropathy.

Vascular Endothelial Growth Factor

The most potent stimulus for angiogenesis is VEGF. If the pathogenesis of diabetic neuropathy goes through loss of vasa nervorum, it is likely that appropriate application of VEGF would reverse the dysfunction. Normally, VEGF activity is induced by tissue hypoxia *(53,54)*. In diabetes it is just such hypoxia that results in increased VEGF activity in the retina, with subsequent pathological angiogenesis *(55)*. Conflicting reports indicated that VEGF in diabetes goes up *(56)* and goes down *(57)*. One possibility to explain this is whether the animals were treated with insulin, which can reduce VEGF expression *(56)*. Only recently it has been demonstrated that there is a reduction in VEGF activity in STZ-diabetic mice that results in failure of neovascularization in hypoxic tissue in the lower limb *(57)*. Furthermore, in the same study it was shown that intramuscular injection of an adenoviral vector encoding for VEGF could induce normal neovascularization in the hindlimb. There have been no human studies of VEGF, and caution is the best approach given the demonstrated pathological effects of VEGF in the retina in diabetes.

Vasodilators

Microvascular insufficiency, endoneurial blood flow, and hemodynamic factors lead to nerve damage in patients with DPN *(58–62)*. Although, the sequence of events is not well understood, investigators propose that microvascular vasoconstriction, edema, and ischemia play a role in DPN development. Endoneurial edema increases endoneurial pressure *(63)*, thereby causing capillary closure and subsequent nerve ischemia and damage *(64,65)*. A diminished regulation of the endoneurial blood flow and ischemia may result from decreased nerve density and innervation of vessels *(66)*, measured with laser Doppler *(67)*. Nerve ischemia stimulates VEGF production exacerbating DPN through overactivation of PKC-β *(56,68–72)*. As a result, ischemia and low blood flow reduces both endothelial dependent and nitric-oxide dependent vasorelaxation nangle

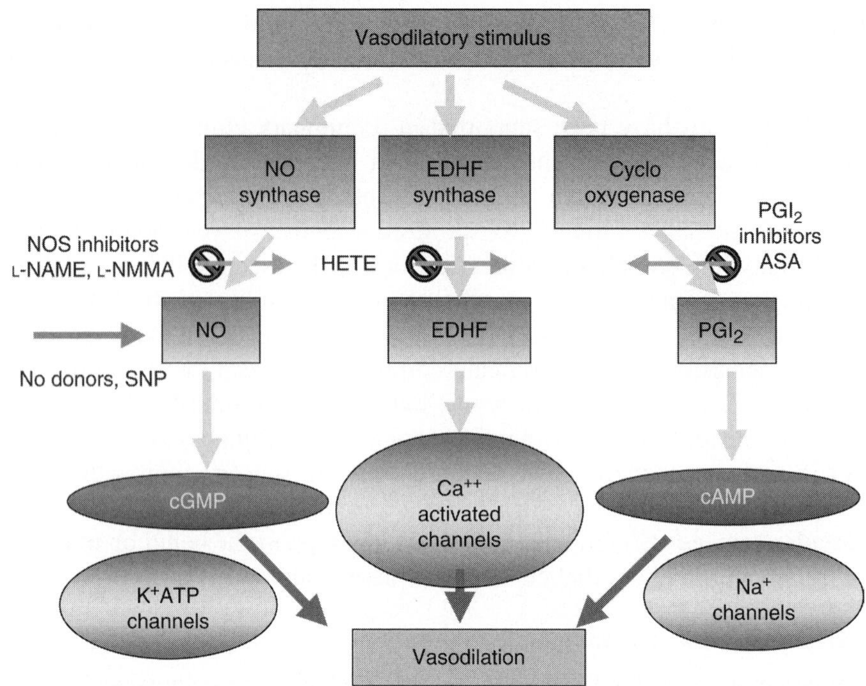

Fig. 3. Mechanisms of peripheral vasodilation and agents being investigated for improving peripheral neurovascular function in diabetes.

(46,73,74). Vascular defects also result in changes in endoneurial vessels. Epineurial changes include arteriolar attenuation, venous distension, arteriovenous shunting that leads to new vessel formation *(75)*. Neural regulation of blood flow is complicated by arteriovenous anastomoses and shunting, which deviate the blood flow from the skin creating an ischemic microenvironment *(76)*. There is thickening and deposition of substances in the vessel wall associated with endothelial cell growth, pericyte loss (in eyes), and occlusion *(77)* Changes in blood flow correlate with changes in oxygen saturation *(60,78)* and reduced sural nerve endoneurial oxygen tension *(79)*. These changes are followed by increased expression or action of vasoconstrictors, such as endothelin and angiotensin and decreased activity of vasodilators, such as prostacyclin, substance P, CGRP, endothelial derived hyperpolarizing factor, and bradykinin *(80,81)*. Based on this theory, investigators have given oxygen and vasodilatory agents to patients, however, these therapies have not improved DPN *(82,83)*. Additionally, methods of assessing skin blood flow have demonstrated that diabetes disturbs microvasculature, tissue PO_2, and vascular permeability. In particular, in patients with DPN there is disruption in vasomotion, the rhythmic contraction exhibited by arterioles, and small arteries *(84,85)*. In Type 2 diabetes, skin blood flow is abnormal and the loss of neurogenic vasodilative mechanism in hairy skin may precede lower limb microangiopathic processes and C-fiber dysfunction *(85,86)*. Changes in endoneurial blood flow often are reflected by changes in nerve conduction *(8,87–89)*. In addition, impaired blood flow can predict ulceration *(2,90–93)*. Therefore, both vascular or endoneural alterations may cause damage over time in the peripheral nerves of patients with diabetes (Fig. 3).

THERAPIES TARGETING AUTOIMMUNITY

Traditional therapies for autoimmune neuropathies have proven beneficial for certain types of diabetic neuropathy *(94)*. Plasmaphoresis and steroidal anti-inflammatories should be considered if the diagnosis is proximal diabetic neuropathy (diabetic amyotrophy) or demyelinating neuropathy. Failure of these treatments or evidence of autoimmunity in typical diabetic polyneuropathy might warrant anti-immune approaches.

Human Intravenous Immunoglobulin

Immune intervention with human intravenous immunoglobulin (IVIg) has become appropriate in some patients with forms of peripheral diabetic neuropathy that are associated with signs of antineuronal autoimmunity *(94,95)*. Chronic inflammatory demyelinating polyneuropathy associated with diabetes is particularly responsive to IVIg infusion. Treatment with immunoglobulin is well tolerated and is considered safe, especially with respect to viral transmission *(96)*. The major toxicity of IVIg has been an anaphylactic reaction, but the frequency of these reactions is now low and confined mainly to patients with immunoglobulin (usually IgA) deficiency. Patients may experience severe headache because of aseptic meningitis, which resolves spontaneously. In some instances, it may be necessary to combine treatment with prednisone and/or azathioprine. Relapses may occur requiring repeated courses of therapy.

THERAPIES FOR NERVE REGENERATION

Neurotrophins

Neurotrophic factors are proteins that promote survival of neurons regulating gene expression through second messenger systems. These proteins may induce morphological changes, nerve differentiation, nerve cell proliferation, and induce neurotransmitter expression and release. Subsequently, reduction in levels of neurotrophic factors *(97)* can lead to neuronal loss, possibly through activation of apoptosis *(98)*. Many proteins have properties and characteristics of neurotrophic factors, including cytokine-like growth factors, TGF-β, NT3, nerve growth factor (NGF), insulin-like growth factor (IGF)-1, and VEGF. Although only a few neurotrophic factors have been extensively investigated, there are number of proteins that have been identified as neurotrophic factors *(31,99)*. Many of these proteins appear to have altered expression in nerves of patients with diabetes *(77)*. For example, interleukin-6, a cytokine-like growth factor may play a role in cell proliferation *(100)*. Although their function is not well understood, IGFs-I and -II have been shown to regulate growth and differentiation of neurons *(101)*. IGF, NGF, and other neurotrophins have been shown to be members of a family of proteins supporting the growth and regeneration of neurons. Often these growth factors are associated with changes in nerve structure through apoptosis or proliferation. The laminin γ gene is upregulated in normal animals undergoing postsection sciatic nerve regeneration *(102,103)*. This process is impaired in diabetes. Other extracellular matrix proteins are also altered in neuropathic nerves *(104)*. Therefore, understanding the role of neurotrophic factors has been the focus of much investigation.

Nerve Growth Factor

Neurons affected in diabetic neuropathy are developmentally dependent on NGF. Therefore, a decline in NGF synthesis in patients with diabetes plays a role in the pathogenesis of neuropathy, especially small fibers *(105)*. More specifically, NGF has been shown to be trophic for sympathetic ganglion neurons and neural crest-derived system *(99)*. Neurotrophins, including NGF, bind to high-affinity receptors, Trk (tropomyosin-related kinases) *(106)* or low-affinity receptors p75 *(107)*; both receptors may activate different signaling cascades.

Neurotrophic proteins are reduced in patients with diabetes. NGF protein levels in the serum of patients with diabetes are suppressed *(108)*. Additionally, diabetes might result in decreased serum IGF and increased IGF-I binding protein-I *(109)* thereby inhibiting the protein's downstream effects. Despite increasing evidence that growth factors are suppressed in patients with diabetes, there is no direct link between neurotrophic factors and the pathogenesis of diabetic neuropathy *(99)* and preliminary studies of both NGF and NT3 treatment have met with limited success.

There is now considerable evidence in animal models of diabetes that decreased expression of NGF and its high-affinity receptor, trk A, reduces retrograde axonal transport of NGF and diminishes support of small unmyelinated neurons and their neuropeptides, such as substance P and CGRP—both potent vasodilators *(110–112)*. Furthermore, recombinant human NGF (rhNGF) administration restores these neuropeptide levels toward normal and prevents the manifestations of sensory neuropathy in animals *(113)*. In a 15 center, double-blind, placebo-controlled study of the safety and efficacy of rhNGF in 250 subjects with symptomatic small fiber neuropathy *(19)*, rhNGF improved the neurological impairment score of the lower limbs, and improved small nerve fiber function cooling threshold (Aδ-fibers) and the ability to perceive heat pain (C-fiber) compared with placebo *(114)*. These results were consistent with the postulated actions of NGF on trk A receptors present on small fiber neurons. This led to two large multicenter studies conducted in the US and the rest of the world. Results of these two studies were presented at the ADA meetings in June 1999 *(115)*. Regrettably, rhNGF was not found to have beneficial effects on and above placebo. The reason for this dichotomy has not been resolved, but this has somewhat dampened the enthusiasm for growth factor therapy of diabetic neuropathy.

ANTICONVULSANT DRUGS

Although the anticonvulsants, including carbamazepine, phenytoin, and gabapentin, have been effective in treating painful diabetic neuropathy (*see* Chapter 21), newer classes of anticonvulsants have shown surprising promise in treating both the symptomatic pain of diabetic neuropathy and the neuronal deficits.

Topiramate

Topiramate is a fructose analog that was initially examined because of its antidiabetic possibilities. Although it is an anticonvulsant used in complex partial seizures, topiramate was recently shown to be efficacious in the management of neuropathic pain *(116)*. Unfortunately, it was first examined only in normal animals and had no hypoglycemic properties. It has now undergone extensive testing for epilepsy, migraine, involuntary movements, central nervous system injury, and neuropathic pain. The first two studies used a titration to 400 mg/day, which was associated with fairly severe central nervous system side effects, which were prohibitive. The studies failed to establish an effect in diabetic neuropathic pain. A third study using different end points, with specificity for the nature and site of the pain and recognizing that a side effect of the drug paresthesia, might be mistaken for pain was successful *(117)*. What has emerged from all the studies is that the drug lowers blood pressure, improves lipid profiles, decreases insulin resistance, and increases nerve fiber regeneration in the skin *(118)*.

Topiramate has the potential to relieve pain by altering the biology of the disease and has now been shown to increase intraepidermal nerve fiber length and density *(118)*. Further, trials are being done. One must start with no more than 15 mg/day, preferably at night and then increase the dose only after the patient can tolerate the drug. A maximum of 200 mg was sufficient to induce nerve fiber recovery.

CONCLUSION

As can be gathered from this list, the pathogenesis of diabetic neuropathy is complex and it is important to understand the underlying pathology leading to the complication in order to best tailor treatment for each individual patient. It is unlikely that reversing any single mechanism will prove sufficient for reversing nerve damage. Several of the drugs mentioned here can have effects on multiple systems that are compromised in diabetic neuropathy, yet even those may not be enough to completely restore neurological function. Combination therapy may prove to be the best long-term approach, and studies of those combinations should prove revealing as to the relative roles of metabolic dysfunction, microvascular insufficiency and autoimmunity in the diabetic neuropathy patient population.

REFERENCES

1. Vinik AI, Pittenger GL, Barlow P, Mehrabyan A. Diabetic Neuropathies: An overview of clinical aspects, pathogenesis, and treatment. In *Diabetes Mellitus: A Fundamental and Clinical Text,* 3rd ed. (LeRoith D, Taylor SI, Olefsky JM, eds.), Philadelphia, PA, Lippincott Williams and Wilkins, 2004.
2. DCCT Research Group. The effect of intensive treatment of diabetes on the development and progression of long-term complications in insulin-dependent diabetes mellitus. *N Engl J Med* 1993;329:977–986.
3. United Kingdom Prospective Diabetes Study Group. United Kingdom prospective diabetes study (UKPDS) 13: relative efficacy of randomly allocated diet, sulphonylurea, insulin, or metformin in patients with newly diagnosed non-insulin dependent diabetes followed for three years. *BMJ* 1995;310:83–88.
4. Ziegler D, Sohr CG, Nourooz-Zadeh J. Oxidative stress and antioxidant defense in relation to the severity of diabetic polyneuropathy and cardiovascular autonomic neuropathy. *Diabetes Care* 2004;27:2178–2183.
5. Vincent AM, Russell JW, Low P, Feldman EL. Oxidative stress in the pathogenesis of diabetic neuropathy. *Endocr Rev* 2004;25:612–628.
6. Cameron NE, Cotter MA, Horrobin DH, Tritschler HJ. Effects of alpha-lipoic acid on neurovascular function in diabetic rats: interaction with essential fatty acids. *Diabetologia* 1998;41:390–399.
7. Stevens MJ, Obrosova I, Cao X, Van Huysen C, Greene DA. Effects of DL-alpha-lipoic acid on peripheral nerve conduction, blood flow, energy metabolism, and oxidative stress in experimental diabetic neuropathy. *Diabetes* 2000;49:1006–1015.
8. Coppey LJ, Gellett JS, Davidson EP, Dunlap JA, Lund DD, Yorek MA. Effect of antioxidant treatment of streptozotocin-induced diabetic rats on endoneurial blood flow, motor nerve conduction velocity, and vascular reactivity of epineurial arterioles of the sciatic nerve. *Diabetes* 2001;50:1927–1937.

9. Ziegler D, Gries FA. Alpha-lipoic acid in the treatment of diabetic peripheral and cardiac autonomic neuropathy. *Diabetes* 1997;46(Suppl 2):S62–66.
10. Ziegler D, Hanefeld M, Ruhnau KJ, et al. Treatment of symptomatic diabetic polyneuropathy with the antioxidant alpha-lipoic acid: a 7-month multicenter randomized controlled trial (ALADIN III Study). ALADIN III Study Group. Alpha-Lipoic Acid in Diabetic Neuropathy. *Diabetes Care* 1999;22:1296–1301.
11. Ziegler D, Schatz H, Conrad F, Gries FA, Ulrich H, Reichel G. Effects of treatment with the antioxidant alpha-lipoic acid on cardiac autonomic neuropathy in NIDDM patients. A 4-month randomized controlled multicenter trial (DEKAN Study). Deutsche Kardiale Autonome Neuropathie. *Diabetes Care* 1997;20:369–373.
12. Jamal GA. The use of gamma linolenic acid in the prevention and treatment of diabetic neuropathy. *Diabet Med* 1994;11:145–149.
13. Keen H, Payan J, Allawi J, et al. Treatment of diabetic neuropathy with gamma-linolenic acid. The gamma-linolenic acid multicenter trial group. *Diabetes Care* 1993;16:8–15.
14. Keen H, Payan J, Allawi J, et al. Treatment of diabetic neuropathy with g-linolenic acid. *Diabetes Care* 1993;16:8–15.
15. Davi G, Ciabattoni G, Consoli A, et al. In vivo formation of 8-iso-prostaglandin f2alpha and platelet activation in diabetes mellitus: effects of improved metabolic control and vitamin E supplementation. *Circulation* 1999;99:224–229.
16. Fuller CJ, Chandalia M, Garg A, Grundy SM, Jialal I. RRR-alpha-tocopheryl acetate supplementation at pharmacologic doses decreases low-density-lipoprotein oxidative susceptibility but not protein glycation in patients with diabetes mellitus. *Am J Clin Nutr* 1996;63:753–759.
17. Ruffini I, Belcaro G, Cesarone MR, et al. Evaluation of the local effects of vitamin E (E-Mousse) on free radicals in diabetic microangiopathy: a randomized, controlled trial. *Angiology* 2003;54:415–421.
18. Beckman JA, Goldfine AB, Gordon MB, Garrett LA, Keaney JF Jr, Creager MA. Oral antioxidant therapy improves endothelial function in Type 1 but not Type 2 diabetes mellitus. *Am J Physiol Heart Circ Physiol* 2003;285:H2392–H2398.
19. Schmidt RE, Dorsey DA, Beaudet LN, Reiser KM, Williamson JR, Tilton RG. Effect of aminoguanidine on the frequency of neuroaxonal dystrophy in the superior mesenteric sympathetic autonomic ganglia of rats with streptozotocin-induced diabetes. *Diabetes* 45 1996;284–290.
20. Miyauchi Y, Shikama H, Takasu T, et al. Slowing of peripheral motor nerve conduction was ameliorated by aminoguanidine in streptozocin-induced diabetic rats. *Eur J Endocrinol* 1996;134:467–473.
21. Vasan S, Zhang X, Kapurniotu A, et al. An agent cleaving glucose-derived protein crosslinks in vitro and in vivo. *Nature* 1996;382:275–278.
22. Oturai PS, Christensen M, Rolin B, Pedersen KE, Mortensen SB, Boel E. Effects of advanced glycation end-product inhibition and cross-link breakage in diabetic rats. *Metabolism* 2000;49:996–1000.
23. Nargi SE, Colen LB, Liuzzi F, Al-Abed Y, Vinik AI. PTB treatment restores joint mobility in a new model of diabetic cheirothropathy. *Diabetes* 1999;48:A17.
24. Vasan S, Foiles P, Founds H. Therapeutic potential of breakers of advanced glycation end product-protein crosslinks. *Arch Biochem Biophys* 2003;419:89–96.
25. Mellor H, Parker PJ. The extended protein kinase C superfamily. *Biochem J* 1998;332 (Pt 2):281–292.
26. Way KJ, Chou E, King GL. Identification of PKC-isoform-specific biological actions using pharmacological approaches. *Trends Pharmacol Sci* 2000;21:181–187.
27. Way KJ, Katai N, King GL. Protein kinase C and the development of diabetic vascular complications. *Diabet Med* 2001;18:945–959.

28. Inoguchi T, Battan R, Handler E, Sportsman JR, Heath W, King GL. Preferential elevation of protein kinase C isoform beta II and diacylglycerol levels in the aorta and heart of diabetic rats: differential reversibility to glycemic control by islet cell transplantation. *Proc Natl Acad Sci USA* 1992;89:11,059–11,063.
29. Nishizuka Y. Intracellular signaling by hydrolysis of phospholipids and activation of protein kinase C. *Science* 1992;258:607–614.
30. Suzuma K, Takahara N, Suzuma I, et al. Characterization of protein kinase C beta isoform's action on retinoblastoma protein phosphorylation, vascular endothelial growth factor-induced endothelial cell proliferation, and retinal neovascularization. *Proc Natl Acad Sci USA* 2002;99:721–726.
31. Leinninger GM, Vincent AM, Feldman EL. The role of growth factors in diabetic peripheral neuropathy. *J Peripher Nerv Syst* 2004;9:26–53.
32. Ishii H, Koya D, King GL. Protein kinase C activation and its role in the development of vascular complications in diabetes mellitus. *J Mol Med* 1998;76:21–31.
33. Bohlen HG, Nase GP. Arteriolar nitric oxide concentration is decreased during hyperglycemia-induced betaII PKC activation. *Am J Physiol Heart Circ Physiol* 2001;280:H621–H627.
34. Nonaka A, Kiryu J, Tsujikawa A, et al. PKC-beta inhibitor (LY333531) attenuates leukocyte entrapment in retinal microcirculation of diabetic rats. *Invest Ophthalmol Vis Sci* 2000;41:2702–2706.
35. Shiba T, Inoguchi T, Sportsman JR, Heath WF, Bursell S, King GL. Correlation of diacylglycerol level and protein kinase C activity in rat retina to retinal circulation. *Am J Physiol* 1993;265:E783–793.
36. Aiello LP, Bursell SE, Clermont A, et al. Vascular endothelial growth factor-induced retinal permeability is mediated by protein kinase C in vivo and suppressed by an orally effective beta-isoform-selective inhibitor. *Diabetes* 1997;46:1473–1480.
37. Ishii H, Jirousek MR, Koya D, et al. Amelioration of vascular dysfunctions in diabetic rats by an oral PKC beta inhibitor. *Science* 1996;272:728–731.
38. Bursell SE, Takagi C, Clermont AC, et al. Specific retinal diacylglycerol and protein kinase C beta isoform modulation mimics abnormal retinal hemodynamics in diabetic rats. *Invest Ophthalmol Vis Sci* 1997;38:2711–2720.
39. Danis RP, Bingaman DP, Jirousek M, Yang Y. Inhibition of intraocular neovascularization caused by retinal ischemia in pigs by PKCbeta inhibition with LY333531. *Invest Ophthalmol Vis Sci* 1998;39:171–179.
40. Nakamura J, Kato K, Hamada Y, et al. A protein kinase C-beta-selective inhibitor ameliorates neural dysfunction in streptozotocin-induced diabetic rats. *Diabetes* 1999;48:2090–2095.
41. Koya D, Haneda M, Nakagawa H, et al. Amelioration of accelerated diabetic mesangial expansion by treatment with a PKC beta inhibitor in diabetic db/db mice, a rodent model for type 2 diabetes. *FASEB J* 2000;14:439–447.
42. Kelly DJ, Zhang Y, Hepper C, et al. Protein kinase C beta inhibition attenuates the progression of experimental diabetic nephropathy in the presence of continued hypertension. *Diabetes* 2003;52:512–518.
43. Cameron NE, Cotter MA. Effects of protein kinase Cbeta inhibition on neurovascular dysfunction in diabetic rats: interaction with oxidative stress and essential fatty acid dysmetabolism. *Diabetes Metab Res Rev* 2002;18:315–323.
44. Efendiev R, Bertorello AM, Pedemonte CH. PKC-beta and PKC-zeta mediate opposing effects on proximal tubule Na^+,K^+-ATPase activity. *FEBS Lett* 1999;456:45–48.
45. Kowluru RA, Jirousek MR, Stramm L, Farid N, Engerman RL, Kern TS. Abnormalities of retinal metabolism in diabetes or experimental galactosemia: V. Relationship between protein kinase C and ATPases. *Diabetes* 1998;47:464–469.
46. Nangle MR, Cotter MA, Cameron NE. Protein kinase C beta inhibition and aorta and corpus cavernosum function in streptozotocin-diabetic mice. *Eur J Pharmacol* 2003;475:99–106.

47. Beckman JA, Goldfine AB, Gordon MB, Garrett LA, Creager MA. Inhibition of protein kinase Cbeta prevents impaired endothelium-dependent vasodilation caused by hyperglycemia in humans. *Circ Res* 2002;90:107–111.
48. Cotter MA, Jack AM, Cameron NE. Effects of the protein kinase C beta inhibitor LY333531 on neural and vascular function in rats with streptozotocin-induced diabetes. *Clin Sci* (Lond) 2002;103:311–321.
49. Kim H, Sasaki T, Maeda K, Koya D, Kashiwagi A, Yasuda H. Protein kinase Cbeta selective inhibitor LY333531 attenuates diabetic hyperalgesia through ameliorating cGMP level of dorsal root ganglion neurons. *Diabetes* 2003;52:2102–2109.
50. Vinik AI, Kles K. Pathophysiology and treatment of diabetic peripheral neuropathy. *Curr Diabetes Rev* 2005 (in press).
51. Vinik AI, Bril V, Litchy WJ, Price KL, Bastyr EJ 3rd, MBBG Study Group. Sural sensory action potential identifies diabetic peripheral neuropathy responders to therapy. *Muscle Nerve* 2005;32:619–625.
52. Vinik AI, Bril V, Kempler P, et al. Treatment of symptomatic diabetic peripheral neuropathy with the protein kinase Cbeta-inhibitor ruboxistaurin mesylate during a 1-year, randomized, placebo-controlled, double-blind clinical trial. *Clin Ther* 2005;27:1164–1180.
53. Shweiki D, Itin A, Soffer D, Keshet E. Vascular endothelial growth factor induced by hypoxia may mediate hypoxia-initiated angiogenesis. *Nature* 1992;359:843–845.
54. Vincent KA, Shyu KG, Luo Y, et al. Angiogenesis is induced in a rabbit model of hindlimb ischemia by naked DNA encoding an HIF-1alpha/VP16 hybrid transcription factor. *Circulation* 2000;102:2255–2261.
55. Aiello LP, Avery RL, Arrigg PG, et al. Vascular endothelial growth factor in ocular fluid of patients with diabetic retinopathy and other retinal disorders. *N Engl J Med* 1994;331: 1480–1487.
56. Samii A, Unger J, Lange W. Vascular endothelial growth factor expression in peripheral nerves and dorsal root ganglia in diabetic neuropathy in rats. *Neurosci Lett* 1999;262:159–162.
57. Rivard A, Silver M, Chen D, et al. Rescue of diabetes-related impairment of angiogenesis by intramuscular gene therapy with adeno-VEGF. *Am J Pathol* 1999;154:355–363.
58. Tesfaye S, Malik R, Ward JD. Vascular factors in diabetic neuropathy. *Diabetologia* 1994;37:847–854.
59. Malik RA, Tesfaye S, Thompson SD, et al. Endoneurial localisation of microvascular damage in human diabetic neuropathy. *Diabetologia* 1993;36:454–459.
60. Tesfaye S, Harris N, Jakubowski JJ, et al. Impaired blood flow and arterio-venous shunting in human diabetic neuropathy: a novel technique of nerve photography and fluorescein angiography. *Diabetologia* 1993;36:1266–1274.
61. Malik RA, Tesfaye S, Thompson SD, et al. Transperineurial capillary abnormalities in the sural nerve of patients with diabetic neuropathy. *Microvascular Res* 1994;48:236–245.
62. Eaton SE, Harris ND, Ibrahim S, et al. Increased sural nerve epineurial blood flow in human subjects with painful diabetic neuropathy. *Diabetologia* 2003;46:934–939.
63. Griffey RH, Eaton RP, Sibbitt RR, Sibbitt WL Jr, Bicknell JM. Diabetic neuropathy. Structural analysis of nerve hydration by magnetic resonance spectroscopy. *JAMA* 1988; 260:2872–2878.
64. Dyck PJ, Hansen S, Karnes J, et al. Capillary number and percentage closed in human diabetic sural nerve. *Proc Natl Acad Sci USA* 1985;82:2513–2517.
65. Myers RR, Powell HC. Galactose neuropathy: impact of chronic endoneurial edema on nerve blood flow. *Ann Neurol* 1984;16:587–594.
66. Teunissen LL, Veldink J, Notermans NC, Bleys RL. Quantitative assessment of the innervation of epineurial arteries in the peripheral nerve by immunofluorescence: differences between controls and patients with peripheral arterial disease. *Acta Neuropathol (Berl)* 2002;103:475–480.

67. Theriault M, Dort J, Sutherland G, Zochodne DW. Local human sural nerve blood flow in diabetic and other polyneuropathies. *Brain* 1997;120:1131–1138.
68. Schratzberger P, Schratzberger G, Silver M, et al. Favorable effect of VEGF gene transfer on ischemic peripheral neuropathy. *Nat Med* 2000;6:405–413.
69. Schratzberger P, Walter DH, Rittig K, et al. Reversal of experimental diabetic neuropathy by VEGF gene transfer. *J Clin Invest* 2001;107:1083–1092.
70. Oosthuyse B, Moons L, Storkebaum E, et al. Deletion of the hypoxia-response element in the vascular endothelial growth factor promoter causes motor neuron degeneration. *Nat Genet* 2001;28:131–138.
71. Williams B, Gallacher B, Patel H, Orme C. Glucose-induced protein kinase C activation regulates vascular permeability factor mRNA expression and peptide production by human vascular smooth muscle cells in vitro. *Diabetes* 1997;46:1497–1503.
72. Koya D, Jirousek MR, Lin YW, Ishii H, Kuboki K, King GL. Characterization of protein kinase C beta isoform activation on the gene expression of transforming growth factor-beta, extracellular matrix components, and prostanoids in the glomeruli of diabetic rats. *J Clin Invest* 1997;100:115–126.
73. Kihara M, Low PA. Impaired vasoreactivity to nitric oxide in experimental diabetic neuropathy. *Exp Neurol* 1995;132:180–185.
74. Cameron NE, Cotter MA, Archibald V, Dines KC, Maxfield EK. Anti-oxidant and pro-oxidant effects on nerve conduction velocity, endoneurial blood flow and oxygen tension in non-diabetic and streptozotocin-diabetic rats. *Diabetologia* 1994;37:449–459.
75. Boulton AJ, Malik RA. Diabetic neuropathy. *Med Clin North Am* 1998;82:909–929.
76. Vinik AI, Erbas T, Stansberry KB, Pittenger GL. Small fiber neuropathy and neurovascular disturbances in diabetes mellitus. *Exp Clin Endocrinol Diabetes* 2001;109(Suppl 2): S451–S473.
77. Boulton AJ, Malik RA, Arezzo JC, Sosenko JM. Diabetic somatic neuropathies. *Diabetes Care* 2004;27:1458–1486.
78. Ibrahim S, Harris ND, Radatz M, et al. A new minimally invasive technique to show nerve ischaemia in diabetic neuropathy. *Diabetologia* 1999;42:737–742.
79. Newrick PG, Wilson AJ, Jakubowski J, Boulton AJ, Ward JD. Sural nerve oxygen tension in diabetes. *Br Med J (Clin Res Ed)* 1986;293:1053–1054.
80. Kakizawa H, Itoh M, Itoh Y, et al. The relationship between glycemic control and plasma vascular endothelial growth factor and endothelin-1 concentration in diabetic patients. *Metabolism* 2004;53:550–555.
81. Schneider JG, Tilly N, Hierl T, et al. Elevated plasma endothelin-1 levels in diabetes mellitus. *Am J Hypertens* 2002;15:967–972.
82. Aydin A, Ozden BC, Karamursel S, Solakoglu S, Aktas S, Erer M. Effect of hyperbaric oxygen therapy on nerve regeneration in early diabetes. *Microsurgery* 2004;24:255–261.
83. Caselli A, Rich J, Hanane T, Uccioli L, Veves A. Role of C-nociceptive fibers in the nerve axon reflex-related vasodilation in diabetes. *Neurology* 2003;60:297–300.
84. Shapiro SA, Stansberry KB, Hill MA, et al. Normal blood flow response and vasomotion in the diabetic Charcot foot. *J Diabetes Complications* 1998;12:147–153.
85. Stansberry KB, Shapiro SA, Hill MA, McNitt PM, Meyer MD, Vinik AI. Impaired peripheral vasomotion in diabetes. *Diabetes Care* 1996;19:715–721.
86. Stansberry KB, Peppard HR, Babyak LM, Popp G, McNitt PM, Vinik AI. Primary nociceptive afferents mediate the blood flow dysfunction in non-glabrous (hairy) skin of type 2 diabetes: a new model for the pathogenesis of microvascular dysfunction. *Diabetes Care* 1999;22:1549–1554.
87. Coppey LJ, Gellett JS, Davidson EP, Dunlap JA, Yorek MA. Changes in endoneurial blood flow, motor nerve conduction velocity and vascular relaxation of epineurial arterioles of the sciatic nerve in ZDF-obese diabetic rats. *Diabetes Metab Res Rev* 2002;18:49–56.

88. Coppey LJ, Gellett JS, Davidson EP, et al. Effect of M40403 treatment of diabetic rats on endoneurial blood flow, motor nerve conduction velocity and vascular function of epineurial arterioles of the sciatic nerve. *Br J Pharmacol* 2001;134:21–29.
89. Coppey LJ, Davidson EP, Dunlap JA, Lund DD, Yorek MA. Slowing of motor nerve conduction velocity in streptozotocin-induced diabetic rats is preceded by impaired vasodilation in arterioles that overlie the sciatic nerve. *Int J Exp Diabetes Res* 2000;1:131–143.
90. Herrmann DN, Griffin JW, Hauer P, Cornblath DR, McArthur JC. Epidermal nerve fiber density and sural nerve morphometry in peripheral neuropathies. *Neurology* 1999;53: 1634–1640.
91. Greene DA, Stevens MJ, Obrosova I, Feldman EL. Glucose-induced oxidative stress and programmed cell death in diabetic neuropathy. *Eur J Pharmacol* 1999;375:217–223.
92. Consensus statement: Report and recommendations of the San Antonio conference on diabetic neuropathy. American Diabetes Association & American Academy of Neurology. *Diabetes Care* 1988;11:592–597.
93. Dyck PJ, Karnes JL, O'Brien PC, Litchy WJ, Low PA, Melton III LJ. The Rochester Diabetic Neuropathy Study: Reassessment of tests and criteria for diagnosis and staged severity. *Neurology* 1992;42:1164–1170.
94. Krendel DA, Costigan DA, Hopkins LC. Successful treatment of neuropathies in patients with diabetes mellitus. *Arch Neurol* 1995;52:1053–1061.
95. Barada A, Reljanovic M, Milicevic Z, et al. Proximal diabetic neuropathy - response to immunotherapy. *Diabetes* 1999;48(Suppl 1):A148.
96. Suez D. Intravenous immunoglobulin therapy: indication, potential side effects and treatment guidelines. *J Intraven Nurs* 1995;18:178–190.
97. Salis MB, Graiani G, Desortes E, Caldwell RB, Madeddu P, Emanueli C. Nerve growth factor supplementation reverses the impairment, induced by Type 1 diabetes, of hindlimb post-ischaemic recovery in mice. *Diabetologia* 2004;47:1055–1063.
98. Srinivasan S, Stevens M, Wiley JW. Diabetic peripheral neuropathy: evidence for apoptosis and associated mitochondrial dysfunction. *Diabetes* 2000;49:1932–1938.
99. Apfel SC. Neurotrophic factors in the therapy of diabetic neuropathy. *Am J Med* 1999; 107(Suppl 2):S34–S42.
100. Knezevic-Cuca J, Stansberry KB, Johnston G, et al. Neurotrophic role of interleukin-6 and soluble interleukin-6 receptors on N1E-115 neuroblastoma cells. *J Neuroimmunol* 2000;102:8–16.
101. Ishii DN, Glazner GW, Whalen LR. Regulation of peripheral nerve regeneration by insulin-like growth factors. *Ann NY Acad Sci* 1993;692:172–182.
102. LeBeau JM, Liuzzi FJ. Laminin B2 mRNA is up-regulated in sensory neurons and Schwann cells during peripheral nerve regeneration. *Soc Neurosci (Abstract)* 1991; 17:1500.
103. LeBeau JM, Liuzzi FJ, Depto AJ, Vinik AI. Up-regulation of laminin B2 gene expression in dorsal root ganglion neurons and non-neuronal cells during sciatic nerve regeneration. *Exp Neurol* 1995;134:150–155.
104. Bradley JL, King RH, Muddle JR, Thomas PK. The extracellular matrix of peripheral nerve in diabetic polyneuropathy. *Acta Neuropathol (Berl)* 2000;99:539–546.
105. Pittenger GL, Vinik AI. Nerve growth factor and diabetic neuropathy. *Exp Diabesity Res* 2003;4:271–285.
106. Klein R, Nanduri V, Jing SA, et al. The trkB tyrosine protein kinase is a receptor for brain-derived neurotrophic factor and neurotrophin-3. *Cell* 1991;66:395–403.
107. Anton ES, Weskamp G, Reichardt LF, Matthew WD. Nerve growth factor and its low-affinity receptor promote Schwann cell migration. *Proc Natl Acad Sci USA* 1994;91: 2795–2799.
108. Faradji V, Sotelo J. Low serum levels of nerve growth factor in diabetic neuropathy. *Acta Neurol Scand* 1990;81:402–406.

109. Crosby SR, Tsigos C, Anderton CD, Gordon C, Young RJ, White A. Elevated plasma insulin-like growth factor binding protein-1 levels in type 1 (insulin-dependent) diabetic patients with peripheral neuropathy. *Diabetologia* 1992;35:868–872.
110. Diemel LT, Stevens JC, Willars GB, Tomlinson DR. Depletion of substance P and calcitonin gene-related peptide in sciatic nerve of rats with experimental diabetes: effects of insulin and aldose reductase inhibition. *Neurosci Lett* 1992;137:253–256.
111. Hellweg R, Hartung HD, Hock C, Whöhrle M, Raivich G. Nerve growth factor (NGF) changes in rat diabetic neuropathy. *Soc Neurosci (Abstract)* 1991;17:1497.
112. Tomlinson DR, Fernyhough P, Diemel LT. Neurotrophins and peripheral neuropathy. *Philos Trans R Soc Lond B Biol Sci* 1996;351:455–462.
113. Apfel SC, Kessler JA. Neurotropic factors in the therapy of peripheral neuropathy. *Bailliere's Clinical Neurology* 1995;4:593–606.
114. Apfel SC, Kessler JA, Adornato BT, Litchy WJ, Sanders C, Rask CA. Recombinant human nerve growth factor in the treatment of diabetic polyneuropathy. NGF Study Group. *Neurology* 1998;51:695–702.
115. Vinik AI. Treatment of diabetic polyneuropathy (DPN) with recombinant human nerve growth factor (rhNGF). *Diabetes* 1999;48(Suppl 1):A54–A55.
116. Raskin P, Donofrio PD, Rosenthal NR, et al. Topiramate vs placebo in painful diabetic neuropathy: analgesic and metabolic effects. *Neurology* 2004;63:865–873.
117. Vinik A, Hewitt D, Xiang J. Topiramate in the treatment of painful diabetic neuropathy: results from a multicenter, randomized, double-blind, placebo-controlled trial. *Neurology* 2003;60(Suppl 1):A154–A155.
118. Vinik AI, Pittenger GL, Anderson SA, Stansberry K, McNear E, Barlow P. Topiramate improves C-fiber neuropathy and features of the dysmetabolic syndrome in type 2 diabetes. *Diabetes* 2003;52(Suppl 1):A130.

20
Pathophysiology of Neuropathic Pain

Misha-Miroslav Backonja, MD

SUMMARY

Cerebral responses to pain are complex and dynamic in nature and in the case of chronic pain, especially neuropathic pain, changes involved are more profound and they are characterized by the involvement of entire pain-related peripheral and central nervous system. Functional magnetic resonance imaging studies identified a number of cerebral, cortical, and subcortical structures that are activated during pain stimuli. Many of those structures are also active in patient with neuropathic pain. While no specific functional magnetic resonance imaging studies were done with patients with diabetic neuropathy, result of the studies with various neuropathic pain disorders that share fundamental characteristics with painful diabetic neuropathy and are through earlier observations expected to apply to patients with painful diabetic neuropathy. Translational pain research is a new field with a few obstacles. Pain research has to rise and they include lack of clinical and pain translational research standards, lack of clear communication among basic scientists and among clinicians as well as between scientists and clinicians, and lack of standard in measurement tools that cross from bench to bedside and vice versa. However there are strong efforts to advance communication and to develop methods relevant to translational neuropathic pain research.

Key Words: Brain imaging; neuropathic pain; painful diabetic neuropathy; peripheral and central sensitization; translational pain research.

INTRODUCTION

Pathophysiology of neuropathic pain in diabetic neuropathy, also called painful diabetic neuropathy (PDN) is not well understood. Neither basic science nor clinical research provides clear insights into the pathophysiology of PDN. Pathology of the PDN has been predominantly studied at the level of the peripheral nervous system and consequently, all of PDN pathophysiological mechanisms are ascribed to the peripheral nervous system. However, it has been postulated that in addition to peripheral mechanisms, central nervous system mechanisms probably play significant role in the overall manifestations of the PDN *(1)*. Diabetes has effects on many aspects of brain function that are probably subtle, but significant *(2–7)*. These include effects on mood *(2,4)*, which are known to influence modulation of pain perception *(8)* and as such would have effect on perception of pain in case of PDN; however, no study has investigated those

From: *Contemporary Diabetes: Diabetic Neuropathy: Clinical Management, Second Edition*
Edited by: A. Veves and R. Malik © Humana Press Inc., Totowa, NJ

aspects of diabetes. Consequently, this chapter reviews what is known about neuropathic pain in general, with the hope that this information can provide insight into PDN.

CHANGES IN BRAIN

Great advances have been made during last couple of decades in our understanding of the pathophysiology of neuropathic pain, as a result of basic scientific findings of the pathological and biochemical changes in the peripheral and central nervous system. The neuronal changes that take place at the level of human brain as the consequence of peripheral neuronal injury, such as in case of PDN, lead to the processes that maintain neuropathic pain known as central sensitization. Examination of the cerebral correlates of central processes related to pain and central sensitization has only been possible during last decade and a half with introduction of neuroimaging. Noninvasive brain imaging technologies provide the opportunity to directly study human clinical conditions. Initially, blood flow based positron emission tomography (PET) scan was utilized *(9)*, but advantages of functional magnetic resonance imaging (fMRI), such as improved temporal and spatial resolution have made it a method of choice for pain studies *(10,11)*. Electrophysiological studies using evoked potentials and magnetoencephalography have also been used to elucidate cerebral mechanisms related to pain *(12)*. This chapter will review what has been learned about changes in brain as the result of neuropathic pain on the basis of fMRI and electrophysiological studies.

Certainly, the role of brain in pain mechanisms is very complex ranging from the perception and experience of pain, to pain modulation, and to formation of behavioral response to pain. Complexity increases in the case of neurological disorders, such as neuropathic pain, when the brain itself undergoes significant changes. This degree of complexity has been appreciated for a long time, but the means to study underlying mechanisms have not been available until recently. At the present time neuroscience is able to address most general aspects of brain mechanisms related to pain, including neuropathic pain, which will be discussed here.

In spite of rapidly increasing number of pain imaging studies, the number of studies specifically focussed on neuropathic pain is a very limited. On the extensive search of published literature no study of painful diabetic neuropathic has been identified. Consequently, discussion in this chapter is presented with the commonly made assumption that findings from other neuropathic pain disorders, which were studied with brain functional imaging, are applicable to PDN. These assumptions are based on the essential clinical similarities of PDN and other painful neuropathic disorders. Certainly, information about the brain-specific changes that occur as a consequence of PDN will come from future functional imaging studies of pain in patients with diabetic neuropathy.

First functional laboratory studies that helped to identify cerebral structures that participate in pain perception will be briefly reviewed, and this will be followed with the review of studies with chronic pain, including neuropathic pain.

Functional Brain Responses to Acute Laboratory Pain

Current functional brain studies utilize stimulation paradigms to identify brain structure involved in physiological processes, such as pain. Numerous pain studies have been conducted using wide variety of stimulation protocols including thermal pulses from heat and cold thermodes, laser heat pulses, limb immersions into cold or hot temperature baths, thermal grill illusion, capsaicin intradermal injections, and distention of internal organs, such as rectum and esophagus *(11,13–18)*. These studies revealed a number of brain structures that are involved in the experience of pain, and a complex (matrix/network instead?) of brain structures that are involved depends on many factors, including the type and length of stimulus used and experimental conditions. Regional cerebral blood flow (rCBF) increases, which reflects increase in neuronal activity of corresponding brain structures, noxious stimuli are most consistently observed in secondary somatic (SII) and insular cortex (IC) region, and in the anterior cingulate cortex (ACC), and less consistently in the contralateral thalamus and the primary somatic cortical area (SI) *(11,17,19–23)*. Activity of the lateral thalamus, SI, SII, and posterior IC are believed to be related to the sensory-discriminative aspects of pain experience, which provides the subject with the ability to localize the site of stimulation and intensity of stimulus. Activity in SI is observed in less than half of the studies and the probability that SI activation is observed appears to be because of influences such as the stimulated body surface, which would represent spatial summation and the attention to or away form the stimulus *(11,17,19–21,24,25)*. A number of studies reported the thalamic responses as bilateral and this observation would probably reflect generalized arousal in reaction to pain *(17,19,26)*. The ACC appears to participate in the affective and attentional components of pain sensation and in selection of the response to the stimulus *(20,21,25,27,28)*. Functional properties of the ACC from imaging studies would suggest that ACC does not code for stimulus intensity or for location of the stimulus. Increased rCBF in the posterior parietal and prefrontal cortices is probably because of activation of attention and memory-related brain structures in response to noxious stimuli. Activation of motor-system related brain structures, such as the striatum, cerebellum, and supplementary motor area are frequently observable, although not frequently commented on, and they are probably involved in motor planning in response to pain and generating pain-related behaviors. Physiologically, a few brain regions are involved in descending pain control and modulation, such as the periaqueductal gray and brainstem nuclei that at times were imaged, but this area is difficult to image, resulting in inconsistent findings. A significant intersubject variability in the activation of any one of the pain-related cerebral regions, particularly during heat- and cold-evoked pain have been noted *(20,29,30)*. In contrast to nonpainful stimuli which showed only transient responses to the onset or offset, painful stimulation was observed to result in a sustained response throughout its duration in the temporoparietal, inferior frontal cortex (IFC), and ACC. These regions therefore show tonic responses to stimuli with ongoing salience *(31)*. The thalamus and putamen also responded throughout tonically painful, but not nonpainful stimulation. These observations would then implicate the basal ganglia in supporting voluntary sustained attention and would suggest that the basal ganglia may play a more general role in supporting sustained attention.

When visceral stimuli are applied and produce an amount of pain that is reported as equivalent to the intensity of pain applied to skin in the same subjects, the similar overall pattern of activation at the SII and parietal cortices, thalamus, basal ganglia, and cerebellum are observed. However, at the insular, primary somatosensory, motor, and prefrontal cortices there are different patterns of activation, suggesting somewhat different brain correlation for cutaneous vs visceral pain experiences *(32–34)*.

Electrophysiological studies, such as evoked potentials have advantage over fMRI because of superior time resolution. Several dipole source analysis as well as subdural recordings have confirmed that the earliest evoked potential following painful laser stimulation of the skin derives from sources in the parietal operculum. Based on imaging and electrophysiological studies in humans it has been concluded that parasylvian cortex is activated by painful stimuli, and this would be one of the first cortical relay stations in the central processing of these stimuli *(35)*. There is evidence for close location but separate representation in parasylvian cortex of pain in a few areas, such as deep parietal operculum and anterior insula and these are distinct from representations for innocuous touch, such as SII and posterior insula. It is likely that some of these areas are involved in sensory-limbic projection pathways that may subserve the recognition of potentially tissue damaging stimuli as well as pain memory *(35)*. With these types of studies it is possible to initiate further analysis of the functional anatomy specific to sensory-discriminative, affective-motivational, and cognitive-evaluative components of pain.

In summary, there is now ample evidence that a well-defined cerebral network participates in human perception of acute pain paradigms. The areas most consistently observed include: SI, SII, ACC, IC, prefrontal cortex (PFC), thalamus, and cerebellum (Fig. 1.).

Changes With Chronic Pain, Including Neuropathic Pain

Manifestations of chronic pain are fundamentally different from acute pain and attempts have been made to identify those differences in functional imaging and electrophysiological studies. There are many conceptual and technical challenges in studying chronic pain, especially, neuropathic pain because of its complexity. Components of neuropathic pain symptoms include spontaneous ongoing pain, spontaneous paroxysms, and stimulus evoked pain *(36,37)*. It is difficult to gain an accurate picture of this range of symptoms with neuroimaging techniques. Spontaneous paroxysms are unpredictable and random by nature and consequently, almost impossible to study. Imaging of spontaneous ongoing pain is difficult because it is necessary to utilize subtraction from nonpain control state for imaging pain studies, so only patients who can achieve a substantial degree of pain relief can be studied with current imaging technology. Even if these conditions are met, it is difficult to know how this report of relief compares to the pain-free state in nonpatient populations and how neuroplastic changes resulting from chronic pain affect either state. Most of the imaging and electrophysiological studies have therefore concentrated on evoked components of pain. Understanding how these results represent the neural changes that underlie the range of symptoms experienced in syndromes like PDN is an ongoing challenge for chronic pain research.

In patients with chronic spontaneous pain, a few pain-imaging studies revealed relative decreases of resting rCBF in contralateral thalamus, when compared with the ipsilateral side *(38,39)*. These findings suggest that ongoing neuropathic pain because of either central or peripheral etiology is linked to thalamic hypoperfusion and that analgesic treatments are mediated through an increase in thalamic blood flow *(38,40,41)*.

One of the aspects of pain most relevant to the study of chronic pain such as PDN are phenomena of hypersensitivity, such as allodynia or hyperalgesia, depending on whether stimulus is innocuous or noxious, respectively. In patients suffering from

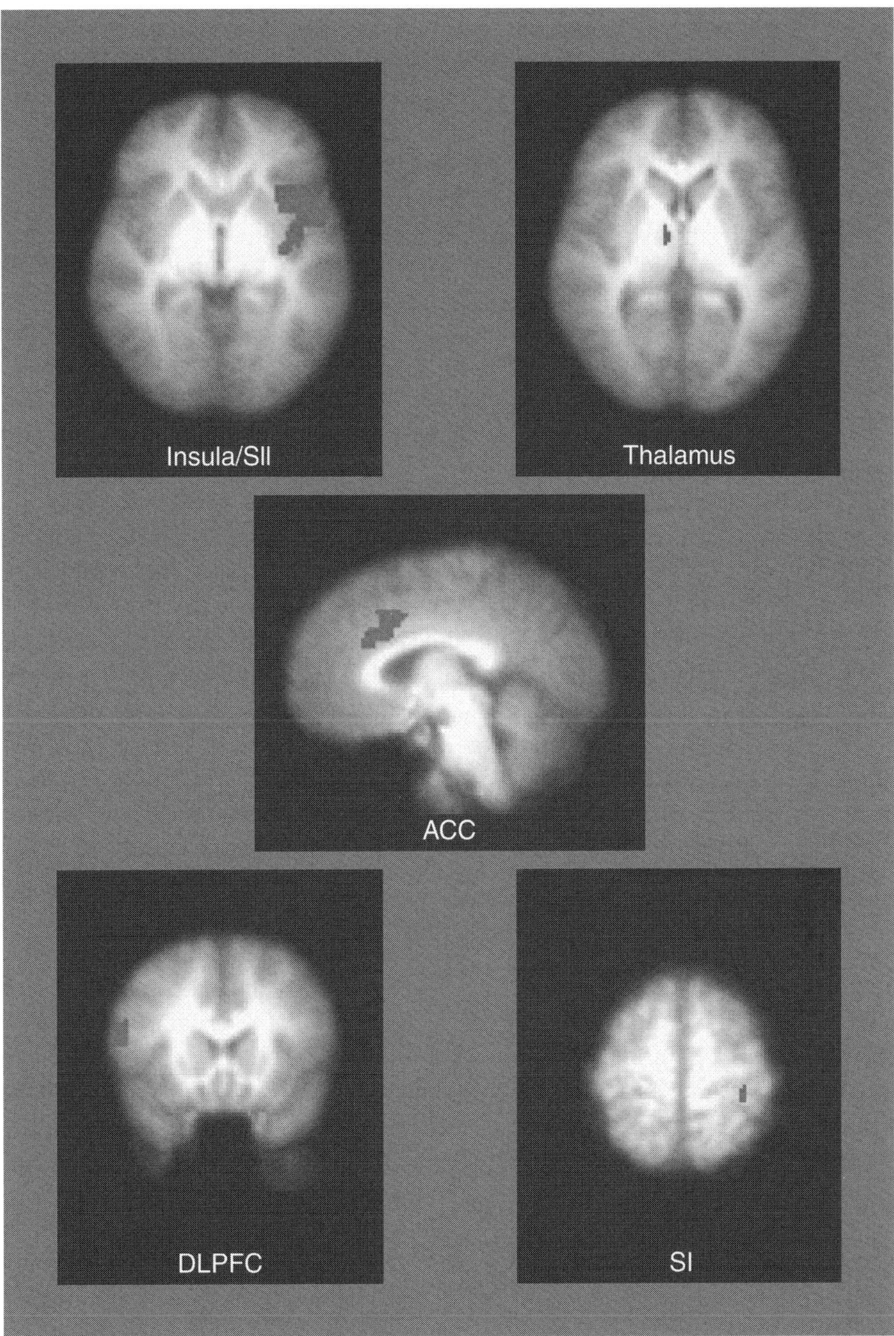

Fig. 1. Regions of brain activated with painful stimuli. Cerebral regions activated by pain are primary somatosensory cortex, secondary sensory cortex/insular cortex, and thalamus seen on horizontal planes, anterior cingulate cortex seen in medial sagittal view and dorsolateral prefrontal cortex on coronal view (Courtesy of Tim Salomons and Regina Lapate, The Waisman laboratory for brain imaging and behavior, University of Wisconsin –Madison).

allodynia, this phenomenon is evoked during PET or fMRI sessions by applying repeated innocuous stimuli. The images from scans obtained during allodynia stimulation are compared either with resting no-stimulation scans, or with an identical stimulation of a nonaffected nonpainful body area.

Brushing the nonpainful limb leads to activations of the contralateral SI, contralateral parietal association cortex (PA), bilateral SII, and contralateral IC, and brushing the skin where patients experience allodynia pain, than cortical responses are partially overlapping with those induced by the nonpainful brush stimulation *(42)*. In addition, the contralateral IFC and the ipsilateral IC are activated. Direct comparison between nonpainful brushing and brush-evoked allodynia revealed significant increases in blood-oxygen-level dependent (BOLD) signals in contralateral SI, PA, IFC, and bilateral SII/IC during allodynia. This study highlights the importance of a cortical network consisting SI, PA, SII/IC, and IFC in the processing of dynamic-mechanical allodynia in the human brain *(42)* and possibly relating to sensory and attentional abnormalities underlying allodynia.

Temporal characteristics of brain responses have also been investigated. The cortical processing of allodynia resulting from neuralgia of the lateral cutaneous femoral nerve was investigated by means of magnetoencephalography *(43,45)*. Brushing the unaffected thigh produced subsequent activation of the contralateral SI with peak latencies of 37 and 56 ms. Allodynic stimulation with brushing of the affected side leads to comparable activation of the contralateral SI cortex but with stronger magnetic fields, and the corresponding equivalent current dipoles located more laterally, suggestive of cortical reorganization and hyperresponsivity. Allodynia is also accompanied by an activation of the cingulate cortex, occurring only 92 ms. after stimulus onset and this observation would suggests that A-β-fiber-mediated neuronal pathways are involved in this type of allodynia. The results cited here support the possibility that cortical reorganization is one of the underlying processes that characterizes allodynia and possibly chronic pain and that early activation of the cingulate cortex may be involved in the cortical processing of allodynia.

When brain activity to acute thermal painful stimuli are examined in chronic pain patients, the resulting pattern is very similar to that seen for acute pain in normal subjects, independent of the type of chronic pain as seen in chronic back pain patients *(46)* and in complex regional pain syndrome patients *(41,47)*. Although chronic pain patients may have various cutaneous sensory abnormalities *(48)*, mapping brain responses to acute pain does not distinguish them from normal subjects. On the other hand, when brain activity specifically related to the chronic pain is isolated then activity seems to be preferentially involving prefrontal cortical regions *(41)*.

Injury of peripheral or central neural tissues leads to long lasting spinal and supraspinal reorganization that includes the forebrain. These forebrain changes may be adaptive and facilitate functional recovery, or they may be maladaptive preventing or prolonging the painful condition and interfering with treatment *(42)*. In an experimental model of heat allodynia, functional brain imaging was used to show that the forebrain activity during heat allodynia is different from that during normal heat pain by increase of dorsolateral prefrontal cortex (DLPFC). Consequently, as it could be argued that during heat allodynia, cortical areas, specifically the DLPFC, can attenuate specific components of the pain experience such as, by reducing the functional connectivity of subcortical pathways. The forebrain of patients with chronic neuropathic pain may undergo pathologically induced changes that can impair the clinical response to treatment *(42)*. Stimuli that are severely painful when applied to the allodynic side, activated regions in the contralateral hemisphere that mirrored the "control" network, with however, lesser activation of the SII and insular cortices in patients with neuropathic pain *(49)*. Increased activation volumes were found in contralateral SI and primary motor cortex, whereas ipsilateral responses appeared very small and restricted after control stimuli, they represented the most salient effect of allodynia and were observed mainly in the ipsilateral parietal operculum of the SI, SII, and insula. Allodynia producing stimuli also recruited additional responses in motor and premotor areas (supplementary motor area), in regions involved in spatial attention (posterior parietal cortices), and in regions linking attention and motor control (mid-ACC) *(49)*.

Series of studies that were conducted not only with fMRI but also using magnetic resonance spectroscopy (MRS) indicate that cortical circuitry underlying chronic pain is distinct from that observed in acute pain, and preferentially involves orbital prefrontal cortex. More specifically regional brain chemistry changes in patients with chronic low back pain were examined and when compared with age- and gendermatched healthy control subjects, these subjects were found to have decreased brain chemical concentrations for multiple chemicals in both DLPFC and orbital frontal cortex and no detectable changes in primary sensory-motor cortex, ACC, insular cortex, or thalamus. Relationships between brain chemicals disrupted in patients with chronic low back pain, in a unique pattern the relation to pain as compared with anxiety were demonstrated in the analysis across number of brain regions. In addition to abnormalities of brain chemistry there was a decreased cortical gray matter size, as well as decreased prefrontal cortical gray matter density. Moreover, chronic pain patients showed a specific cognitive deficit, which is consistent with the brain activity observed in such patients along with the observed chemical and morphological abnormalities as well. Therefore, it could be concluded that chronic pain is reflected at the cortical level, and is associated with cortical reorganization and perhaps even neurodegeneration.

In summary, cerebral responses to pain are complex and dynamic in nature and in the case of chronic pain, especially neuropathic pain, changes involve more profound characterized by the involvement of entire pain-related network and some of the elements undergo significant reorganization and possibly neurodegeneration. All of these observations have significant implication for development of treatment strategies. As stated in the introduction of this section, the above discussed findings were result of studies with various neuropathic pain disorders which share fundamental characteristics with PDN, and it would be expected that many of the observations above would apply to patients with PDN.

Pain Models and Translational Neuropathic Pain Research

Models of diabetic neuropathy and translational research related to diabetic neuropathy, including painful neuropathies, are also discussed in previous chapters of this book, so to avoid repetition this chapter will concentrate on neuropathic pain in more general terms. Certainly, the appropriate reference to diabetic neuropathy will be made.

Major advances in understanding of neuropathy have been achieved during last couple of decades primarily because of development and from results of studies of animal models that mimic human neuropathic pain *(50,51)*. First animal models utilized nerve trauma such as constriction *(52)* or partial nerve cut *(53)* or nerve root cut *(50)*, as the mechanisms of nerve insult, however, other disease processes were utilized to induce nerve injury, such as diabetes *(1,55–57)* and chemotherapy *(58)*. On the basis of these studies, a wealth of information about underlying mechanisms was obtained and one of the main conclusions is that neuropathic pain is a complex and dynamic disease process. Although injury can be limited to the peripheral nerves, the pain system along the entire neuroaxis is affected, from the receptors, to primary afferents, dorsal horn, spinothalamic tract, brainstem nuclei with discending modulatory projection pathways, to thalamus and brain. Pathophysiological processes that characterize neuropathic pain include peripheral and central sensitization, which are manifestations of a complex interaction between increased excitability, decreased inhibition and activation of immune responses. The degree of complexity of neuropathic pain indicates that neuropathic pain is a disordered system, rather than a disfunction of particular pain system component. This view could than explain the complexity of PDN, and also the possibility that peripheral nerve injury because of diabetes could than be maintained by central processes as suggested by Calcutt *(1,54)*.

In addition to animal models, advances in neuropathic pain were possible because of the increased sophistication of human laboratory studies in patients with neuropathic pain. Although basic concept of quantitative sensory testing (QST) have been known for more than a century and applied to various neuropathic pain disorders such as postherpetic neuralgia and PDN for decades, expanding the number of testing methods during QST and combining QST with questionnaires provides opportunity for further investigation of neuropathic pain disorders.

Neuropathic pain research is of recent inception and as a field is still evolving. This is reflected also in rudimentary efforts in translational pain research, which is an important engine for advancements in more mature areas of medical research, such as oncology and cardiology. Development of new tools, specifically biochemistry and genetics *(59)*, as well as imaging as discussed earlier, provide new opportunities for the further advancements in pain research but complexity of neuropathic pain and especially its dynamic nature poses significant obstacle. Translational neuropathic pain research requires conceptual models that would respect complex and dynamic nature of neuropathic pain and guide progress, but those models are currently lacking. Attempts have been made to chart the course of translational pain research *(60)* but at this point in time there is no specific example of successful model of translational neuropathic pain research and specifically there is no model of translational pain research related to PDN.

There are a few obstacles that have been mentioned earlier, which pain research has to overcome and they include lack of clinical and pain translational research standards, lack of clear communication among basic scientists and among clinicians as well as between scientists and clinicians, and lack of standard in measurement tools that cross from bench to bedside and vice versa. However, there are strong efforts to advance communication and to develop methods relevant to translational neuropathic pain research.

REFERENCES

1. Calcutt NA. Potential mechanisms of neuropathic pain in diabetes. *Int Rev Neurobiol* 2002;50:205–228.
2. McCall AL. Cerebral glucose metabolism in diabetes mellitus. *Eur J Pharmacol* 2004; 490(1–3):147–158.
3. Evans ML, Sherwin RS. Blood glucose and the brain in diabetes: between a rock and a hard place? *Curr Diabetes Rep* 2002;2(2):101–102.

4. Jacobson AM, Samson JA, Weinger K, Ryan CM. Diabetes, the brain, and behavior: is there a biological mechanism underlying the association between diabetes and depression? *Int Rev Neurobiol* 2002;51:455–479.
5. Gispen WH, Biessels GJ. Cognition and synaptic plasticity in diabetes mellitus. *Trends in Neurosci* 2000;23(11):542–549.
6. Newman JC, Holden RJ. The "cerebral diabetes" paradigm for unipolar depression. *Med Hypotheses* 1993;41(5):391–408.
7. McCall AL. The impact of diabetes on the CNS. *Diabetes* 1992;41(5):557–570.
8. Ploghaus A, Narain C, Beckmann CF, et al. Exacerbation of pain by anxiety is associated with activity in a hippocampal network. *J Neurosci* 2001;21(24):9896–9903.
9. Talbot JD, Marrett S, Evans AC, Meyer E, Bushnell MC, Duncan GH. Multiple representations of pain in human cerebral cortex (*see* comments). Comment in: *Science* 1992; 255(5041):215–216; *Science* 1991;251(4999):1355–1358.
10. Jones AK, Kulkarni B, Derbyshire SW. Functional imaging of pain perception. *Curr Rheumatol Rep* 2002;4(4):329–333.
11. Peyron R, Laurent B, Garcia-Larrea L. Functional imaging of brain responses to pain. A review and meta-analysis. *Neurophysiol Clin* 2000;30(5):263–288.
12. Flor H, Elbert T, Knecht S, et al. Phantom-limb pain as a perceptual correlate of cortical reorganization following arm amputation. *Nature* 1995;375(6531):482–484.
13. Coghill RC, Gilron I, Iadarola MJ. Hemispheric lateralization of somatosensory processing. *J Neurophysiol* 2001;85(6):2602–2612.
14. Craig AD, Reiman EM, Evans A, Bushnell MC. Functional imaging of an illusion of pain. *Nature* 1996;384(6606):258–260.
15. Malisza KL, Docherty JC. Capsaicin as a source for painful stimulation in functional MRI. *J Magne Reson Imaging* 2001;14(4):341–347.
16. Casey Kl, Minoshima S, Morrow TJ, Koeppe RA. Comparison of human cerebral activation pattern during cutaneous warmth, heat pain, and deep cold pain. *J Neurophysiol* 1996; 76(1):571–581.
17. Casey KL, Minoshima S, Morrow TJ, Koeppe RA. Comparison of human cerebral activation pattern during cutaneous warmth, heat pain, and deep cold pain. *J Neurophysiol* 1996;76(1):571–581.
18. Aziz Q, Andersson Jl, Valind S, et al. Identification of human brain loci processing esophageal sensation using positron emission tomography. *Gastroenterol* 1997;113(1): 50–59.
19. Casey KL, Minoshima S, Morrow TJ, Koeppe RA, Frey KA. Imaging the Brain in Pain: Potentials, Limitations, and Implications. in *Pain and the Brain: From Nociception to Cognition* (Bromm B, Desmedt JE, eds.), New York, Raven Press, 1995, pp. 201–211.
20. Davis KD. The neural circuitry of pain as explored with functional MRI. *Neurol Res* 2000;22(3):313–317.
21. Davis KD. Neurophysiological and anatomical considerations in functional imaging of pain. *Pain* 2003;105(1–2):1–3.
22. Rainville P, Carrier B, Hofbauer RK, Bushnell MC, Duncan GH. Dissociation of sensory and affective dimensions of pain using hypnotic modulation. *Pain* 1999;82(2):159–171.
23. Tolle TR, Kaufmann T, Siessmeier T, et al. Region-specific encoding of sensory and affective components of pain in the human brain: a positron emission tomography correlation analysis. *Annals Neurol* 1999;45(1):40–47.
24. Bushnell MC, Duncan GH, Hofbauer RK, Ha B, Chen JI, Carrier B. Pain perception: is there a role for primary somatosensory cortex? *Proc Natl Acad Sci USA* 1999;96(14): 7705–7709.
25. Vogt BA, Derbyshire S, Jones AK. Pain processing in four regions of human cingulate cortex localized with co-registered PET and MR imaging. *Eur J Neurosci* 1996;8(7):1461–1473.

26. Derbyshire SW, Vogt BA, Jones AK. Pain and Stroop interference tasks activate separate processing modules in anterior cingulate cortex. *Exp Brain Res* 1998;118(1):52–60.
27. Casey KL. Forebrain mechanisms of nociception and pain: analysis through imaging. *Proc Natl Acad Sci USA* 1999;96(14):7668–7674.
28. Davis KD, Hutchison WD, Lozano AM, Tasker RR, Dostrovsky JO. Human anterior cingulate cortex neurons modulated by attention-demanding tasks. *J Neurophysiol* 2000; 83(6):3575–3577.
29. Davis KD. Cold-induced pain and prickle in the glabrous and hairy skin. *Pain* 1998; 75(1):47–57.
30. Davis KD, Pope GE. Noxious cold evokes multiple sensations with distinct time courses. *Pain* 2002;98(1–2):179–185.
31. Downar J, Mikulis DJ, Davis KD. Neural correlates of the prolonged salience of painful stimulation. *Neuroimage* 2003;20(3):1540–1551.
32. Baciu MV, Bonaz BL, Papillon E, et al. Central processing of rectal pain: a functional MR imaging study. AJNR: *Am J Neuroradiol* 1999;20(10):1920–1924.
33. Bernstein CN, Frankenstein UN, Rawsthorne P, Pitz M, Summers R, McIntyre MC. Cortical mapping of visceral pain in patients with GI disorders using functional magnetic resonance imaging. *Am J Gastroenterol* 2002;97(2):319–327.
34. Derbyshire SW. A systematic review of neuroimaging data during visceral stimulation. *Am J Gastroenterol* 2003;98(1):12–20.
35. Treede RD, Apkarian AV, Bromm B, Greenspan JD, Lenz FA. Cortical representation of pain: functional characterization of nociceptive areas near the lateral sulcus. *Pain* 2000;87(2): 113–119.
36. Backonja MM, Galer BS. Pain assessment and evaluation of patients who have neuropathic pain. *Neurol Clin North Am* 1998;16(4):775–790.
37. Backonja MM. Defining neuropathic pain. *Anesthe Analge* 2003;97(3):785–790.
38. Hsieh JC, Belfrage M, Stone-Elander S, Hansson P, Ingvar M. Central representation of chronic ongoing neuropathic pain studied by positron emission tomography. *Pain* 1995; 63(2):225–236.
39. Iadarola MJ, Max MB, Berman KF, et al. Unilateral decrease in thalamic activity observed with positron emission tomography in patients with chronic neuropathic pain. *Pain* 1995; 63(1):55–64.
40. Jones AK, Qi LY, Fujirawa T, et al. In vivo distribution of opioid receptors in man in relation to the cortical projections of the medial and lateral pain systems measured with positron emission tomography. *Neurosci Lett* 1991;126:25–28.
41. Apkarian AV, Thomas PS, Krauss BR, Szeverenyi NM. Prefrontal cortical hyperactivity in patients with sympathetically mediated chronic pain. *Neurosci Lett* 2001;311(3):193–197.
42. Casey KL, Lorenz J, Minoshima S. Insights into the pathophysiology of neuropathic pain through functional brain imaging. *Exp Neurol* 2003;184(Suppl 1):S80–S88.
43. Baumgartner U, Vogel H, Ellrich J, Gawehn J, Stoeter P, Treede RD. Brain electrical source analysis of primary cortical components of the tibial nerve somatosensory evoked potential using regional sources. *Electroencephalogr Clin Neurophysiol* 1998;108(6):588–599.
44. Schaefer M, Muhlnickel W, Grusser SM, Flor H. Reliability and validity of neuroelectric source imaging in primary somatosensory cortex of human upper limb amputees. *Brain Topogr* 2002;15(2):95–106.
45. Peyron R, Frot M, Schneider F, et al. Role of operculoinsular cortices in human pain processing: converging evidence from PET, fMRI, dipole modeling, and intracerebral recordings of evoked potentials. *Neuroimage* 2002;17(3):1336–1346.
46. Derbyshire SW, Jones AK, Creed F, et al. Cerebral responses to noxious thermal stimulation in chronic low back pain patients and normal controls. *Neuroimage* 2002;16(1):158–168.

47. Apkarian AV, Krauss BR, Fredrickson BE, Szeverenyi NM. Imaging the pain of low back pain: functional magnetic resonance imaging in combination with monitoring subjective pain perception allows the study of clinical pain states. *Neurosci Lett* 2001;299(1–2):57–60.
48. Petzke F, Clauw DJ, Ambrose K, Khine A, Gracely RH. Increased pain sensitivity in fibromyalgia: effects of stimulus type and mode of presentation (*see* comment). *Pain* 2003;105(3):403–413.
49. Peyron R, Schneider F, Faillenot I, et al. An fMRI study of cortical representation of mechanical allodynia in patients with neuropathic pain. *Neurol* 2004;63(10):1838–1846.
50. Bennett GJ. Animal models of pain. in *Methods in Pain Research* (Krueger L, ed.), CRC Press, Boca, Raton, 2001, pp. 67–91.
51. Vierck CJ Jr, Siddall P, Yezierski RP. Pain following spinal cord injury: animal models and mechanistic studies. *Pain* 2000;89(1):1–5.
52. Bennett GJ, Xie YK. A peripheral mononeuropathy in rat that produces disorders of pain sensation like those seen in man. *Pain* 1988;33:87–107.
53. Decosterd I, Woolf CJ. Spared nerve injury: an animal model of persistent peripheral neuropathic pain. *Pain* 2000;87(2):149–158.
54. Kim SH, Chung JM. An experimental model for peripheral neuropathy produced by segmental spinal nerve ligation in the rat. *Pain* 1992;50(3):355–363.
55. Calcutt NA. Experimental models of painful diabetic neuropathy. *J Neurol Sci* 2004;220(1–2): 137–139.
56. Powell HC, Costello ML, Myers RR. Endoneurial fluid pressure in experimental models of diabetic neuropathy. *J Neuropathol Exp Neurol* 1981;40(6):613–624.
57. Simmons Z, Feldman EL. Update on diabetic neuropathy. *Curr Opin Neurol* 2002;15(5): 595–603.
58. Pisano C, Pratesi G, Laccabue D, et al. Paclitaxel and Cisplatin-induced neurotoxicity: a protective role of acetyl-L-carnitine. *Clin Cancer Res* 2003;9(15):5756–5767.
59. Ji RR, Strichartz G. Cell signaling and the genesis of neuropathic pain. *Sci Stke* 2004; 2004(252):RE14.
60. Woolf CJ, Bennett GJ, Doherty M, et al. Towards a mechanism-based classification of pain? *Pain* 1998;77(3):227–229.

21
Treatment of Painful Diabetic Neuropathy

Andrew J. M. Boulton, MD, DSc(hon), FRCP

SUMMARY

Up to 50% of patients with chronic sensorimotor diabetic neuropathy will experience painful or uncomfortable symptoms, and of these a significant minority may require pharmacological therapy. As painful symptomatology may be worsened by a sudden change in glycaemic control, the first step in management should be the quest for stable, near normal glycaemic control avoiding glycaemic flux. Of all the disease-modifying treatments, only alpha-lipoic acid appears to be promising in the management of neuropathic pain, although this only licensed in certain European countries. Several groups of pharmacological agents have been proved to be efficacious in symptomatic relief in diabetic neuropathy: these include the tricyclic drugs, a number of anti-convulsants, and certain other pharmacological treatments. Although helpful in many cases, the tricyclic drugs are plagued by frequent and predictable side effects. The anti-convulsants, gabapentin and pregabalin are useful in the management of neuropathic pain, and the dual 5-HT and norepinephrine reuptake inhibitor duloxetine has also demonstrated efficacy. Although many topical and non-pharmacological treatments have been proposed, few have proven efficacy in appropriately designed controlled trials.

Key Words: Diabetic neuropathy; pain; tricyclic drugs; anti-convulsants.

INTRODUCTION

The painful symptomatology of diabetic neuropathy has been recognized for many years and one of the first descriptions of neuropathic pain is attributed to Rollo *(1)*, who described pain and paraesthesiae in the legs of a diabetic patient in the 18th century. Painful symptoms are common in many of the neuropathic syndromes of diabetes described elsewhere in this book: these include both focal and multifocal neuropathies, proximal motor neuropathy or amytrophy, and the symmetrical sensory polyneuropathies. A simple definition of diabetic neuropathy, agreed by an international consensus group, is "the presence of symptoms and/or signs of peripheral nerve dysfunction in people with diabetes after exclusion of other causes" *(2)*. This definition refers to the chronic sensorimotor diabetic neuropathy, which is truly a paradoxical condition as up to 50% of patients might experience painful or uncomfortable symptomatology, whereas the remaining 50% might experience no pain whatsoever putting them at risk of foot ulceration and other late sequalae of neuropathy including Charcot neuroarthropathy *(3)*. Thus, one patient

From: *Contemporary Diabetes: Diabetic Neuropathy: Clinical Management, Second Edition*
Edited by: A. Veves and R. Malik © Humana Press Inc., Totowa, NJ

Table 1
Diabetic Neuropathies Associated With Pain

Focal and multifocal neuropathies
Cranial, for example, third or sixth nerve
Focal limb, for example, entrapment or spontaneous mononeuropathy
Amyotrophy (proximal motor neuropathy)
Truncal radiculoneuropathy
Generalized symmetrical polyneuropathies
Acute sensory (invariably accompanied by pain)
Chronic sensorimotor

with sensorimotor neuropathy might experience severe pain vividly described by Pavy *(4)* in 1887 as being "of a burning and unremitting character," whereas another patient with the same deficit might be completely asymptomatic: patients such as the latter one lack what Dr. Paul Brand described as "the gift of pain" *(5)*.

In this chapter, after a brief description of those neuropathies associated with painful symptoms, the methods of assessment of neuropathic pain will be discussed. This will be followed by a description of the impact of painful neuropathy on quality of life (QoL) and then some of the problems and pitfalls of clinical trial design for studies of new therapies for painful neuropathy. Subsequently, the role of blood glucose control in the management of painful neuropathy will be followed by a discussion of pharmacological treatments and finally by nonpharmacological therapies, such as acupuncture and topical therapies.

In medicine there are few cures, but many treatments, so it is hoped that by the end of this chapter the reader will appreciate that the question asked in an editorial in 1983 "can we do anything about diabetic neuropathy or do we just have to document it and commiserate with the patient?" *(6)*, is no longer rhetorical: there are indeed a number of effective therapies for the painful symptomatology of diabetic neuropathy.

NEUROPATHIES ASSOCIATED WITH PAIN

As stated earlier, a number of the neuropathic syndromes associated with diabetes may be accompanied by painful symptomatology: these are summarized in Table 1.

Focal and Multifocal Neuropathies

Although discussed in detail in Chapter 22, a brief description of those associated with painful symptomatology is provided here *(7,8)*. Those cranial mononeuropathies affecting the nerves supplying the external ocular muscles typically present with sudden onset of diplopia and an ipsilateral headache often described as a dull pain coming from behind the eye. Similarly, many of the focal limb neuropathies including entrapment neuropathies *(7)* might present with painful symptoms in the area supplied by the individual nerve. The tarsal tunnel syndrome, which is analogous to the carpal tunnel syndrome in the upper limbs, may present with localized foot pain, which should be distinguished from the pain of the diffuse sensorimotor neuropathy.

Other focal limb neuropathies presenting with painful symptoms include meralgia paraesthetica: in this condition, which involves compression of the lateral cutaneous nerve of thigh, neuropathic symptoms occur in the lateral area of the thigh. Diabetic

Table 2
Contrasts Between Acute Sensory and Chronic Sensorimotor Neuropathies

	Acute sensory	Chronic sensorimotor
Mode of onset	Relatively rapid	Gradual, insidious
Symptoms	Severe burning pain, aching: weight loss usual	Burning pain, paresthesiae, numbness: weight loss unusual
Symptom severity	+++	0 to ++
Associated features	Depression, erectile dysfunction	
Signs	Mild sensory in some motor unusual	Stocking and glove sensory loss: ankle reflexes
Other diabetic complications	Unusual	Increased prevalence
Electrophysiological investigations	May be normal or minor abnormalities	Abnormalities unusual in motor and sensory nerves
Natural history	Complete recovery within 12 months	Symptoms might persist for years

amyotrophy (otherwise known as proximal motor neuropathy) typically occurs in older patients with type 2 diabetes and can present with severe neuropathic pain affecting one or both lower extremities, particularly in the thigh region. The pain might be extremely troublesome with marked nocturnal exacerbation and sleep disruption. A history, together with clinical features of weakness and wasting in the proximal thigh muscles, is usually suggestive of this condition although the exclusion of malignant disease and other treatable neuropathies, such as chronic inflammatory demyelinating neuropathy (CIDP) (Chapters 1 and 13) is recommended. One of the principal features of the truncal neuropathies is that of pain usually described as being of a burning or aching quality, and frequently accompanied by lancinating stabbing discomfort with cutaneous hyperaesthesiae and nocturnal exacerbation.

Generalized Symmetrical Polyneuropathy

Acute painful sensory neuropathy has been described as a separate clinical entity *(9)*, and appears to be a distinctive variant of symmetrical polyneuropathy that warrants a separate discussion. Although many of the symptoms of acute and chronic sensorimotor neuropathy are similar if not identical, there are clear differences in the mode of onset, accompanying signs, symptom severity, and prognosis that are summarized in Table 2. The outstanding complaint in acute sensory neuropathy is one of severe neuropathic pain with marked sleep disturbance. Weight loss, depression, and frequently in the male, erectile dysfunction, are common accompanying features, although the clinical exam of the lower limbs is often unremarkable with preserved reflexes and few sensory signs. This acute neuropathy is associated with poor glycemic control and may follow an episode of ketoacidosis and has been associated with weight loss and eating disorders *(10)*.

Chronic Sensorimotor Neuropathy

This is by far, the most common manifestation of all the diabetic neuropathies and as noted elsewhere, might be present at the diagnosis of type 2 diabetes. In many ways

Table 3
Characteristics of Neuropathic Pain Characteristics of Neuropathic Pain

Dysesthetic	Nociceptive or nerve-trunk
Unfamiliar	Familiar to patient
Burning, "on fire"	Aching, tender, like toothache
Throbbing, prickling	Knife-like
Electrical shock-like	
Knife-like	
Allodynia (nonnoxious stimulus giving rise to pain)	
Hyperesthesia (increased sensitivity)	

chronic sensorimotor neuropathy manifests a spectrum of symptomatic involvement: at one end of the spectrum there are patients with persistent troublesome neuropathic symptoms and evidence of sensory and motor dysfunction on examination of the lower limbs, whereas at the other end, the patient might be completely asymptomatic and still have a significant neuropathic deficit on examination. Intermediate between these two extremes are patients with moderate, but intermittent symptomatology (sometimes painless, but may be with "negative" symptoms, such as numbness, feet feel dead, and so on) and neurological abnormalities on examination of the feet. Even more confusing for the patient is the "painful–painless" foot. In these patients, there might be spontaneous painful symptomatology, but on examination there is marked loss of pain vibration, and other sensory modalities.

ASSESSMENT OF NEUROPATHIC PAIN

It is important to emphasize the difficulties in the description and in the assessment of painful symptoms. Pain is a very personal experience and there is marked variation in the description of symptoms between patients with similar pathological lesions. This has important implications for trials of therapies for neuropathy and, as stated by Huskison *(11)*: "pain is a personal psychological experience and an observer can play no legitimate part in its direct management." Thus, any trial of treatments for pain must rely upon the patients' response to questions, questionnaires, or other measures. This principle has not been followed in all trials: for example, it is inadmissible to rely on the "physician's overall impression" of the patient's response as was the case in one trial *(12)*. In recent years, a number of valid measures for the assessment of chronic neuropathic pain and for the evaluation of treatment responses have been developed and tested. One or more of the following methods are usually used in clinical trials of new treatments for painful neuropathy (Table 3).

Visual Analog and Verbal Descriptor Scales

One of the most common measures of neuropathic pain in clinical trials is the visual analog scale (VAS), originally described by Scott and Huskison *(13)*. The VAS is a straight line the ends of which are the extreme limits of the sensation being assessed. The VAS has been shown to be a satisfactory method for assessing pain or the relief of pain. The line is normally 10 cm in length and is frequently referred to as the 10 cm VAS. A VAS with descriptive terms placed along the length of the line is known as a verbal descriptor scale. Thus a 10 cm VAS with the terms "mild, moderate, and severe" along the base of the line is known as a 10 cm verbal descriptor scale.

Mcgill Pain Questionnaire

There are three major classes of word descriptors in the Mcgill pain questionnaire (MPQ) originally described by Melzack *(14)*: sensory qualities, affective qualities, and evaluative words. The MPQ was originally designed to provide more quantitative measures of clinical pain, changes which can be evaluated statistically. Masson et al. *(15)* later showed that the MPQ was a useful aid in the differential diagnosis of painful diabetic neuropathic symptomatology.

Neuropathic Pain Scale

Galer and Jensen *(16)* developed a neuropathic pain scale as they felt that previous measures, such as the VAS did not adequately assess the experience of neuropathic pain. Therefore, this scale includes two items that assess the overall dimension of pain intensity and pain unpleasantness.

Other Methods of Assessment

A number of simple symptom screening questionnaires are available to record symptom quality and severity. These include a simplified neuropathy symptom score that was used in European prevalence studies and might also be useful in clinical practice *(17,18)*, and the Michigan neuropathy screening instrument, which is a brief 15 item questionnaire that can be administered to patients as a screening tool for neuropathy *(19)*. Other similar symptom scoring systems have also been described *(20)*. Finally, some of the newer condition specific QoL measures also include symptom scoring scales as described in the following paragraph.

QoL AND NEUROPATHIC PAIN

It is well-recognized that painful symptomatology, and also neuropathic deficits, might have an adverse effect on the QoL in diabetic neuropathy *(21,22)*. It is increasingly recognized that QoL, rather than being a mere rating of health status, is actually a uniquely personal experience, representing the way that individuals perceive and react to their health status *(23)*. This increasing recognition emphasizes the need to address the patient's perspective, rather than the researchers' views when measuring QoL.

Until recently, the studies which reported that neuropathy can have a negative impact on the functioning and QoL relied upon generic instruments, which do not describe the condition-specific features of neuropathy. Thus, Vileikyte et al. *(24)* developed the first neuropathy-specific QoL instrument, NeuroQoL, which investigates the impact of symptoms and/or foot ulceration as a consequence of neuropathy on QoL. The results of this study demonstrated that patients experiencing neuropathic symptoms reported severe restrictions in activities of daily living (e.g., leisure, daily tasks), problems with interpersonal relationships, and changes in self perception. It therefore appears that neuropathic pain and changes in self perception as a result of foot complications have the most devastating effect on the individual's QoL. Finally, recent research suggests that not only do painful neuropathic symptoms have an effect on qualify of life, but also generate symptoms of anxiety *(23)*.

CLINICAL TRIAL DESIGN FOR PAINFUL NEUROPATHY TRIALS

A number of considerations must be taken into account in the design of clinical trials to assess potential therapies for chronic painful sensorimotor neuropathy:

1. Is this chronic neuropathy? As noted earlier, there are two main types of painful symmetrical diabetic neuropathy: acute painful neuropathy, which is relatively rare and typically presents after a period of poor glycemic control with severe symptoms and few signs. The natural history of this condition is one of improvement of symptoms during a period of months *(9)*. In contrast, chronic painful neuropathy is of insidious onset and although the symptoms are similar in character to those of acute neuropathy, on examination there is usually a peripheral sensory loss to multiple modalities and absent ankle reflexes. The natural history of this condition is that whereas the symptoms may wax and wane and persist for several years, the disappearance of symptoms is not necessarily a sign of improvement but might represent progression to the insensitive foot *(25)*. It is clearly important in view of the difference in natural history, that trials of any potential new treatments should only include patients with the chronic sensorimotor neuropathy. If patients with acute neuropathy were included, improvement might be because of the natural history of the disease and not necessarily to a therapeutic effect of the agent under investigation.
2. Is the symptomatic neuropathy secondary to diabetes? There are numerous causes of painful sensory neuropathy *(26)*, and Dyck et al. *(27)* have estimated that more than 5% of neuropathy in patients with diabetes is of nondiabetic causation. Moreover, the symptomatology of diabetic neuropathy can be relatively nonspecific, and a recent community study demonstrated that almost 5% of patients without diabetes reported neuropathic pain *(28)*. A further study reported that chronic foot pain is common in the community with more than 20% of men and women reporting foot pain in the month before the survey, and almost 10% of patients reporting disabling foot pain *(29)*.
3. Other considerations. A number of other considerations need to be taken into account in the design of clinical trials. Important among these is of course the measures used for symptom assessment as discussed earlier. A further question is "should the agent under investigation be compared against a placebo or against another commonly used and proven drug for symptomatic neuropathy?" Unfortunately, the vast majority of studies have the new agent compared against placebo: this probably relates to the fact that most such trials are sponsored by the pharmaceutical industry. Finally, the trial design should account for potential confounding variables, the most important of which is the level of glycemic control. As blood glucose flux might be important in the genesis of neuropathic pain, the stability of daily glycemic control is important if the agent under investigation is to be properly assessed.

TREATMENT OF PAINFUL DIABETIC NEUROPATHY

Under this section the many different approaches to the management of symptoms in those with distal sensory neuropathy will be considered. First, the role of blood glucose control in the prevention and management of painful neuropathy will be discussed followed by a description of the various pharmacological treatments that have been proposed. This section will be divided into those purely symptomatic treatments and those symptoms that target the underlying pathogenesis of neuropathy and might in addition be useful for symptoms. Finally, a number of varied nonpharmacological treatments will be discussed.

Glycemic Control and Painful Diabetic Neuropathy

A number of studies have confirmed the major contribution of prolonged hyperglycemia in the pathogenesis of neuropathy and neuropathic pain *(30–33)*. More recent studies in patients with idiopathic painful neuropathies further support the relationship between hyperglycemia and painful neuropathy. In the study of Singleton et al. *(34)*, impaired glucose tolerance was more common in patients with idiopathic painful neuropathy than the general population. Thus, achieving near normoglycemia should be the primary aim in both the prevention of and the first step in the management of generalized peripheral neuropathy.

A number of small open-label uncontrolled studies have suggested that achieving stable near-normoglycemia is helpful in the management of painful neuropathic symptoms. In one such study *(35)*, patients with painful neuropathy were treated with continuous subcutaneous insulin infusion for a period of 4 months. As well as resulting in the relief of neuropathic pain, improvements were also noted in quantitative measures of nerve function. Improvement of blood glucose control in this study was assessed by glycated hemoglobin as well as by regular home blood glucose monitoring. The fact that blood glucose flux was reduced in this early study might explain the symptomatic benefits of this treatment in light of more recent observations *(33)*. In this latter study, Oyibo et al. compared patients with painful and painless neuropathy: those with painful symptoms had poorer control, more excursions to hyper and hypoglycemic levels and greater blood glucose flux as assessed by a number of measures. It therefore appears that the stability of glycemic control is equally important as the level of achieved control. It might be that biochemical changes associated with blood glucose flux result in spontaneous firing in nociceptive afferent fibres of diseased sensory neurones. Despite the lack of appropriately designed controlled trials in this area, generally, it is accepted that intensive diabetes therapy aimed at stable near-normoglycemia should be the first step in the treatment of any form of diabetic neuropathy.

Disease-Modifying Treatments

A number of agents aimed at correcting the underlying pathogenesis of diabetic neuropathy are currently under investigation, but none is licensed for use in the United States by the Food and Drug Administration (FDA).

Aldose Reductase Inhibitors

As discussed in Chapter 18, the aldose reductase inhibitors block the rate-limiting enzyme, aldose reductase, in the polyol pathway. Numerous aldose reductase inhibitors have been studied for the last 20 years in the management of neuropathy, but with the exception of *epalrestat,* which is marketed in Japan, presently none is available in any country. Of the many published studies, symptomatic relief was reported in a large multicenter study using the now withdrawn drug *tolrestat (36)*, and pain relief was also reported with *epalrestat* in a 12-week controlled study *(37)*.

α-Lipoic Acid

There is accumulating evidence to support the role of oxidative stress in the pathogenesis of neuropathy. Studies with the antioxidant α-lipoic acid have provided evidence of potential efficacy for this agent which might well be beneficial both for neuropathic symptom relief, and for modifying the natural history of neuropathy *(38,39)*.

PKC-β Inhibition

Preliminary data suggest that treatment with the PKC-β inhibitor, *Ruboxistaurin,* might ameliorate some of the symptoms of diabetic neuropathy *(40)*.

Table 4
Initial Management of Symptomatic Neuropathy

Exclude nondiabetic causes
Malignant disease (e.g., bronchogenic carcinoma)
Metabolic
Toxic (e.g., alcohol)
Infective (e.g., HIV infection)
Iatrogenic (e.g., isoniazid, vinca alkaloids)
Medication related (chemotherapy, HIV treatment)
Explanation, support and practical measures, for example, bed cradle to lift bedclothes off hyperaesthetic skin
Assess level of blood glucose control
Regular self glucose monitoring (possibly continuous glucose monitoring)
Glycated hemoglobin
Aim for optimal, stable control
Consider pharmacological or physical therapy

A number of other agents are currently under investigation as reported in recent reviews *(6,41)*.

Symptomatic Pharmacological Treatment of Painful Neuropathy

This section will discuss the pharmacological management of painful neuropathic symptoms. Most of the pharmacological interventions described here have no effect on the natural history of neuropathy which is one of the progressive loss of nerve function. Before considering pharmacological treatment, the initial approach to the management of a patient with symptomatic neuropathy is summarized in Table 4. A large number of therapeutic agents have been used in the management of painful symptoms: some of the more commonly used ones are listed in Table 5. Although some have advocated the use of nonsteroidal, anti-inflammatory drugs as the first treatment for neuropathy, there is little evidence to support their use. Moreover, these agents should be used with caution in neuropathic patients with diabetes many of whom will have renal impairment as a consequence of nephropathy, a contra indication to nonsteroidal drug usage in most cases.

Tricyclic Drugs

Several randomized clinical trials have supported the use of these agents in the management of neuropathic pain. Putative mechanisms by which these drugs relieve pain include inhibition of norepinephrine and/or serotonin reuptake at synapses of central descending pain control systems and more recently, the antagonism of *N*-methyl-D-aspartate receptors, which mediate hyperalgesia and allodynia *(42)*. Most experience has been achieved with amitriptyline and imipramine. The dosage of both of these agents required for symptomatic relief is similar (25–150 mg daily), although in older patients it can be useful to start at 10 mg daily. To avoid undue drowsiness, the dose can be taken once daily usually in the evening or bedtime. The usefulness of these agents in neuropathic pain was confirmed in the systematic review performed by McQuay et al. *(43)*. However, the major problem with these agents remains the frequency of side

Table 5
Commonly Used Pharmacological Therapies for Painful Diabetic Neuropathy

Drug class	Drug	Daily dose (mg)	Side-effects	References
Tricyclics	Amitriptyline	25–150	++++	*42,43*
	Imipramine	25–150	++++	*42,43*
	Desipramine	25–150	++++	*42*
SSRIs	Citalopram	40	+++	*45*
	Paroxitene	40	+++	*44*
Anticonvulsants	Carbamazepine	200–800	+++	*46*
	Gabapentin	900–3600	++	*47,48*
	Pregabalin	150–600	++	*49*
Opioids	Tramadol	50–400	+++	*53,54*
	Oxycodone-CR	10–60	++++	*55,56*

affects, which are predictable. Although drowsiness and lethargy are common, the anticholinergic side affects, particularly dry mouth, are most troublesome.

Selective Serotonin-Reuptake Inhibitors

The selective serotonin-reuptake inhibitors inhibit presynaptic reuptake of serotonin but not norepinephrine. Studies suggest that treatment with *paroxetine (44)* and *citalopram (45)* both at 40 mg per day, are efficacious in relieving neuropathic pain.

Anticonvulsants

Anticonvulsants have been used in the management of neuropathic pain for many years *(8)*. Limited evidence exists for the efficacy of phenytoin and carbamazepine in painful neuropathy. Carbamazepine proved to be successful in the management of trigeminal neuralgia and following this was used in painful neuropathy. Of the few small clinical trials in diabetic neuropathy, the one by Rull et al. *(46)* did report quite a number of adverse events. It is the frequency of adverse events, particularly central (somnolence, dizziness), together with a lack of clinical trial data that limits the use of this agent.

GABAPENTIN

Gabapentin is now widely used for the relief of neuropathic pain and is specifically licensed for this indication in certain European countries. It is structurally related to the neurotransmitter γ-aminobutyric acid (GABA) and was first introduced as an anticonvulsant for complex partial seizures. In a large controlled trial of Gabapentin in symptomatic diabetic neuropathy, significant pain relief together with reduced sleep disturbance was reported using dosages of 900–3600 mg daily *(47)*. In a recent review of all the trials of Gabapentin for neuropathic pain, it was concluded that dosages of 1800–3600 mg per day of this agent were effective: the side effect profile also seems superior to that of the tricyclic drugs *(48)*.

PREGABALIN

Pregabalin, which is structurally related to Gabapentin, has recently been confirmed to be useful in painful diabetic neuropathy in a randomized controlled trial *(49)*.

In contrast to Gabapentin, which is usually given three times daily, Pregabalin is effective when given twice daily. This agent was recently licensed for the indication of neuropathic pain by the FDA.

Other Anticonvulsants

In recent years, controlled trial evidence has also been published for a number of other anticonvulsant treatments including oxcarbazepine, sodium valproate, topiramate, and lamotrigine *(8,50–52)*.

Opioids

The weak opioid-like centrally acting agent tramadol has been shown to be useful in the management of patients with painful neuropathy in a randomized controlled trial *(53)*. A follow-up study to the original trial suggested that symptomatic relief could be maintained for at least 6 months' usage *(54)*. More recently, two randomized trials have confirmed the efficacy of controlled-relief oxycodone for neuropathic pain in diabetes *(55,56)*. It is advised that opioids such as oxycodone-CR should be considered as add-on therapies for patients failing to respond to nonopioid medications.

Other Pharmacological Treatments

Mexiletine is a Class 1B antiarrhythmic agent and is a structural analog of lignocaine. Its efficacy in neuropathic pain has been confirmed in controlled trials *(57)*. However, in this review of seven controlled trials of mexiletine, it was suggested that it only provided a modest analgesic effect *(57)*. Regular EKG monitoring is essential and its short-term use should be reserved for patients who have failed to respond to other agents.

The 5-hydroxytryptamine and norepinephrine reuptake inhibitor *duloxetine* was licensed by the FDA for usage in neuropathic pain in late 2004. This is an interesting agent as it has analgesic and antidepressant effects, but at the time of writing, evidence for the efficacy of this agent was only available in abstract form *(41)*. Preliminary studies using two inhibitors of *N*-methyl-D-Aspartate (NMDA) receptors provide preliminary evidence for efficacy of these agents. A small study of the NMDA receptor antagonist *dextromethorphan (58)* and a larger study of *memantine (59)* suggest that this class of drugs might prove to be useful in treating neuropathic pain in the future. Table 6 lists the number needed to treat for some of the more commonly used agents described in this section.

Topical and Nonpharmacological Treatments of Painful Neuropathy

Topical Agents

Capsaicin

Capsaicin, which is the "hot" ingredient of red chilli pepper, depletes tissue of substance P and reduces chemically-induced pain. There have been a number of controlled studies of topically-applied capsaicin cream (0.075%) in the treatment of painful diabetic neuropathy. Although a meta-analysis *(60)* did suggest overall efficacy from a number of trials, the most recent trial failed to demonstrate any pain relief with capsaicin *(61)*. A potential problem with all trials of capsaicin is the difficulty in ensuring that it is truly blinded, as topical capsaicin itself gives rise to transient local hyperalgesia (usually a mild burning sensation) in many patients.

Table 6
Number Needed to Treat Successfully and Number Needed to Induce a Harmful Effect

Drug	NNT (CI)	NNH (CI)
Carbamazepine	3.3 (2–9.4)	1.9 (1.4–2.8)
Gabapentin	3.7 (2.4–8.3)	2.7 (2.2–3.4)
Mexiletine	10 (3–∞)	5–10
Phenytoin	2.1 (1.5–3.6)	9.5 (4.9–130)
Pregabalin	3.3 (2.3–5.9)	3.7
TCAs	2.4 (2–3)	2.7 (2.1–3.9)
Topiramate	3 (2.3–4.5)	9
Tramadol	3.4 (2.3–6.4)	7.8

NNT, numbers needed to treat to achieve pain relief in 1 patient;
NNH, numbers needed to treat to harm in 1 patient; CI, 95% confidence interval.

TOPICAL NITRATE

A controlled study suggested that the local application to the feet of isosorbide dinitrate spray was effective in relieving overall pain and a burning discomfort of painful neuropathy *(62)*. More recently, the use of nitrate patches has also been shown to be useful *(63)*. However, both of these studies were small and single center and a multicenter trial is now indicated for this agent.

LIDOCAINE

A preliminary study of topically-applied 5% lidocaine by a patch demonstrated improvements in pain and QoL outcomes during a 3-week treatment period *(64)*. However, as this was not a controlled trial, a properly designed study is required before this can be recommended.

Psychological Support/Counselling

It is vital to provide all patients with a full explanation of their condition, to allay the fear and misconception often that they have some underlying malignancy, and informing them that the natural history might well be that the pain resolves in due course and that specific treatments are available for the pain in the short term, can be extremely helpful *(23)*. Further evidence emphasizing the importance of comfort and support to improve painful symptomatology was provided in some preliminary observations of Kaye et al. *(65)* who also demonstrated that disappointment and failure of health care can result in intensification of painful symptomatology.

Acupuncture

Several uncontrolled studies report significant benefits of acupuncture in the relief of painful symptomatology. In the most recent of these, a 10-week uncontrolled study of up to six courses of traditional Chinese acupuncture, resulted in 77% of patients experiencing significant pain relief and during a follow-up of up to 1 year, the majority of patients were able to stop or significantly reduce their other pain medication *(66)*. Although, controlled trials are needed to confirm the benefits of acupuncture which appears to be free of side-effects, these are difficult to design because of the problems encountered with finding the correct site for "sham" acupuncture.

Other Physical Therapies

Many other physical therapies have been proposed, but most are supported by small single-center studies, thus, indicating the need for proper multicenter-controlled trials. The efficacy of pulsed-dose electrical stimulation through stocking electrodes in the treatment of painful diabetic neuropathy that was previously supported in an open-labelled study was not confirmed to be efficacious in a recent randomized cross-over trial *(67)*.

A number of other physical therapies have been proposed and do have support from small-controlled trials: these include low-intensity laser therapy *(68)*, monochromatic infrared light treatment *(69)*, percutaneous electrical nerve stimulation *(70)*, and static magnetic field therapy *(71)*. For patients with the most severe painful neuropathy in unresponsive to conventional therapy, the use of electrical spinal cord stimulation was proposed in a small case series *(72)*. However, although this cannot be generally recommended except in very resistant cases as it is invasive, expensive, and unproven in controlled studies, a recent follow-up of patients suggested that long-term symptomatic relief can be achieved *(73)*.

CONCLUSION

The treatment of painful diabetic distal polyneuropathy remains a daunting challenge to the physicians. Major problems in this area remain the paucity of large multicenter conclusive trials, the frequency of side-effects, and particularly the lack of controlled trials using comparator therapies rather than a placebo. Before embarking on a pharmacological therapy, the importance of a thorough history and examination together with an understanding approach, and a serious attempt to stabilize glycemic control cannot be overemphasized. Finally, it must be remembered that all patients with distal sensory polyneuropathy are at potential risk of foot ulceration and should receive preventative foot care education as outlined in Chapter 28 of this volume.

REFERENCES

1. Rollo J. *Cases of Diabetes Mellitus*. 2nd ed. Dilly, London, 1798, pp. 17–62.
2. Boulton AJM, Gries FA, Jervell JA. Guidelines for the diagnosis and outpatient management of diabetic peripheral neuropathy. *Diabetic Med* 1998;15:508–514.
3. Boulton AJM, Kirsner RS, Vileikyte L. Neuropathic diabetic foot ulcers. *N Engl J of Med* 2004;351:48–55.
4. Pavy FW. Address on diabetes, Washington International Congress. Medical News, Philadelphia, 1887, p. 357.
5. Boulton AJM. The diabetic foot – from art to science. *Diabetologia* 2004;47:1343–1353.
6. Editorial. Diabetic neuropathy: where are we now? *Lancet* 1983;1366–1367.
7. Vinik AI, Mehrabyon A, Colen L, Boulton AJ. Focal entrapment neuropathies in diabetes. *Diabetes Care* 2004;27:1783–1788.
8. Boulton AJM, Malik RA, Arezzo JS, Sosenko JM. Diabetic somatic neuropathies. *Diabetes Care* 2004;27:1458–1486.
9. Archer AG, Watkins PJ, Thomas PK, et al. The natural history of acute Painful neuropathy in diabetes mellitus. *J Neurol Neurosurg Psychiatry* 1983;46:491–499.

10. Steel JM, Young RJ, Lloyd GG, Clarke BF. Clinical apparent eating disorders in young diabetic women: associations with painful neuropathies and other complications. *Br Med J* 1987;294:859–862.
11. Huskisson EC. Measurement of pain. *Lancet* 1974;ii:1127–1131.
12. Tandan R, Lewis GA, Krusinksi PB, et al. Topical Capsaicin in painful Neuropathy: controlled trial with long-term follow-up. *Diabetes Care* 1992;15:8–14.
13. Scott J, Huskisson EC. Graphic representation of pain. *Pain* 1976;2:175–184.
14. Melzack R. The McGill Pain Questionnaire: major properties and scoring Methods. *Pain* 1975;1:277–299.
15. Masson EA, Hunt L, Gem JM, et al. A novel approach to the diagnosis and Assessment of symptomatic diabetic neuropthy. *Pain* 1989;38:25–28.
16. Galer BS, Jensen MP. Development and preliminary validation of a pain measure specific to neuropathic pain: the Neuropathic Pain Scale. *Neurology* 1997;48:328–332.
17. Young MJ, Boulton AJM, MacLeod AF, et al. A multicentre study of the prevalence of diabetic peripheral neuropathy in the United Kingdom hospital clinic population. *Diabetologia* 1993;36:150–154.
18. Cabezas-Cerrato J. The prevalence of clinical diabetic polyneuropathy in Spain: study in primary care and hospital clinic groups. Neuropathy Spanish Study Group of the Spanish Diabetes Society (SDS). *Diabetologia* 1998;41:1263–1269.
19. Feldman EL, Stevens MJ, Thomas PK, et al. A practice two-step quantitative Clinical and electrophysiological assessment for the diagnosis and staging of diabetic neuropathy. *Diabetes Care* 1996;19:1881–1889.
20. Meijer JW, Smit AJ, Sondersen EV, et al. Symptom scoring systems to diagnose distal polyneuropathy in diabetes: the Diabetic Neuropathy Symptom Score. *Diabetes Med.* 2002;19:962–965.
21. Benbow SJ, Wallymahmed ME, McFarlane IA. Diabetic peripheral Neuropathy and quality of life. *QJM* 1998;91:733–737.
22. Vileikyte L. Psychological aspects of diabetic peripheral neuropathy. *Diabetes Reviews* 1999;7: 387–394.
23. Vileikyte L, Rubin RR, Leventhal H. Psychological aspects of diabetic neuropathic foot complications. *Diabetes Metab Res Rev* 2004;20(Suppl 1):S13–S17.
24. Vileikyte L, Peyrot M, Bundy C, et al. The development and validation of a neuropathy—and foot ulcer—specific quality of life instrument. *Diabetes Care* 2003;2549–2555.
25. Boulton AJM, Scarpello JHB, Armstrong WD, et al. The natural history of Painful diabetic neuropathy – a 4-year study. *Postgrad Med J* 1983;59:556–559.
26. Mendell JR, Sahenk Z. Painful sensory neuropathy. *N Engl J Med* 2003;348:1243–1255.
27. Dyck PJ, Katz KM, Karnes JL, et al. The prevalence by staged severity of various types of diabetic neuropathy, retinopathy and nephropathy in a population-based cohort: the Rochester Diabetic Neuropathy Study. *Neurology* 1993;43:817–824.
28. Daousi C, MacFarlane IA, Woodward A, et al. Chronic painful peripheral neuropathy in an urban community controlled comparison of people with and without diabetes. *Diabetic Med* 2004;976–982.
29. Garrow AP, Silman AJ, MacFarlane GJ. The classification foot pain and disability survey: a population survey assessing prevalence and associations. *Pain* 2004;110:378–384.
30. DCCT Research Group. The effect of intensive diabetes therapy on the development and progression of neuropathy. *Annals of Internal Med* 1995;122:561–568.
31. Partanen J, Niskanen L, Lehtinen J, et al. Natural history of peripheral neuropathy in patients with non-insulin dependent diabetes. *N Engl J of Med* 1995;333:39–84.
32. Tesfaye S, Stevens LK, Stephenson JM, EuroDiab IDDM study group. Prevalence of diabetic peripheral neuropathy and its relation to glycaemic control and potential risks: the EuroDiab IDDM complication study. *Diabetologia* 1996;39:1377–1386.

33. Oyibo S, Prasad YD, Jackson NJ, Jude EB, Boulton AJM. The relationship between blood glucose excursions and painful diabetic peripheral neuropathy: a pilot study. *Diabetic Med* 2002;19:870–873.
34. Singleton JR, Smith AG, Bromberg MB. Painful sensory polyneuropathy associated with impaired glucose tolerance. *Muscle Nerve* 2001;24:1109–1112.
35. Boulton AJM, Drury J, Clarke B, Ward JD. Continuous subcutaneous insulin infusion in the management of painful diabetic neuropathy. *Diabetes Care* 1982;16:1446–1452.
36. Boulton AJM, Levin S, Comstock JA. A multicentre trial of the aldose-Reductase inhibitor, tolrestat, in patients with symptomatic diabetic Neuropathy. *Diabetologia* 1990;33:431–437.
37. Goto Y, Hotta N, Shigeta Y, et al. Effects of aldose-reductase inhibitor, Epalrestat, on diabetic neuropathy. Clinical benefit and indication for the Drug assessed from the results of a placebo-controlled double-blind study. *Biomed Pharmacother* 1995;49:269–277.
38. Ziegler D, Reljanovic M. Mehnert H, et al. Alpha-lipoic acid in the treatment of diabetic polyneuropathy in Germany: current evidence from clinical trials. *Exp Clin Endocrinol Diabetes* 1999;107:42–430.
39. Ametov AS, Barinov A, Dyck PJ, et al. SYDNEY Trial Study Group: the sensory symptoms of diabetic polyneuropathy are improved with a-lipoic acid: the SYDNEY trial. *Diabetes Care* 2003;26:770–776.
40. Vinik A, Tesfaye S, Hand D, Bastyr E. LY333531 treatment improves diabetic peripheral neuropathy with symptoms (Abstract). *Diabetes* 2002;51(Suppl 2):A79.
41. Boulton AJM, Vinik AJ, Arezzo JC, et al. Diabetic Neuropathies: a Statement by the American Diabetes Association. *Diabetes Care* 2005;28:955–962.
42. Max MB, Lynch SA, Muir J, et al. Effects of despiramine, Amitriptyline and fluoxetine on pain relief in diabetic in diabetic neuropathy. *N Engl J Med* 1996;326:1250–1256.
43. McQuay H, Tramer M, Nye BA. A systematic review of antidepressants in neuropathic pain. *Pain* 1996;68:217–227.
44. Sindrup SH, Gram LF, Brosen K, et al. The SSRI Paroxetine is effective in the treatment of diabetic neuropathy symptoms. *Pain* 1990;42:135–144.
45. Sindrup SH, Bjerre U, Dejgaard A, et al. The selective serotonin reuptake inhibitor Citalopram relieves the symptoms of diabetic neuropathy. *Clin Pharmacol Ther* 1992;53:547–552.
46. Rull JA, Quibrera R, Gonzalex-Millan H, et al. Symptomatic treatment of peripheral diabetic neuropathy with Carbamazepine (Tegretol): double blind crossover trial. *Diabetologia* 1969;5:215–218.
47. Backonja M, Beydoun A, Edward KR, et al. Gabapentin for the Symptomatic treatment of painful neuropathy in patients with diabetes Mellitus: a randomized controlled trial. *JAMA* 1998;280:1831–1836.
48. Backonja M, Glazman RL. Gabapentin dosing for neuropathic pain: evidence from randomized placebo controlled clinical trials. *Clin Ther* 2003;25:81–104.
49. Rosenstock J, Tuchman M, LaMoreau L, et al. Pregabalin for the treatment of painful diabetic neuropathy: a randomized, controlled trial. *Pain* 2004;110:628–634.
50. Beydoun A, Kobetz SA, Carrazana EJ. Efficacy of oxcarbazepine in the treatment of diabetic neuropathy. *Clin J Pain* 2004;20:174–178.
51. Kochar DK, Rawat N, Agrawal RP, et al. Sodium valproate for painful diabetic neuropathy: a randomized double-blind trial. *QJM* 2004;97:33–38.
52. Raskin P, Donofrio PD, Rosenthal NR, et al. Topiramate vs placebo in Painful diabetic neuropathy: analgesic and metabolic effects. *Neurology* 2004;63:865–873.
53. Harati Y, Gooch C, Swenson M, et al. Double-blind randomized trial of tramadol for the treatment of the pain of diabetic neuropathy. *Neurology* 1998;50:1841–1846.
54. Harati Y, Gooch C, Swenson M, Edelman SV, et al. Maintenance of the long-term effectiveness of tramadol in treatment of the pain of diabetic neuropathy. *J Diabetes Compl* 2000;14:65–70.

55. Gimbel JS, Richards P, Portenoy RK. Controlled-release oxycodone for pain in diabetic neuropathy: a randomized controlled trial. *Neurology* 2003;60:927–934.
56. Watson CPN, Moulin D, Watt-Watson J, et al. Controlled-release oxycodone relieves neuropathic pain: a randomized controlled trial in painful diabetic neuropathy. *Pain* 2003;105: 71–78.
57. Jarvis B, Coukell AJ. Mexilitene: a review of its therapeutic use in Painful diabetic neuropathy. *Drugs* 1998;56:691–708.
58. Nelson KA, Park KM, Robinovitz E, et al. High-dose oral dextromethorphan versus placebo in painful diabetic neuropathy and postherpetic neuralgia. *Neurology* 1997; 48:1212–1218.
59. Kirby LC. Memantine in the treatment of diabetic patients with painful peripheral neuropathy: a double-blind placebo-controlled phase IIB trial. *Pain Med* 2002;3:182–183.
60. Zhang WY, Wan Po AL. The effectiveness of topically applied capsaicin: a meta-analysis. *Eur J Clin Pharm* 1994;45:517–522.
61. Low PA, Opfer-Gehrking TL, Dyck PJ, et al. Double-blind placebo- Controlled study of capsaicin cream in chronic distal painful Polyneuropathy. *Pain* 1995;62:163–168.
62. Yuen KC, Baker NR, Rayman G. Treatment of chronic painful diabetic neuropathy with isosorbide dinitrate spray: a double-blind placebo- controlled cross-over study. *Diabetes Care* 2002;25:1699–1703.
63. Rayman G, Baker NR, Krishnan ST. Glyceryl trynitrate patches as an alternative to isosorbide dinitrate spray in the treatment of painful neuropathy. *Diabetes Care* 2003;26: 2697–2698.
64. Barbano RL, Herrmann DN, Hart SG, et al. Effectiveness, tolerability and impact on quality of life of the 5% Lidocaine patch in diabetic polyneuropathy. *Arch Neurol* 2004;61: 914–918.
65. Kaye G, Wollitzer AO, Jovanovic L. Comfort and support improve painful diabetic neuropathy whereas disappointment and frustration deteriorate the metabolic and neuropathic status. *Diabetes Care* 2003;26:2478–2479.
66. Abusaisha BB, Constanzi JB, Boulton AJM. Acupuncture for the treatment of chronic painful diabetic neuropathy: a long-term study. *Diabetes Res Clinl Practice* 1998;39: 115–121.
67. Oyibo S, Breislin K, Boulton AJM. Electrical stimulation therapy through stocking electrodes for painful diabetic neuropathy: a double- blind controlled crossover study. *Diabetic Med* 2004;21:940–944.
68. Zinman LH, Ngo M, Ng ET, et al. Low-intensity laser therapy for painful symptoms of diabetic sensorimotor polyneuropathy: a controlled trial. *Diabetes Care* 2004;27:921–924.
69. Leonard DR, Farooqu MH, Myers S. Restoration of sensation, reduced pain, and improved balance in subjects with diabetic peripheral neuropathy: a double-blind, randomized placebo-controlled study with monochromatic infrared treatment. *Diabetes Care* 2004; 27:168–172.
70. Hamza MA, White PF, Craig WF, et al. Percutaneous electrical nerve stimulation: a novel analgesic therapy for diabetic neuropathic pain. *Diabetes Care* 2000;23:365–370.
71. Weintraub MI, Wolfe GI, Barohn RA, et al. Static magnetic field therapy for symptomatic diabetic neuropathy: a randomized, double-blind, placebo-controlled trial. *Arch of Phys Med Rehab* 2003;86:736–746.
72. Tesfaye S, Watt J, Benbow SJ, et al. Electrical spinal-cord stimulation for painful diabetic peripheral neuropathy. *Lancet* 1996;348:1696–1701.
73. Daousi C, Benbow SJ, Macfarlane IA. Electrical spinal cord stimulation in the long-term treatment of chronic painful diabetic neuropathy. *Diabet Med* 2005;25:393–398.

22
Focal and Multifocal Diabetic Neuropathy

Gérard Said, MD

SUMMARY

Diabetic neuropathy is currently the most common neuropathy in the world, and it is associated with a wide range of clinical manifestations. The vast majority of patients with clinical diabetic neuropathy have a distal symmetrical form of the disorder that progresses following a fiberlength-dependent pattern, with sensory and autonomic manifestations predominating. Occasionally, patients with diabetes can develop focal and multifocal neuropathies that include cranial nerve involvement and limb and truncal neuropathies. This neuropathic pattern tends to occur after 50 years of age, and mostly in patients with long-standing diabetes mellitus. Length-dependent diabetic polyneuropathy does not show any trend towards improvement, and either relentlessly progresses or remains relatively stable over a number of years. Conversely, the focal diabetic neuropathies, which are often associated with inflammatory vasculopathy on nerve biopsies, remain self-limited, sometimes after a relapsing course. Other causes of neuropathies must be excluded in diabetic patients with focal neuropathies, and treatable causes must always be sought in diabetic patients with disabling motor deficit.

Key Words: Proximal diabetic neuropathy; diabetic ophthalmoplegia; thoracic neuropathy; inflammatory diabetic neuropathy; nerve biopsy.

INTRODUCTION

Diabetic neuropathy is the most common neuropathy in industrialized countries, with a remarkable range of clinical manifestations. More than 80% of the patients with clinical diabetic neuropathy have a distal sy mmetrical form, with predominant or isolated sensory and autonomic manifestations *(1,2)*. In the others, and usually in association with symptomatic or latent distal symmetrical sensory polyneuropathy, patients with diabetes might develop a focal neuropathy that includes cranial nerve involvement, limb and truncal neuropathies, and proximal diabetic neuropathy (PDN) of the lower limbs. In this group of neuropathies the disorder tends to occur both in men and women more than 50 years of age, most with longstanding type 1 and type 2 diabetes. The long-term prognosis of focal neuropathy is good in most cases, but sequelae occur. The occurrence of focal neuropathy in patients with diabetes requires first to exclude a nerve lesion owing to a superimposed cause by appropriate investigations. Then, to consider the occurrence of nondiabetic neuropathies more common

From: *Contemporary Diabetes: Diabetic Neuropathy: Clinical Management, Second Edition*
Edited by: A. Veves and R. Malik © Humana Press Inc., Totowa, NJ

in patients with diabetes, before concluding that the patient is suffering from a focal diabetic neuropathy and discussing which treatment, if any, is needed in addition to control of diabetes.

CRANIAL DIABETIC NEUROPATHY

Oculomotor nerve palsies are the most common if not the only cranial neuropathy observed in patients with diabetes.

Historical Background

Ogle in 1866, was the first author to mention the occurrence of diabetic ophthalmoplegia *(3)*. In 1905, Dieulafoy published a series of 58 personal cases, in which most of the clinical characteristics of diabetic ophthalmoplegia were described *(4)*. In 1935, Waite and Beetham *(5)* performed the first epidemiological study on the subject in which they compared the occurrence of oculomotor palsy in 2002 diabetic patients with 457 patients without diabetes. A series of other clinical reports have refined our knowledge on the subject but pathological studies remain scanty with only a few autopsy cases studied *(6–8)* and the pathophysiology of oculomotor palsies in patients with diabetes remains a matter of discussion.

Epidemiology

Such as focal neuropathy observed in other sites of the body, diabetic ophthalmoplegia is uncommon in diabetic patients. In 1933, Gray *(9)* observed two patients with ophthalmoplegia among 500 diabetic patients examined and Waite and Beetham *(5,10)* estimated the incidence of oculomotor palsy among patients with diabetes to be 0.8–1.8%. It is interesting to note that in this study, the frequency of oculomotor palsy was 0.8% in patients of less than 45 years of age, against 2.1% after 45 years.

Frequency of involvement of the different oculomotor nerves: the sixth and the third cranial nerves are most commonly affected. In a series of 58 cases of diabetic ophthalmoplegia, Dieulafoy *(4)* reported 35 cases of sixth nerve palsy, 12 cases of third nerve palsy, five cases of fourth nerve palsy, and six cases of external ophthalmoplegia. The sixth cranial nerve was more often affected than the third one in two series *(5,11)*. Conversely, in other series the third nerve is predominantly affected as the 14 patients reported by Weinstein and Dolger *(12)*, included seven cases of third nerve palsy, six of sixth nerve involvement, and one with simultaneous involvement of both nerves. In an analysis of 811 cases of oculomotor palsies, diabetes accounted for 2.6% of third nerve palsy, 1.9% of sixth nerve palsy, and 0.6% of fourth nerve palsy *(13)*. Finally, in Zorrilla and Kozak's series of 24 cases, 17 patients had an involvement of the third nerve, including two bilaterally, and seven cases of sixth nerve palsy, but no fourth nerve involvement *(14)*.

Clinical Manifestations

In virtually all cases diabetic ophthalmoplegia occurs in patients with diabetes with more than 50 years of age, both in type 1 and type 2 diabetes. Rare cases have been reported in younger patients or even in children *(15)*. The onset is rapid, within a day or two. In many cases, the patient experiences pains a few hours to a few days before noticing diplopia. Pain thus preceded the onset of diplopia in 14 out of the 25 patients reported by Green et al. *(16)* and in 18 out of the 22 episodes of oculomotor palsy that occurred in the 20 patients reported by Goldstein and Cogan *(17)*. Pain seems common when the third cranial nerve is affected than when the sixth nerve is involved *(14)*. Pain is usually aching behind or above the eye, and sometimes more diffuse, but always homolateral to the oculomotor palsy. Pain is often attributed to the involvement of the first and second divisions of the trigeminal nerve within the cavernous sinus *(14)*, whereas others suggest a role for activation of pain-sensitive endings within the sheath of the third nerve as it traverses the cavernous sinus *(8,18)*. Pain does not persist after the onset of diplopia.

Oculomotor dysfunction is often incomplete when the third nerve is involved, one or two muscles might only be paralyzed. In their series of 22 episodes of ophthalmoplegia observed in 20 patients, Goldstein and Cogan *(17)* mentioned 12 episodes of complete dysfunction, three episodes of nearly complete dysfunction, and three of partial paralysis. Ptosis is marked, the eye is deviated outward when the internal rectus muscle is affected; the patient is unable to move the eye medially, upward, or downward. Pupillary innervation is often spared, as in 75% of the cases in *(17)*, whereas massive pupillar paralysis was observed in only two out of 20 patients. In another study *(16)* pupillary function was spared in 68% of cases, whereas Rucker *(13)* observed pupillary dysfunction in three out of 21 cases of third nerve palsy. Sparing of pupillary function permits differentiation of third nerve palsy of diabetic origin from third nerve palsy, resulting from compression of the nerve by an aneurysm of the posterior communicating artery in which pupillary dilatation is very common. The centrofascicular lesion found by Asbury and coworkers *(8)* at an autopsy of a patient with third nerve palsy accounts for sparing of pupillary function because of the relative sparing of pupillomotor fibers, which are peripherally placed in the third nerve *(18)*. However, it has been suggested recently that isolated third nerve lesions in patients with diabetes, with or without pupillary sparing, could result from mesencephalic infarcts *(19)*. In any case, brain magnetic resonance imaging should be performed to exclude a tumor, an aneurysm, or a hematoma.

Spontaneous complete recovery invariably occurs within an average 2–3 months, independently of the quality of control of hyperglycemia. Aberrant regeneration and synkinesis, which are so common after facial nerve palsy of different origin, do not disturb recovery of diabetic ophthalmoplegia.

Pathology

Two serial section studies performed in patients with third cranial nerve palsy demonstrated a centrofascicular lesion of the nerve in its intracavernous portion *(7,8)*. In the latter report, the axons were relatively spared on silver-stained sections. The myelin destructive lesion was 6–7 mm in length and the fibers placed at the periphery of the nerve trunk were relatively spared, which accounted for the pupillary sparing. The authors found no occluded vessel either intraneurally or in the nutrient vessels supplying the third nerve. In both reports the authors agreed that the observed centrofascicular lesions of the third nerve were most likely ischemic in origin. However, it must be noted that nerve ischemia usually induce axonal nerve lesions, and not demyelinative ones. An inflammatory process of the type observed in biopsy specimens of the femoral nerve with partial ischemic lesions should also be considered.

FOCAL AND MULTIFOCAL LIMB NEUROPATHY

Isolated involvement of peripheral nerve of the limbs including radial, median, and ulnar nerves in the upper limbs and of the peroneal nerve for the lower limbs, occurs in patient with diabetes. It is sometimes, difficult to know whether it is a manifestation of increased liability of nerves to pressure palsy in common sites of entrapment in patients with diabetes, or a specific diabetic neuropathy. In other cases development of a sensorimotor deficit in the territory of one or several nerve trunks occur without evidence of a superimposed cause for neuropathy. Such cases are extremely rare considering the frequency of distal symmetrical diabetic neuropathy and should always be investigated as in patients without diabetes. In particular, it is necessary to perform electrophysiological testings to enable a more accurate localization of the lesions, and when clinical and electrophysiological data point to spinal root lesions, magnetic resonance imaging of the spine has to be performed, or any other investigation needed to exclude another cause of neuropathy. When nerve trunks are clearly affected clinically and electrophysiologically, a nerve and muscle biopsy in an affected territory should be considered to exclude such causes as necrotizing arthritis, sarcoidosis, or leprosy. In some cases however, no other cause than diabetes is found and the diagnosis of diabetic neuritis is likely. In the lower limbs, the most common pattern of focal neuropathy is that of proximal sensory and motor manifestations. It is worth noting that markers of systemic inflammation are normal in diabetic multifocal neuropathy, but dramatic weight loss is common.

PDN of the Lower Limbs

Patients with diabetes, usually more than 50 years of age, might also present with proximal neuropathy of the lower limbs characterized by a variable degree of pain and sensory loss associated with uni- or bilateral proximal muscle weakness and atrophy. This syndrome, which was originally described by Bruns in 1890 *(20)* has been subsequently reported under the terms of diabetic myelopathy *(21)*, diabetic amyotrophy *(22)*, femoral neuropathy *(23,24)*, PDN *(25,26)*, femoral-sciatic neuropathy *(27)*, and the Bruns–Garland syndrome *(28,29)*. The neurological picture is limited to the lower limbs and is usually asymmetrical *(30)*. Clinically, the different patterns and the course of PDN strikingly differ from those of DSSP, suggesting different pathophysiological features. In a recent study with 27 patients *(31)*, 24 with type 2 diabetes and 3 with type 1 diabetes had a mean age at diagnosis of 62 years (range 46–71) and the male : female ratio was 16 : 11.

The onset of the neuropathy is acute or subacute. The patient complains of numbness or pain of the anterior aspect of the thigh, often of the burning type and worse at night. Difficulty in walking and climbing stairs occurs because of weakness of the quadriceps and iliopsoas muscles. Muscle wasting is also an early and common phenomenon, which is often easier to palpate than to observe in fatter patients. The patellar reflex is decreased or more often abolished. The syndrome progresses during weeks or months in most cases, then stabilizes and spontaneous pains decrease, sometimes rapidly. In many instances, as in those originally reported, there is no any marked or sensory loss, as emphasized by Garland *(22)* who found inconstant extensor plantar response and increased cerebrospinal fluid (CSF) protein content, felt that they resulted from a metabolic myelopathy in patients who were treated for diabetes, but not under full diabetic control. In approximately, one-third of the patients there is a definite sensory loss on the anterior aspect of the thigh, and in the others a painful contact dysesthesia in the distribution of the cutaneous branches of the femoral nerve, without definite sensory loss.

Bruns *(20)* who had described this condition, found in 1890 that the disorder was reversible only by dietetic restriction. Garland *(22)* also noticed that in four of his five patients there had been a striking recovery of power, with less obvious improvement of muscle wasting. Most of the features identified by Garland were subsequently confirmed, including the usual good long-term prognosis, independently of the quality of diabetic control.

In most cases, the patient's condition improves after months, but sequelae including disabling weakness and amyotrophy, sensory loss, and patellar areflexia are common *(31,32)*. In a recent survey of long-term follow-up of upto 14 years, recovery began after a median interval of 3 months (range 1–12 months) *(31)*. Pain was the first symptom to improve, resolution being comparatively rapid, beginning within a few weeks and being almost completed by 12 months. Residual discomfort in the patients of Coppack and Watkins took up to 3 years to subside. Motor recovery was satisfactory and none of their 27 cases showed disabling residual deficits, but seven complained of some persisting weakness and significant wasting of the thigh was evident in half of the cases *(31)*. Denervation atrophy found in the muscle samples fits well with the long-term, or permanent weakness and amyotrophy that often affected distal muscles. Relapses on the other side are common, sometimes in spite of good diabetic control. In one-fifth of the patients that were investigated for this syndrome relapses occurred on the other side within a few months, the same proportion as in *(31)*. Thus, the clinical features of PDN with frequent motor involvement, asymmetry of the deficit, gradual yet often incomplete spontaneous recovery, markedly differ from those of DSSP in which the length dependent symmetrical sensory deficit is associated with motor signs only in extreme cases and which virtually never improves spontaneously. In the syndrome described by Garland as "diabetic amyotrophy" motor manifestations are more prominent and both sides are affected, but the syndrome is a variant of PDN, as lesions of the sensory branch of the femoral nerve are also present in patients who have no sensory signs or symptoms *(32)*.

Electrophysiological Studies

Needle electromyography reveals signs of denervation in affected muscles with spontaneous fibrillation, usually bilaterally even in cases with weakness restricted to one side. In more severe cases there may be evidence of widespread denervation affecting distal leg muscles as well and also those innervated by the lower thoracic spinal roots. In cases of long duration, motor unit potentials are of increased amplitude, reflecting reinnervation by collateral sprouting from surviving motor axons. The motor action potentials might be polyphasic and of low amplitude leading to the suspicion of myopathy *(33)*. Nerve conduction studies indicate axonal loss rather than demyelination *(26)* and the compound muscle action potential in the quadriceps muscles on femoral nerve stimulation is reduced in amplitude. The F wave latencies to distal muscles *(34,35)* are difficult to interpret in view of the frequent coexistence of a distal polyneuropathy *(26,36,37)*.

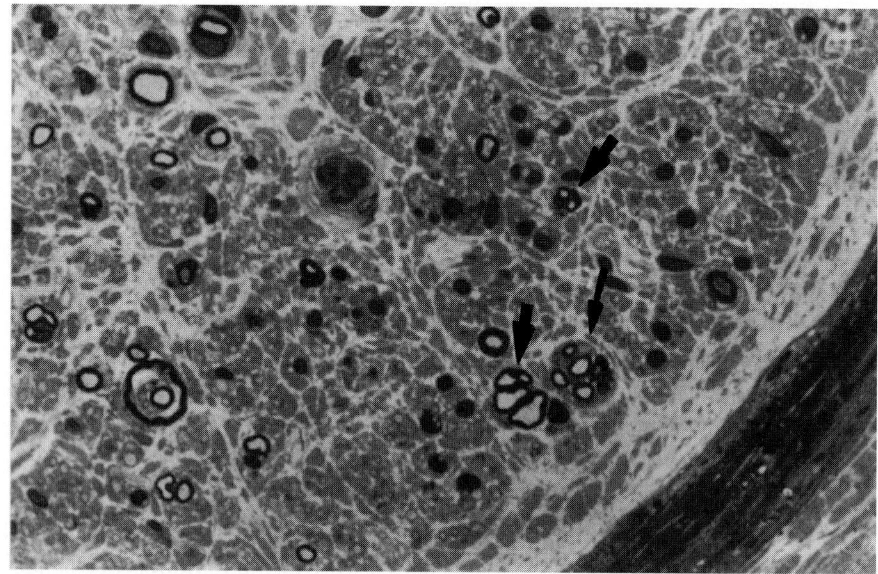

Fig. 1. One micron thick cross section of a biopsy specimen of the intermediate cutaneous nerve of the thigh from a patient with NIDDM who presented with proximal, purely motor, neuropathy of the lower limbs. There was no sensory loss upon examination. Note the striking reduction in the density of nerve fibers with several regenerating axons forming clusters (arrows). Thionin blue staining. Magnification: ×1000.

Pathological Aspects of PDN

In a recent pathological study of biopsy specimens of the intermediate cutaneous nerve of the thigh, a sensory branch of the femoral nerve, which conveys sensation from the anterior aspect of the thigh, a territory commonly involved in PDN it is found that the pathology of proximal nerves varied with the clinical aspects of the neuropathy *(32)*. Patients with the most severe sensory and motor deficit examination of the biopsy specimen revealed lesions characteristic of severe nerve ischemia, including total axon loss in two patients with the most severe deficit, and centrofascicular degeneration of fibers associated with a large number of regenerating fibers in one (Fig. 1), following a pattern of axonal loss observed in clinical and experimental nerve ischemia *(38,39)*. Lesions of nerve fibers coexisted with occlusion of a perineurial blood vessel in one of the patients, in keeping with the only detailed postmortem study of PDN available *(40)* in which the authors found a small infiltration with mononuclear cells associated with the occlusion of an interfascicular artery of the obturator nerve in a patient with proximal and distal deficit of the left lower limb. In a patient who developed a rapid, asymmetrical, distal, sensorimotor deficit shortly after the onset of the proximal deficit, recent occlusion of a perineurial blood vessel and perivascular, perineurial, and subperineurial inflammatory infiltration with mononuclear cells were demonstrated, along with axonal degeneration of the majority of nerve fibers of the superficial peroneal nerve. In the other patients, lesions of nerve fibers and of endoneurial capillaries were similar to those observed in the sural nerve in diabetic patients with symptomatic DSSP. Mixed, axonal, and demyelinative nerve lesions were associated with increased

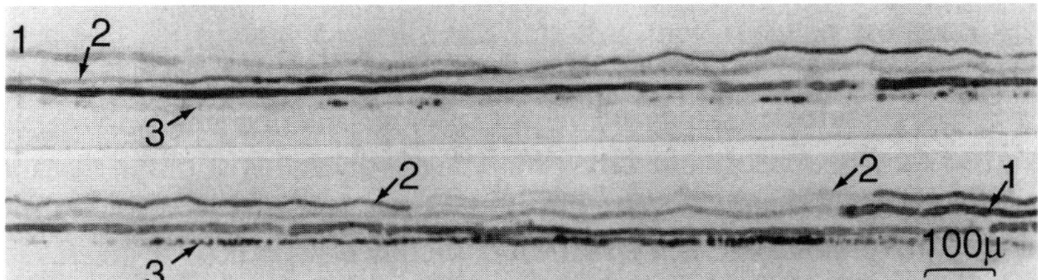

Fig. 2. Consecutive segments of groups of teased nerve fibers to illustrate the mixture of axonal degeneration (fiber 3) and segmental demyelination (fiber 2) and remyelination (fiber 1) observed in the intermediate cutaneous nerve of the thigh from a patient with clinically purely motor proximal diabetic neuropathy.

endoneurial cellularity made of mononuclear cells that suggested the presence of a low grade endoneurial inflammatory process in four of them (Fig. 2). In a recent study of patients with extremely painful PDN, similar inflammatory lesions with B and T lymphocytes mixed with macrophages were found *(41)*. The patients who were already treated with insulin for weeks or months, became painless within days after performance of the biopsy, without additional treatment (Fig. 3). These observations show that the presence of inflammatory infiltrates does not preclude spontaneous recovery *(41)*.

The relationship between the occurrence of inflammatory infiltrates, vasculitis, and diabetes is not clear. Small inflammatory infiltrates have been occasionally encountered in sural nerve biopsy specimens of patients with diabetes with neurological deficit *(42)* and in autonomic nerve bundles and ganglia *(43)*. Lesions of nerve fibers and of blood vessels because of diabetes might trigger an inflammatory reaction and reactive vasculitis in some patients; alternatively diabetes might make the nerves more susceptible to intercurrent inflammatory or immune processes. In both cases, lesions of epi- or perineurial blood vessels can induce ischemic nerve lesions responsible for severe proximal sensory and motor deficits. Conversely, in milder forms the lesions are more reminiscent of those observed in distal symmetrical polyneuropathy.

Multifocal Diabetic Neuropathy

In a small proportion of patients with diabetes a multifocal neuropathy is observed, with successive or simultaneous involvement during weeks or months of roots and nerves of the lower limbs, the trunk, and upper extremities. Prospectively, 22 consecutive patients with diabetes were studied with MDN for which other causes of neuropathy were excluded by appropriate investigations, including biopsy of a recently affected sensory nerve *(44)*. Three patients had a relapsing course, the others an unremitting subacute-progressive course. Painful multifocal sensory-motor deficit progressed during 2–12 months. Distal lower limbs were involved in all patients, unilaterally in seven, bilaterally in the others, with an asynchronous onset in most cases. In addition, proximal deficit of the lower limbs was present on one side in seven patients, on both sides in six. Thoracic radiculoneuropathy was present bilaterally in two patients, unilaterally in one. The ulnar nerve was involved in one patient, the radial nerve in two. The cerebrospinal fluid protein ranged from 0.40 to 3.55 g/L; mean: 0.87 g/L. Electrophysiological testing showed severe, multifocal, axonal nerve lesions in all cases. MDN is comparable with

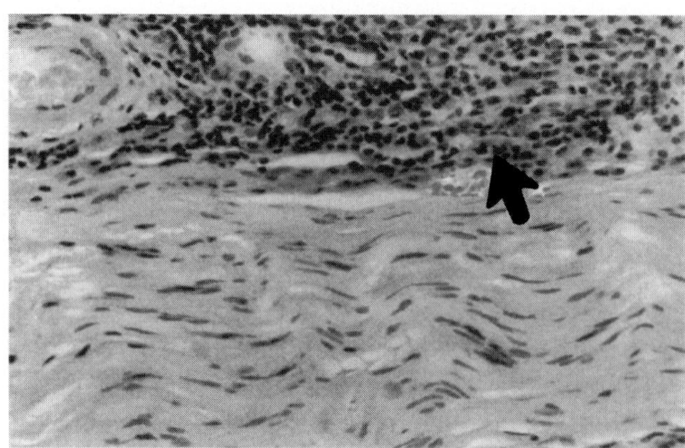

Fig. 3. Paraffin section of the a nerve specimen from a patient with painful proximal diabetic neuropathy who recovered spontaneously after performance of the biopsy of the intermediate cutaneous nerve of the thigh. Note the conspicuous inflammatory infiltration of the epineurium and perineurium (arrow). Immunolabeling showed a mixture of B and T lymphocytes with a few macrophages. H&E staining. Magnification: ×250.

the lumbosacral radiculoplexus neuropathy *(45)*. However, because this subacute neuropathy can also affect territories beyond the lumbosacral area, multifocal neuropathy seems more appropriate. It is also obvious that multifocal neuropathy or lumbosacral radiculoplexopathy is not specific to patients with diabetes, as further shown *(46)*, which underlines the need to exclude other causes of neuropathy in this setting, including a superimposed cause in patients with diabetes, such as necrotizing arthritis or chronic inflammatory demyelinating polyneuropathy that require specific treatment *(47)*.

Pathological Aspects of PDN

Asymmetrical axonal lesions were present in all nerve specimens of patients with MDN. The mean density of myelinated and of umyelinated axons was reduced to 1340 per mm^2 of endoneurial area and to 5095 per mm^2 (extremes: 0–26,600), respectively. On teased fiber preparations one-third of the fibres were at different stages of axonal degeneration, whereas 7% showed segmental demyelination or remyelination. Necrotizing vasculitis of perineurial and endoneurial blood vessels were found in six patients. Evidence of present or past endoneurial bleeding that included seepage of red cells, haemorrhage, and/or ferric iron deposits were found in the majority of the specimens. Perivascular mononuclear cell infiltrates were present in the nerve specimens of 21/22 patients, prominently in 4 patients. In comparison, nerve biopsy specimens of 30 patients with severe DSSP showed mild epineurial mononuclear cell infiltrate in one patient and endoneurial seepage of red cells in one. Thus, it is believed that MDN is related to precapillary blood vessel involvement in older patients with diabetes with a secondary inflammatory response.

Besides the high frequency both of endoneurial bleeding and of inflammatory infiltrates, occlusion of small- and middle-sized epineurial and perineurial arteries differentiate MDN from DSP. The intensity and distribution of the lesions seemed more severe in MDN than in PDN, but both patterns can be included in multifocal diabetic neuropathies. The outcome is better in MDN than in DSP. Improvement occurs in all patients after a few months, but sequelae are common.

Focal Neuropathy of the Upper Limbs

Focal nerve lesions of the upper limbs are very uncommon in diabetes, and another cause must always be looked for in this setting. They occurred in the setting of MDN in 3/22 patients of our series. Besides these patients only two patients were seen with painful ulnar nerve involvement, two patients with a radial nerve palsy, and one patient who developed brachial neuritis after a proximal neuropathy of the lower limbs, which could be attributed to diabetes. Proximal weakness of the upper limbs, as it appears in the lower limbs, is very uncommon, and seems to affect predominantly muscles supplied by the C5–C6 spinal roots *(48)*.

Truncal Neuropathy

Trunk or thoracoabdominal neuropathy affects almost only older subjects with diabetes *(49)*. It is unilateral or predominantly so. The onset is abrupt or rapid, with pains or dysesthesiae as the main feature. The pain might have a radicular distribution and is made worse by contact and at night. Weakness of abdominal muscles occurs *(50)*. Thoracic or truncal neuropathy should not be confused with sensory loss that affects the anterior aspect of the trunk in severe forms of length dependent neuropathy, which is virtually never painful on the trunk *(51)*.

NONDIABETIC NEUROPATHIES MORE COMMON IN PATIENTS WITH DIABETES

In addition to specific neuropathies, patients with diabetes appear more prone to develop some types of neuropathy than patients without diabetes.

Increased Liability to Pressure Palsy

Pressure palsy is more common in diabetic individuals *(52)*. Carpal tunnel syndrome occurs in 12% of diabetic patients *(53)* and the incidence of ulnar neuropathy because of microlesions at the elbow level is high in patients with diabetes too *(54)*.

Acquired Inflammatory Demyelinative Polyneuropathy

Inflammatory, predominantly demyelinative neuropathy also must be differentiated from diabetic polyneuropathy, and may occur with a greater frequency in this population. This diagnosis must be suspected when an acute or subacute, often predominantly motor, demyelinating polyneuropathy occurs in a patient with diabetes. Electrophysiological features are those of a demyelinating neuropathy *(55)*. The course and response to treatments are the same as in patients without diabetes.

Mucormycosis

This rare condition is an acute disease that affects successively the air cavities of the face, the orbit, and the brain, in relation to proliferation of a fungus of the class *Phycomyceta (56)*. In 36% of cases it is associated with diabetes, especially in patients with diabetes with ketoacidosis. After an episode of rhinological involvement with epistaxis, a patient with diabetes in acidosis manifests violent headaches and orbitonasal pains with swelling of the lids and ophthalmoplegia. The disease spreads to the meninges and to the brain through the arteries, inducing thrombosis of the ophthalmic then of the internal carotid artery with subsequent hemiplegia. The prognosis is extremely poor.

The diagnosis should be made very early by biopsy of the nasal lesions, which allows identification of the causative phycomycete allowing immediate treatment.

DIFFERENTIAL DIAGNOSIS

In focal neuropathy, occurring in patients with diabetes, a neuropathy of another origin must always be excluded. In patients with ophthalmoplegia, preservation of pupillary function in a nearly complete third nerve palsy strongly suggests a diabetic origin, however, even in such cases, it is wiser to perform a noninvasive investigation of the area. Magnetic resonance angiography will permit exclusion of a compressive lesion of the third nerve by a large aneurysm of the carotid artery within the cavernous sinus, of the posterior communicating artery, or a fusiform aneurysm of the top of the basilar artery. Imaging will also permit to exclude tumors occurring at the base of the brain or in the basal skull. In patients with progressive involvement of several cranial nerves without imaging abnormalities, examination of the CSF might detect malignant cells characteristic of a carcinomatous meningitis. In patients with diabetes who develop a focal or multifocal neuropathy of the limbs, causes other than diabetes should be considered. The first step in this context is to determine if the lesions are located in the spinal roots or in the peripheral nerves, a distinction which might be difficult clinically and electrophysiologically. In addition, the lesions might be mixed. A nerve and a muscle biopsy might be considered, especially when another cause of focal or multifocal neuropathy is considered. When a patient with diabetes develops proximal weakness without much pain, a superimposed cause of motor neuropathy or of motor neuron disease must be considered, and appropriate investigations undertaken.

TREATMENT OF FOCAL DIABETIC NEUROPATHIES

Cranial nerve palsies improve spontaneously and do not require specific treatment. PDN is often very painful and should be treated, for example, with paracetamol (acetaminophen) and codeine. As some patients with disabling painful proximal neuropathy responded only to corticosteroids, this treatment should be considered in severe forms *(32)*. This will require adjustment of diabetic control with insulin in most cases. Others have suggested the use of immunosuppressive or immunomodulators, like intravenous immunoglobulins *(42)*, but it should be kept in mind that the overall spontaneous prognosis of focal diabetic neuropathies is good.

REFERENCES

1. De Freitas MR, Nascimento OJ, Chimelli L, et al. Neuropatia diabética. I - Conceito; Epidemiologia, Classificaçao, Quadro Clinico E Electroneuromiografico. Estudo De 210 Casos. *Rev Bras Neurol* 1992;28:69–73.
2. Llewelyn JG, Tomlinson DR, Thomas PK. Diabetic neuropathies, in *Peripheral Neuropathy*, vol 2, (Dyck PJ, Thomas PK, eds.), Elsevier Saunders, Philadelphia, 2005, pp. 1951–1991.
3. Man HX. Aspects neuro-ophtalmologiques du diabète sucré, in: *Journées de Diabétologie de l'Hôtel Dieu*. Editions Médicales Flammarion. Paris, 1967, pp. 83–100.
4. Dieulafoy G. *Clinique Médicale de l'Hotel-Dieu de Paris* 1905–1906. Masson et Cie, Paris, 1906, pp. 130–154.
5. Waite JH, Beetham VP. The visual mechanisms in diabetes mellitus (a comparative study of 2002 diabetics and 457 non diabetics). *New Engl J Med* 1935;212:429–443.

6. Weber RB, Daroff RB, Mackey EA. Pathology of oculomotor nerve palsy in diabetes. *Neurology* 1970;20:835.
7. Dreyfus PM, Hakim S, Adams RD. Diabetic ophthalmoplegia. *Arch Neurol Neurosurg Psychiatr* 1957;77:337–349.
8. Asbury AK, Aldredge H, Hershberg R, Fischer CM. Oculomotor palsy in diabetes mellitus: a clinico-pathological study. *Brain* 1970;93:555–566.
9. Gray WA. Ocular conditions in diabetes mellitus. *Brit J Ophtha* 1933;17:577–620.
10. Dollfus M. Examen ophtalmologique de 1300 diabétiques. XVII congrès international d'Ophtalmologie, *Acta Concil* 1954;119–127.
11. Collier J. Paralysis of the oculomotor nerve trunks in diabetes. *Proc Roy Soc Med* 1929; 23:627–630.
12. Weinstein EA, Dolger H. External ocular muscle palsies occurring in diabetes mellitus. *Arch Neurol Psychiatr (Chicago)* 1948;60:597–603.
13. Rucker CW. Paralysis of the third, fourth and sixth cranial nerves. *Am J Ophthal* 1958;46:787–794.
14. Zorrilla E, Kozak GP. Ophthalmoplegia in diabetes mellitus. *Ann Intern Med* 1967; 5:968–977.
15. Jackson WP. Ocular nerve palsy with severe headache in diabetes. *Br Med J* 1955;2:408.
16. Green WR, Hackett R, Schlezinger NS. Neuro-ophthalmologic evaluation of oculomotor nerve paralysis. *Arch Ophthal* 1964;72:154–167.
17. Goldstein JE, Cogan DG. Diabetic ophthalmoplegia with special reference to the pupil. *Arch Ophthal* 1960;64:592–600.
18. Sunderland S, Hughes ESR. The pupilloconstrictor pathway and the nerves to the ocular muscles in man. *Brain* 1946;69:301.
19. Hopf HC, Gutmann L. Diabetic third nerve palsy: evidence for a mesencephalic lesion. *Neurology* 1990;40:1041.
20. Bruns L. Ueber neuritische Lähmungen beim diabetes mellitus. *Berl Klin Wochenscher* 1890;27:509–515.
21. Garland HT, Taverner D. Diabetic myelopathy. *Br Med J* 1953;1:1505.
22. Garland HT. Diabetic amyotrophy. *Br Med J* 1955;2:1287–1290.
23. Goodman JI. Femoral neuropathy in relation to diabetes mellitus: report of 17 cases. *Diabetes* 1954;3:266–273.
24. Calverley JR, Mulder DW. Femoral neuropathy. *Neurology* (*Minneap.*) 1960;10:963–967.
25. Asbury AK. Proximal diabetic neuropathy. *Ann Neurol* 1977;2:179.
26. Subramony SH, Wilbourn AJ. Diabetic proximal neuropathy. Clinical and electromyographic studies. *J Neurol Sci* 1982;53:293.
27. Skanse B, Gydell K. A rare type of femoral-sciatic neuropathy in diabetes mellitus. *Acta Med Scand* 1956;155:463–468.
28. Barohn RJ, Sahenk Z, Warmolts JR, Mendell JR. The Bruns-Garland syndrome (Diabetic amyotrophy) revisited 100 years later. *Arch Neurol* 1991;48:1130–1135.
29. Chokroverty S, Reyes MG, Rubino FA. Bruns-Garland syndrome of diabetic amyotrophy. *Trans Am Neurol Assoc* 1977;102:1–4.
30. Asbury AK. Focal and multifocal neuropathies of diabetes, in *Diabetic Neuropathy* (Dyck PJ, et al. eds.), Saunders, Philadelphia, 1987, pp. 43–55.
31. Coppack SW, Watkins PJ. The natural history of diabetic femoral neuropathy. *Q J Med* 1991;79:307–313.
32. Said G, Goulon-Goeau C, Lacroix C, Moulonguet A. Nerve biopsy findings in different patterns of proximal diabetic neuropathy. *Ann Neurol* 1994;35:559–569.
33. Lamontagne A, Buchthal F. Electrophysiological studies in diabetic neuropathy. *J Neurol Neurosurg Psychiatr* 1970;33:442–452.

34. Williams IR, Mayer RF. Subacute proximal diabetic neuropathy. *Neurology* 1976;26: 108–116.
35. Chokroverty S. Proximal nerve dysfunction in diabetic proximal amyotrophy. *Arch Neurol* 1982;39:403–407.
36. Isaacs H, Gilchrist G. Diabetic amyotrophy. *S Afr Med J* 1960;134:768–773.
37. Bastron JA, Thomas JE. Diabetic polyradiculopathy: clinical and electromyographic findings in 105 patients. *Mayo Clin Proc* 1981;56:725–732.
38. Fujimura H, Lacroix C, Said G. Vulnerability of nerve fibers to ischaemia. *Brain* 1991; 114:1929–1942.
39. Nukada H, Dyck PJ. Microsphere embolization of nerve capillaries and fiber degeneration. *Am J Path* 1984;115:275–287.
40. Raff MC, Sangalang V, Asbury AK. Ischemic mononeuropathy and mononeuropathy multiplex in diabetes mellitus. *Arch Neurol* 1968;18:487–499.
41. Said G, Elgrably F, Lacroix C, et al. Painful Proximal diabetic neuropathy: Inflammatory nerve lesions and spontaneous favourable outcome. *Ann Neurol* 1997;41:762–770.
42. Krendel DA, Costigan DA, Hopkins LC. Successful treatment of neuropathies in patients with diabetes mellitus. *Arch Neurol* 1995;52:1053–1061.
43. Duchen LW, Anjorin A, Watkins PJ, Mackay JD. Pathology of autonomic neuropathy in diabetes mellitus. *Ann Int Med* 1980;92:301–303.
44. Said G, Lacroix C, Lozeron P, Ropert A, Planté V, Adams D. Inflammatory vasculopathy in multifocal diabetic neuropathy. *Brain* 2003;126:376–385.
45. Dyck PJ, Norell JE, Dyck PJ. Microvasculitis and ischemia in diabetic lumbosacral radiculoplexus neuropathy. *Neurology* 1999;10:2113–2121.
46. Dyck PJ, Norell JE, Dyck PJ. Non-diabetic lumbosacral radiculoplexus neuropathy: natural history, outcome and comparison with the diabetic variety. *Brain* 2001;124:1197–1207.
47. Lozeron P, Nahum L, Lacroix C, Ropert A, Guglielmi JM, Said G. Symptomatic diabetic and non-diabetic neuropathies in a series of 100 diabetic patients. *J Neurol* 2002;249: 569–575.
48. Wilbourn AJ. Diabetic neuropathies, in *Clinical Electromyography* (Brown WF, Bolton CF, eds.), 2nd ed. Butterworth-Heinemann, Boston, 1993, pp. 477–516.
49. Ellenberg M. Diabetic truncal mononeuropathy: a new clinical syndrome. *Diabetes Care* 1978;1:10–13.
50. Boulton AJ, Angus E, Ayyar DR, Weiss R. Diabetic thoracic polyradiculopathy presenting as an abdominal swelling, *B Med J* 1984;289:798–799.
51. Said G, Slama G, Selva J. Progressive centripetal degeneration of axons in small fibre type diabetic polyneuropathy. A clinical and pathological study. *Brain* 1983;106:791–807.
52. Mulder DW, Lambert EH, Bastron JA, Sprague RG. The neuropathies associated with diabetes: a clinical and electromyographic study of 103 unselected diabetic patients. *Neurology (Minneap.)* 1961;11:275–284.
53. Palumbo PJ, Elveback LR, Whisnant JP. Neurologic complications of diabetic mellitus: transient ischemic attack, stroke and peripheral neuropathy, in *Advances in Neurology* (Schoenberg BS, ed.), Raven Press, New York, 1978, Vol. 19, pp. 593–601.
54. Fraser DM, Campbell IW, Ewing DJ, et al. Mononeuropathy in diabetes mellitus. *Diabetes* 1979;28:96.
55. Cornblath D, Drachman DB, Griffin JW. Demyelinating motor neuropathy in patients with diabetic polyneuropathy. *Ann Neurol* 1987;22:126–132.
56. Dhermy P. Phycomycosis (Mucormycosis), in *Handbook of Clinical Neurology* (Vinken PJ, Bruyn GW, eds.), North Holland Publishing Company, Amsterdam, 1978, Vol. 35, pp. 541–555.

23
Hypoglycemia and the Autonomic Nervous System

Roy Freeman, MD

SUMMARY

Widespread implementation of regimens to rigorously control blood sugar in patients with diabetes has led to an increased incidence of severe iatrogenic hypoglycemic events with substantial morbidity and mortality. Hypoglycemia provokes a sequence of counterregulatory metabolic, neural, and clinical responses. Insulin secretion decreases whereas glucagon, epinephrine, norepinephrine, pancreatic polypeptide, cortisol, and growth hormone increase. The sympathetic, parasympathetic, and sympatho-adrenal divisions of the autonomic nervous system are activated in response to the falling blood sugar. The spectrum of reduced counterregulatory hormone responses (in particular epinephrine) and decreased symptom perception of hypoglycemia because of decreased autonomic nervous system activation following recent antecedent hypoglycemia has been termed "hypoglycemia induced autonomic failure." This leads to a vicious cycle of hypoglycemia unawareness that induces a further decrease in counterregulatory hormone responses to hypoglycemia. This vicious cycle occurs commonly in diabetic subjects in strict glycemic control. The reduced epinephrine response to antecedent hypoglycemia occurs in the absence of diabetic autonomic neuropathy as measured by standard tests of autonomic function. The presence of autonomic neuropathy, however, further attenuates the epinephrine response to hypoglycemia in diabetic subjects after recent hypoglycemic exposure. The mechanisms of hypoglycemia induced autonomic failure are not fully elucidated.

Key Words: Autonomic failure; autonomic neuropathy; counterregulation; hypoglycemia; hypothalamus sympathetic nervous system.

INTRODUCTION

Results from the Diabetes Control and Complications Trial, *(1)* the United Kingdom Prospective Diabetes Study *(2)* and other studies of type 1 *(3,4)* and type 2 *(5,6)* diabetes mellitus have consistently documented that improved glycemic control decreases the incidence and progression of retinopathy, nephropathy, and neuropathy in subjects with diabetes. The widespread implementation of regimens to rigorously control blood sugar in patients with diabetes has led to an increased incidence of severe iatrogenic hypoglycemic events. The annual incidence of severe hypoglycemia and coma is increased threefold in intensively treated patients *(1,7)*. This complication of intensive treatment has limited rigorous glycemic management of diabetes.

From: *Contemporary Diabetes: Diabetic Neuropathy: Clinical Management, Second Edition*
Edited by: A. Veves and R. Malik © Humana Press Inc., Totowa, NJ

The counterregulatory response is triggered by specialized glucose-sensing neurons within the brain and, to a lesser extent, the portal venous system *(8)*. The brain regions that play a critical role in the detection of incipient hypoglycemia localize to the ventromedial hypothalamus—in particular the ventromedial and arcuate nuclei *(9,10)*, and brainstem *(11)*. The molecular mechanisms whereby these neurons detect fluctuations in glucose levels are not fully elucidated. It is suggested that this kinase functions as a intracellular fuel gauge *(12)* that becomes activated by a decrease in the ATP-to-ADP ratio *(13)*.

Deficient secretion of glucagon and catecholamines is in large part responsible for the morbidity and mortality associated with iatrogenic hypoglycemia. The glucagon response to hypoglycemia is irreversibly attenuated after several years of type 1 diabetes and the adrenergic response becomes the critical defense mechanism against insulin induced hypoglycemia *(14)*. Numerous studies have documented that antecedent hypoglycemia is a primary cause of the impaired adrenergic response to insulin-induced hypoglycemia. The mechanisms whereby this impairment occurs are not fully elucidated *(15,16)*.

Glucose Counterregulation

Hypoglycemia provokes a sequence of metabolic, neural, and clinical responses *(17,18)*. Insulin secretion decreases whereas glucagon, epinephrine, norepinephrine, pancreatic polypeptide, cortisol, and growth hormone increase. The sympathetic, parasympathetic, and sympatho-adrenal divisions of the autonomic nervous system are activated in response to the falling blood sugar. The autonomic clinical features associated with these metabolic and neural changes include tremor, palpitations, anxiety, diaphoresis, hunger, and paresthesias. Hypoglycemia also impairs neuronal function leading to fatigue, weakness, dizziness, and cognitive and behavioural symptoms. Lower blood sugar levels may cause seizures, coma, and death *(19–22)*.

Studies carried out in several different laboratories have confirmed that diabetic subjects in strict glycemic control or on insulin pump therapy exhibit decreased counterregulatory responses to hypoglycemia *(23–29)*. In these individuals perception of hypoglycemic symptoms is reduced *(27–31)* and the glucose threshold at which symptoms of hypoglycemia are perceived is lowered (i.e., a lower blood glucose level is required to elicit symptoms of hypoglycemia) *(20,21,28)*. These adaptations lead to impaired glucose counterregulation and contribute to the increased incidence of severe hypoglycemia during intensive diabetes treatment *(30,32)*. Furthermore, defective counterregulatory hormone responses can be partially restored by the meticulous avoidance of hypoglycemia in intensively treated patients with short duration *(33–36)* and long duration diabetes *(37,38)*.

These studies suggest that an increased incidence of recurrent hypoglycemia is responsible for the induction of altered hormonal counterregulation and symptom perception in patients with diabetes in strict glycemic control. This assertion was confirmed in studies of normal humans without diabetes who were exposed to recurrent hypoglycemia. These studies showed that recurrent hypoglycemia induced defective hormonal counterregulation, lowered glucose thresholds for symptom perception, and impaired symptom responses to hypoglycemia is similar to those seen in strictly controlled subjects with diabetes *(39–43)*. Similarly, subjects with hypoglycemia because of insulinoma also exhibit blunted counterregulatory responses to hypoglycemia *(44)*. This altered counterregulation was reversed following removal of the insulinoma *(44,45)*.

Compared with men, women demonstrate a significantly lower counterregulatory response to the same hypoglycemic stimulus. Specifically, during hypoglycemia, epinephrine, glucagon, and growth hormone levels in the circulation are lower in women than men. Muscle sympathetic nerve activity and metabolic counterregulatory responses are also reduced in women during hypoglycemia *(46)*. In aggregate these counterregulatory responses to hypoglycemia are 50% greater in men than in women. However, antecedent hypoglycemia produces less blunting of the counterregulatory response to subsequent hypoglycemia in women than in men *(46)*. The gender differences in counterregulation in response to hypoglycemia are not attributable to gender-mediated differences in glycemic thresholds, as both men and women have a glycemic threshold for release of neuroendocrine hormones between 71 and 78 mg/dL *(47)*.

Hypoglycemic Autonomic Failure

The spectrum of reduced counterregulatory hormone responses (in particular epinephrine) and decreased symptom perception of hypoglycemia because of decreased autonomic nervous system activation following recent antecedent hypoglycemia has been termed "hypoglycemia induced autonomic failure" *(48–50)*. This leads to a vicious cycle of hypoglycemia unawareness that induces a further decrease in counterregulatory hormone responses to hypoglycemia. This vicious cycle occurs commonly in subjects with diabetes in strict glycemic control. The reduced epinephrine response to antecedent hypoglycemia occurs in the absence of diabetic autonomic neuropathy as measured by standard tests of autonomic function *(32,49,51)* (*see* Figs. 1 and 2).

However, the presence of autonomic neuropathy further attenuates the epinephrine response to hypoglycemia in subjects with diabetes after recent hypoglycemic exposure *(52–54)*. The additional downregulation of the epinephrine response is present in patients with parasympathetic nervous system involvement even in the absence of significant sympathetic nervous system deficits *(52)*. This interaction between autonomic neuropathy and the counterregulatory response is seen in most but not all studies *(49)*. Furthermore, patients with abnormal autonomic function have a greater risk for severe hypoglycemia; the odds ratio for severe hypoglycemia in people with abnormal responses in heart rate and blood pressure to standing compared with those with normal responses, was 1.7 (95% confidence interval 1.3, 2.2) after controlling for age, duration of diabetes, glycemic control, and study centre *(55)*.

Although there is consistent evidence that the antecedent hypoglycemia attenuates the sympathoadrenal (epinephrine) and parasympathetic hormonal (pancreatic polypeptide) responses to subsequent hypoglycemia *(39,43,49)*, there is conflicting evidence as to the effect of recent hypoglycemia on sympathetic neural responses. Davis and coworkers reported that antecedent hypoglycemia reduces peroneal muscle sympathetic nerve activity measured with microneurography during subsequent hypoglycemia *(43,56,57)*. In contrast, Paramore and colleagues *(58)* using another measure of sympathetic activity, forearm norepinephrine spillover rates, observed that antecedent hypoglycemia does not attenuate sympathetic activity during subsequent hypoglycemia. It is possible that differential control of the autonomic nervous

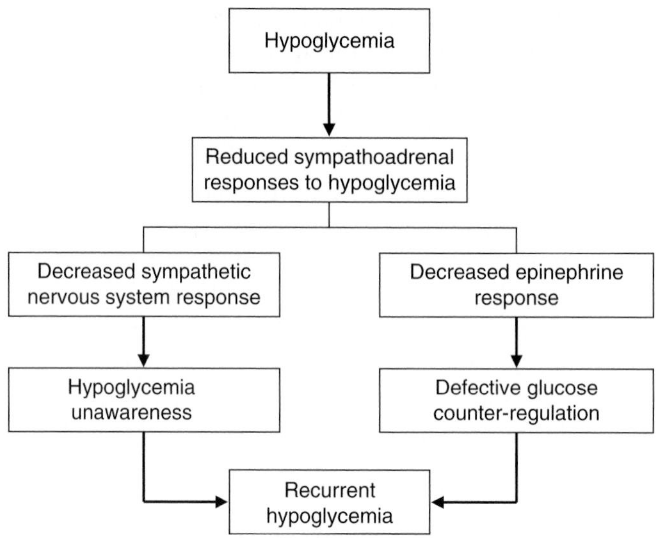

Fig. 1. Hypoglycemia-associated autonomic failure in diabetes. Adapted from ref. *14*.

system outflow in response to different stimuli is responsible for these conflicting results *(59)*.

The studies described earlier have established that recent antecedent iatrogenic hypoglycemia impairs some autonomic responses to subsequent hypoglycemia. It is not clear whether antecedent hypoglycemia has more general effects on autonomic nervous system function, impairing the response to nonhypoglycemic stimuli. Ratarsan and coworkers reported the autonomic impairment was specific to hypoglycemic stimuli. In a study of subjects with type 1 diabetes they observed that, following antecedent hypoglycemia, the epinephrine responses to exercise, standing, and a meal, and the norepinephrine responses to standing and exercise were intact *(60)*. In contrast, data from Kinsley and colleagues from a study of subjects with type1 diabetes suggested that the deficit was more generalized. These investigators noted that the epinephrine and norepinephrine response to a cold pressor test was reduced in well-controlled subjects with type 1 diabetes in comparison with controls *(61)*.

More recently, Davis and coworkers reported that antecedent hypoglycemia reduces the normal exercise-induced rise in epinephrine, norepinephrine, glucagon, growth hormone, pancreatic polypeptide, and cortisol in healthy individuals *(62)*. These data lend further support to the view that the effects of antecedent hypoglycemia on the autonomic nervous system are more generalized and not specific to subsequent hypoglycemic stimuli. Furthermore, antecedent exercise in normal subjects (two bouts of earlier exercise for 90 minutes at 50% VO2max and for 60 minutes at 70% VO2max attenuate the counterregulatory responses to subsequent next-day hypoglycemia occurring in nondiabetic subjects *(63)*. A similar although more restricted effect was found by McGregor et al. *(64)*, using a different experimental design (two bouts of cycle exercise at approximately 70% peak oxygen consumption for 1 hour separated by 180 minutes) was associated with reduced epinephrine response to subsequent hypoglycemia (but not norepinephrine, neurogenic symptom, pancreatic polypeptide, or glucagons *(64)*.

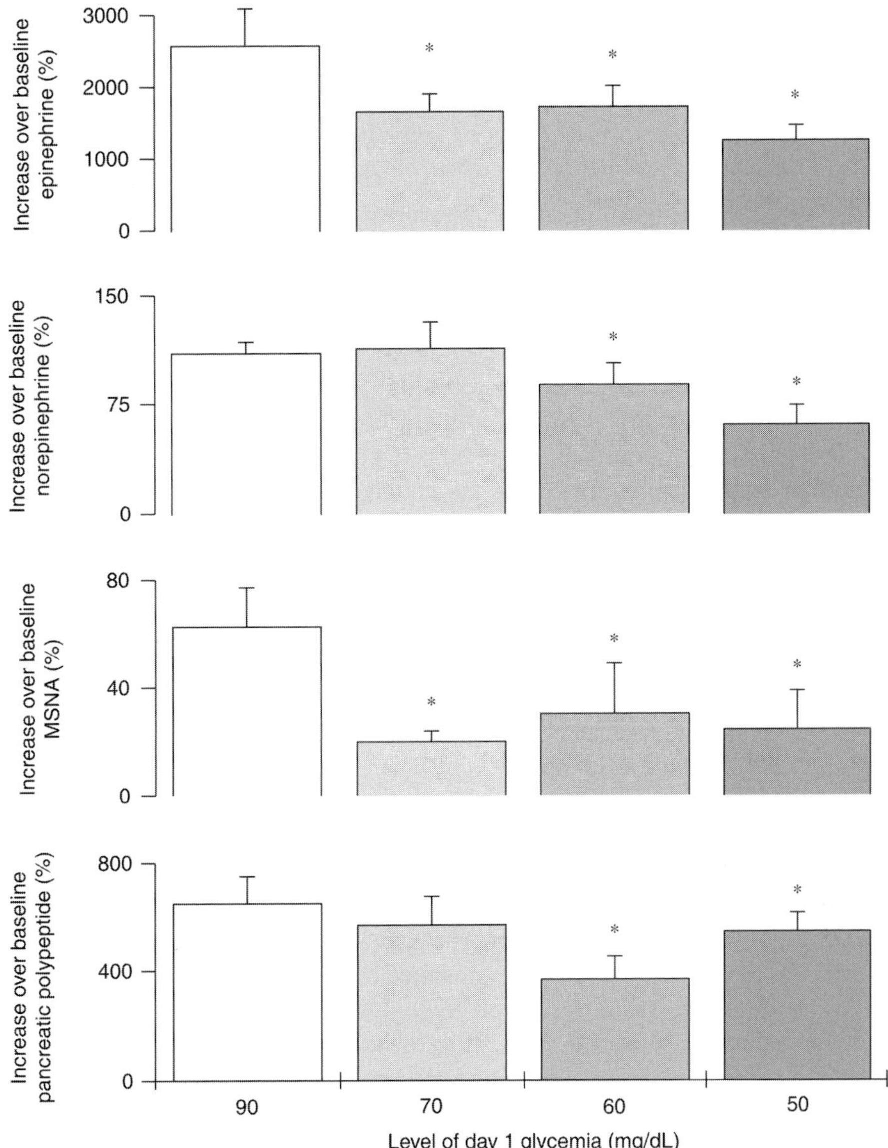

Fig. 2. The percentage increase over baseline of plasma epinephrine, norepinephrine, muscle sympathetic nerve activity and pancreatic polypeptide in healthy males during the last 30 minutes of a 2-hour hypoglycemic clamp at 50 mg/dL. Subjects were exposed on the previous day, to either euglycemia, or hypoglycemia of 70, 60, or 50 mg/dL. Data are group means ± SEM. * = $p < 0.05$ vs 90 mg/dL. From ref. *16*.

Similar findings may be present in individuals with type 1 diabetes that may play a role in exercise-induced hypoglycemia. The autonomic response (epinephrine, pancreatic polypeptide, and muscle sympathetic nerve activity) and hypoglycemic symptom response to subsequent hypoglycemia was attenuated after two bouts of low-intensity (90 minutes at 30% VO2max) and moderate-intensity (90 minutes at 50% VO2max) exercise separated by 180 mins *(65)*. In contrast, Rattarasarn et al. *(60)* found that a

60-minutes bout of exercise at 60% VO2max did not attenuate the autonomic response to subsequent hypoglycemia in subjects with type1 diabetes. The differences in experimental design may be responsible for the different results.

The Etiology of Hypoglycemia Induced Impairment in the Counterregulatory Response and Hypoglycemia Induced Autonomic Failure

The etiology of hypoglycemia-induced impairment in the counterregulatory response to repeat hypoglycemia has not been established, but does not appear to be because of changes in glucose uptake by the brain *(66)*. A series of studies by Davis and others suggest that the increase in cortisol that occurs during hypoglycemia plays an important role in development of impaired counterregulation to repeat hypoglycemia. Administration of Adrenocorticotropic hormone (ACTH) or cortisol intravenously to achieve blood levels of cortisol similar to those observed during hypoglycemia blunts the counterregulatory response to subsequent hypoglycemia *(56,67)*. Raising cortisol levels through exercise may also blunt the counterregulatory response to subsequent hypoglycemia *(63)*. Finally, patients with Addison's disease who are unable to increase cortisol in response to a hypoglycemic stress, do not show impairment of the counterregulatory response to repeat hypoglycemia *(57)*.

These results have not been replicated consistently. Whereas, increased endogenous cortisol secretion elicited by an infusion of a pharmacological dose of α-(1–24)-ACTH, which raised plasma cortisol levels to approximately 45 ug/dL, reduced the adrenomedullary (epinephrine), sympathetic (norepinephrine) and parasympathetic (pancreatic polypeptide), and autonomic symptom response to subsequent hypoglycemia *(67)*. However, elevations of antecedent cortisol levels more comparable with those that occur during hypoglycemia were not found to reduce adrenomedullary epinephrine or hypoglycemia neurogenic symptoms in response to subsequent hypoglycemia *(68)*.

Other elements of the hypothalamic-pituitary-adrenal axis (HPA) axis may be implicated too. Studies in a rodent model support a role for corticotrophin releasing hormone (CRH). Animals pretreated with CRH had impaired release of epinephrine, norepinephrine and glucagon following insulin induced hypoglycemia. This downregulation of the sympathoadrenal response was not present following pretreatment with ACTH or corticosterone. The impaired release of catecholamines and glucagon was abolished by simultaneous administration of a CRHr1 antagonist with CRH *(69)*.

REFERENCES

1. The effect of intensive treatment of diabetes on the development and progression of long-term complications in insulin-dependent diabetes mellitus. The Diabetes Control and Complications Trial Research Group. *N Engl J Med* 1993;329(14):977–986.
2. Intensive blood-glucose control with sulphonylureas or insulin compared with conventional treatment and risk of complications in patients with type 2 diabetes (UKPDS 33). UK Prospective Diabetes Study (UKPDS) Group. *Lancet* 1998;352(9131):837–853.
3. Reichard P, Britz A, Carlsson P, et al. Metabolic control and complications over 3 years in patients with insulin dependent diabetes (IDDM): the Stockholm Diabetes Intervention Study (SDIS). *J Intern Med* 1990;228(5):511–517.
4. Reichard P, Nilsson BY, Rosenqvist U. The effect of long-term intensified insulin treatment on the development of microvascular complications of diabetes mellitus. *N Engl J Med* 1993;329(5):304–309.

5. Ohkubo Y, Kishikawa H, Araki E, et al. Intensive insulin therapy prevents the progression of diabetic microvascular complications in Japanese patients with non-insulin- dependent diabetes mellitus: a randomized prospective 6-year study. *Diabetes Res Clin Pract* 1995; 28(2):103–117.
6. Gaede P, Vedel P, Parving HH, Pedersen O. Intensified multifactorial intervention in patients with type 2 diabetes mellitus and microalbuminuria: the Steno type 2 randomised study. *Lancet* 1999;353(9153):617–622.
7. Epidemiology of severe hypoglycemia in the diabetes control and complications trial. The DCCT Research Group. *Am J Med* 1991;90(4):450–459.
8. Donovan CM, Hamilton-Wessler M, Halter JB, Bergman RN. Primacy of liver glucosensors in the sympathetic response to progressive hypoglycemia. *Proc Natl Acad Sci USA* 1994;91(7):2863–2867.
9. Borg WP, During MJ, Sherwin RS, Borg MA, Brines ML, Shulman GI. Ventromedial hypothalamic lesions in rats suppress counterregulatory responses to hypoglycemia. *J Clin Invest* 1994;93(4):1677–1682.
10. Borg WP, Sherwin RS, During MJ, Borg MA, Shulman GI. Local ventromedial hypothalamus glucopenia triggers counterregulatory hormone release. *Diabetes* 1995;44(2):180–184.
11. Ritter S, Llewellyn-Smith I, Dinh TT. Subgroups of hindbrain catecholamine neurons are selectively activated by 2-deoxy-D-glucose induced metabolic challenge. *Brain Res* 1998; 805(1–2):41–54.
12. Hardie DG, Carling D. The AMP-activated protein kinase—fuel gauge of the mammalian cell? Eur J Biochem 1997;246(2):259–273.
13. McCrimmon RJ, Fan X, Ding Y, Zhu W, Jacob RJ, Sherwin RS. Potential role for AMP-activated protein kinase in hypoglycemia sensing in the ventromedial hypothalamus. *Diabetes* 2004;53(8):1953–1958.
14. Cryer PE. Diverse causes of hypoglycemia-associated autonomic failure in diabetes. *N Engl J Med* 2004;350(22):2272–2279.
15. Cryer PE, Davis SN, Shamoon H. Hypoglycemia in diabetes. *Diabetes Care* 2003; 26(6):1902–1912.
16. Diedrich L, Sandoval D, Davis SN. Hypoglycemia associated autonomic failure. *Clin Auton Res* 2002;12(5):358–365.
17. Gerich JE, Langlois M, Noacco C, Karam JH, Forsham PH. Lack of glucagon response to hypoglycemia in diabetes: evidence for an intrinsic pancreatic alpha cell defect. *Science* 1973;182(108):171–173.
18. Rizza RA, Cryer PE, Gerich JE. Role of glucagon, catecholamines, and growth hormone in human glucose counterregulation. Effects of somatostatin and combined alpha- and beta-adrenergic blockade on plasma glucose recovery and glucose flux rates after insulin-induced hypoglycemia. *J Clin Invest* 1979;64(1):62–71.
19. Cryer PE, Binder C, Bolli GB, et al. Hypoglycemia in IDDM. *Diabetes* 1989;38(9): 1193–1199.
20. Mitrakou A, Ryan C, Veneman T, et al. Hierarchy of glycemic thresholds for counterregulatory hormone secretion, symptoms, and cerebral dysfunction. *Am J Physiol* 1991; 260(1 Pt 1):E67–E74.
21. Schwartz NS, Clutter WE, Shah SD, Cryer PE. Glycemic thresholds for activation of glucose counterregulatory systems are higher than the threshold for symptoms. *J Clin Invest* 1987;79(3):777–781.
22. de Feo P, Perriello G, Torlone E, et al. Contribution of adrenergic mechanisms to glucose counterregulation in humans. *Am J Physiol* 1991;261(6 Pt 1):E725–E736.
23. White NH, Skor DA, Cryer PE, Levandoski LA, Bier DM, Santiago JV. Identification of type I diabetic patients at increased risk for hypoglycemia during intensive therapy. *N Engl J Med* 1983;308(9):485–491.

24. Simonson DC, Tamborlane WV, DeFronzo RA, Sherwin RS. Intensive insulin therapy reduces counterregulatory hormone responses to hypoglycemia in patients with Type I diabetes. *Ann Intern Med* 1985;103:184–190.
25. Amiel SA, Tamborlane WV, Simonson DC, Sherwin RS. Defective glucose counterregulation after strict glycemic control of insulin-dependent diabetes mellitus. *N Engl J Med* 1987;316(22):1376–1383.
26. Bolli GB, de Feo P, De Cosmo S, et al. A reliable and reproducible test for adequate glucose counterregulation in type I diabetes mellitus. *Diabetes* 1984;33(8):732–737.
27. Heller SR, Macdonald IA, Herbert M, Tattersall RB. Influence of sympathetic nervous system on hypoglycaemic warning symptoms. *Lancet* 1987;2:359–363.
28. Amiel SA, Sherwin RS, Simonson DC, Tamborlane WV. Effect of intensive insulin therapy on glycemic thresholds for counterregulatory hormone release. *Diabetes* 1988;37(7): 901–907.
29. Hepburn DA, Patrick AW, Brash HM, Thomson I, Frier BM. Hypoglycaemia unawareness in type 1 diabetes: a lower plasma glucose is required to stimulate sympatho-adrenal activation. *Diabet Med* 1991;8(10):934–945.
30. Ryder RE, Owens DR, Hayes TM, Ghatei MA, Bloom SR. Unawareness of hypoglycaemia and inadequate hypoglycaemic counterregulation: no causal relation with diabetic autonomic neuropathy. *BMJ* 1990;301(6755):783–787.
31. Clarke WL, Gonder-Frederick LA, Richards FE, Cryer PE. Multifactorial origin of hypoglycemic symptom unawareness in IDDM. Association with defective glucose counterregulation and better glycemic control. *Diabetes* 1991;40(6):680–685.
32. Hepburn DA, Patrick AW, Eadington DW, Ewing DJ, Frier BM. Unawareness of hypoglycaemia in insulin-treated diabetic patients: prevalence and relationship to autonomic neuropathy. *Diabet Med* 1990;7(8):711–717.
33. Fanelli CG, Epifano L, Rambotti AM, et al. Meticulous prevention of hypoglycemia normalizes the glycemic thresholds and magnitude of most of neuroendocrine responses to, symptoms of, and cognitive function during hypoglycemia in intensively treated patients with short-term IDDM. *Diabetes* 1993;42(11):1683–1689.
34. Davis M, Mellman M, Friedman S, Chang CJ, Shamoon H. Recovery of epinephrine response but not hypoglycemic symptom threshold after intensive therapy in type 1 diabetes. *Am J Med* 1994;97(6):535–542.
35. Dagogo-Jack S, Rattarasarn C, Cryer PE. Reversal of hypoglycemia unawareness, but not defective glucose counterregulation, in IDDM. *Diabetes* 1994;43(12):1426–1434.
36. Lingenfelser T, Buettner UW, Uhl H, et al. Recovery of hypoglycaemia-associated compromised cerebral function after a short interval of euglycaemia in insulin-dependent diabetic patients. *Electroencephalogr Clin Neurophysiol* 1994;92(3):196–203.
37. Cranston I, Lomas J, Maran A, Macdonald I, Amiel SA. Restoration of hypoglycaemia awareness in patients with long-duration insulin-dependent diabetes. *Lancet* 1994;344(8918): 283–287.
38. Fanelli C, Pampanelli S, Epifano L, et al. Long-term recovery from unawareness, deficient counterregulation and lack of cognitive dysfunction during hypoglycaemia, following institution of rational, intensive insulin therapy in IDDM. *Diabetologia* 1994;37(12): 1265–1276.
39. Heller SR, Cryer PE. Reduced neuroendocrine and symptomatic responses to subsequent hypoglycemia after 1 episode of hypoglycemia in nondiabetic humans. *Diabetes* 1991; 40(2):223–226.
40. Davis MR, Shamoon H. Counterregulatory adaptation to recurrent hypoglycemia in normal humans. *J Clin Endocrinol Metab* 1991;73(5):995–1001.
41. Veneman T, Mitrakou A, Mokan M, Cryer P, Gerich J. Induction of hypoglycemia unawareness by asymptomatic nocturnal hypoglycemia. *Diabetes* 1993;42(9): 1233–1237.

42. Davis MR, Shamoon H. Deficient counterregulatory hormone responses during hypoglycemia in a patient with insulinoma. *J Clin Endocrinol Metab* 1991;72(4):788–792.
43. Davis SN, Shavers C, Mosqueda-Garcia R, Costa F. Effects of differing antecedent hypoglycemia on subsequent counterregulation in normal humans. *Diabetes* 1997;46(8):1328–1335.
44. Maran A, Taylor J, Macdonald IA, Amiel SA. Evidence for reversibility of defective counterregulation in a patient with insulinoma. *Diabet Med* 1992;9(8):765–768.
45. Mitrakou A, Fanelli C, Veneman T, et al. Reversibility of unawareness of hypoglycemia in patients with insulinomas. *N Engl J Med* 1993;329(12):834–839.
46. Davis SN, Shavers C, Costa F. Gender-related differences in counterregulatory responses to antecedent hypoglycemia in normal humans. *J Clin Endocrinol Metab* 2000;85(6): 2148–2157.
47. Davis SN, Shavers C, Costa F. Differential gender responses to hypoglycemia are due to alterations in CNS drive and not glycemic thresholds. *Am J Physiol Endocrinol Metab* 2000;279(5):E1054–E1063.
48. Cryer PE. Iatrogenic hypoglycemia as a cause of hypoglycemia-associated autonomic failure in IDDM. A vicious cycle. *Diabetes* 1992;41(3):255–260.
49. Dagogo-Jack SE, Craft S, Cryer PE. Hypoglycemia-associated autonomic failure in insulin-dependent diabetes mellitus. Recent antecedent hypoglycemia reduces autonomic responses to, symptoms of, and defense against subsequent hypoglycemia. *J Clin Invest* 1993;91(3):819–828.
50. Cryer PE. Hypoglycemia-associated autonomic failure in diabetes. *Am J Physiol Endocrinol Metab* 2001;281(6):E1115–E1121.
51. Hoeldtke RD, Boden G. Epinephrine secretion, hypoglycemia unawareness, and diabetic autonomic neuropathy. *Ann Intern Med* 1994;120(6):512–517.
52. Bottini P, Boschetti E, Pampanelli S, et al. Contribution of autonomic neuropathy to reduced plasma adrenaline responses to hypoglycemia in IDDM: evidence for a nonselective defect. *Diabetes* 1997;46(5):814–823.
53. Fanelli C, Pampanelli S, Lalli C, et al. Long-term intensive therapy of IDDM patients with clinically overt autonomic neuropathy: effects on hypoglycemia awareness and counterregulation. *Diabetes* 1997;46(7):1172–1181.
54. Meyer C, Grossmann R, Mitrakou A, et al. Effects of autonomic neuropathy on counterregulation and awareness of hypoglycemia in type 1 diabetic patients. *Diabetes Care* 1998; 21(11):1960–1966.
55. Stephenson JM, Kempler P, Perin PC, Fuller JH. Is autonomic neuropathy a risk factor for severe hypoglycaemia? The EURODIAB IDDM Complications Study. *Diabetologia* 1996;39(11):1372–1376.
56. Davis SN, Shavers C, Costa F, Mosqueda-Garcia R. Role of cortisol in the pathogenesis of deficient counterregulation after antecedent hypoglycemia in normal humans. *J Clin Invest* 1996;98(3):680–691.
57. Davis SN, Shavers C, Davis B, Costa F. Prevention of an increase in plasma cortisol during hypoglycemia preserves subsequent counterregulatory responses. *J Clin Invest* 1997; 100(2):429–438.
58. Paramore DS, Fanelli CG, Shah SD, Cryer PE. Hypoglycemia per se stimulates sympathetic neural as well as adrenomedullary activity, but, unlike the adrenomedullary response, the forearm sympathetic neural response is not reduced after recent hypoglycemia. *Diabetes* 1999;48(7):1429–1436.
59. Morrison SF. Differential control of sympathetic outflow. *Am J Physiol Regul Integr Comp Physiol* 2001;281(3):R683–R698.
60. Rattarasarn C, Dagogo-Jack S, Zachwieja JJ, Cryer PE. Hypoglycemia-induced autonomic failure in IDDM is specific for stimulus of hypoglycemia and is not attributable to prior autonomic activation. *Diabetes* 1994;43(6):809–818.

61. Kinsley BT, Widom B, Utzschneider K, Simonson DC. Stimulus specificity of defects in counterregulatory hormone secretion in insulin-dependent diabetes mellitus: effect of glycemic control. *J Clin Endocrinol Metab* 1994;79(5):1383–1389.
62. Davis SN, Galassetti P, Wasserman DH, Tate D. Effects of antecedent hypoglycemia on subsequent counterregulatory responses to exercise. *Diabetes* 2000;49(1):73–81.
63. Galassetti P, Mann S, Tate D, et al. Effects of antecedent prolonged exercise on subsequent counterregulatory responses to hypoglycemia. *Am J Physiol Endocrinol Metab* 2001; 280(6):E908–E917.
64. McGregor VP, Greiwe JS, Banarer S, Cryer PE. Limited impact of vigorous exercise on defenses against hypoglycemia: relevance to hypoglycemia-associated autonomic failure. *Diabetes* 2002;51(5):1485–1492.
65. Sandoval DA, Guy DL, Richardson MA, Ertl AC, Davis SN. Effects of low and moderate antecedent exercise on counterregulatory responses to subsequent hypoglycemia in type 1 diabetes. *Diabetes* 2004;53(7):1798–1806.
66. Segel SA, Fanelli CG, Dence CS, et al. Blood-to-brain glucose transport, cerebral glucose metabolism, and cerebral blood flow are not increased after hypoglycemia. *Diabetes* 2001;50(8):1911–1917.
67. McGregor VP, Banarer S, Cryer PE. Elevated endogenous cortisol reduces autonomic neuroendocrine and symptom responses to subsequent hypoglycemia. *Am J Physiol Endocrinol Metab* 2002;282(4):E770–E777.
68. Raju B, McGregor VP, Cryer PE. Cortisol elevations comparable to those that occur during hypoglycemia do not cause hypoglycemia-associated autonomic failure. *Diabetes* 2003;52(8):2083–2089.
69. Flanagan DE, Keshavarz T, Evans ML, et al. Role of corticotrophin-releasing hormone in the impairment of counterregulatory responses to hypoglycemia. *Diabetes* 2003; 52(3):605–613.

24
Cardiovascular Autonomic Neuropathy

Martin J. Stevens, MD

SUMMARY

Cardiovascular autonomic neuropathy (CAN) is a common but frequently overlooked complication of diabetes, which can lead to a diverse spectrum of disabling clinical manifestations ranging from mild exercise intolerance to sudden cardiac death. Although traditionally diagnosed using indirect cardiovascular reflex tests, new direct scintigraphic imaging techniques have demonstrated that a cardiac "dysinnervation" can occur early in the course of diabetes, which may have considerable implications for myocardial stability and function. Indeed recent studies have demonstrated that cardiovascular sympathetic tone may be altered very early in the cause of diabetes, and can be associated with altered myocardial blood flow regulation and impaired left ventricular (LV) function. Although convincing evidence has yet to be generated that any therapeutic intervention is capable of reversing CAN complicating diabetes once established, the development and progression of CAN has recently been shown to be sensitive to the simultaneous management of multiple cardiovascular risk factors. This chapter will review the clinical importance of CAN in diabetes, with a particular focus on its impact on the heart.

Key Words: Cardiac; diabetes; neuropathy; imaging; scintigraphy; autonomic.

INTRODUCTION

Diabetes is reaching epidemic proportions in many parts of the world with the number of subjects with diabetes expected to double during the next 30 years *(1)*. In concert with the rising prevalence of diabetes, the impact of its chronic complications is expected to have a major impact on health care resources utilization during the same time period. Cardiovascular autonomic neuropathy (CAN) is a common but frequently overlooked complication of diabetes, which can lead to a diverse spectrum of clinical manifestations ranging from impairment of exercise tolerance to sudden cardiac death *(2)*. New scintigraphic imaging techniques have demonstrated that cardiac dysinnervation can occur early in the course of diabetes and is often asymptomatic, but can rapidly progress with poor metabolic control and result in a complex array of clinical outcomes *(3)*. Although the impact of cardiac dysinnervation on myocardial stability and function remains unclear and somewhat controversial, recent data have highlighted its role in the development of altered myocardial blood flow regulation, impaired left ventricular (LV) function, and potentially in the development of diabetic cardiomyopathy *(4–6)*. Although the sensitivity

From: *Contemporary Diabetes: Diabetic Neuropathy: Clinical Management, Second Edition*
Edited by: A. Veves and R. Malik © Humana Press Inc., Totowa, NJ

of CAN to intensified glycemic control has been inconsistent, the simultaneous management of multiple cardiovascular risk factors in subjects with diabetes appears to have salutary effects in halting its development and progression *(7)*. This chapter will consider the clinical importance of CAN complicating diabetes, with a particular focus on its impact on the heart.

EPIDEMIOLOGY

Difficulties in accurate estimates of the prevalence of CAN reflect a number of factors including variations in the populations studied, the source of the patients within these populations, individual patient characteristics, choice of test utilized, and the diagnostic criteria. In 1988, in order to reduce some of these variabilities, the San Antonio Conference on Diabetic Neuropathy made a number of recommendations, including the choice of tests to be performed as well as recommending that autonomic function data should be standardized by the development of reference ranges in the local population as well as by reporting absolute data *(8)*. As described later, indirect assessment of CAN utilizing more indirect reflex tests tend to yield lower overall estimates of CAN prevalence compared with newer direct scintigraphic methodology.

CAN is usually detected using widely available indirect standardized cardiovascular reflex tests, which evaluate the integrity of complex reflex arcs. These assessments in general, identify abnormalities of cardiovascular innervation in 16–20% of subjects with diabetes *(9–15)*. In the Eurodiab IDDM Complications Study, for example, altered heart rate variability (HRV) was detected in approximately 19% of subjects *(14)*. In another study of more than 600 subjects with type 1 diabetes approximately 25% of subjects had abnormalities of at least two autonomic function tests *(16)*. However, in the diabetes control and complication trial of type 1 diabetes in the primary prevention cohort, deficits of HRV were found less than 2% *(17)*. In subjects with microvascular complications at baseline, this prevalence increased to approximately 6% *(18,19)*. Despite some earlier controversy, it is now widely recognized that type 2 diabetes is also frequently complicated by the development of CAN. In the French multicenter study of type 1 and type 2 diabetes, for example, approximately 25% of subjects had symptoms consistent with autonomic neuropathy *(20)*. CAN was found to be the most common (51%) diabetes complication with rates of moderate and more severe CAN being higher in type 1 than in type 2 subjects. CAN correlated with diabetes duration and retinopathy and was independently associated with obesity in type 2 diabetes *(20)*. The frequency of parasympathetic CAN has been reported to be 20% at 5 years and 65% at 10 years *(21)*, and sympathetic CAN 7% at 5 years and 24% at 10 years.

Recently, CAN has also been extensively evaluated using more direct, but expensive techniques involving radiolabeled analogs of norepinephrine, which are actively taken up by cardiac sympathetic nerve terminals (*see* next) *(3–6,22–33)*. These techniques have identified a specific cardiac sympathetic dysinnervation complicating diabetes, and proven useful in not only determining the prevalence of cardiac sympathetic dysinnervation, but have also been utilized to follow its progression and its response to therapeutic intervention. Both [^{131}I] *meta*iodobenzylguanidine (MIBG) and [^{11}C] *meta*hydroxyephedrine (HED) have been extensively utilized to assess the integrity of cardiac sympathetic innervation.

In cross-sectional studies, LV [^{123}I] MIBG and [^{11}C]-HED retention deficits have been identified in subjects with type 1 and type 2 diabetes even in the absence of

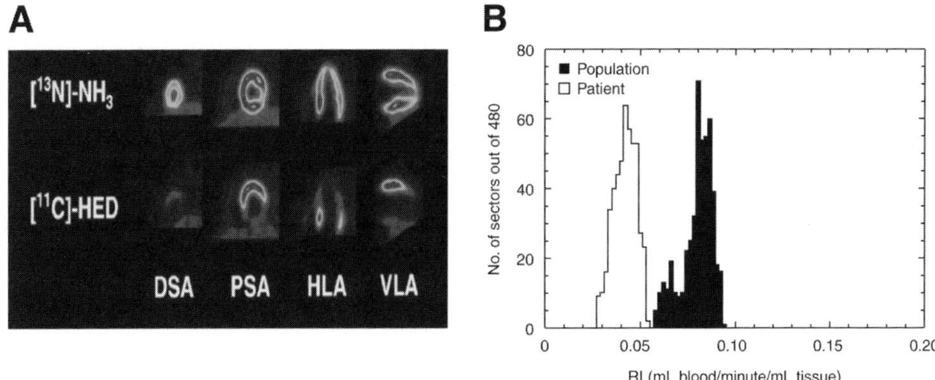

Fig. 1. HED-PET images demonstrating advanced cardiac sympathetic dysinnervation. **(A)** Top panels show the blood flow images, which are normal. However in the lower panels, the [^{11}C]HED retention deficits are extensive with only the proximal cardiac segments demonstrating retained tracer retention, consistent with "islands" of innervation. **(B)** Retention of LV [^{11}C]HED is globally decreased in a subject with microangiopathy. Retention of LV [^{11}C]HED (expressed as a Retention Index [RI]) is globally reduced in a subject early background retinopathy and normal autonomic reflex tests (open plot), compared with the values obtained in a healthy nondiabetic control population (shaded plot).

abnormalities of autonomic reflex testing *(23,27,29)*. Retention of [^{123}I]-MIBG in the heart can be abnormal in metabolically compromised newly diagnosed subjects with type 1 diabetes, which are partially correctable by intensive insulin therapy *(32)*. These defects most likely reflect acute neuronal dysfunction. In contrast, there are significantly fewer reports utilizing [^{11}C]HED, and these are mostly restricted to subjects with type 1 diabetes. In type 1 diabetes, deficits of [^{11}C]HED retention effecting upto about 10% of the left ventricle have been reported in 40% of healthy subjects without deficits of autonomic reflex testing *(29)*. These small deficits typically begin distally in the LV in the infero-lateral walls, and with progression of CAN spread proximally and circumferentially, and might in some subjects eventually result in islands of basal increased [^{11}C]HED retention *(29)* (Fig. 1, Panel A). However, a different pattern of reduced [^{11}C]HED retention has recently been reported in a subset of asymptomatic subjects with type 1 diabetes *(4)*. In these subjects, extensive global deficits of LV [^{11}C]HED retention were observed, despite good glycemic control indicating an etiology other than neuronal loss or acute hyperglycemia-induced neuronal dysfunction (Fig. 1, Panel B).

NATURAL HISTORY OF CAN

The natural history of CAN has been extensively evaluated utilizing standardized cardiovascular reflex tests, and to a much lesser extent utilizing scintigraphic techniques. Comparison of these two methodologies is hindered by the relative difficulty of reflex testing to sensitively detect the progression of sympathetic deficits and the inability of current scintigraphic tracers to safely map human cardiovascular parasympathetic integrity. Abnormalities in the sensitive parasympathetic cardiovascular reflex tests might be present at diagnosis of diabetes *(16)* even in children *(33)*, but the importance of this abnormality is unclear as clinical symptoms are rare and it might not predict the development of complications. The beneficial effects of improved glycemic control on the progression of peripheral somatic neuropathy *(17–19)*, neuropathic symptoms *(34)*, electrophysiological deficits *(18,34)*, and vibration perception thresholds *(18,35)* are now beyond dispute. However, the relationship of metabolic control to progression of autonomic dysfunction has been less clear. The inconsistent effects of improved metabolic control on the progression of CAN could reflect a number of factors including the inability of some studies to sufficiently improve HbA1c, too advanced CAN at initiation of the study, insufficient study duration or insensitivity of autonomic testing to detect a change. Scintigraphic studies have also been utilized to directly explore the effect of glucose control on cardiac autonomic function. These techniques have shown that poor glycemic control can result in progression of LV sympathetic dysinnervation, which can be prevented *(30)* or reversed *(31)* by the institution of near-euglycemia.

Tests of cardiovascular autonomic function often deteriorate at a faster rate in patients with diabetes compared with age-matched nondiabetic individuals, with beat-to-beat variability reported to decrease at one beat per minute per year (three times the rate of normal subjects) *(36)*. The Valsalva ratio has been reported to decrease at a rate of 0.015 per year in type 1 diabetes, which might be twice that observed in the normal nondiabetic population *(37)*. In a recently reported 14 year prospective study of subjects with type 1 diabetes, autonomic nerve function was also found to progressively deteriorate *(38)*. Additionally, autonomic neuropathy and the presence of abnormal orthostatic diastolic blood pressure were associated with future renal complications *(38)*. However, clinical symptoms of autonomic dysfunction might correlate poorly with changes in reflex tests, might be intermittent, and not progress *(3,35)*.

With the progression of CAN and the development of sympathetic deficits and disabling symptoms such as orthostatic hypotension, a poor prognosis has been reported with up to a 60% 5 year mortality *(39)*. However, other studies have not predicted such a dire outlook, as 90% of asymptomatic subjects with reduced HRV without the presence of symptoms were still alive after 10 years *(36)*. However, the presence of symptoms, (again in particular postural hypotension) was associated with reduced survival (73% alive after 10 years). The precise cause of death in these subjects is controversial: most probably reflect coexistent renal and cardiovascular disease, but a small number of deaths remain unexplained and the potential causes are discussed (*see* Cardiac Denervation Syndrome).

METHODS OF ASSESSMENT

Cardiovascular Autonomic Reflex Tests

CAN might be classified as being subclinical or clinical, dependent upon whether clinical manifestations are present. Subclinical autonomic neuropathy usually accompanies distal symmetrical polyneuropathy, but might only be evident by cardiovascular reflex testing (Table 1). Conventionally, the integrity of autonomic function is assessed indirectly by assessing cardiovascular reflexes. A consensus statement of the American Diabetes Association and the American Academy of Neurology in 1988 recommended that a battery of tests should be performed to assess autonomic function *(8)*. Although the precise choice of tests remains debated, these might include HRV to deep respiration and the change in heart rate on assuming upright posture (predominantly tests of parasympathetic function), the change in systolic and diastolic blood pressure on standing,

Table 1
Commonly Used Techniques to Diagnose CAN

Tests of predominantly parasympathetic integrity

Heart rate variability to deep breathing (usually at six breaths per minute): Assessments include standard deviation, coefficient of variation, expiratory: inspiratory difference and ratio, mean circular resultant of vector analysis, spectral analysis (mid [0.05–0.15 Hz] and high [0.15–0.5 Hz] frequency fluctuations)

Heart rate response on standing: Assessments include maximum/minimum 30:15 ratio (i.e., longest and shortest R–R intervals at about beat 30 and 15, respectively), or the longest and shortest R–R intervals between beats 20–40 and 5–25, respectively

Tests of predominantly sympathetic integrity

Postural systolic blood pressure fall: Assessed by a systolic blood pressure fall ≥20 mmHg or a diastolic blood pressure fall ≥10 mmHg together with symptoms within 2 minutes of standing upright

Spectral analysis: low (0.01–0.05 Hz) frequency fluctuations

Blood pressure response to sustained handgrip: Assessed using a handgrip dynamometer held at 30% maximum for 5 minutes (abnormality is a rise of diastolic blood pressure of <10 mmHg)

Head up tilt table testing: Assessed by measured heart rate response and blood pressure change to a 60° head up tilt

Quantitative sudomotor axon reflex test: Assessed using a cholinergic agonist to test skin postganglionic sudomotor function

Plasma norepinephrine: supine and standing

Scintigraphic techniques:

Positron emission tomography using [^{11}C] *meta*hydroxyephedrine

Single photon emission tomography using [^{123}I] *meta*iodobenzylguanidine

Tests of both parasympathetic and sympathetic integrity

Valsalva ratio: Assessed by maintaining an exhaling pressure of 40 mmHg for 15 seconds and calculating the ratio of the longest R–R interval after the manoeuvre to the shortest interval during the manoeuvre

---

the blood pressure response to sustained handgrip (predominantly tests of sympathetic function), and the Valsalva ratio (tests both parasympathetic as well as sympathetic integrity) *(40)*. These tests can be utilized to stage the severity of CAN, with the mildest degree consisting isolated deficits in heart rate response to deep breathing, and the most severe when postural hypotension is also present (these stages correlate well with the impact of CAN on patient outcome in longitudinal studies). In 1992, the recommendations were updated to recommend that the heart rate response to deep respiration, the Valsalva ratio, and the blood pressure response to standing were suitable for the assessment of longitudinal progression of CAN *(41)*.

There are many different methods for assessing HRV *(15)*. Perhaps the "gold standard" measure is power spectral analysis, which can indirectly quantify defects in sympathetic and vagal innervation of the heart. The power spectral density of the R–R interval time series can be measured by a 256-point fast-Fourier transformation and can be determined in low (0.01–0.05 Hz), mid (0.05–0.15 Hz), and high (0.15–0.5 Hz) frequency ranges. The low and high frequency components are thought to reflect primarily sympathetic and parasympathetic integrity, respectively. Sympathetic nervous system responsiveness can also be explored by evaluating heart rate frequency responses on head up tilt table testing. The postural responses are determined by evaluating the difference between measurements made in the supine and the tilt positions *(42)*. HRV during standardized head up tilt table testing under paced breathing has demonstrated that increased postural change (supine to upright) in the low-frequency component power predicted an increased risk for cardiac death *(42)*, consistent with a detrimental effect of augmented sympathetic nervous system tone and/or reactivity.

Scintigraphic Characterization of Cardiac Sympathetic Integrity

As discussed earlier, CAN has also been evaluated using more direct techniques utilizing radiolabeled analogs of norepinephrine, which are actively taken up by cardiac sympathetic nerve terminals (Fig. 2). The most widely utilized tracer is MIBG *(43–45)*, a guanethidine derivative. This nonmetabolized tracer is taken up into the postganglionic presynaptic sympathetic nerve terminals and stored in synaptic vesicles *(46)* and (Fig. 2) its retention can be assessed by single photon emission computed tomography. [^{123}I]-MIBG uptake in the heart can be quantified in counts per minute per mL tissue, which is normalized to injected dose and body weight. [^{123}I]-MIBG uptake is calculated in myocardial regions of interest *(25)* and normalized to the highest pixel value in the LV and expressed as a percentage of this value. A semiquantitative analysis can then be performed, which involves blinded observers scoring images using a scoring system for each segment, which might range from no detectable tracer to normal tracer retention and a "defect score" obtained.

HED also undergoes highly specific and rapid uptake into sympathetic nerve varicosities through norepinephrine transporters (uptake-1) (Fig. 2). Like MIBG, HED is metabolically stable, is not metabolized but is continuously recycled into and out of the neuron *(46)*. Its neuronal retention requires intact vesicular storage and is also potentially susceptible to changes in synaptic norepinephrine levels making it a useful tool to assess cardiac sympathetic nerve fiber integrity and potentially tone. [^{11}C]-HED has been extensively evaluated in both subjects with diabetes *(26,29,31)* and in subjects with neuronal loss secondary to ischemic heart disease *(47)*. The myocardial retention of [^{11}C]-HED can be performed semiquantitatively or quantitatively. In subjects with diabetes, the heterogeneity of regional LV [^{11}C]-HED retention can be compared with the normal nondiabetic values by calculating a z-score with sectors that have a z-score higher than a predefined cut-off value (often 2.5) being defined as abnormal. An increase of heterogeneity is consistent with LV denervation *(26,29,31)*. The "extent" of the heterogeneity is usually expressed as the percentage of sectors that are abnormal. Additionally, changes in absolute regional [^{11}C]-HED retention can be quantified using a "retention index" approach *(29)*, which corrects [^{11}C]-HED retention for myocardial tracer delivery. Unfortunately, direct comparison of [^{11}C]-HED and [^{123}I]-MIBG to detect CAN complicating diabetes has not been reported.

Although both scintigraphic techniques are clearly able to detect early cardiac CAN and accurately chart its progression, the significance of early deficits detected by this methodology remains unclear. For example, the natural history of small (<10%) distal deficits of LV sympathetic innervation which have been identified in many patients with diabetes is not well-understood, and extensive age-adjusted normative databases are not

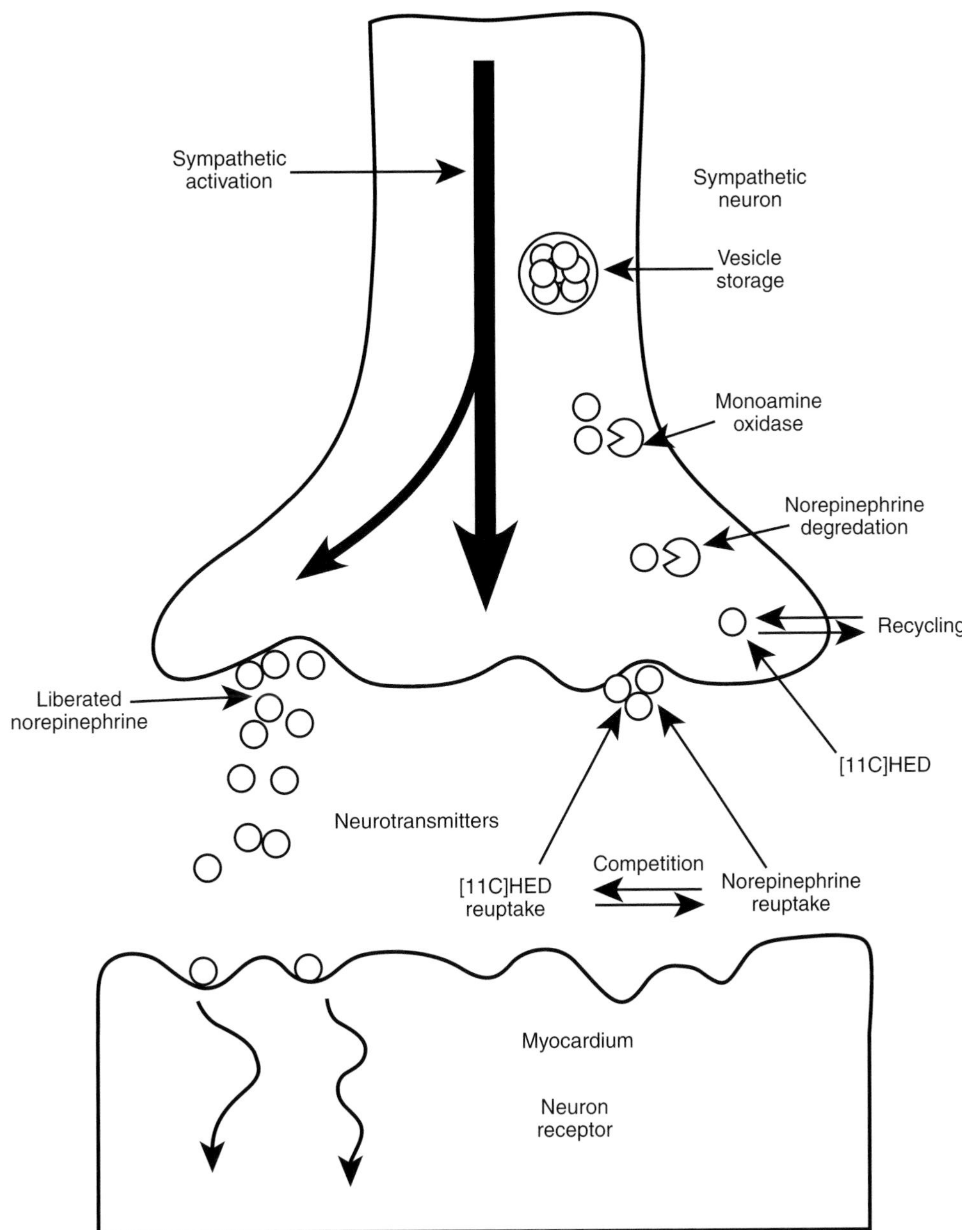

Fig. 2. Imaging the cardiac sympathetic nerve terminal using positron emission tomography and [^{11}C]*meta*hydroxyephedrine ([^{11}C]HED). [^{11}C]HED undergoes highly specific and rapid uptake into sympathetic nerve varicosities through norepinephrine transporters (uptake-1) and is continuosly recycled. Unlike norepinephrine, [^{11}C]HED is not metabolized by monoamine oxidase but its neuronal retention requires intact vesicular storage. As it competes with norepinephrine for neuronal reuptake, it is also potentially susceptible to changes in synaptic norepinephrine levels making it a useful tool to assess both cardiac sympathetic nerve fiber integrity and potentially tone.

Table 2
Clinical and Subclinical Manifestations of Cardiovascular Autonomic Neuropathy

Clinical	Subclinical
Resting and fixed tachycardia	Increased resting myocardial blood flow Increased cardiac sympathetic tone
Abnormal exercise tolerance	Impaired cardiac ejection fraction, abnormal systolic function, decreased diastolic filling, LV hypertrophy, myocardial apoptosis
Orthostatic and postprandial hypotension	Failure to augment heart rate. Pooling of splanchnic blood
Supine hypertension	Reduction of diurnal blood pressure variation, relative nocturnal sympathetic predominance and incipient nephropathy
Hemodynamic instability during anesthesia	
Cardiac denervation syndrome Silent myocardial ischemia Sudden cardiac death in patients with and without myocardial ischemia	QT prolongation, altered ventricular repolarization, heterogeneous cardiac sympathetic tone

yet available. Hence, the utility of these tools is undoubtedly mostly for research purposes to determine the pathophysiological effects of cardiac sympathetic dysinnervation complicating diabetes and to quantitate the effects of therapeutic interventions in randomized clinical trials.

The interpretation of findings using sympathetic neurotransmitter analogs is also complicated by the fact that in addition to being a marker for nerve fiber dysfunction or loss, alterations in sympathetic nervous system tone may also profoundly affect the retention of these tracers. For example, in the isolated rat heart model, elevated concentrations of norepinephrine in the perfusion increase neuronal HED clearance rates, suggesting that neuronal "recycling" of HED can be disrupted by high synaptic norepinephrine levels *(48)*. Additionally, myocardial retention of MIBG has been reported to be inversely related to plasma catecholamines in subjects with pheochromocytoma *(49)*. These findings were proposed to reflect competition with endogenous catecholamines for uptake into neuronal storage vesicles *(50)*. Therefore, increased synaptic norepinephrine might be a potential explanation for the reduction of cardiac [^{11}C]HED retention in these subjects. Direct measurement of cardiac norepinephrine spill-over will be required to confirm the etiology of this defect.

CLINICAL IMPLICATIONS

Cardiovascular denervation can give rise to a number of clinical syndromes including impaired exercise-induced cardiovascular performance, orthostatic hypotension, and the cardiac denervation syndrome (Table 2).

Abnormal Cardiovascular Exercise Performance

Advanced CAN might impair cardiovascular performance during exercise *(51)*, which might be subclinical *(52,53)*. CAN might be accompanied by impaired LV function, which encompasses a spectrum of different deficits (*see* Cardiac Denervation Syndrome) *(4,54–57)*. In diabetes complicated by autonomic dysfunction, resting heart is increased (and might reach 120 beats per minute, but then declines with the progression of CAN). The precise etiology of these temporal changes in heart rate is not certain, but has been proposed to reflect decreased parasympathetic tone accompanied by augmented sympathetic activity. This resting tachycardia is typically unresponsive to mild exercise, and any exercise-induced rise in cardiac output is proportional to the resting vagal tone. In CAN complicated by resting tachycardia, resting myocardial perfusion is increased, but vasodilatory reserve is impaired in response to stress *(22)*. Consideration needs to be given to the impairment of exercise capacity and silent myocardial ischemia when prescribing exercise regimens in these subjects.

Orthostatic Hypotension

Orthostatic hypotension (defined as a fall in systolic or diastolic blood pressure in excess of 20 mmHg or 10 mmHg, respectively with symptoms *[58]*) is a consequence of cardiovascular denervation and might reflect the consequences of a fixed resting heart rate and impaired visceral and lower limb vascular tone. The normal increase of plasma norepinephrine on standing is often attenuated in CAN *(59)*. Symptoms can vary from intermittent dizziness, to visual impairment, and syncope. The diurnal variation of blood pressure is decreased in CAN subjects, and may contribute to nocturnal supine hypertension and nephropathy *(60)*.

The Risks of Anesthesia and Surgery

Subjects with CAN might have greater hemodynamic instability during anesthesia, which might increase risk and require greater therapeutic intervention. For example, intraoperative reductions in blood pressure requiring assistance *(61)* and impaired respiratory drive *(62)* have been reported to be more frequent in subjects with CAN. These deficits might eventually contribute to poorer postoperative outcomes.

Cardiac Denervation Syndrome

The precise metabolical, physiological, and functional consequences of advanced cardiac dysinnervation are of great interest, but poorly understood. Cardiac dysinnervation complicating diabetes can result in abnormal myocardial blood flow regulation, cardiovascular instability during anesthesia, silent myocardial ischemia, and potentially increased susceptibility to cardiac arrhythmias and sudden death.

Implications for Enhanced Cardiovascular Risk

CAN has for many years been invoked as a cause of sudden cardiac death in diabetes *(63)*. Many studies have demonstrated increased mortality of subjects with diabetes postmyocardial infarction *(64–70)*, which might reflect increased susceptibility to a number of triggering factors including autonomic imbalance, particularly when CAN is manifested as increased sympathetic and reduced parasympathetic tone. Indeed, in diabetes complicated by myocardial infarction, CAN is predictive of both increased mortality and LV failure *(71)*. A meta-analysis of diabetic patients demonstrated that the mortality of CAN-free subjects during 5.5 years is approximately 5%, and increased to 27% in the presence of abnormal cardiovascular reflex tests *(71)*. In general, mortality risk increases in proportion to the severity of CAN. For example, in moderately advanced CAN, 5 year mortality approaches 30% *(72,73)*. In advanced CAN subjects, this rate increases to 53% with the highest mortality associated with advanced cardiovascular sympathetic denervation when accompanied by symptoms and orthostatic hypotension *(42,63)*. A similar relationship between CAN, orthostatic hypotension, and mortality was also recently reported in subjects with type 2 diabetes *(74)*. Increased cerebrovascular risk, potentially reflecting impaired cerebral autoregulation *(75)* also contributes to the detrimental effects of CAN. In normotensive and hypertensive patients with type 2 diabetes enrolled in the Appropriate Blood Pressure Control in Diabetes Trial, CAN (defined as a borderline or abnormal E/I ratio) was found to be a significant independent risk factor for the occurrence of stroke *(76)*.

The precise role of CAN *per se* in directly contributing to overall risk remains uncertain and controversial, as CAN is often associated with other advanced complications of diabetes, such as cardiovascular or renal disease. For example, diabetes, hypertension, and/or cardiovascular disease complicated by impaired autonomic function, has recently been shown to double the risk of all cause and cardiovascular mortality, a relationship not observed in the absence of these risk factors *(77)*. In the Rochester Diabetic Neuropathy Study, sudden cardiac death correlated with ischemic heart disease and nephropathy, and to a lesser degree with CAN—a relationship which became insignificant after adjusting for nephropathy *(78)*. Finally, the Pittsburgh Epidemiology of Diabetes Complications Study *(79)*, failed to find a significant association of CAN with mortality in type 1 diabetes, after adjusting for cardiovascular and renal disease.

However, other studies have demonstrated an association of CAN with increased mortality even in patients without other risk factors *(80)*. Indeed in subjects with diabetes with coronary artery disease, CAN has been found to be a significant predictor for death and cardiac events, even after correction was made for myocardial perfusion deficits and additional prognostic information was provided *(81)*. Finally, a recent meta-analysis explored the relationship of CAN and mortality complicating diabetes in 15 separate studies *(2)*. Total mortality rates were higher in CAN subjects with a statistically significant difference identified in 11 of these studies with a pooled estimate of the relative risk of 2.14.

The potential mechanisms whereby CAN might increase mortality rates in subjects with diabetes is not clear. Potential mechanisms invoked include deficits in the regulation of respiration provoking respiratory arrest *(82)*, susceptibility to severe hypoglycemia *(83)*, and arrhythmias, resulting in sudden cardiac death *(42,80)*. Some studies have identified an association of QT prolongation and CAN in subjects with diabetes *(84,85)* and/or abnormalities of ventricular repolarization *(86)*. Perhaps, electrophysiological deficits attributable to CAN complicating diabetes are of most importance as a contributing factor to the increased mortality after myocardial infarction observed in subjects with diabetes *(71,87)*.

Subjects with diabetes might have an altered circadian pattern of fibrinolytic activity and hemostasis, which in concert with changes in autonomic tone can contribute to changed pattern of myocardial ischemia, as the incidence of myocardial infarction is relatively decreased in the morning, but increased in the evening *(88)*. This might reflect impaired evening parasympathetic tone and relative predominance of sympathetic tone coupled with decreased fibrinolytic activity *(89)*. Many ischemic events in subjects with

CAN might not be associated with the development of classical symptoms *(2,90–92)*, although symptoms might persist even in advanced CAN *(93)*.

An obvious candidate to explain enhanced cardiac risk associated with CAN is abnormal myocardial electrical activity, which has been most extensively evaluated by assessing QT prolongation and altered ventricular repolarization *(94)*. Prolongation of the QT interval has been associated with cardiac death in subjects with diabetes *(95)*. In the EURODIAB Type 1 Complications Study, the prevalence of QT prolongation was 16% (11% in men, 21% in women *[85]*). In normoalbuminuric subjects with type 1 diabetes, increased Corrected QT interval (QTc) dispersion was found to be associated with reduced fall in the nocturnal blood pressure and altered sympathovagal balance *(96)*. Another report identified an association of vagal dysfunction with QT prolongation, whereas sympathetic and vagal dysfunction were most closely related to increased QT dispersion in subjects with type 2 diabetes *(97)*. However, despite these reports of an association of abnormal cardiac electrical activity and CAN, no irrefutable evidence has emerged definitively linking CAN (uncomplicated by myocardial ischemia) with the development of malignant arrhythmias. Therefore, it seems reasonable to assume that in subjects with CAN, additional provocation such as strenuous exercise or hypoglycemia (which activates the sympathetic nervous system) might be required to promote arrythmogenesis. However, a recent report examined QTc during controlled hypoglycemia using a hyperinsulinemic clamp, and failed to identify abnormal cardiac repolarization during hypoglycemia and even suggested that there was some degree of protection afforded by CAN *(98)*. These studies therefore confirm that the effect of CAN on myocardial electrical stability and the potential for arrhythmogenesis remains unresolved.

The potential mechanisms whereby cardiac dysinnervation might increase the risk of myocardial instability have begun to be addressed using scintigraphic techniques. The retention of [^{123}I]-MIBG is reduced in the inferior and posterior LV in subjects with both silent *(99,100)* or symptomatic *(100)* myocardial ischemia. Altered myocardial [^{123}I]-MIBG uptake has been shown to correlate with alterations of the QT interval *(101)* and QT dispersion *(102,103)*. Abnormal retention of LV [^{123}I]-MIBG in subjects with diabetes has also been found to be predictive of sudden death *(104)*.

Studies using the sympathetic tracer [^{11}C]HED have shown that abnormalities of LV sympathetic innervation begin distally in the LV, spread circumferentially, and proximally involving anterior, inferior, and lateral ventricular walls, reflecting a proximal–distal progression in the severity of neuropathy *(22,29,31)*. Interestingly, despite extensive cardiac denervation, islands of proximal myocardial sympathetic "hyperinnervation" have been identified in which [^{11}C]HED retention is increased by 30% above values in CAN-free subjects *(29)*. Distally, [^{11}C]HED retention is decreased in these subjects by about 30%, resulting in a dramatic gradient of sympathetic innervation, which could potentially destabilize the myocardium *(29)*. Distally the denervated myocardium might demonstrate evidence of insulin resistance, as uptake of glucose is decreased compared with the innervated proximal myocardium (MJS, personal observations).

Effect of CAN on Myocardial Blood Flow Regulation and LV Function in Diabetes

Scintigraphy has been used to explore myocardial blood flow/innervation relationships in subjects with type 1 diabetes. Reduced myocardial blood flow reserve has been found in subjects with both type 2 diabetes *(105,106)* and type 1 diabetes *(22,106–108)*

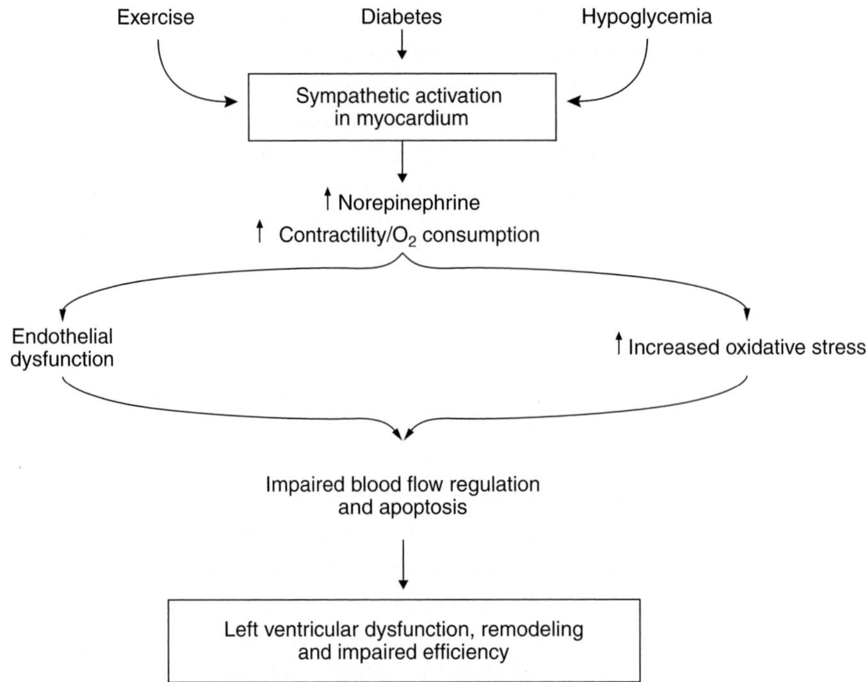

Fig. 3. In diabetes, sympathetic activation might lead to deficits in left ventricular structure and performance. In early CAN, cardiac sympathetic tone might be elevated which might result in increased oxidative stress, abnormal myocardial blood flow regulation and apoptosis, which predisposes to left ventricular structural and functional deficits.

and has been associated with impaired glucose control *(109)*. CAN is also associated with impaired vasodilation of coronary resistance vessels *(22,108)*. Interestingly, maximally impaired vasodilatory capacity in response to adenosine stress in advanced diabetic CAN *(22)* and to cold pressor testing in subjects with diabetes with normal cardiovascular reflex tests *(4)* occurs in the proximal myocardial segments *(4,22)*. Although the etiology of this deficit is unknown, endothelial dysfunction in concert with decreased myocardial vascularity (a cardiac microangiopathy) *(22,110)* might be important contributing factors.

In diabetes alterations of cardiac sympathetic tone in concert with abnormal myocardial blood flow regulation might profoundly impact myocardial structure, efficiency, and ultimately stability and function (Fig. 3). Alterations of diastolic *(54,92,111)* and systolic *(112)* function are widely reported in healthy subjects with diabetes and might predate the development of other complications. Although the etiology of LV dysfunction is poorly understood, a contribution from CAN has been proposed by a number of different investigators. For example, in diabetes, CAN has been reported to be accompanied by diastolic dysfunction *(4,113,114)*, impaired LV ejection fraction *(115,116)*, LV hypertrophy *(113)*, and LV hypercontractility *(114)*. LV dysfunction has been shown to correlate with abnormal cardiac [^{123}I] MIBG retention *(117,118)*.

Recently, the relationships of early diabetic microangiopathy (manifested as background diabetic retinopathy or microalbuminuria) to alterations of cardiac sympathetic tone and LV function in healthy subjects with stable type 1 diabetes were explored *(4)*. Deficits of LV [^{11}C]HED retention were extensive and global in the subjects with preclinical microangiopathy despite preservation of cardiovascular autonomic reflex tests. In the subjects with early microangiopathy, systemic plasma levels of norepinephrine at rest were unaltered, but norepinephrine excursions in response to a cold pressor test were exaggerated, a finding consistent with enhanced cardiovascular sympathetic nervous system reactivity. Moreover, diastolic dysfunction was detected by two-dimensional echocardiography in five out of eight of these subjects, but in none of the diabetic subjects without HED deficits or increased sympathetic responsiveness.

Adrenergic activity is a major determinant of vascular tone and altered adrenergic activity might contribute to abnormalities of regional blood flow regulation and myocardial microvascular disease complicating diabetes. In general, most studies have not identified a change in basal sympathetic nerve activity in diabetes, before the development of CAN *(119,120)*. In contrast, in diabetes, responsiveness to infused norepinephrine tends to be increased *(121–123)*. Exercise-provoked excursions of circulating norepinephrine are more pronounced in subjects with diabetes irrespective of the complication status, although the change in systolic blood pressure response might be higher in subjects with diabetic microangiopathy *(124)*. Impaired glycemic control might also exert its detrimental effect on the heart in part by augmenting sympathetic responsiveness *(120,125)*. However, with the progression of CAN the epinephrine and norepinephrine responsiveness become attenuated *(126)*. Therefore, it is tempting to speculate that augmented cardiac sympathetic tone or reactivity might contribute to early myocardial injury in diabetes.

Impaired LV function complicating diabetes has been linked to the development of a cardiomyopathy consisting myocardial interstitial and perivascular fibrosis *(127)*, and apoptosis *(128)*. These histopathological defects resemble those observed in arrhythmogenic right ventricular cardiomyopathy *(129)*, a condition, which is characterized by increased cardiac sympathetic nervous system activity *(129–131)* (in the absence of increased systemic sympathetic nerve activity) and clinically by ventricular tachycardia, sudden death, and cardioprotection from β-adrenergic receptor (β-AR) blockade *(129–131)*, implicating an important role of elevated cardiac sympathetic nervous system activity in myocardial injury and arrhythmogenesis. Additionally, increased cardiac sympathetic tone can increase myocardial reactive oxygen species production *(132)*, perturb intracellular signaling *(133)*, and accelerate apoptosis *(128,133)*. Adrenergic stimulation also impairs myocardial efficiency *(134)* and promotes myocardial remodeling *(134,135)*.

Paradoxically, progressive distal cardiac sympathetic denervation is also likely to contribute to myocardial dysfunction. For example, in experimentally denervated dogs, positron emission tomography has demonstrated that denervation can upregulate β-ARs *(136)* and facilitate a shift from β_1- to β_2-AR subtype (β_2-ARs are principally coupled to adenylyl cyclase) *(137)*, which might therefore augment denervation supersensitivity. In concert, denervation might promote insulin resistance *(138,139)* and increase myocardial fatty acid metabolism *(140)*. Because fatty acids are an inefficient substrate in comparison with glucose, in diabetic CAN, myocardial efficiency might also be impaired in the distal denervated segments.

MANAGEMENT

There is no therapy currently available for the treatment of CAN. Therefore, treatment mostly focuses upon management of a number of modifiable risk factors, which can significantly reduce the risk of developing CAN. In the European Diabetes Prospective Complications Study (EURODIAB), which enrolled 1172 patients with type 1 diabetes, the incidence of neuropathy was associated with a poor glycemic control, elevated triglyceride levels, increased body-mass index, smoking, and hypertension *(141)*. Initially, treatment should focus upon improving overall cardiovascular fitness. Indeed, an exercise program has been shown to be able to improve early CAN *(142)*. However, because CAN might impair exercise tolerance *(51,57)* and mask myocardial ischemia *(25,90–92)*, subjects with CAN should be considered for a cardiac stress study before undertaking an exercise program.

In the Diabetes Control and Complication Trial study, an HbA1c difference of 1.9% decreased the risk of development of confirmed clinical neuropathy (diagnosed by neurological history and physical examination and confirmed by nerve conduction or autonomic function studies at year five) by 60% *(17–19)*. More recently, multifactorial risk factor intervention (primarily glucose, blood pressure, and lipid control) were found to reduce the risk of CAN in type 2 diabetes by 63% *(7)*. The individual contribution of agents, such as angiotensin converting enzyme inhibitors and statins to these salutary effects remains uncertain *(143,144)*. Perhaps, if additional studies confirm an important role for sympathetic activation early in the development of abnormal blood flow regulation and myocardial damage complicating diabetes, consideration should be given to the use of β-AR blockade before the development of hypertension (particularly as newer agents such as carvedilol appear to reduce oxidative stress, microalbumuria, and insulin resistance in subjects with type 2 diabetes *[145]*). In any event, these studies are highly supportive of the importance of multiple risk factor management in delaying the development and slowing the progress of CAN (and its down-stream consequences) complicating diabetes and may be particularly important in the high-risk patient with established myocardial ischemia in whom CAN appears to further augment risk.

Increased oxidative stress has emerged as a leading candidate in the pathogenesis of experimental diabetic neuropathy, with a direct relationship between measures of oxidative stress and the development of nerve blood flow and nerve conduction deficits *(146–148)*. In diabetic rodents, measures of oxidative stress, including increased nerve conjugated dienes *(148)* and reduced levels of nerve superoxide dismutase *(146,149)*, glutathione peroxidase *(150)*, glutathione *(151)*, and norepinephine *(152)* are closely associated with the development of neuropathy. In concert, oxidative stress has also been implicated in the development of cardiomyopathy *(120,153)* and a contributing factor to endothelial dysfunction *(154,155)* and changes in acute phase reactants *(156)*. Increases in reactive oxygen species can stimulate apoptosis in cardiac myocytes *(157,158)* potentially resulting in myocardial dysfunction *(159)*. In the heart, chronic oxidative stress might also impair neurotrophism by depleting nerve growth factor (NGF) *(160)* and may downregulate NGF receptor expression, sensitivity, and transport in the myocardium *(160,161)* of diabetic rats *(162)*. The chain breaking antioxidant, α-lipoic acid as well as the beta amino acid and endogenous antioxidant taurine *(163)* may stimulate NGF synthesis *(164)* and can prevent NGF protein depletion in sciatic nerve *(161,163)* and myocardium of diabetic rats *(162)*.

Many studies have shown that oxidative stress is increased in subjects with diabetes before the development of diabetic complications *(4,165,166)*, and recently studies have reported that oxidative stress is further increased in the presence of diabetic neuropathy *(4,167)* including CAN *(4)*. Finally, activation of the aldose reductase pathway impairs antioxidant defense and promotes oxidative stress and has been implicated for many years in the pathogenesis of the chronic complications of diabetes including neuropathy *(168,169)*. Aldose reductase-mediated oxidative stress is multifactorial, mediated by oxidizing the $NADP^+$/NADPH and GSH/GSSG redox couples and by causing the compensatory depletion of taurine *(163,169)*.

In subjects with diabetes and CAN and abnormal LV function measured during maximal bicycle exercise by gated radionuclide ventriculography (but without coronary heart disease), 1-year treatment with the aldose reductase inhibitor zopolrestat was shown to stabilize or reverse these functional deficits *(115)*. In another study, a trend toward improvement of HRV was found after 4 months of oral treatment with α-lipoic acid (800 mg per day) in patients with type 2 diabetes with CAN *(170)*. Most recently, 120 subjects with diabetic neuropathy were administered either α-lipoic acid 600 mg intravenously for 5 days per week for 14 treatments or a placebo. Treatment with α-lipoic acid resulted in significant improvements in total symptom score and in one attribute of nerve conduction, but did not improve quantitative sensory testing or cardiovascular reflex measures of autonomic function *(171)*. These studies suggest that a single interventional therapy might be insufficient to reverse CAN. In order to test the contribution of oxidative stress to the development and progression of CAN complicating diabetes, a 2-year prospective clinical trial is currently in progress exploring the ability of a combination of antioxidant approaches to reverse established cardiac sympathetic denervation assessed using HED and positron emission tomography.

In summary, CAN is a common but frequently overlooked complication of diabetes, with multiple subclinical and clinical cardiac manifestations ranging from impairment of exercise tolerance to sudden cardiac death. The advent of cardiac scintigraphy has allowed direct characterization of cardiac sympathetic dysinnervation complicating diabetes, and should greatly facilitate the elucidation of its metabolic and functional consequences. The salutary effects of multiple risk factor management in preventing the development and/or the progression of CAN underlines the importance of intensification of metabolic control early in the course of diabetes before the development of cardiovascular denervation. For individuals with already established CAN, the ability of combination antioxidant therapy to reinnervate the heart is currently being evaluated.

ACKNOWLEDGMENTS

This work was supported in part by grants from the Juvenile Diabetes Research Foundation, the National Institutes of Health R01-DK54916-05, R01AT002146-01A1 and an American Diabetes Association Research Award.

REFERENCES

1. Wild S, Roglic G, Green A, Sicree R, King H. Global prevalence of diabetes: estimates for the year 2000 and projections for 2030. *Diabetes Care* 2003;27:1047–1053.
2. Vinik AI, Maser RE, Mitchell BD, Freeman R. Diabetic autonomic neuropathy. *Diabetes Care* 2003;26:1553–1579.

3. Stevens MJ. New imaging techniques for cardiovascular autonomic neuropathy: a window on the heart. *Diab Technol Ther* 2001;3:9–22.
4. Pop-Busui R, Kirkwood I, Schmid H, et al. Sympathetic dysfunction in type 1 diabetes: association with impaired myocardial blood flow reserves and diastolic dysfunction. *J Am Coll Cardiol* 2004;44:2368–2374.
5. Kreiner G, Wolzt M, Fasching P, et al. Myocardial m-[123I]iodobenzylguanidine scintigraphy for the assessment of adrenergic cardiac innervation in patients with IDDM. Comparison with cardiovascular reflex tests and relationship to left ventricular function. *Diabetes* 1995; 44:543–549.
6. Mustonen J, Mantysaari M, Kuikka J, et al. Decreased myocardial 123I-metaiodobenzylguanidine uptake is associated with disturbed left ventricular diastolic filling in diabetes. *Am Heart J* 1992;123:804–805.
7. Gaede P, Vedel P, Larsen N, Jensen GV, Parving HH, Pedersen O. Multifactorial intervention and cardiovascular disease in patients with type 2 diabetes. *N Engl J Med* 2003;348: 383–393.
8. American Diabetes Association and American Academy of Neurology. Report and recommendations of the San Antonio Conference on diabetic neuropathy (Consensus Statement) *Diabetes* 1988;37:1000–1004.
9. Hilsted J, Jeensen SB. A simple test for autonomic neuropathy in juvenile diabetics. *Acta Med Scand* 1979;205:385–387.
10. Dyberg T, Benn J, Christiansen JS, Hilsted J, Nerup J. Prevalence of diabetic autonomic neuropathy measured by simple bedside tests. *Diabetologia* 1981;20:190–194.
11. Ewing DJ, Martyn CN, Young RJ, Clarke BF. The value of cardiovascular autonomic function tests: 10 years experience in diabetes. *Diabetes Care* 1985;8:491–498.
12. Kennedy WR, Navarro X, Sakuta M, Mandell H, Knox C, Sutherland DE. Physiological and clinical correlates of cardiovascular reflexes in diabetes mellitus. *Diabetes Care* 1989;12:399–408.
13. Neil HA, Thomson AV, John S, McCarty ST, Mann JL. Diabetic autonomic neuropathy: the prevalence of impaired heart rate variability in a geographically defined population. *Diabet Med* 1989;6:20–24.
14. Eurodiab IDDM Complication Group. Microvascular and acute complications in IDDM patients: the EURODIAB IDDM complications study. *Diabetologia* 1994;37:278–285.
15. Ziegler D, Dannehl K, Muhlen H, Spuler M, Gries FA. Prevalence of cardiovascular autonomic dysfunction assessed by spectral analysis, vector analysis, and standard tests of heart rate variation and blood pressure responses at various stages of diabetic neuropathy. *Diabet Med* 1992;9:806–814.
16. Ziegler D, Gries FA, Spuler M, Lessmann F. Diabetic Cardiovascular Autonomic Neuropathy Multicenter Study Group: The epidemiology of diabetic neuropathy. *J Diab Compl* 1992;6:49–57.
17. The DCCT Research Group. Factors in the development of diabetic neuropathy: baseline analysis of neuropathy in the feasibility phase of the Diabetes Control and Complications Trial (DCCT). *Diabetes* 1988;37:476–481.
18. The Diabetes Control and Complications Trial Research Group. The effect of intensive diabetes therapy on the development and progression of neuropathy. *Ann Intern Med* 1995;122:561–568.
19. The Diabetes Control and Complications Trial Research Group. The effect of intensive diabetes therapy on measures of autonomic nervous system function in the Diabetes Control and Complications Trial (DCCT). *Diabetologia* 1998;41:416–423.
20. Valensi P, Paries J, Attali JR. French Group for Research and Study of Diabetic Neuropathy. Cardiac autonomic neuropathy in diabetic patients: influence of diabetes duration, obesity, and microangiopathic complications—the French multicenter study. *Metab Clin Exp* 2003;52:815–820.

21. Toyry JP, Niskanen LK, Mantysaari MJ, Lansimies EA, Uusitupa MI. Occurrence, predictors and clinical significance of autonomic neuropathy in NIDDM. *Diabetes* 1996;45:308–315.
22. Stevens MJ, Dayanikli F, Raffel DM, et al. Scintigraphic assessment of regionalized defects in myocardial sympathetic innervation and blood flow regulation in diabetic patients with autonomic neuropathy. *J Am Coll Cardiol* 1998;31:1575–1584.
23. Mantysaari M, Kuikka J, Mustonen J, et al. Noninvasive detection of cardiac sympathetic nervous dysfunction in diabetic patients using [^{123}I] metaiodobenzylguanidine. *Diabetes* 1992;41:1069–1075.
24. Kreiner G, Wolzt M, Fasching P, et al. Myocardial m-[^{123}I] iodobenzylguanidine scintigraphy for the assessment of adrenergic cardiac innervation in patients with IDDM. *Diabetes* 1995; 44:543–549.
25. Langer A, Freeman ME, Josse RG, Armstrong PW. Metaiodobenzylguanidine imaging in diabetes mellitus: assessment of cardiac sympathetic denervation and its relation to autonomic dysfunction and silent myocardial ischemia. *J Am Coll Cardiol* 1995;25:610–618.
26. Allman KC, Stevens MJ, Wieland DM, et al. Noninvasive assessment of cardiac diabetic neuropathy by C-11 hydroxyephedrine and positron emission tomography. *J Am Coll Cardiol* 1993;22:1425–1432.
27. Schnell O, Kirsch CM, Stemplinger J, Haslbeck M, Standl E. Scintigraphic evidence for cardiac sympathetic dysinnervation in long-term IDDM patients with and without ECG-based autonomic neuropathy. *Diabetologia* 1995;38:1345–1352.
28. Schnell O, Muhr D, Weiss M, Dresel S, Haslbeck M, Standl E. Reduced myocardial ^{123}I-metaiodobenzylguanidine uptake in newly diagnosed IDDM patients. *Diabetes* 1996; 45:801–805.
29. Stevens MJ, Raffel DM, Allman K, et al. Cardiac sympathetic dysinnervation in diabetes-an explanation for enhanced cardiovascular risk? *Circulation* 1998;98:961–968.
30. Ziegler D, Weise F, Langen KJ, et al. Effect of glycemic control on myocardial sympathetic innervation assessed by [^{123}]metaiodobenzylguanidine scintigraphy: a 4-year prospective study in IDDM patients. *Diabetologia* 1998;41:443–451.
31. Stevens MJ, Raffel DM, Allman KC, Schwaiger M, Wieland DM. Regression and progression of cardiac sympathetic dysinnervation in diabetic patients with autonomic neuropathy. *Metabolism* 1999;48:92–101.
32. Schnell O, Muhr D, Weiss M, Dresel S, Haslbeck M, Standl E. Reduced myocardial ^{123}I-metaiodobenzylguanidine uptake in newly diagnosed IDDM patients. *Diabetes* 1996; 45:801–805.
33. Verrotti A, Chiarelli F, Blasetti A, Morgese G. Autonomic neuropathy in diabetic children. *J Paediatr Child Health* 1995;31:545–548.
34. Ziegler D, Dannehl K, Wiefels K, Gries FA. Differential effects of near-normoglycaemia for 4 years on somatic nerve dysfunction and heart rate variation in type I diabetic patients. *Diabet Med* 1992;9:622–629.
35. Jakobsen J, Christiansen JS, Kristoffersen I, et al. Autonomic and somatosensory nerve function after 2 years of continuous subcutaneous insulin infusion in type 1 diabetes. *Diabetes* 1988;37:452–455.
36. Sampson MJ, Wilson S, Karagiannis P, Edmonds M, Watkins PJ. Progression of diabetic autonomic neuropathy over a decade of insulin-dependent diabetics. *Q J Med* 1990;75:635–646.
37. Levitt NS, Stansberry KB, Wynchank S, Vinik AI. The natural progression of autonomic neuropathy and autonomic function tests in a cohort of people with IDDM. *Diabetes Care* 1996;19:751–754.
38. Forsen A, Kangro M, Sterner G, et al. A 14-year prospective study of autonomic nerve function in Type 1 diabetic patients: association with nephropathy. *Diabet Med* 2004;21: 852–858.

39. Ewing DJ, Campbell IW, Clarke BF. The natural history of diabetic autonomic neuropathy. *Q J Med* 1980;49:95–108.
40. Ewing DJ. Cardiovascular reflexes and autonomic neuropathy. *Clin Sci Mol Med* 1978;55:321–327.
41. American Diabetes Association and American Academy of Neurology. Proceedings of a consensus development conference on standardized measures in diabetic neuropathy. *Diabetes Care* 1992;15:1080–1107.
42. Hayano J, Mukai S, Fukuta H, Sakata S, Ohte N, Kimura G. Postural response of low-frequency component of heart rate variability is an increased risk for mortality in patients with coronary artery disease. *Chest* 2001;120:1942–1952.
43. Wieland DM, Brown LE, Tobes MC, et al. Imaging the primate adrenal medulla with [I-^{123}] and [I-^{131}] metaiodobenzylguanidine: concise communication. *J Nucl Med* 1981;22:358–364.
44. Sisson JC, Wieland DM, Mangner TJ, Tobes MC, Jacques S. Metaiodobenzylguanidine as an index of the adrenergic system integrity and function. *J Nucl Med* 1987;28:1620–1624.
45. Glowniak JV. Cardiac studies with metaiodobenzylguanidine: a critique of methods and interpretation of results. *J Nucl Med* 1995;36:2133–2137.
46. Raffel DM, Corbett JR, Schwaiger M, Wieland DM. Mechanism-based strategies for mapping heart sympathetic function. *Nucl Med Biol* 1995;22:1019–1026.
47. Allman KC, Wieland DM, Muzik O, DeGrado TR, Wolfe ER, Schwaiger M. Carbon-11 hydroxyephedrine with positron emission tomography for serial assessment of cardiac adrenergic neuronal function after acute myocardial infarction in humans. *J Am Coll Cardiol* 1993;22:368–375.
48. DeGrado TR, Hutchins GD, Toorongian SA, Wieland DM, Schwaiger M. Myocardial kinetics of carbon-11-meta-hydroxyephedrine (HED): retention mechanisms and effects of norepinephrine. *J Nucl Med* 1993;34:1287–1293.
49. Nakajo M, Shapiro B, Glowniak J, Sisson JC, Beierwaltes WH. Inverse relationship between cardiac accumulation of meta-[^{131}I]iodobenzylguanidine (I-^{131} MIBG) and circulating catecholamines in suspected pheochromocytoma. *J Nucl Med* 1983;24:1127–1134.
50. Gasnier B, Roisin MP, Scherman D, Coornaert S, Desplanches G, Henry JP. Uptake of meta-iodobenzylguanidine by bovine chromaffin granule membranes. *Mol Pharmacol* 1986;29:275–280.
51. Vinik AI, Erbas T. Neuropathy, in *Handbook of Exercise in Diabetes* (Ruderman N, Devlin JT, Schneider SH, Kriska A, eds.), Alexandria, VA, 2002, pp. 463–496.
52. Vinik AI, Park TS, Stansberry KB, Pittenger GL. Diabetic neuropathies. *Diabetologia* 2000;43:957–973.
53. Hilsted J. Pathophysiology in diabetic autonomic neuropathy: Cardiovascular, hormonal, and metabolic studies. *Diabetes* 1982;31:730–737.
54. Zola B, Kahn JK, Juni JE, Vinik AI. Abnormal cardiac function in diabetic patients with autonomic neuropathy in the absence of ischemic heart disease. *J Clin Endocrinol Metab* 1986;63:208–214.
55. Willenheimer RB, Erhardt LR, Nilsson H, Lilja B, Juul-Moller S, Sundkvist G. Parasympathetic neuropathy associated with left ventricular diastolic dysfunction in patients with insulin-dependent diabetes mellitus. *Scand Cardiovasc J* 1998;32:172–180.
56. Dhalla NS, Liu X, Panagia V, Takeda N. Subcellular remodelling and heart dysfunction in chronic diabetes. *J Cardiovasc Res* 1988;40:239–247.
57. Roy TM, Peterson HR, Snider HL, et al. Autonomic influence on cardiovascular performance in diabetic subjects. *Am J Med* 1989;87:382–388.
58. Position paper. Orthostatic hypotension, multiple system atrophy (the Shy Drager syndrome) and pure autonomic failure. *J Auton Nerv Syst* 1996;58:123–124.
59. Hilsted J, Parving HH, Christensen NJ, Benn J, Galbo H. Hemodynamics in diabetic orthostatic hypotension. *J Clin Invest* 1981;68:1427–1434.

60. Hornung RS, Mahler RF, Raftery EB. Ambulatory blood pressure and heart rate in diabetic patients: an assessment of autonomic function. *Diabet Med* 1989;6:579–585.
61. Burgos LG, Ebert TJ, Asiddao C, et al. Increased intraoperative cardiovascular morbidity in diabetics with autonomic neuropathy. *Anesthesiology* 1989;70:591–597.
62. Sobotka PA, Liss HP, Vinik AI. Impaired hypoxic ventilatory drive in diabetic patients with autonomic neuropathy. *J Clin Endocrinol Metab* 1986;62:658–663.
63. Ewing DJ, Campbell IW, Clarke BF. Assessment of cardiovascular effects in diabetic autonomic neuropathy and prognostic implications. *Ann Int Med* 1980;92:308–311.
64. Hjalmarson A, Elmfeldt D, Herlitz J, et al. Effect on mortality of metoprolol in acute myocardial infarction, a double-blind randomized trial. *Lancet* 1981;ii:123–127.
65. Beta-blocker Heart Attack Trial Research Group. A randomized trial of propranolol in patients with acute myocardial infarction. I. Mortality results. *JAMA* 1982;247:1707–1714.
66. Norwegian Multicentre Study Group. Timolol-induced reduction in mortality and reinfarction in patients surviving acute myocardial infarction. *N Engl J Med* 1981;304: 801–807.
67. Australian and Swedish Pindolol Study Group. The effect of pindolol on the two year mortality after complicated myocardial infarction. *Eur Heart J* 1983;4:367–375.
68. Jaffe AS, Spadaro JJ, Schectman K, Roberts R, Geltman EM, Sobel BE. Increased congestive heart failure after myocardial infarction of modest extent in patients with diabetes mellitus. *Am Heart J* 1984;108:31–37.
69. Gundersen T, Kjekshus JT. Timolol treatment after myocardial infarction in diabetic patients. *Diabetes Care* 1983;6:285–290.
70. Smith JW, Marcus FI, Serokman R. With the Multicentre Postinfarction Research Group. Prognosis of patients with diabetes mellitus after acute myocardial infarction. *Am J Cardiol* 1984;54:718–721.
71. Fava S, Azzopardi J, Muscatt HA, Fenech FF. Factors that influence outcome in diabetic subjects with myocardial infarction. *Diabetes Care* 1993;16:1615–1618.
72. Ziegler D. Cardiovascular autonomic neuropathy: clinical manifestations and measurement. *Diabetes Rev* 1999;7:342–357.
73. Kennedy WR, Navarro X, Sakuta M, Mandell H, Knox CK, Sutherland DE. Physiological and clinical correlates of cardiovascular reflexes in diabetes mellitus. *Diabetes Care* 1989;12:399–408.
74. Chen HS, Hwu CM, Kuo BI, et al. Abnormal cardiovascular reflex tests are predictors of mortality in Type 2 diabetes mellitus. *Diabete Med* 2001;18:268–273.
75. Mankovsky BN, Piolot R, Mankovsky OL, Ziegler D. Impairment of cerebral autoregulation in diabetic patients with cardiovascular autonomic neuropathy and orthostatic hypotension. *Diabete Med* 2003;20:119–126.
76. Cohen JA, Estacio RO, Lundgren RA, Esler AL, Schrier RW. Diabetic autonomic neuropathy is associated with an increased incidence of strokes. *Aut Neurosci Basic Clin* 2003; 108:73–78.
77. Gerritsen J, Dekker JM, ten Voorde BJ, et al. Impaired autonomic function is associated with increased mortality, especially in subjects with diabetes, hypertension, or a history of cardiovascular disease: the Hoorn Study. *Diabetes Care* 2001;24:1793–1798.
78. Suarez GA, Clark VM, Norell JE, et al. Sudden cardiac death in diabetes mellitus: risk factors in the Rochester diabetic neuropathy study. *J Neurol Neurosurg Psych* 2005;76: 240–245.
79. Orchard TJ, Lloyd CE, Maser RE, Kuller LH. Why does diabetic autonomic neuropathy predict IDDM mortality? An analysis from the Pittsburgh Epidemiology of Diabetes Complications Study. *Diabetes Res Clin Pract* 1996;34(Suppl):S165–S171.
80. Rathman W, Ziegler D, Jahnke M, Haastert B, Gries FA. Mortality in diabetic patients with cardiovascular autonomic neuropathy. *Diabet Med* 1993;10:820–824.

81. Lee KH, Jang HJ, Kim YH, et al. Prognostic value of cardiac autonomic neuropathy independent and incremental to perfusion defects in patients with diabetes and suspected coronary artery disease. *Am J Cardiol* 2003;92:1458–1461.
82. Page MM, Watkins PJ. Cardiorespiratory arrest and diabetic autonomic neuropathy. *Lancet* 1978;1:14–16.
83. Meyer C, Grossmann R, Mitrakou A, et al. Effects of autonomic neuropathy on counterregulation and awareness of hypoglycemia in type 1 diabetic patients. *Diabetes Care* 1998;21:1960–1966.
84. Sivieri R, Veglio M, Chinaglia A, Scaglione P, Cavallo-Perin P. Prevalence of QT prolongation in a type 1 diabetic population and its association with autonomic neuropathy. *Diabet Med* 1993;10:920–924.
85. Veglio M, Borra M, Stevens LK, Fuller JH, Perin PC. The relation between QTc interval prolongation and diabetic complications: the EURODIAB IDDM Complications Study Group. *Diabetologia* 1999;42:68–75.
86. Valensi PE, Johnson NB, Maison-Blanche P, Extramania F, Motte G, Coumel P. Influence of cardiac autonomic neuropathy on heart rate dependence of ventricular repolarization in diabetic patients. *Diabetes Care* 2002;25:918–923.
87. Miettinen H, Lehto S, Salomaa V, et al. Impact of diabetes on mortality after the first myocardial infarction: The FINMONICA Myocardial Infarction Register Study Group. *Diabetes Care* 1998;21:69–75.
88. Morning peak in the incidence of myocardial infarction: experience in the ISIS-2 trial. ISIS-2 (Second International Study of Infarct Survival) Collaborative Group. *Eur Heart J* 1992;13:594–598.
89. Aronson D, Weinrauch LA, D'Elia JA, Tofler GH, Burger AJ. Circadian patterns of heart rate variability, fibrinolytic activity, and hemostatic factors in type I diabetes mellitus with cardiac autonomic neuropathy. *Am J Cardiol* 1999;84:449–453.
90. Valensi P, Sachs RN, Harfouche B, et al. Predictive value of cardiac autonomic neuropathy in diabetic patients with or without silent myocardial ischemia. *Diabetes Care* 2001;24:339–343.
91. Milan Study on Atherosclerosis and Diabetes (MiSAD) Group. Prevalence of unrecognized silent myocardial ischemia and its association with atherosclerotic risk factors in noninsulin-dependent diabetes mellitus. *Am J Cardiol* 1997;79:134–139.
92. Zarich S, Waxman S, Freeman RT, Mittleman M, Hegarty P, Nesto RW. Effect of autonomic nervous system dysfunction on the circadian pattern of myocardial ischemia in diabetes mellitus. *J Am Coll Cardiol* 1994;24:956–962.
93. Campbell IW, Ewing DJ, Clarke BF. Painful myocardial infarction in severe diabetic autonomic neuropathy. *Acta Diabetol Lat* 1978;15:210–214.
94. Sawickim PT, Kiwitt S, Bender R, Berger M. The value of QT interval dispersion for identification of total mortality risk in non-insulin-dependent diabetes mellitus. *J Intern Med* 1998;24:49–56.
95. Naas AA, Davidson NC, Thompson C, et al. QT and QTc dispersion are accurate predictors of cardiac death in newly diagnosed non-insulin dependent diabetes: cohort study. *BMJ* 1998;316:745–746.
96. Poulsen PL, Ebbehoj E, Arildsen H, et al. Increased QTc dispersion is related to blunted circadian blood pressure variation in normoalbuminuric type 1 diabetic patients. *Diabetes* 2001;50:837–842.
97. Takahashi N, Nakagawa M, Saikawa T, et al. Regulation of QT indices mediated by autonomic nervous function in patients with type 2 diabetes. *Int J Cardiol* 2004;96:375–379.
98. Lee SP, Yeoh L, Harris ND, et al. Influence of autonomic neuropathy on QTc interval lengthening during hypoglycemia in type 1 diabetes. *Diabetes* 2004;53:1535–1542.

99. Matsuo S, Takahashi M, Nakamura Y, Kinoshita M. Evaluating of cardiac sympathetic innervation with iodine-123-metaiodobenzylguanidine imaging in silent myocardial ischemia. *J Nucl Med* 1996;37:712–717.
100. Koistinen MJ, Airaksinen KE, Huikuri HV, et al. No difference in cardiac innervation of diabetic patients with painful and asymptomatic coronary artery disease. *Diabetes Care* 1996;19:231–235.
101. Langen K-J, Ziegler D, Weise F, et al. Evaluation of QT interval length, QT dispersion and myocardial m-iodobenzylguanidine uptake in insulin-dependent diabetic patients with autonomic neuropathy. *Clin Sci* 1997;92:325–333.
102. Shimabukuro M, Chibana T, Yoshida H, Nagamine F, Komiya I, Takasu N. Increased QT disperson and cardiac adrenergic dysinnervation in diabetic patients with autonomic neuropathy. *Am J Cardiol* 1996;78:1057–1059.
103. Hara M, Sakino H, Katsuragi I, Tanaka K, Yoshimatsu H. Regulation of QT indices mediated by autonomic nervous function in patients with type 2 diabetes. *Int J Cardiol* 2004; 96:375–379.
104. Kahn JK, Sisson JC, Vinik AI. Prediction of sudden cardiac death in diabetic autonomic neuropathy. *J Nucl Med* 1988;29:1605–1606.
105. Nitenberg A, Valensi P, Sachs R, Dali M, Aptecar E, Attali JR. Impairment of coronary vascular reserve and ACh-induced coronary vasodilation in diabetic patients with angiographically normal coronary arteries and normal left ventricular systolic function. *Diabetes* 1993;42:1017–1025.
106. Di Carli MF, Janisse J, Grunberger G, Ager J. Role of chornic hyperglycemia in the pathogenesis of coronary microvascular dysfunction in diabetes. *J Am Coll Cardiol* 2003; 41:1387–1393.
107. Pitkanen OP, Nuutila P, Raitakari OT, et al. Coronary flow reserve is reduced in young men with IDDM. *Diabetes* 1998;47:248–54.
108. Di Carli MF, Bianco-Batlles D, Landa ME, et al. Effects of autonomic neuropathy on coronary blood flow in patients with diabetes mellitus. *Circulation* 1999;100:813–819.
109. Yokoyama I, Ohtake T, Momomura S, et al. Hyperglycemia rather than insulin resistance is related to reduced coronary flow reserve in NIDDM. *Diabetes* 1998;47:119–124.
110. Torry RJ, Connell PM, O'Brien DM, Chilian WM, Tomanek RJ. Sympathectomy stimulates capillary but not precapillary growth in hypertrophic hearts. *Am J Physiol* 1991;260: H1515–H1521.
111. Fang ZY, Yuda S, Anderson V, Short L, Case C, Marwick TH. Echocardiographic detection of early diabetic myocardial disease. *J Am Coll Cardiol* 2003;41:611–617.
112. Vered A, Battler A, Segal P, et al. Exercise-induced left ventricular dysfunction in young men with asymptomatic diabetes mellitus (diabetic cardiomyopathy). *Am J Cardiol* 1984; 54:633–637.
113. Taskiran M, Rasmussen V, Rasmussen B, et al. Left ventricular dysfunction in normotensive Type 1 diabetic patients: the impact of autonomic neuropathy. *Diab Med* 2004;21:524–530.
114. Didangelos TP, Arsos GA, Karamitsos DT, Athyros VG, Karatzas ND. Left ventricular systolic and diastolic function in normotensive type 1 diabetic patients with or without autonomic neuropathy: a radionuclide ventriculography study. *Diabetes Care* 2003;26:1955–1960.
115. Johnson BF, Nesto RW, Pfeifer MA, et al. Cardiac abnormalities in diabetic patients with neuropathy: effects of aldose reductase inhibitor administration. *Diabetes Care* 2004; 27:448–454.
116. Bristow MR. beta-adrenergic receptor blockade in chronic heart failure. *Circulation* 2000;101:558–569.
117. Sugiyama T, Kurata C, Tawarahara K, Nakano T. Is abnormal iodine-123-MIBG kinetics associated with left ventricular dysfunction in patients with diabetes mellitus? *J Nucl Cardiol* 2000;7:562–568.

118. Nakata T, Wakabayashi T, Kyuma M, et al. Prognostic implications of an initial loss of cardiac metaiodobenzylguanidine uptake and diabetes mellitus in patients with left ventricular dysfunction. *J Card Fail* 2003;9:113–121.
119. Hogikyan RV, Galecki AT, Halter JB, Supiano MA. Heightened norepinephrine-mediated vasoconstriction in type 2 diabetes. *Metabolism* 1999;48:1536–1541.
120. Christensen NJ. Plasma norepinephrine and epinephrine in untreated diabetics, during fasting and after insulin administration. *Diabetes* 1974;23:1–8.
121. Eckberg DL, Harkins SW, Fritsch JM, Musgrave GE, Gardner DF. Baroreflex control of plasma norepinephrine and heart period in healthy subjects and diabetic patients. *J Clin Invest* 1986;78:366–374.
122. Eichler HG, Blaschke TF, Kraemer FB, Ford GA, Blochl-Daum B, Hoffman BB. Responsiveness of superficial hand veins to alpha-adrenoceptor agonists in insulin-dependent diabetic patients. *Clin Sci (Lond)* 1992;82:163–168.
123. Weidmann P, Beretta-Piccoli C, Trost BN. Pressor factors and responsiveness in hypertension accompanying diabetes mellitus. *Hypertension* 1985;7:1133–1142.
124. Hoogenberg K, Dullaart RP. Abnormal plasma noradrenaline response and exercise induced albuminuria in type 1 (insulin-dependent) diabetes mellitus. *Scand J Clin Lab Invest* 1992; 52:803–811.
125. Tamborlane WV, Sherwin RS, Koivisto V, Hendler R, Genel M, Felig P. Normalization of the growth hormone and catecholamine response to exercise in juvenile-onset diabetic subjects treated with a portable insulin infusion pump. *Diabetes* 1979;28:785–788.
126. Meyer C, Grossmann R, Mitrakou A, et al. Effects of autonomic neuropathy on counterregulation and awareness of hypoglycemia in type 1 diabetic patients. *Diabetes Care* 1998; 21:1960–1966.
127. Francis GS. Diabetic cardiomyopathy: fact or fiction? *Heart* 2001;85:247–248.
128. Frustaci A, Kajstura J, Chimenti C, et al. Myocardial cell death in human diabetes. *Circ Res* 2000;87:1123–1132.
129. Thiene G, Nava A, Corrado D, Rossi L, Pennelli N. Right ventricular cardiomyopathy and sudden death in young people. *N Engl J Med* 1988;318:129–133.
130. Marcus FI, Fontaine GH, Guiraudon G, et al. Right ventricular dysplasia: a report of 24 adult cases. *Circulation* 1982;65:384–398.
131. Mallat Z, Tedgui A, Fontaliran F, Frank R, Durigon M, Fontaine G. Evidence of apoptosis in arrhythmogenic right ventricular dysplasia. *N Engl J Med* 1996;335:1190–1196.
132. Givertz MM, Sawyer DB, Colucci WS. Antioxidants and myocardial contractility: illuminating the "Dark Side" of beta-adrenergic receptor activation? *Circulation* 2001;103: 782–783.
133. Communal C, Singh K, Pimentel DR, Colucci WS. Norepinephrine stimulates apoptosis in adult rat ventricular myocytes by activation of the beta-adrenergic pathway *Circulation* 1998;98:1329–1334.
134. Eichhorn EJ, Bristow MR. Medical therapy can improve the biological properties of the chronically failing heart. A new era in the treatment of heart failure. *Circulation* 1996;94: 2285–2296.
135. Gambardella S, Frontoni S, Spallone V, et al. *Am J Hypertens* 1993;6:97–102.
136. Valette H, Deleuze P, Syrota A, et al. Canine myocardial beta-adrenergic, muscarinic receptor densities after denervation: a PET study. *J Nucl Med* 1995;36:140–146.
137. Van der Vusse GJ, Dubelaar ML, Coumans WA, et al. Depletion of endogenous dopamine stores and shift in beta-adrenoceptor subtypes in cardiac tissue following five weeks of chronic denervation. *Mol Cell Biochem* 1998;183:215–219.
138. Brown M, Marshall DR, Sobel BE, Bergmann SR. Delineation of myocardial oxygen utilization with carbon-11-labeled acetate. *Circulation* 1987;76:687–696.
139. Buxton DB, Schwaiger M, Nguyen A, Phelps ME, Schelbert HR. Radiolabeled acetate as a tracer of myocardial tricarboxylic acid cycle flux. *Circ Res* 1988;63:628–634.

140. Drake-Holland AJ, Van der Vusse GJ, Roemen TH, et al. *Cardiovasc Drugs Ther* 2001; 15:111–117.
141. Tesfaye S, Chaturvedi N, Eaton SE, et al. Vascular risk factors and diabetic neuropathy. *N Engl J Med* 2005;352:341–350.
142. Howorka K, Pumprla J, Haber P, Koller-Strametz J, Mondrzyk J, Schabmann A. Effects of physical training on heart rate variability in diabetic patients with various degrees of cardiovascular autonomic neuropathy. *Cardiovascular Res* 1997;34:206–214.
143. Kontopoulos AG, Athyros VG, Didangelos TP, et al. Effect of chronic quinapril administration on heart rate variability in patients with diabetic autonomic neuropathy. *Diabetes Care* 1997;20:355–361.
144. Malik RA, Williamson S, Abbott C, et al. Effect of angiotensin-converting-enzyme (ACE) inhibitor trandolapril on human diabetic neuropathy: randomised double-blind controlled trial. *Lancet* 1998;352:1978–1981.
145. Bakris GL, Fonseca V, Katholi RE, et al. Metabolic effects of carvedilol vs metoprolol in patients with type 2 diabetes mellitus and hypertension: a randomized controlled trial. *JAMA* 2004;292:2227–2236.
146. Stevens MJ, Obrosova I, Cao X, Van Huysen C, Greene DA. Effects of DL-a-lipoic acid on peripheral nerve conduction, blood flow, energy metabolism, and oxidative stress in experimental diabetic neuropathy. *Diabetes* 2000;49:1006–1015.
147. Cameron NE, Cotter MA, Archibald V, Dines KC, Maxfield EK. Anti-oxidant and pro-oxidant effects on nerve conduction velocity, endoneurial blood flow and oxygen tension in non-diabetic and streptozotocin-diabetic rats. *Diabetologia* 1994;37:449–459.
148. Low PA, Nickander KK. Oxygen free radical effects in sciatic nerve in experimental diabetes. *Diabetes* 1991;40:873–877.
149. Loven D, Schedl H, Wilson H, et al. Effect of insulin and oral glutathione on glutathione levels and superoxide dismutase activities in organs of rats with streptozocin- induced diabetes. *Diabetes* 1986;35:503–507.
150. Godin DV, Wohaieb SA, Garnett ME, Doumeniouk AD. Antioxidant enzyme alterations in experimental and clinical diabetes. *Mol Cell Biochem* 1988;84:223–231.
151. Bravenboer B, Kappelle AC, Hamers FP, van Buren T, Erkelens DW, Gispen WH. Potential use of glutathione for the prevention and treatment of diabetic neuropathy in the streptozotocin-induced diabetic rat. *Diabetologia* 1992;35:813–817.
152. Ward KK, Low PA, Schmelzer JD, Zochodne DW. Prostacyclin and noradrenaline in peripheral nerve of chronic experimental diabetes in rats. *Brain* 1989;112:197–208.
153. Kajstura J, Fiordaliso F, Andreoli AM, et al. IGF-1 overexpression inhibits the development of diabetic cardiomyopathy and angiotensin II-mediated oxidative stress. *Diabetes* 2001; 50:1414–1424.
154. Tesfamariam B, Cohen RA. Free radicals mediate endothelial cell dysfunction caused by elevated glucose. *Am J Physiol* 1992;263:H321–H326.
155. Ting HH, Timimi FK, Boles KS, Creager SJ, Ganz P, Creager MA. Vitamin C improves endothelium-dependent vasodilation in patients with non-insulin-dependent diabetes mellitus. *J Clin Invest* 1996;97:22–28.
156. Upritchard JE, Sutherland WH, Mann JI. Effect of supplementation with tomato juice, vitamin E, and vitamin C on LDL oxidation and products of inflammatory activity in type 2 diabetes. *Diabetes Care* 2000;23:733–738.
157. Cook SA, Sugden PH, Clerk A. Regulation of bcl-2 family proteins during development and in response to oxidative stress in cardiac myocytes: association with changes in mitochondrial membrane potential. *Circ Res* 1999;85:940–949.
158. von Harsdorf R, Li P, Dietz R. Signaling pathways in reactive oxygen species-induced cardiomyocyte apoptosis. *Circulation* 1999;99:2934–2941.
159. Bisognano JD, Weinberger HD, Bohlmeyer TJ, et al. Myocardial-directed overexpression of the human beta(1)-adrenergic receptor in transgenic mice. *J Mol Cell Cardiol* 2001;32:817–830.

160. Naveilhan P, Neveu I, Jehan F, Baudet C, Wion D, Brachet P. Reactive oxygen species influence nerve growth factor synthesis in primary rat astrocytes. *J Neurochem* 1994; 62:2178–2186.
161. Garrett NE, Malcangio M, Dewhurst M, Tomlinson DR. α-lipoic acid corrects neuropeptide deficits in diabetic rats via induction of trophic support. *NeurosciLett* 1997;222:191–194.
162. Schmid H, Forman LA, Cao X, Sherman PS, Stevens MJ. Heterogeneous cardiac sympathetic denervation and decreased myocardial nerve growth factor in streptozotocin diabetic rats: implications for cardiac sympathetic dysinnervation complicating diabetes. *Diabetes* 1999;48:603–608.
163. Obrosova IG, Fathallah L, Stevens MJ. Taurine counteracts oxidative stress and nerve growth factor deficits in early experimental diabetic neuropathy. *Exp Neurol* 2001;172: 211–219.
164. Murase K, Hattori A, Kohno M, Hayashi K. Stimulation of nerve growth factor synthesis/ secretion in mouse astroglial cells by coenzymes. *Biochem Mol Biol Int* 1993;30:615–621.
165. Ghiselli A, Serafini M, Maiani G, Azzini E, Ferro-Luzzi A. A fluorescence-based method for measuring total plasma antioxidant capability. *Free Radic Biol Med* 1995;18:29–36.
166. Ceriello A, Bortolotti N, Falleti E, et al. Total radical-trapping antioxidant parameter in NIDDM patients. *Diabetes Care* 1997;20:194–197.
167. Ziegler D, Sohr CG, Nourooz-Zadeh J. Oxidative stress and antioxidant defense in relation to the severity of diabetic polyneuropathy and cardiovascular autonomic neuropathy *Diabetes Care* 2004;27:2178–2183.
168. Stevens MJ, Feldman EL, Thomas TP, Greene DA. The pathogenesis of diabetic neuropathy, in *Clinical Management of Diabetic Neuropathy* (Veves A, Conn PMC, eds.), Humana, Totowa, NJ, 1997, pp. 13–47.
169. Obrosova IG, Van Huysen C, Fathallah L, Cao X, Greene DA, Stevens MJ. Evaluation of aldose reductase inhibitior on nerve blood flow, conduction, metabolism, and antioxidant defense in streptozotocin-diabetic rats: an intervention study. *FASEB J* 2002;16:123–125.
170. Ziegler D, Schatz H, Conrad F, et al. Effects of treatment with the antioxidant α-lipoic acid on cardiac autonomic neuropathy in NIDDM patients. A 4-month randomized controlled multicenter trial (DEKAN study). *Diabetes Care* 1997;20:369–373.
171. Ametov AS, Barinov A, Dyck PJ, et al. The sensory symptoms of diabetic polyneuropathy are improved with alpha-lipoic acid: The Sydney trial. *Diabetes Care* 2003;26:770–776.

25
Postural Hypotension and Anhidrosis

Phillip A. Low, MD

SUMMARY

Orthostatic hypotension (OH) occurs in 10–20% of patients seen in diabetic practice. Patients can be asymptomatic or manifest symptoms of cerebral hypoperfusion, such as lightheadedness or weakness, or less common symptoms of sympathetic overactivity. Syncope can occur. Symptoms correlate with autonomic deficits. Autonomic laboratory evaluation demonstrates early impairment of cardiovagal and distal postganglionic sudomotor function, eventually leading to generalized autonomic failure. Treatment of OH consists nonpharmacological and pharmacological therapy. The former involves patient education, management of salt, fluids, sleeping with head of the bed elevated, compression garments, and physical countermaneuvers. Pharmacological therapy with midodrine is efficacious but aggravates supine hypertension. Pyridostigmine will improve OH without aggravating supine hypertension although its effects are the modest. Sudomotor failure is the rule, manifests initially as distal anhidrosis followed by regional, multifocal, and other patterns of sweat loss. Sudomotor symptoms include regional hyperhidrosis and heat intolerance.

Key Words: Adrenergic; anhidrosis; baroreflex; cardiovagal; denervation; gustatory; hypovolemia; midodrine; orthostatic hypotension; vasomotor.

INTRODUCTION

Autonomic failure can occur as part of diabetic and other autonomic neuropathies. Although, cardiovagal impairment is well-recognized, sudomotor impairment occurs just as early if sensitive and quantitative tests are used to detect anhidrosis *(1)*. Manifestations of sympathetic failure include a loss of baroreflex function and loss of sweating. This chapter will focus on orthostatic hypotension (OH) and anhidrosis.

WHAT IS OH?

Consensus criteria for definition of OH is a reduction of systolic blood pressure (BP) of at least 20 mmHg or diastolic BP of at least 10 mmHg within 3 minutes after standing up *(2)*. The use of a tilt table in the head-up position at an angle of at least 60° was accepted as an alternative. The consensus conference recommended that the confounding variables of food ingestion, time of day, state of hydration, ambient temperature, recent recumbency, postural deconditioning, hypertension, medications, sex, and age be considered. OH may be symptomatic or asymptomatic. If the patient has

From: *Contemporary Diabetes: Diabetic Neuropathy: Clinical Management, Second Edition*
Edited by: A. Veves and R. Malik © Humana Press Inc., Totowa, NJ

symptoms suggestive of, but does not have documented OH, BP measurements should be repeated.

The values chosen are reasonable screening values, but are associated with 5% false-positive values. A value of 30-mmHg decrease in systolic BP would reduce the frequency of false-positive values to 1% *(3)*. Preferably, an autonomic laboratory study should be performed to confirm the presence of adrenergic failure. The clinician should further characterize OH in terms of frequency and severity of symptoms, standing time before the onset of symptoms, and presyncope and its influence on activities of daily living. Additionally, it is desirable to document whether OH is associated with supine hypertension and if there is a loss of diurnal variation in BP.

The prevalence of OH is not certainty known. For adults who have diabetes mellitus (combined type 1 and type 2 diabetes) from 1987 to 1997, 10% of patients with OH were evaluated. The mean age of the Rochester Diabetic Cohort over this decade was 60.6 ± 11.7 years.

REGULATION OF BLOOD PRESSURE

The maintenance of postural normotension without an excessive heart rate increment requires an adequate blood volume and the integration of reflex and humoral systems in several key vascular beds. These include striated muscle, splanchnic-mesenteric, and cerebrovascular beds. An adequate blood volume is essential. Hypovolemia regularly causes OH, even if vascular reflexes are intact. Hypovolemia can also be relative. Adrenergic denervation decreases vascular tone and increases vascular capacity, so that these patients are relatively hypovolemic, although plasma volume is normal. A decreased red cell mass or normocytic normochromic anemia of chronic autonomic failure aggravates OH. Correcting anemia with erythropoietin improves orthostatic intolerance *(4)*.

Vasomotor tone is controlled by two sets of baroreflexes, the arterial (or high-pressure) and venous (or low-pressure) baroreflexes. When BP falls, baroreceptors are unloaded in the carotid sinus and aortic arch *(5)*. These are arterial baroreceptors. Afferents through the IX and X cranial nerves synapse in the nucleus of the tractus solitarius. From this nucleus, a polysynaptic cardiovagal pathway travels to the nucleus ambiguus and dorsal motor nucleus of the vagus and hence, through the vagus nerve to the sinoatrial node to control heart rate. Sympathetic function is regulated by the rostroventrolateral nucleus of medulla, which projects to the intermediolateral column of the thoracic spinal cord that in turn provides sympathetic innervation to the heart and periphery (arterioles and venules) *(6)*. In addition to arterial baroreceptors, there are low-pressure baroreceptors, that respond to a decrease in central venous pressure. Cardiopulmonary receptors in the heart and lungs send mainly nonmyelinated vagal fibers to the nucleus of the tractus solitarius. The central pathways and efferents are the same as for arterial baroreceptors. Baroreflexes are often referred to as "buffer" nerves as they maintain BP constant in all positions. Baroreflex failure results in the triad of OH, supine hypertension, and loss of diurnal variation in BP. In normal subjects BP is lower at night than during the day. The converse occurs in baroreflex failure *(7)*.

The splanchnic-mesenteric capacitance bed is a large-volume, low-resistance system of great importance in the maintenance of postural normotension in humans. It constitutes 25–30% of the total blood volume *(8)*. Unlike muscle veins, splanchnic veins have an abundance of smooth muscle and a rich sympathetic innervation. The mesenteric capacitance bed is markedly responsive to both arterial and venous baroreflexes. Venoconstriction is mediated by α-adrenergic receptors *(9)*. The nerve supply to the mesenteric bed is mostly from preganglionic axon in the greater splanchnic nerve, with cell bodies in the intermediolateral column (mainly T4–T9) that synapse in the celiac ganglion from where postganglionic adrenergic fibers supply effector cells. Abnormalities in the splanchnic autonomic outflow have been found in human diabetic neuropathy, indicating that preganglionic fibers can be affected *(10)*.

Cerebral vasoregulation is important for ensuring adequate and stable flow to the brain in spite of changing systemic BP. The maintenance of constant blood flow in spite of variations in BP is termed autoregulation *(11)*. Within a mean BP range of approximately 50–150 mmHg, a change in BP produces insignificant change in cerebral perfusion. Previous studies of patients with OH demonstrated an expansion of the autoregulated range at both the upper and lower limits, so that cerebral perfusion remained relatively constant with the patient supine (when supine hypertension might be present) and in response to standing (when OH occurs) *(11–14)*.

DIABETIC OH

OH is relatively common in patients with diabetic neuropathy *(10,15,16)*, although the frequency reflects referral bias. OH was found in 43% of 16 patients *(10)* and 26% of 73 patients *(1)*. Mulder et al. *(17)* found OH in 18 of 103 unselected patients with diabetes of whom 43 had polyneuropathy. Veglio et al. *(16)* reported orthostatic intolerance in 34% of 221 patients with NIDDM patients. In some studies clinical failure is very uncommon. For instance, Young et al. *(18)* in a study of teenagers, did not find any symptoms of autonomic failure. The prevalence of symptomatic OH is less than 1% in population based studies *(19)*, but if asymptomatic OH is considered the prevalence, might be about 10% (ongoing Rochester diabetic study of PJ Dyck).

The mechanism of diabetic OH is multiplex. There is denervation of postganglionic adrenergic nerve fibers that innervate arterioles and venules that occurs as an integral part of diabetic peripheral neuropathy *(3)*. As a result, the adrenergic sympathetic component of the baroreflex arc is defective and arteriolar vasoconstriction fails to occur; and total systemic resistance fails to increment. In the Autonomic laboratory, this is manifested as an exaggerated fall in BP during the Valsalva maneuver with failure of reflex vasoconstriction (loss of late phase II and IV and delayed BP recovery). Reflex changes in heart rate fail to occur because of cardiovagal failure. An important additional mechanism is the consistent and early degeneration of sympathetic pre- and postganglionic fibers supplying the splanchnic mesenteric bed *(10,20)*. The autonomic denervation of the muscle resistance bed is also present, but in humans sustained postural normotension is more dependent on the splanchnic system, whereas innervation of skeletal muscle is important in the regulation of moment to moment adjustments *(21)*. Plasma volume, cardioacceleration, and central blood volume are normal or near-normal in diabetic OH *(20)*. Subcutaneous vasoconstrictor function is impaired *(10,20)*.

Limited information is available on recording of the splanchnic-mesenteric bed in diabetic neuropathy patients. It is possible to measure superior mesenteric artery flow using a duplex scanner *(22)*. Normal subjects undergo a two- to threefold increase in superior mesenteric flow with a meal, and splanchnic capacitance falls with tilt-up.

Patients with neurogenic OH are reported to undergo a normal increase in capacity postprandially, and hypotension develops because of failure of muscle arteriolar vasoconstriction *(23)*. Some workers have reported similar responses to tilt and a meal in diabetic neuropathy patients when compared with controls and conclude that the splanchnic bed may be less important than was assumed *(24)*. One possible explanation is that there is heterogeneity of responses in patients with diabetic neuropathy *(22)*.

CLINICAL MANIFESTATIONS OF OH

OH is manifested as a constellation of symptoms that develop on standing and dissipates on lying back down. Lightheadedness is common, but other symptoms are also very common. These include a sense of weakness, especially of the legs, and difficulty thinking clearly. Pain in the neck and trapezii (coat hanger headache) occurs in about 20% of patients. It was evaluated in a prospective study, 90 patients with symptomatic OH, 60 patients with symptoms but without laboratory confirmation of OH, and 5 patients with asymptomatic OH. Although lightheadedness is common about 50% of patients more than the age of 60 have problems of cognitive impairment on standing that clears on sitting or lying down *(25)*. Cognitive problems are typically more obvious to the companion than the patient, although not infrequently the patient will use terms like "I feel goofy," at least in Minnesota. Some patients complain of a retrocollic heaviness or headache on continued standing *(26)*. The patient may feel faint only under certain conditions. Many patients complain of weakness, especially in the legs on standing. Some patients develop ataxia when their BP falls. Aggravating symptoms need to be sought. Apart from continued standing other orthostatic stressors include exercise, environmental warming, or food ingestion. Standing time is most commonly less than 1 minute before the onset of symptoms. Indeed, an increase in standing time by 1–2 minutes results in a dramatic increase in activities of daily living. Although it is well known that patients are often worse on first awakening in the morning, the most common time of day when orthostatic intolerance is worse is not particular. It should be emphasized that, although the patients were highly symptomatic about 75% having frequent symptoms, the majority of patients do not have syncope, suggesting that these patients either have sufficient warning to avert syncope or have sufficient compensatory mechanisms to avoid syncope.

It is important to obtain an estimate of the severity and its effect on the patient's activities encountered in daily living. An orthostatic intolerance grade has been generated that grades patients by the severity of symptoms, standing time, and interference with ability to perform activities of daily living (Table 1) *(27)*. This scale was validated against comprehensive autonomic function tests in 145 patients, 97 (67%) of whom had OH. The 5-item scale demonstrated strong internal consistency (coefficient $\alpha = .91$). Patients with OH had significantly higher scores on each questionnaire item and the composite autonomic severity score (CASS) subscores than those without OH. The scale items correlated significantly with each of the CASS subscores, maximally with the CASS adrenergic subscore. Based on this evaluation, the following conclusions were made. OH is not the only cause of reduced orthostatic tolerance, and some patients may have OH, but be asymptomatic. Results of this study indicate that this 5-item questionnaire is a reliable and valid measure of the severity of symptoms of OH and that it can supplement laboratory-based measures

Table 1
Symptom Scale for Evaluation of Autonomic Symptoms

1. Frequency of orthostatic symptoms
   0. I *never or rarely* experience orthostatic symptoms when I stand up
   1. I *sometimes* experience orthostatic symptoms when I stand up
   2. I *often* experience orthostatic symptoms when I stand up
   3. I *usually* experience orthostatic symptoms when I stand up
   4. I *always* experience orthostatic symptoms when I stand up
2. Severity of orthostatic symptoms
   0. I *do not* experience orthostatic symptoms when I stand up
   1. I experience *mild* orthostatic symptoms when I stand up
   2. I experience *moderate* orthostatic symptoms when I stand up and *sometimes* have to sit down for relief
   3. I experience *severe* orthostatic symptoms when I stand up and *frequently* have to sit back down for relief
   4. I experience *severe* orthostatic symptoms when I stand up and *regularly faint* if I do not sit back down
3. Conditions under which orthostatic symptoms occur
   0. I *never or rarely* experience orthostatic symptoms under any circumstances
   1. I *sometimes* experience orthostatic symptoms under certain conditions, such as prolonged standing, a meal, exertion (e.g., walking), or when exposed to heat (e.g., hot day, hot bath, hot shower)
   2. I *often* experience orthostatic symptoms under certain conditions, such as prolonged standing, a meal, exertion (e.g., walking), or when exposed to heat (e.g., hot day, hot bath, hot shower)
   3. I *usually* experience orthostatic symptoms under certain conditions, such as prolonged standing, a meal, exertion (e.g., walking), or when exposed to heat (e.g., hot day, hot bath, hot shower)
   4. I *always* experience orthostatic symptoms when I stand up; the specific conditions do not matter
4. Activities of daily living
   0. My orthostatic symptoms *do not interfere* with activities of daily living (e.g., work, chores, dressing, bathing)
   1. My orthostatic symptoms *mildly interfere* with activities of daily living (e.g., work, chores, dressing, bathing)
   2. My orthostatic symptoms *moderately interfere* with activities of daily living (e.g., work, chores, dressing, bathing)
   3. My orthostatic symptoms *severely interfere* with activities of daily living (e.g., work, chores, dressing, bathing)
   4. My orthostatic symptoms *severely interfere* with activities of daily living (e.g., work, chores, dressing, bathing). *I am bed or wheelchair bound because of my symptoms.*
5. Standing time
   0. On most occasions, I can stand as long as necessary without experiencing orthostatic symptoms
   1. On most occasions, I can stand *more than 15 minutes* before experiencing orthostatic symptoms
   2. On most occasions, I can stand *5–14 minutes* before experiencing orthostatic symptoms
   3. On most occasions, I can stand *1–4 minutes* before experiencing orthostatic symptoms
   4. On most occasions, I can stand *less than 1 minute* before experiencing orthostatic symptoms

Table 2
Studies for the Patient With Suspected OH

1. Autonomic reflex screen
   - Quantitative sudomotor axon reflex test
   - Tests of cardiovagal function
   - Beat-to-beat BP responses to the Valsalva maneuver
   - BP and heart rate response to HUT
2. Thermoregulatory sweat test
3. Plasma catecholamines—supine/standing
4. 24-hour urinary sodium excretion

to provide a rapid, more complete clinical assessment. This questionnaire would also be useful as a brief screening device for orthostatic intolerance to aid physicians in identifying patients who may have OH.

LABORATORY EVALUATION

The patient with OH should be subjected to a full autonomic evaluation in order to determine the severity and distribution of autonomic failure. The recommended panel is shown in Table 2. The autonomic reflex screen evaluates the severity and distribution of postganglionic sudomotor, cardiovagal, and adrenergic failure. The thermoregulatory sweat test is a useful test in diabetic autonomic neuropathy, as the sweat loss has a number of different patterns *(10,28)*. These can be multifocal, distal, regional, or generalized.

In the evaluation of adrenergic function, the beat-to-beat BP (BP_BB) responses to the Valsalva maneuver and to HUT are the most sensitive and useful tests. There are four main phases in the Valsalva maneuver *(29–31)*. In phase I, there is a transient rise in BP because of increased intrathoracic and intra-abdominal pressure causing mechanical compression of the aorta *(32)*. In early phase II (phase II_E), the reduced preload (venous return) *(33)* and reduced stroke volume *(34)* lead to a fall in cardiac output in spite of tachycardia caused by a withdrawal of cardiovagal influence. Total peripheral resistance increases as a result of efferent sympathetic discharge to muscle *(35)* and within 4 seconds after the increase in sympathetic discharge the fall in BP is arrested. This is late phase II (II_L). In normal subjects phase II_L is so efficient that by the beginning of phase III, MAP is at the resting MAP level or above. Phase III like phase I is mechanical, lasting 1 to 2 seconds during which BP falls. The major mechanism is the sudden fall in intrathoracic pressure. There is a further burst of sympathetic activity during this phase. In phase IV, venous return *(36)* and cardiac output *(34)* have returned to normal whereas the arteriolar bed remains vasoconstricted, hence the overshoot of BP above baseline values. In the clinical autonomic laboratory setting, with studies done on the patients lying supine, phase IV may be more dependent on cardiac adrenergic tone than on systemic peripheral resistance. Intravenous phentolamine 10 mg resulted in the expected elimination of late phase II, but augmented rather than blocked phase IV. In contrast, 10 mg intravenous propranolol completely blocked phase IV *(30)*. The use of the phases of the Valsalva maneuver to evaluate adrenergic function has been validated in using pharmacological dissection *(30)* and by studying its effect on normal subjects and patients with different severities of autonomic failure a CASS has been generated

Table 3
Nonpharmacological Management of OH

1. Patient education
2. Raise head of bed 4 inches
3. Increase salt and fluid intake
4. Compression of capacitance bed with compression garments
5. Physical countermaneuvers to raise orthostatic BP
6. Water bolus therapy

that corrects the confounding effects of age and gender *(37)*. The most reliable phases of the maneuver are late phase II and IV. More recently, it has been demonstrated that BP recovery time defined as the duration from phase III to baseline may be a better index *(38)*. It is free of the limitations of late phase II that is lost with even moderate autonomic failure.

Orthostatic BP recordings to tilt are recorded using BP_BB and with a sphygmomanometer cuff with the patient supine and following tilt to 70° using an automated tilt-table. Cuff recordings are obtained at 1 and 5 minutes after tilt up. It is important to perform the upright tilt procedure at a standard time after lying down because the orthostatic reduction in BP is higher following 20 minutes of preceding rest as compared with 1 minute. During upright tilt, normal individuals undergo a transient reduction in systolic, mean, and diastolic BP followed by recovery within 1 minute. The decrement is modest (<10 mmHg, mean BP). Normative data, based on 270 normal subjects aged 10–83 years have been obtained *(3)*. Patients with adrenergic failure have a marked and progressive reduction in BP and pulse pressure. The heart rate response is typically attenuated, but in patients whose cardiac adrenergic innervation is spared, heart rate response is intact and may be increased.

TREATMENT OF OH

The goal of treatment is to improve standing BP, minimize symptoms, and improve orthostatic quality of life without causing excessive supine hypertension. In this chapter, nonpharmacological and pharmacological approaches to therapy will be covered. OH and supine hypertension that occurs under specific conditions will also be addressed.

NONPHARMACOLOGICAL TREATMENT OF OH

Nonpharmacological approaches are extremely important (Table 3).

Patient Education

Patient education is extremely important. The patient should understand in simple terms the maintenance of postural normotension. They need to understand the orthostatic stressors and their mechanisms. Important items of education include the following.

1. Advice on handling early morning and postprandial worsening of OH.
2. Instructions on how to keep a BP log. The patient or caregiver should learn to use an automated sphygmomanometer to measure BP with the patient supine and after standing for 1 minute. It is helpful to the physician if, for 2 or 3 days before a visit, recordings have been

taken and recorded on awakening, after a meal, during a time of maximal orthostatic tolerance, during a time of poor orthostatic tolerance, and before and 1 hour after medication.

3. Salt and volume expansion. All patients with neurogenic OH require generous fluid intake of five to eight 8-ounce glasses of fluid each day. Salt supplementation is essential. Most patients manage with added salt with their meals. Occasionally, patients prefer to use salt tablets (available as 0.5 g tablets). Adequate salt and fluid intake can be verified by checking the 24-hour urinary volume and concentration of sodium. Patients who have a value less than 170 mmol/24 hours can be given supplemental sodium, 1–2 g three times daily *(39)*. Their weight, symptoms, and urinary concentration of sodium should be checked 1 or 2 weeks later.
4. Oral water bolus. The imbibing of a moderate volume of water results in a reduction in OH that lasts for about 2 hours. In a recent study, rapid water drinking (480 mL) increased BP by a mean of over 30 mmHg in patients with multiple system atrophy and pure autonomic failure *(40)*. The pressor response was evident within 5 minutes after drinking started, reached a maximum after 30–35 minutes, and was sustained for 1–2 hours. The practical application of this observation is that the patient who needs to be subjected to sustained orthostatic stress should drink two 8-ounce glasses of water 10–20 minutes before such activity.
5. Raise head of bed. The head of the bed is elevated four inches for two reasons. First, it reduces nocturia, probably by stimulating renin release. Second, it reduces supine hypertension. During the day, it is important to maintain adequate orthostatic stress. If patients are tilted up repeatedly, OH gradually attenuates. This likely result from the release of renin and arginine vasopressin, which requires more sustained or repetitive orthostatic stress. Another mechanism that has been suggested is extravasated plasma around veins providing a vascular cuff, increasing venomotor tone.
6. Compression garments. For some patients, wearing a tightly fitting body stocking ameliorates OH and associated symptoms. These stockings have to be well-fitted and put on before arising. They work by reducing the venous capacitance bed. Their disadvantages are the cumbersome application and discomfort in hot weather. Calf compression alone confers minimal benefit, but a reasonable substitute to Jobst compression is the use of a tightly fitting abdominal binder, which confers about two-thirds of the benefit *(41)*.
7. Physical countermaneuvers. Physical counter-maneuvers that involve the contraction of certain muscle groups of the lower extremities decrease venous capacitance and increase venous return *(42)*. These maneuvers, which once learned can substantially prolong standing time, include crossing of the legs and contracting the leg muscles of one leg against the other, slow stepping or marching on the spot, propping the leg up on a chair, or contraction of the thigh muscles *(43)*.

PHARMACOLOGICAL MANAGEMENT

Drug treatment is an important part of the overall therapeutic regimen and, if used well, greatly enhances BP control *(44)*. The main drugs are midodrine, pyridostigmine, and possibly fludrocortisone.

Midodrine

The optimal approach, with the availability of midodrine, is to expand plasma volume modestly with increased salt and fluid intake without aggravating supine hypertension and to add midodrine during the waking period to reduce OH. The safest approach to volume expansion is oral salt supplementation. The best guide to adequate salt intake is the 24-hour urinary sodium. The patient has a normal plasma volume and adequate salt intake if the 24-hour urine sodium is at or slightly exceeds 170 mequivalents per 24 hours. Patients who achieve this excretion have normal measured plasma volumes *(39)*. To ensure adequate fluid intake, it is optimal to aim for a volume of 1500–2500 mL in 24 hours.

Midodrine is a directly acting α-agonist *(45)*. The minimal effective dose of midodrine is 5 mg. Most patients respond best to 10 mg. The duration of action is between 2 and 4 hours, corresponding to the blood levels of midodrine and its active metabolite desglymidodrine *(46)*. The onset of action is between 30 minutes and 1 hour. In some patients, the duration of action of midodrine is short, less than 4 hours. Because one of the mechanisms of hypertensive swings is severe hypotension, it is best to increase the frequency of dosing to every 3 hours during the period of maximal orthostatic stress. Patients should generally avoid midodrine after 6 PM so as not to aggravate supine nocturnal hypertension. The main limiting factor is the worsening of supine BP. The drug dose-dependently increases both supine and standing BP *(46)*.

Pyridostigmine

As baroreflex activity is modest with the patient supine and increases proportional to orthostatic stress, a novel approach in treatment is to enhance ganglionic transmission (through autonomic ganglia) by acetylcholinesterase inhibition *(47)*. Pyridostigmine has minimal effect on supine BP, but improves standing BP (by enhancing standing baroreflex-mediated vasoconstriction). It functions as a smart drug, improving OH without aggravating supine hypertension (Fig. 1). The preferred dose is 180 mg per day as the time span. To minimize cholinergic side effect, the drug can be started as 30 mg morning and noon and slowly increased.

Fludrocortisone

For patients who cannot take enough salt or who do not have an adequate response to midodrine, fludrocortisone, 0.1 mg once or twice daily, can be added to provide volume expansion and to sensitize vascular smooth muscle. This approach of reducing dependence on fludrocortisone and avoiding nocturnal midodrine substantially reduces supine hypertension. Uncommonly, the dose of fludrocortisone may be increased to 0.4 or 0.6 mg daily for patients with refractory OH. Because the regulatory reflexes are greatly impaired, it is necessary to overexpand the plasma volume slightly in these patients. A reasonable clue for adequate volume expansion is a weight gain of 3–5 pounds. Mild dependent edema is to be expected. The potential risks are congestive heart failure and excessive supine hypertension. Two weeks after starting treatment with fludrocortisone, patients should have their BP checked while supine and standing.

TREATMENT FOR PERIODS OF ORTHOSTATIC DECOMPENSATION

Patients who have restricted autonomic neuropathy and associated postural tachycardia have periods of orthostatic decompensation. Patients with generalized autonomic failure also have episodes of apparent decompensation when they have greater OH or less response to pressor agents. These patients need to be evaluated for a cause of decompensation. The causes include fluid deficit, hypokalemia, anemia, deconditioning related to a recent period of recumbency, and another illness (including pump [cardiac]

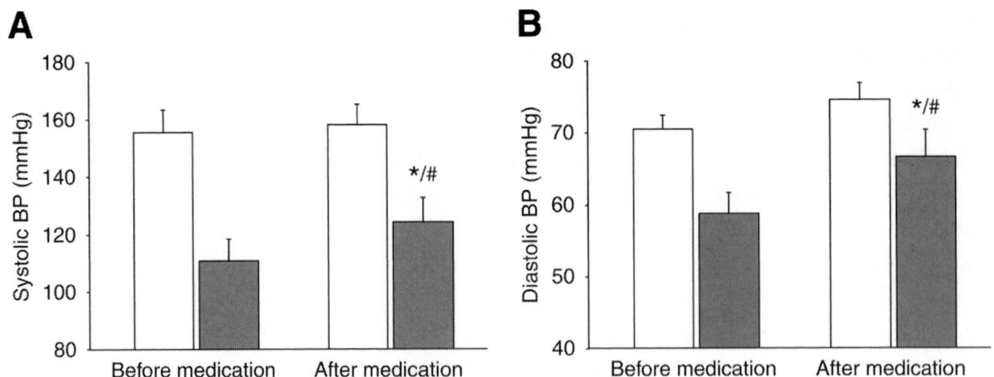

Fig. 1. Systolic **(A)** and diastolic **(B)** blood pressure in the supine position (light bars) and during head-up tilt (dark bars) before and after medication. * = significant difference ($p < 0.05$) comparing parameters for the same body position before and after medication, # = significant difference ($p < 0.05$) comparing position-induced changes before and after medication.

failure). Often, however, no cause is found. The patient appears to respond to management with volume expansion. The first approach is the "bouillon treatment." The patient makes one of these extremely salty soups and drinks about five 8-ounce servings in half a day. An alternative is supplemental sodium chloride, 2 g three times daily, and a minimum of eight 8-ounce servings of fluids daily for 2 days. If the patient does not have improvement with this regimen or reports that fluid is not being retained, desmopressin, one puff each nostril at bedtime, is taken for 1 week. The dose of vasoconstrictor can be adjusted upward. This is when a tight-fitting body stocking (e.g., Jobst) can be beneficial. Fludrocortisone, 0.2 mg three times daily, can be taken for 1 week. The drug is traditionally considered to be slowly cumulative in its action; however, recent studies have suggested that it also has a rapid mode of action. If all these measures are unsuccessful, the treatment is isotonic saline, 1–2 L, given intravenously.

HOSPITAL MANAGEMENT OF SEVERE OH

Some patients with severe OH need acute hospital management. In addition to a search for the cause of OH and specific treatment, management is aimed at improving orthostatic tolerance to the degree that subsequent management can be continued on an outpatient basis. A regimen of treatment extending for approximately 3 days is suggested. These patients are volume-depleted, either absolutely or relatively (because of increased capacity as a result of denervation). Intravenous infusion of 1–2 L of isotonic saline is needed to expand plasma volume. Early volume expansion is critically important because hypovolemia greatly reduces the effectiveness of vasoconstrictors in increasing BP, markedly affecting the sensitivity of cardiopulmonary, but not carotid-cardiac baroreflex responses to α-agonists *(48)*. In elderly patients, care needs to be exercised to avoid heart failure. Postural training is needed. The head of the bed is elevated 4 inches or at an angle of 10–30°. The patient spends an increasing period of time seated and standing. Treatment with fludrocortisone, 0.2 mg per day, is commenced, as is sodium chloride, 1 g three times daily, and high fluid intake. During this time, the patient is educated about dietary salt content, maintenance of postural normotension, physical countermaneuvers, management of periods of increased orthostatic stress, and supine hypertension. Blood pressure is measured with the patient supine and standing 1 minute before and 1 hour after 10 mg of midodrine, and the supine and standing values are recorded hourly to establish the optimal dose and duration of action.

TREATMENT OF EARLY MORNING OH

The most common time of day that OH is worse is on awakening. In some patients, this occurs because of excessive nocturia. For many patients, the situation is improved by sleeping with the head of the bed elevated (reducing nocturia). A common routine is to drink two cups of strong coffee (250 mg caffeine), to take vasoconstrictors, and to read the newspaper before getting up.

TREATMENT OF POSTPRANDIAL OH

Patients often have postprandial accentuation of OH. This can occur with any type of neurogenic OH, but is particularly common with diabetic autonomic neuropathy. It often occurs on the background of gastrointestinal autonomic neuropathy, highlighting the great importance of the splanchnic-mesenteric bed in orthostatic BP control. This is a large-volume (20–30% of total blood volume) capacitance bed that, unlike other venous beds, is exquisitely baroreflex responsive. Some patients with mild postprandial OH discover that the worsening can be reduced by frequent small meals, and some find that certain foods are most troublesome and should be avoided. Some patients report that hot drinks or hot food need to be avoided. Carbohydrates are especially troublesome. Ibuprofen, 400–800 mg, or indomethacin, 25–50 mg, with the meal is well-tolerated and should be tried. The next step is the administration of a vasoconstrictor such as midodrine, 10 mg. A problem with vasoconstrictors is the aggravation of gastroparesis. Rarely, symptoms suggestive of gut ischemia may occur. If all the approaches are inadequate, the somatostatin analog octreotide can be administered with the meal. The dose is 25 μg by subcutaneous injection. The dose can be increased if necessary to 100–200 μg. This is the most efficacious agent but requires parenteral administration.

TREATMENT OF NOCTURNAL HYPERTENSION

Normal subjects have a diurnal variation in BP, with lower nocturnal BP. Patients with neurogenic OH have nocturnal hypertension. To minimize the problems of nocturnal hypertension, pressor medications should not be taken after 6 PM. The head of the bed should be elevated, resulting in lower intracranial BP. A nighttime snack with a glass of fluids (not coffee or tea) results in some postprandial hypotension, and can be used to increase fluid intake and decrease nocturnal hypertension. Patients who enjoy a glass of wine should drink it at this time for its vasodilator effect. Occasionally, it is not possible to control OH without marked nocturnal hypertension. For these patients, hydralazine (Apresoline), 25 mg, can be given at night. Because this drug has sodium-retaining properties, it is especially suitable. Alternatives include the angiotensin-converting enzyme inhibitor nifedipine (Procardia), 10 mg, or a nitroglycerin patch.

ERYTHROPOIETIN

Mild-to-moderate normocytic, normochromic anemia is not uncommon. After it has been determined that iron stores are adequate, the patient can be given erythropoietin. The anemia may be because of renal denervation, resulting in a decrease in renin. A typical dose of erythropoietin, administered subcutaneously three times weekly, is 50 U/kg until reticulocytosis and an increase in the hematocrit occur *(4,49)*. The duration of treatment is 3–10 weeks.

DIABETIC SUDOMOTOR DISORDERS

Sudomotor Symptoms

Sudomotor symptoms are common, but do not usually command much attention. Initially, there may be hyperhidrosis of the feet associated with coldness (I can't keep my feet warm). This is followed by anhidrosis and vasomotor alterations, which can be variable, with venous congestion and a purple discoloration being common. Some patients will have alternating warming and cooling. Infrequently, widespread anhidrosis results in heat intolerance. In these patients, a high ambient temperature and sustained physical exertion results in overheating. In most patients, the diabetic state results in a significant impairment in exercise capacity, and heat intolerance does not develop.

Gustatory sweating commonly occurs in diabetics with cervical sympathetic denervation. The patient has excessive facial sweating in response to food, especially spicy food. The suggested mechanism is denervation of postganglionic sudomotor fibers with faulty reinnervation, although some evidence suggests a more dynamic metabolic mechanism and an association with nephropathy.

Sudomotor Failure

Sudomotor deficits are very common if quantitative approaches are used to detect autonomic sudomotor impairment. It is important to detect the severity and distribution of sudomotor deficit. The most commonly used tests to evaluate sudomotor function are as follows:

1. Quantitative Sudomotor Axon Reflex Test (QSART).
2. Thermoregulatory sweat test.
3. Sympathetic skin response (SSR).
4. Skin biopsy.

QSART

QSART evaluates postganglionic sudomotor function. It probably evaluates the distal ends of the postganglionic axon *(50)*. The test is quantitative, reproducible, and noninvasive with a coefficient of variation of 8% *(51)*. QSWEAT is the commercial counterpart, modeled after the Mayo Clinic system.

The neural pathway consists of an axon "reflex" mediated by the postganglionic sympathetic sudomotor axon. The axon terminal is activated by acetylcholine. The impulse travels antidromically, reaches a branch-point, then orthodromically to release acetylcholine from nerve terminal. Acetylcholine traverses the neuroglandular junction and binds to M3 muscarinic receptors on eccrine sweat glands to evoke the sweat response *(52)*. Acetylcholinesterase in subcutaneous tissue cleaves acetylcholine to acetate and choline, resulting in its inactivation and cessation of the sweat response. The test is usually done on one arm and three lead sites *(37)*.

QSART recordings have been performed in many neuropathies including diabetic neuropathy *(1)*. Distal sympathetic and vagal function were measured in 73 consecutive patients with diabetic neuropathy seen at the Mayo Autonomic Reflex Laboratory. Postganglionic sympathetic failure measured proximally within the foot occurred as commonly as vagal failure (58 and 55%, respectively) and occurred much more frequently than did OH (26%). This study found that distal sympathetic sudomotor failure and vagal failure occur with equal frequency when sensitive and quantitative recording methods are used. This pattern of distal sudomotor loss is the most common pattern seen in diabetes. It is often associated with the burning feet syndrome in diabetes and idiopathic neuropathies *(53)*. There is a progressive loss of sweating with increasing duration and severity of neuropathy. Early on, there can be an exaggerated forearm (proximal) volume response *(54)*.

QSART sweating is cholinergic. Of interest is that, during development sweating is under adrenergic control, with an adrenergic to cholinergic switch occurring, so that, in postnatal humans only 20% of sweating is under adrenergic control. There is some evidence that in neuropathic pain states, there may be a reversion back to predominantly adrenergic sweating *(55)*. Whether that occurs in diabetic distal small fiber neuropathy is not known.

Thermoregulatory Sweat Test

The thermoregulatory sweat test (TST) is a sensitive qualitative test of sudomotor function that provides important information on the pattern and distribution of sweat loss. The presence of sweating causes a change in the indicator from brown to a violet color. The subject is heated in a sweat cabinet *(10,28)*. The value of the test can be enhanced and rendered semiquantitative by measuring the percent of anterior body surface anhidrosis *(56)*.

Certain sweat patterns are recognizable in human diabetic neuropathy *(28)*. Of 51 patients suspected of having neuropathy on the basis of a clinical examination, 48 (94%) had unequivocal abnormalities on the TST. Pathological loss of sweating occurred distally in 65%, segmentally in 25%, and only in isolated dermatomes in 25%; 78% of patients had a combination of two or more patterns. Global anhidrosis was noted in eight patients (16%), all of whom had profound autonomic neuropathy, and in the entire group, the percentage of body surface anhidrosis correlated with the degree of clinical dysautonomia (rank correlation coefficient = 0.77; $p < 0.01$). Major advantages of the method are its simplicity, sensitivity, the ability to recognize patterns of anhidrosis, including mixed patterns, and its semiquantitative nature. The disadvantages are its inability to distinguish between postganglionic, preganglionic, and central lesions, the discomfort, the qualitative nature of the information obtained, and the staining of clothing.

SSR

Skin potential recordings can be used to detect sympathetic sudomotor deficit in the peripheral neuropathies and central autonomic disorders *(57,58)*. The recording electrodes are commonly electrode pairs 1 cm in diameter applied to the dorsal and ventral surfaces of the foot, the hand, or thigh. The stimulus might be an inspiratory gasp, a cough, a loud noise, or an electric shock. The sources of the skin potential are the sweat gland and the epidermis *(59)*. A reasonable interpretation of studies in mammals, including humans, is that a component of the skin potential (early fast changes) is related to sweating, but that the later changes are because of skin potential changes. The latter can occur in patients who have congenital absence of sweat glands *(60–63)*. The major advantage of the method is its simplicity so that it can be used in any electromyography (EMG) lab. The disadvantages are its enormous variability and the tendency of the responses to habituate, although claims for low coefficient of variation have appeared, and attempts have been made to reduce variability by using magnetic stimulation *(64)*. The responses vary with the recording system, composition of the electrolyte paste, stimulus frequency, age, temperature, stress, status of central structures, and the effects of hormones and drugs *(65)*. Following peripheral nerve section, skin potentials are no longer obtainable in the affected dermatome on direct and reflex stimulations. There was usually associated hypothermia and anhidrosis. Following sympathectomy, skin potentials are also lost, but only temporarily, returning in 4–6 months *(66)*.

Skin potential recordings to detect sympathetic sudomotor deficit in the peripheral neuropathies and central autonomic deficits have been popularized *(58)*. There is general agreement that a loss of SSR is abnormal. There is some controversy concerning whether a reduction of skin potential and a change in latency are reliable abnormalities *(67)*. There is some evidence that unmyelinated fibers conduct without slowing or not at all *(68)*. The test has been reported to correlate well with QSART *(69)*, but in our experience is often present when QSART is clearly impaired. Potentials are reported to become reduced with aging *(70)*.

SSR has been utilized in the evaluation of the peripheral neuropathies, especially diabetic neuropathy *(71,72)*. The SSR deficit in amplitude and volume is reported to worsen with increasing duration of diabetes and correlates with sweatspot values *(64)* and clinical neuropathy *(73)*. Both amplitude reduction and latency prolongation were seen and abnormalities may precede clinical neuropathy *(73)*. In patients with well-established neuropathy, SSR in the foot is abnormal or absent in the majority of patients *(72,74)*. For instance, in a study of 72 patients with diabetes with electrophysiologically confirmed sensorimotor peripheral neuropathy, SSR was absent in 83%. Statistically significant correlation was found between the Valsalva test abnormality, the degree of peripheral neuropathy, and the SSR *(74)*. Its sensitivity and specificity to detect early abnormalities or improvement in clinical trials have not been established.

GUSTATORY SWEATING

Gustatory sweating was first linked to diabetes mellitus by Watkins *(75)*, and is now known to occur quite commonly in patients with either diabetic nephropathy or neuropathy *(76)*. The syndrome consists of localized hyperhidrosis of the face during meals. The mechanism of gustatory sweating is not proven, but is considered to be because of sympathetic postganglionic denervation followed by aberrant reinnervation by parasympathetic fibers. It is suggested that sympathetic cholinergic fibers to eccrine sweat gland are lesioned. These denervated sweat glands are thought to become reinnervated by misdirected cholinergic parasympathetic fibers. Evidence cited usually emanate from surgical lesions *(77)*. In diabetic autonomic neuropathy, the sympathetic denervation that occurs in sweat glands might be compensated by reinnervation of aberrant parasympathetic fibers stemming from the minor petrous nerve, and normally innervating the parotid gland through the auriculotemporal and facial nerve, after being relayed in the otic ganglion *(78)*. Thus, sweating occurs in the reinnervated area when salivation is induced on cholinergic stimulation (food ingestion).

The symptom can be troublesome and embarrassing. Occasionally it affects food intake to the degree that it could make glycemic control difficult. As sweating is controlled by sympathetic cholinergic pathways, treatment has traditionally involved oral anticholinergic drugs, but the acceptability of these to patients is low because of systemic side effects. Topical antimuscarinic agents, such as glycopyrrolate, have been demonstrated to be effective in controlling gustatory sweating caused by parotid surgery and in diabetic gustatory sweating *(79,80)*. Gustatory sweating and flushing within and surrounding the cutaneous distribution of the auriculotemporal nerve (Frey's syndrome), can develop after surgery or trauma to parotid gland. Surgery as resection of the glossopharyngeal nerve (which supplies the otic ganglion and hence the auriculotemporal and buccal nerves with parasympathetic fibers) abolishes the syndrome *(81,82)*. A better approach is the injection of botulinum toxin into the symptomatic skin to treat pathological gustatory sweating *(83,84)*. This obviously is a major advance in treatment because it is far simpler and less invasive than sectioning parasympathetic nerves intracranially *(85)*. Botulinum toxin enters cholinergic neuron terminals and prevents the exocytotic release of acetylcholine. As parasympathetic secretomotor fibers use acetylcholine as a neurotransmitter, and sweat glands have cholinergic muscarinic receptors, botulinum toxin abolishes the cholinergic activation of sympathetically-denervated sweat glands during salivation.

PATTERNS OF ANHIDROSIS IN DIABETIC NEUROPATHY

There are a number of patterns of anhidrosis in diabetic neuropathy. A full appreciation of these patterns requires the administration of the thermoregulatory sweat test, a method that is not under widespread clinical use. Several well characterized patterns are described.

Distal Small Fiber Neuropathy

Perhaps, the most common pattern of anhidrosis is distal anhidrosis. The "burning feet" syndrome is perhaps the most common presentation of diabetic neuropathy. These patients have distal involvement with burning, prickling, and some stabbing discomfort with variable allodynia, and most have normal motor function. There is a subset of patients with completely normal motor function, intact tendon reflexes, and nerve conduction studies that are normal or near-normal. For this pattern of neuropathy, the underlying neuropathy has been assumed to be a length-dependent distal small fiber neuropathy demonstrable on skin biopsy *(86)*. Autonomic fibers are presumed to be involved as well because these patients will usually have vasomotor symptoms, manifest as excessive coldness, discoloration, or sometimes erythromelalgia *(53,87)*. Hyper- and hypohidrosis can also be a feature. When sudomotor testing is used, approximately 80% of patients have abnormal QSART responses *(53,88)*. There is good agreement between loss of intraepidermal fibers (somatic C fiber involvement) and QSART loss (autonomic C fiber involvement) *(89)*.

Multifocal Sweating Loss

A common and characteristic pattern of anhidrosis in diabetic neuropathy is that of multifocal regions of sweat loss *(10,28)*, which differs in distribution to other neuropathies *(10)*. These patients have anhidrosis that affects parts of the body in the distribution of specific nerve trunks, plexus, or regions in the distribution of autonomic ganglia. The value of this test is that this pattern of loss reduces the number of likely causes. Apart from diabetes, this pattern is seen with autoimmune autonomic neuropathy and angiopathic neuropathy (although regional anhidrosis is usually not seen in this group of neuropathies).

Generalized Anhidrosis

An unusual pattern of anhidrosis is that of generalized anhidrosis, where there is total or subtotal anhidrosis (>70%). This pattern is seen in diabetic neuropathy, autoimmune autonomic neuropathy, chronic idiopathic anhidrosis, pure autonomic failure, and multiple system atrophy. In diabetes, percent anhidrosis provides one index of autonomic failure.

REFERENCES

1. Low PA, Zimmerman BR, Dyck PJ. Comparison of distal sympathetic with vagal function in diabetic neuropathy. *Muscle Nerve* 1986;9:592–596.
2. Anonymous. Consensus statement on the definition of orthostatic hypotension, pure autonomic failure, and multiple system atrophy. The Consensus Committee of the American Autonomic Society and the American Academy of Neurology. *Neurology* 1996;46:1470.
3. Low PA, Denq JC, Opfer-Gehrking TL, Dyck PJ, O'Brien PC, Slezak JM. Effect of age and gender on sudomotor and cardiovagal function and blood pressure response to tilt in normal subjects. *Muscle Nerve* 1997;20:1561–1568.
4. Hoeldtke RD, Streeten DH. Treatment of orthostatic hypotension with erythropoietin. *N Engl J Med* 1993;329:611–615.
5. Korner PI, West MJ, Shaw J, Uther JB. "Steady-state" properties of the baroreceptor-heart rate reflex in essential hypertension in man. *Clin Exp Pharmacol Physiol* 1974;1:65–76.
6. Joyner MJ, Shepherd JT. Autonomic regulation of circulation, in *Clinical Autonomic Disorders: Evaluation and Management* (Low PA, ed.), Lippincott-Raven, Philadelphia, 1997, pp. 61–71.
7. Carvalho MJ, van Den Meiracker AH, Boomsma F, et al. Diurnal blood pressure variation in progressive autonomic failure. *Hypertension* 2000;35:892–897.
8. Rowell LB. Regulation of splanchnic blood flow in man. *Physiologist* 1973;16:127–142.
9. Thirlwell MP, Zsoter TT. The effect of propranolol and atropine on venomotor reflexes in man. Venous reflexes—effect of propranolol and atropine. *J Med* 1972;3:65–72.
10. Low PA, Walsh JC, Huang CY, McLeod JG. The sympathetic nervous system in alcoholic neuropathy. A clinical and pathological study. *Brain* 1975;98:357–364.
11. Novak V, Novak P, Spies JM, Low PA. Autoregulation of cerebral blood flow in orthostatic hypotension. *Stroke* 1998;29:104–111.
12. Depresseux JC, Rousseau JJ, Franck G. The autoregulation of cerebral blood flow, the cerebrovascular reactivity and their interaction in the Shy-Drager syndrome. *Eur Neurol* 1979;18:295–301.
13. Brooks DJ, Redmond S, Mathias CJ, Bannister R, Symon L. The effect of orthostatic hypotension on cerebral blood flow and middle cerebral artery velocity in autonomic failure, with observations on the action of ephedrine. *J Neurol Neurosurg Psychiatry* 1989;52:962–966.
14. Novak V, Gordon V, Novak P, LowPA. Altered cerebral autoregulation in patients with orthostatic hypotension. *Neurology* 1997;48:A131.
15. Rundles RW. Diabetic neuropathy. General review with report of 125 cases. *Medicine* 1945;24:111–160.
16. Veglio M, Carpano-Maglioli P, Tonda L, et al. Autonomic neuropathy in non-insulin-dependent diabetic patients: correlation with age, sex, duration and metabolic control of diabetes. *Diabete Metab* 1990;16:200–206.

17. Mulder DW, Lambert EH, Bastron JA, Sprague RG. The neuropathies associated with diabetes mellitus: a clinical and electromyographic study of 103 unselected diabetic patients. *Neurology* 1961;11:275–284.
18. Young RJ, Ewing DJ, Clarke BF. Nerve function and metabolic control in teenage diabetics. *Diabetes* 1983;32:142–147.
19. Palumbo PJ, Elveback LR, Whisnant JP. Neurologic complications of diabetes mellitus: transient ischemic attack, stroke, and peripheral neuropathy. *Adv Neurol* 1978;19:593–601.
20. Hilsted J, Parving HH, Christensen NJ, Benn J, Galbo H. Hemodynamics in diabetic orthostatic hypotension. *J Clin Invest* 1981;68:1427–1434.
21. Mancia G, Grassi G, Ferrari A, Zanchetti A. Reflex cardiovascular regulation in humans. *J Cardiovasc Pharmacol* 1985;7:S152–S159.
22. Fujimura J, Camilleri M, Low PA, Novak V, Novak P, Opfer-Gehrking TL. Effect of perturbations and a meal on superior mesenteric artery flow in patients with orthostatic hypotension. *J Auton Nerv Syst* 1997;67:15–23.
23. Kooner JS, Raimbach S, Watson L, Bannister R, Peart S, Mathias CJ. Relationship between splanchnic vasodilation and postprandial hypotension in patients with primary autonomic failure. *J Hypertens Suppl* 1989;7:S40–S41.
24. Purewal TS, Goss DE, Zanone MM, Edmonds ME, Watkins PJ. The splanchnic circulation and postural hypotension in diabetic autonomic neuropathy. *Diabetes Med* 1995;12:513–522.
25. Low PA, Opfer-Gehrking TL, McPhee BR. Prospective evaluation of clinical characteristics of orthostatic hypotension. *Mayo Clin Proc* 1995;70:617–622.
26. Robertson D, Kincaid DW, Robertson RM. The head and neck discomfort of autonomic failure: an unrecognized etiology of headache. *Clin Auton Res* 1994;4:99–103.
27. Schrezenmaier C, Gehrking JA, Hines SM, Low PA, Benrud-larson LM, Sandroni P. Evaluation of orthostatic hypotension: relationship of a new self-report instrument to laboratory-based measures. *Mayo Clin Proc* 2005;80:330–334.
28. Fealey RD, Low PA, Thomas JE. Thermoregulatory sweating abnormalities in diabetes mellitus. *Mayo Clin Proc* 1989;64:617–628.
29. Benarroch EE, Opfer-Gehrking TL, Low PA. Use of the photoplethysmographic technique to analyze the Valsalva maneuver in normal man. *Muscle Nerve* 1991;14:1165–1172.
30. Sandroni P, Benarroch EE, Low PA. Pharmacological dissection of components of the Valsalva maneuver in adrenergic failure. *J Appl Physiol* 1991;71:1563–1567.
31. Sandroni P, Novak V, Opfer-Gehrking TL, Huck CA, Low PA. Mechanisms of blood pressure alterations in response to the Valsalva maneuver in postural tachycardia syndrome. *Clin Auton Res* 2000;10:1–5.
32. Corbett JL, Frankel HL, Harris PJ. Cardiovascular changes associated with skeletal muscle spasm in tetraplegic man. *J Physiol* 1971;215:381–393.
33. Candel S, Ehrlich DE. Venous blood flow during the Valsalva experiment including some clinical applications. *Am J Med* 1953;15:307–315.
34. Brooker JZ, Alderman EL, Harrison DC. Alterations in left ventricular volumes induced by Valsalva manoeuvre. *Br Heart J* 1974;36:713–718.
35. Delius W, Hagbarth KE, Hongell A, Wallin BG. Manoeuvres affecting sympathetic outflow in human muscle nerves. *Acta Physiol Scand* 1972;84:82–94.
36. Wexler L, Bergel DH, Gabe IT, Makin GS, Mills CJ. Velocity of blood flow in normal human venae cavae. *Circ Res* 1968;23:349–359.
37. Low PA. Composite autonomic scoring scale for laboratory quantification of generalized autonomic failure. *Mayo Clin Proc* 1993;68:748–752.
38. Vogel ER, Sandroni P, Low PA. Blood pressure recovery from Valsalva maneuver in patients with autonomic failure. *Neurology* 2005;65:1517.
39. El-Sayed H, Hainsworth R. Salt supplementation increases plasma volume and orthostatic tolerance in patients with unexplained syncope. *Heart* 1996;75:134–140.

40. Jordan J, Shannon JR, Black BK, et al. The pressor response to water drinking in humans: a sympathetic reflex? *Circulation* 2000;101:504–509.
41. Denq JC, Opfer-Gehrking TL, Giuliani M, Felten J, Convertino VA, Low PA. Efficacy of compression of different capacitance beds in the amelioration of orthostatic hypotension. *Clin Auton Res* 1997;7:321–326.
42. Ten Harkel AD, van Lieshout JJ, Wieling W. Effects of leg muscle pumping and tensing on orthostatic arterial pressure: a study in normal subjects and patients with autonomic failure. *Clin Sci* 1994;87:553–558.
43. Bouvette CM, McPhee BR, Opfer-Gehrking TL, Low PA. Role of physical countermaneuvers in the management of orthostatic hypotension: Efficacy and biofeedback augmentation. *Mayo Clin Proc* 1996;71:847–853.
44. Fealey RD, Robertson D. Management of orthostatic hypotension, in *Clinical Autonomic Disorders: Evaluation and Management* (Low PA, ed.), Lippincott-Raven, Philadelphia, 1997, pp. 763–775.
45. Low PA, Gilden JL, Freeman R, Sheng KN, McElligott MA. Efficacy of midodrine vs placebo in neurogenic orthostatic hypotension. A randomized, double-blind multicenter study. Midodrine Study Group. *JAMA* 1997;277:1046–1051.
46. Wright RA, Kaufmann HC, Perera R, et al. A double-blind, dose-response study of midodrine in neurogenic orthostatic hypotension. *Neurology* 1998;51:120–124.
47. Singer W, Opfer-Gehrking TL, McPhee BR, Hilz MJ, Bharucha AE, Low PA. Acetylcholinesterase inhibition: a novel approach in the treatment of neurogenic orthostatic hypotension. *J Neurol Neurosurg Psychiatry* 2003;74:1294–1298.
48. Thompson CA, Tatro DL, Ludwig DA, Convertino VA. Baroreflex responses to acute changes in blood volume in humans. *Am J Physiol* 1990;259:R792–R798.
49. Perera R, Isola L, Kaufmann H. Effect of recombinant erythropoietin on anemia and orthostatic hypotension in primary autonomic failure. *Clin Auton Res* 1995;5:211–213.
50. Low PA, Opfer-Gehrking TL Kihara M. In vivo studies on receptor pharmacology of the human eccrine sweat gland. *Clin Auton Res* 1992;2:29–34.
51. Low PA, Caskey PE, Tuck RR, Fealey RD, Dyck PJ. Quantitative sudomotor axon reflex test in normal and neuropathic subjects. *Ann Neurol* 1983;14:573–580.
52. Low PA, Zimmerman IR. Development of an autonomic laboratory, in *Clinical Autonomic Disorders: Evaluation and Management* (Low PA, ed.), Little Brown and Company, Boston, 1993, pp. 345–354.
53. Stewart JD, Low PA, Fealey RD. Distal small fiber neuropathy: results of tests of sweating and autonomic cardiovascular reflexes. *Muscle Nerve* 1992;15:661–665.
54. Hoeldtke RD, Bryner KD, Horvath GG, Phares RW, Broy LF, Hobbs GR. Redistribution of sudomotor responses is an early sign of sympathetic dysfunction in type 1 diabetes. *Diabetes* 2001;50:436–443.
55. Chemali KR, Gorodeski R, Chelimsky TC. Alpha-adrenergic supersensitivity of the sudomotor nerve in complex regional pain syndrome. *Ann Neurol* 2001;49:453–459.
56. Fealey RD. Thermoregulatory sweat test, in *Clinical Autonomic Disorders: Evaluation and Management* (Low PA, ed.), Lippincott-Raven, Philadelphia, 1997, pp. 245–257.
57. Schondorf R. The role of sympathetic skin responses in the assessment of autonomic function, in *Clinical Autonomic Disorders: Evaluation and Management* (Low PA, ed.), Little, Brown and Company, Boston, 1993, pp. 231–241.
58. Shahani BT, Halperin JJ, Boulu P, Cohen J. Sympathetic skin response—a method of assessing unmyelinated axon dysfunction in peripheral neuropathies. *J Neurol Neurosurg Psychiatry* 1984;47:536–542.
59. Edelberg R. Electrical properties of the skin, in *Methods in Psychophysiology* (Brown CC, ed.), Williams and Wilkins, Baltimore, 1967, pp. 1–52.
60. Lloyd D. Action potential and secretory potential of sweat glands. *Proc Natl Acad Sci USA* 1961;47:351–362.

61. Morimoto T, Imai Y, Watari H. Skin potential response and sweat output of the cat foot pad. *Jpn J Physiol* 1974;24:205–215.
62. Richter CP. A study of the electrical skin resistance and the psychogalvanic reflex in a case of unilateral sweating. *Brain* 1927;50:216–235.
63. Shaver BA, Brusilow SW, Cooke RE. Origin of the galvanic skin response. *Proc Soc Exp Biol Med* 1962;110:559–564.
64. Levy DM, Reid G, Rowley DA, Abraham RR. Quantitative measures of sympathetic skin response in diabetes: relation to sudomotor and neurological function. *J Neurol Neurosurg Psychiatry* 1992;55:902–908.
65. Low PA. Quantitation of autonomic function, in *Peripheral Neuropathy* (Dyck, PJ, Thomas, PK, Lambert, EH, and Bunge, R, eds.), WB Saunders, Philadelphia, 1984, pp. 1139–1165.
66. Sourek K. The nervous control of skin potentials in man. Rozpravy Ceskoslovenske Akademie Ved Roenik 75–Sesit 1, Prague, 1965;1–97.
67. Arunodaya GR, Taly AB. Sympathetic skin response: a decade later. *J Neurol Sci* 1995; 129:81–89.
68. Tzeng SS, Wu ZA, Chu FL. The latencies of sympathetic skin responses. *Eur Neurol* 1993;33:65–68.
69. Maselli RA, Jaspan JB, Soliven BC, Green AJ, Spire JP, Arnason BGW. Comparison of sympathetic skin response with quantitative sudomotor axon reflex test in diabetic neuropathy. *Muscle Nerve* 1989;12:420–423.
70. Drory VE, Korczyn AD. Sympathetic skin response: age effect. *Neurology* 1993;43:1818–1820.
71. Knezevic W, Bajada S. Peripheral autonomic surface potential. A quantitative technique for recording sympathetic conduction in man. *J Neurol Sci* 1985;67:239–251.
72. Soliven B, Maselli R, Jaspan J, et al. Sympathetic skin response in diabetic neuropathy. *Muscle Nerve* 1987;10:711–716.
73. Braune HJ, Horter C. Sympathetic skin response in diabetic neuropathy: a prospective clinical and neurophysiological trial on 100 patients. *J Neurol Sci* 1996;138:120–124.
74. Niakan E, Harati Y. Sympathetic skin response in diabetic peripheral neuropathy. *Muscle Nerve* 1988;11:261–264.
75. Watkins PJ. Facial sweating after food: a new sign of diabetic autonomic neuropathy. *Br Med J* 1973;1:583–587.
76. Shaw JE, Parker R, Hollis S, Gokal R, Boulton AJ. Gustatory sweating in diabetes mellitus. *Diabet Med* 1996;13:1033–1037.
77. Kurchin A, Adar R, Zweig A, Mozes M. Gustatory phenomena after upper dorsal sympathectomy. *Arch Neurol* 1977;34:619–623.
78. Restivo DA, Lanza S, PattiF, et al. Improvement of diabetic autonomic gustatory sweating by botulinum toxin type A. *Neurology* 2002;59:1971–1973.
79. Atkin SL, Brown PM. Treatment of diabetic gustatory sweating with topical glycopyrrolate cream. *Diabet Med* 1996;13:493–494.
80. Shaw JE, Abbott CA, Tindle K, Hollis S, Boulton AJ. A randomised controlled trial of topical glycopyrrolate, the first specific treatment for diabetic gustatory sweating. *Diabetologia* 1997;40:299–301.
81. Glaister DH, Hearnshaw JR, Heffron PF, Peck AW. The mechanism of post-parotidectomy gustatory sweating (the auriculotemporal syndrome). *Br Med J* 1958;2:942–946.
82. Gardner WJ, McCubbin JW. Auriculotemporal syndrome: gustatory sweating due to misdirection of regenerated nerve fibers. *JAMA* 1956;160:272–277.
83. von Lindern JJ, Niederhagen B, Berge S, Hagler G, Reich RH. Frey syndrome: treatment with type A botulinum toxin. *Cancer* 2000;89:1659–1663.
84. Beerens AJ, Snow GB. Botulinum toxin A in the treatment of patients with Frey syndrome. *Br J Surg* 2002;89:116–119.
85. Drummond PD. Mechanism of gustatory flushing in Frey's syndrome. *Clin Auton Res* 2002; 12:144–146.

86. Periquet MI, Novak V, Collins MP, et al. Painful sensory neuropathy: prospective evaluation using skin biopsy. *Neurology* 1999;53:1641–1647.
87. Sandroni P, Davis MDP, Harper CM Jr, et al. Neurophysiologic and vascular studies in erythromelalgia: A retrospective analysis. *J Clin Neuromusc Dis* 1999;1:57–63.
88. Novak V, Freimer ML, Kissel JT, et al. Autonomic impairment in painful neuropathy. *Neurology* 2001;56:861–868.
89. Singer W, Spies JM, McArthur J, et al. Prospective evaluation of somatic and autonomic small fibers in selected autonomic neuropathies. *Neurology* 2004:62:612–618.

26
Gastrointestinal Syndromes Due to Diabetes Mellitus

Juan-R. Malagelada, MD

SUMMARY

Diabetes mellitus is a condition that might result in a variety of derangements of gastrointestinal (GI) structure and function. Disturbances may manifest as symptoms and metabolic changes that in turn, might impich in the management of the patient with diabetes. The present chapter describes the pathophysiology, clinical findings, and management options dealing with the main clinical syndromes associated with disturbances of GI physiology in diabetics. It deals with esophageal dysfunction, sometimes subclinical, but often a source of bothersome upper GI symptoms and also, describes the gastroparesis syndrome, arguably the most characteristic form of gastroduodenal dysfunction in the diabetic. It deals as well with the complex issue of diarrhea in the diabetic patient, often multifactorial and sometimes resulting from a mixture of pathophysiological abnormalities related to diabetic sequela and association with common GI ailments, such as irritable bowel syndrome. Similarly, some space is dedicated to the issue of constipation and fecal incontinence in the patient with diabetes, a particularly troublesome problem quite common in long-standing diabetics. The chapter also provides advice about indications and interpretation of various diagnostic test and reviews the main drugs now available or expected in the future for dealing with these various clinical problems.

Key Words: Diabetic diarrhea; dysphasia; gastroparesis; intestinal neuropathy; esophageal dysmotility; diabetic incontinence; gut autonomic dysfunction.

INTRODUCTION

In a patient with diabetes, gastrointestinal (GI) symptoms may be caused by the same spectrum of disorders as in the general population or by disturbances that arise as a complication of diabetes. The prevalence of GI symptoms in diabetics is not well-established, but appears to be substantially higher than in the general population. As many as 60–75% of patients visiting diabetes clinics report significant GI symptoms *(1,2)*. Bytzer et al. *(3)* on the basis of a population-based survey of 15,000 adults, showed that the prevalence of a variety of upper and lower GI symptoms and symptom complexes in diabetics was increased. Interestingly, abnormalities in GI function, particularly motor function, are not invariably symptomatic. Annese et al. *(4)* studied esophageal, gastric, and gallbladder motor function in a group of patients with type 2 diabetes mellitus (most with autonomic neuropathy) and detected esophageal motor

From: *Contemporary Diabetes: Diabetic Neuropathy: Clinical Management, Second Edition*
Edited by: A. Veves and R. Malik © Humana Press Inc., Totowa, NJ

abnormalities and delayed gastric emptying of solids in about 50% of the group, and impaired gallbladder emptying in two-thirds. In total, 74% of the patients had at least one of the three organs affected although, only 26% had all three involved. About two-thirds had GI symptoms, although these could not always be related to specific organ dysfunction. Sometimes even asymptomatic patients might show evidence of digestive tract dysfunction when tested *(5)*, but again precise prevalence figures are not known because population-based studies have not been performed.

The pathogenesis of gut disturbances that arise as a complication of diabetes is likely to be multifactorial and is incompletely understood. In 1945, Rundles *(6)* recognized autonomic neuropathy as one of the etiological factors involved. However, other factors such as metabolic alterations (hyperglycemia, hypokalemia), vascular changes (microangiopathy), altered hormonal control, and increased susceptibility to infections might play an important role. Primary smooth muscle dysfunction is considered unlikely, because motility is restored with parenterally administered prokinetic drugs such as erithromycin or metoclopramide *(7)*.

From a pathophysiological standpoint, alterations in gut motor, secretory, and absorptive functions may be observed in the diabetic gut. Sometimes alteration of one of these functions predominates the others, but mixed disturbances are quite common. Furthermore, abnormal function, i.e., motility, might affect predominantly one region of the gut, manifesting itself clinically as a regional disturbance (Fig. 1). However, when the appropriate tests are performed, multiple levels of the gut are most often found to be affected. In this chapter the different levels of gut dysfunction that might occur in patients with diabetes will be described separately; however, this subdivision is adopted only for organizational purposes.

ESOPHAGEAL DYSFUNCTION

Pathogenesis

Autonomic neuropathy is the main pathogenetic suspect. Neuropathological esophageal abnormalities have been reported by Smith *(8)*, who observed swelling, irregularity of caliber, and disruption of parasympathetic fibers in the esophageal wall and in the extrinsic trunks. The myenteric plexus appeared normal except for a lymphocytic infiltration within the ganglia. Hyperglycemia might also be involved, it will be shown later for a number of motor gut disturbances.

Clinical Findings and Evaluation

Esophageal motor dysfunction is common in patients with diabetes, but is usually asymptomatic (Table 1). The most frequent complaints are heartburn and dysphagia, but these symptoms are evidently nonspecific. Nishida et al. *(9)* reported that 25.3% of a group of 241 patients with diabetes mellitus had symptomatic gastroesophageal reflux disease (GERD) symptoms against 9.5% of a control group of patients with chronic hepatitis C. This figure approximates the 28% prevalence of abnormally elevated gastroesophageal reflux in diabetics, based on pHmetry studies, reported by Lluch et al. *(10)*, although most patients in the latter group appeared to be asymptomatic. In any case, the presence of abnormal gastroesophageal reflux was associated with cardiovascular autonomic neurophathy *(10)*. However, on the issue of reflux

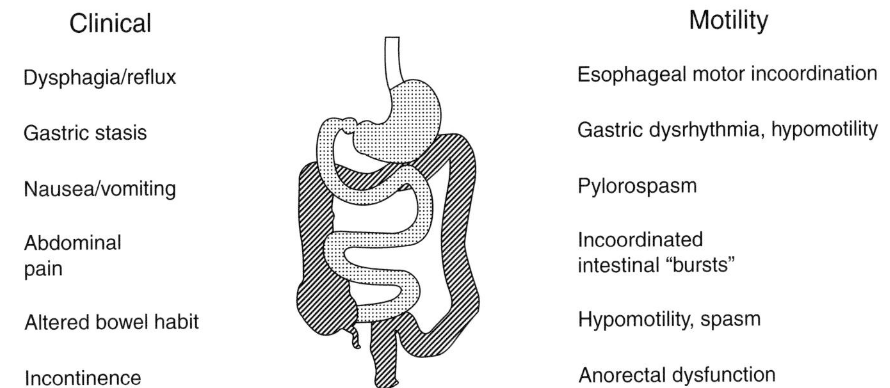

Fig. 1. Diagramatic representation of various gastrointestinal syndromes related to diabetes mellitus. Approximate symptom–regional relationships are noted.

Table 1
Evaluation of Upper Gut Symptoms in a Patient With Diabetes

Esophageal symptoms
Radiographic studies
Endoscopy
Scintigraphy (esophageal transit or clearance)
Esophageal manometry
Psychological assessment
Gastroparesis syndrome
Upper GI X-rays (only useful if showing manifest retention)
Gastroduodenoscopy, to exclude mechanical obstruction and to show retained residue
Gastric emptying studies: radioscintigraphic (liquid and/or solid component); breath test; ultrasound
Upper gut manometry
Electrogastrography (unproven reliability)

and autonomic neuropathy there are some conflicting reports. Jackson et al. *(11)* observed that among symptomatic GERD patients, those with diabetes mellitus often have normal 24-hour pHmetry, but abnormal autonomic functioning. In contrast to nondiabetics in whom the correlation between GERD symptoms and abnormal esophageal pHmetry is closer. It is quite possible that abnormal esophageal motility or sensitivity, or both, produce symptoms in diabetics with autonomic neuropathy that mimic acid reflux, but are not directly related to acid. This possibility should be considered in patients who do not respond as well as expected to antisecretory pharmacological therapy. These issues were also explored by Antwi et al. *(12)* who observed that endoscopic esophagitis was more prevalent among diabetics with autonomic neuropathy than without, whereas reflux like symptoms were similar with or without neuropathy. Further insight was provided by Kinekawa et al. *(13)* who showed that abnormal acid reflux on the basis of esophageal pHmetry correlated with motor nerve conduction velocity, although not with the coefficient of variation of R–R intervals on the electrocardiogram.

Esophageal dysmotility usually consists of reduced or absent primary peristaltic waves, sporadic tertiary contractions, and delayed esophageal clearance. However, Loo et al. *(14)* were more impressed with the finding of multipeaked peristaltic wave complexes than with the aforementioned abnormalities, which they regarded as nonspecific. Esophageal motor dysfunction, measured manometrically, also appears to correlate with test evidence of neuropathy *(13)*. Holloway et al. *(15)* explored the relationship between esophageal transit and esophageal dysmotility in patients with long-standing diabetes mellitus. He concurrently performed esophageal manometry and radionucleide transit measurement of solids and liquids in the esophagus. They observed a high prevalence of transit hold-ups in diabetics, significantly higher than in controls (both young and elderly, the latter being afflicted by a higher prevalence of dysmotility on account of presbiesophagus). The major mechanism responsible for esophageal bolus hold up in diabetics was peristaltic failure or focal low amplitude pressure waves, demonstrated manometrically.

Pitfalls in interpreting esophageal motor dysfunction as a cause of patients' symptoms do abound. A recent report of unsatisfactory symptomatic response to laparoscopic myotomy in a patient with diabetes with apparent achalasia diagnosed by manometry should be considered *(16)*. Psychosomatic factors in the genesis of esophageal motor incoordination have also been postulated *(17)*.

GASTRODUODENAL DYSFUNCTION (THE GASTROPARESIS SYNDROME)

Pathogenesis

Diabetic gastroparesis is an electromechanical motility disorder that in many instances involves not only the stomach, but also the upper small bowel. The molecular pathophysiology of diabetic gastroparesis is unknown. In fact, a variety of pathogenetic factors may be implicated in most patients. Animal studies point to a defect in the enteric nervous system characterized by a loss of nitric oxide signals from nerves to gut smooth muscle *(18,19)*. Interstitial cells of Cajal might also be disrupted *(20)*. "Vagal denervation" by autonomic neuropathy is probably relevant and in turn might induce changes in postprandial hormone profile, including gastrin levels *(21)*. Prostaglandin overproduction in gastric smooth muscle has been linked to gastric slow-wave disruption *(22)*. Interestingly, in animal models of diabetic gastroparesis there is evidence that homeostatic mechanisms are activated in the enteric nervous system to compensate for the loss of extrinsic innervation *(20)*.

Acute hyperglycemia might play an important pathogenetic role *(23)*. Antral motility decreases with postprandial glucose levels more than 9.7 mmol/L *(2)*. In 10 patients with type 1 diabetes mellitus and sensory motor neuropathy, Flowaczny and coworkers *(24)* showed that when plasma glucose concentrations were controlled by permanent iv administration of insulin, gastric emptying rates were near normal. Nevertheless, although achieving and sustaining normoglycemia is undoubtedly important, in clinical practice symptomatic patients with gastroparesis still require prokinetic therapy for satisfactory results *(2)*. However, to further complicate matters, it has been shown that the accelerating effect of prokinetics, such as cisapride and erithromycin is in turn significantly dampened by hyperglycemia *(25)*. Thus, good glycemic control is an inevitable premise to successful management of diabetic gastroparesis.

Another possible connection between diabetes mellitus and the GI tract can be infrequent autoimmune disease associated with type 1 diabetes mellitus, such as celiac disease, autoimmune chronic pancreatitis, and autoimmune gastropathy *(2)*. Indeed, about 15–20 of patients with type 1 diabetes mellitus exhibit parietal cell antibodies *(26)*, but on the other hand no clear-cut relationship has been found between parietal cell antibody titers and delayed gastric emptying *(26)*. Finally, the finding of gastroparesis associated with autonomic neuropathy in a diabetic should not preclude the possibility of coexistent mechanical factors contributing to the apparent motor abnormality *(27)*. First assessing the possibility of mechanical obstruction remains a key premise to diagnosing a gut motor disorder under any circumstances.

Clinical Findings and Evaluation

Both acute and chronic gastroparesis are relatively common occurrences (Table 1). Gastric emptying of solids is delayed in 30–50% of patients with diabetes mellitus *(23,26,28,29)*. Another 20% might in fact present accelerated gastric emptying *(29)*. Although, many such patients experience upper GI symptoms that impair their quality of life, others are asymptomatic. Thus, the concept that symptoms are the direct outcome of delayed gastric emptying or conversely that delayed gastric emptying might be associated with clinical symptoms is now recognized as overly simplistic. Lack of correlation between gastric emptying rates and GI symptoms has been evidenced by numerous studies *(26)*. In contrast, the potential impact of gastroparesis on oral drug absorption and blood glucose control in diabetics has probably been underestimated *(28)*. Indeed, gastroparesis should be suspected in individuals with erratic glucose control *(23,30)* and timing insulin regarding gastric emptying rates might be helpful. A hypothesis has been put forward that improving gastric emptying in diabetics with gastroparesis with the use of prokinetics would regularize duodenal nutrient delivery rates and achieve better glycemic control. Although seemingly logical and attractive, experimental studies in human diabetics have not shown enough supportive evidence to justify it as clinically relevant *(31,32)*.

Gastroparesis affects both type 1 and type 2 forms of diabetes *(13)*. Diabetic neuropathy is present in about two-thirds of gastroparetic patients with type 1 and about one-fifth with type 2 diabetes *(2)*. One study *(33)* examined the relationship between gastric emptying parameters, gastric symptoms, and cardiovascular autonomic function. In addition, they found no significant relationship between the prevalence of GI symptoms and abnormalities in gastric emptying. Neither there was any significant relationship between delayed gastric emptying and cardiovascular autonomic neuropathy in their group of patients *(33)*.

This is a particularly contentious issue as other studies' results are discrepant. Tomi et al. *(29)* found an association between abnormalities in gastric emptying (delayed or accelerated) and cardiovascular autonomic neuropathy, although not with symptoms. De Block et al. *(26)* also found an association between delayed gastric emptying and autonomic nerve function (Ewing tests). Similarly, other investigators *(34)* found a strong correlation between diabetic gastroparesis and cardiac autonomic denervation, nephropathy, and retinopathy. Huszno et al. *(35)* also explored the potential concordance between diabetic gastroparesis and cardiovascular neuropathy in 42 subjects with type 1 diabetes mellitus. Their results show a trend toward a higher prevalence of established cardiovascular neuropathy in patients with diabetic gastroparesis as opposed to those with normal or accelerated emptying, but considerable overlap was apparent. These authors concluded that diabetic autonomic neuropathy tends to be disseminated and does not invariably affect and alter the function of a particular organ in the body.

Gastric emptying abnormalities, including both solid and liquid components of a test meal, remain rather stable for long periods of time (mean 12.3 ± 3.1 years of follow-up (SD) in one study *[36]*). Neither there was much change in the GI symptom pattern during such long follow-up *(36)*. As expected, the prevalence of autonomic neuropathy did increase during the years from an initial 35% at baseline to 80% at follow-up *(36)*.

When it comes to specific abnormalities in upper gut function as responsible for gastroparesis, the thinking has fluctuated considerably during the decades. Antral hypomotility with failure to grind and propel mixed chyme into the duodenum has been traditionally accepted as a major pathophysiological factor. However, animal models, suggest that proximal gastric hypomotility and pyloric hypercontractility are more relevant *(37)*. Indeed, quite early, in the laboratory it was recognized that some patients with diabetic gastroparesis presented manometric evidence of hyperactivity at the pylorus (Fig. 2) *(38)*. In other patients, delayed gastric emptying might be caused or aggravated by intestinal dysmotility *(39)*. Finally, in some patients with chronic nausea, gastric stasis may be owing in part to centrally relayed reflexes triggered by gastric dysrhythmia or other visceral afferent signals.

When symptomatic, gastroparesis manifests by episodes of nausea and vomiting (fasting as well as postprandial) that are often, but not invariably associated with upper abdominal pain. Dyspeptic symptoms such as early satiety, frequent belching as well as bloating might be present. On abdominal examination, a gastric splash might be detected, but it is rare. The episodes of nausea and vomiting tend to follow a variable course and might be self-limited, recurrent, or unrelenting. In severe cases, the gastroparesis syndrome might lead to malnutrition or serious complications, such as bleeding from Mallory–Weiss tears secondary to repeated bouts of retching or vomiting. Symptoms tend to be worse during periods of diabetic decompensation and in fact the prototypic patient with symptomatic diabetic gastroparesis has poorly controlled, longstanding, insulin-dependent diabetes. Peripheral neuropathy and other manifestations of autonomic dysfunction (orthostatic hypotension, impotence, bladder dysfunction, sweat abnormality) are frequently, but not invariably associated.

In evaluating a patient with suspected diabetic gastroparesis, gastroduodenoscopy, and at least upper GI radiology should be performed first to exclude pyloric or any other type of mechanical obstruction. A careful history about medications (e.g., psychotropic drugs, anticholinergics, ganglion-blocking agents, and so on) should also be obtained. Radiological signs of gastric stasis, such as dilatation of the stomach with retained food and secretions are useful if present in the absence of demonstrable mechanical lesion. However, the sensitivity of radiology in detecting GI motor dysfunction is low. Therefore, a normal barium series does not exclude diabetic gastric dysmotility.

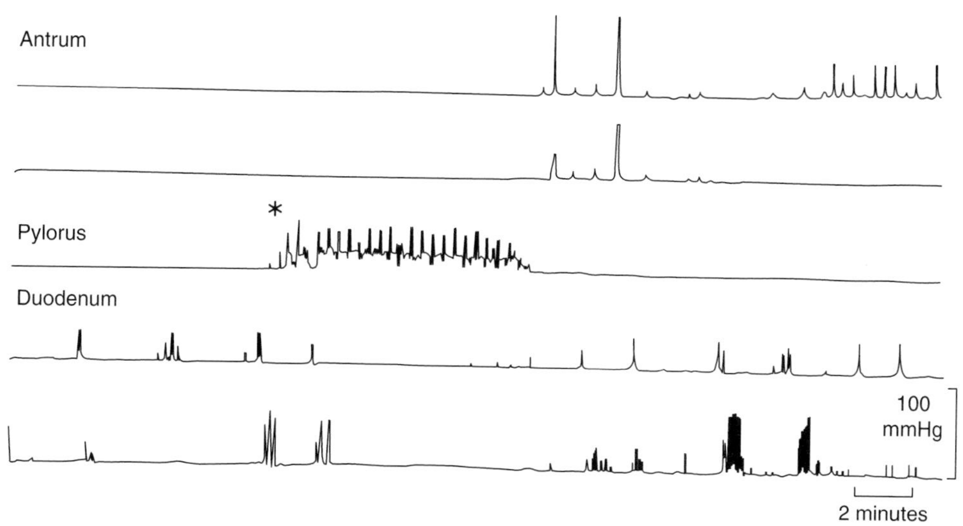

Fig. 2. Example of pyloric tonic activity recorded manometrically in a patient with diabetic gastroparesis. *Note* the prolongad tonic closure of the pylorus (pylorospasm). (Reproduced from ref. *38*.)

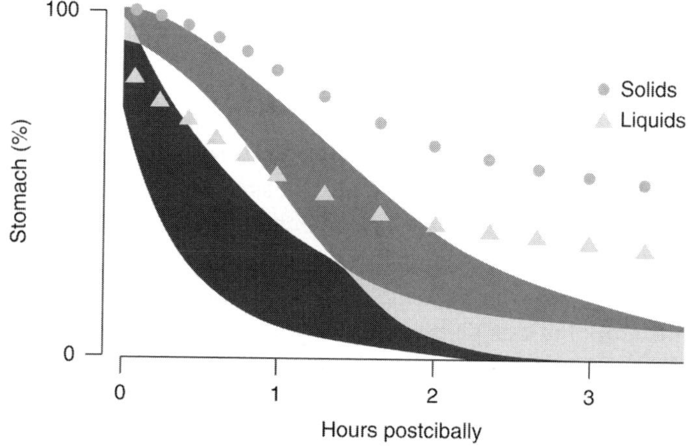

Fig. 3. Example of radioscintigraphic gastric emptying measurements for solids and liquids in a patient with diabetic gastroparesis. *Note* shaded areas representing normal ranges and lines representing patient data.

Several methods with higher sensitivity to assess gastric motor function are nowadays available. Gastric emptying time is best evaluated using radioscintigraphic techniques that differentiate between emptying of the solid and the liquid phases of a meal (double-isotope scintigraphy). Measurement of gastric emptying rates by a radionucleide study remains the gold standard for assessment of gastroparesis (Fig. 3). Alternatives include the ^{13}C-octanoic acid breath test and ultrasonographic measurement of gastric emptying. The ^{13}C-octanoic acid breath test has been compared with radionucleide emptying test in diabetics *(17)* and has been shown to constitute a suitable method for diagnostic purposes with good correlation observed between both tests.

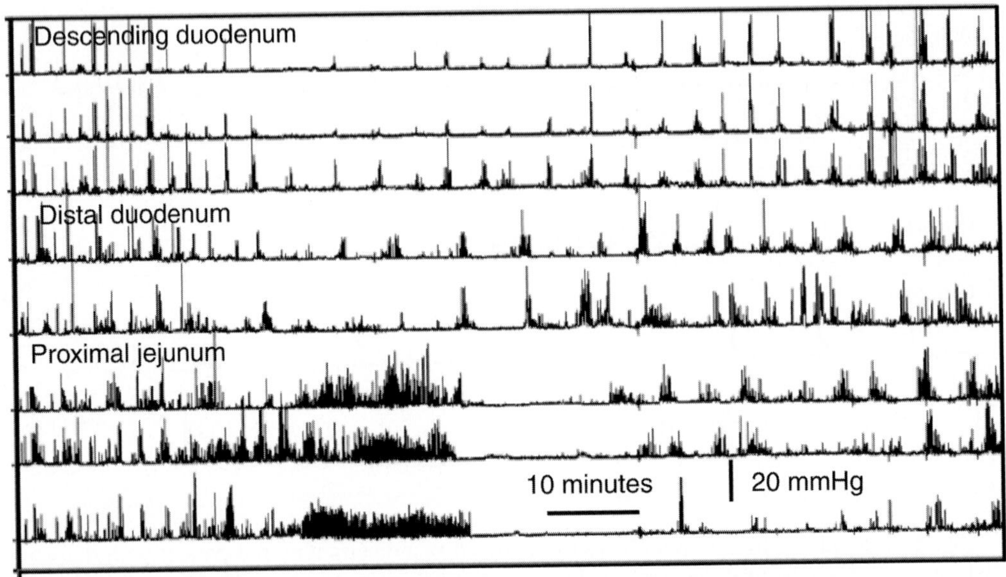

Fig. 4. Manometric abnormalities recorded during the postprandial period in a diabetic patient with gastroparesis and diarrea. *Note* burst activity interrupting the otherwise normal postprandial irregular sustained contractile activity of the small bowel.

Real-time ultrasonographic measurement of gastric emptying of a semisolid meal has also shown a reasonably good correlation with the conventional scintigraphic test *(40)*. The ultrasonographic method does not actually measure disappearance of meal from the stomach, but the reduction in antral cross-sectional area as the stomach empties. Electrogastrography has also been suggested as a diagnostic method for gastric motor disturbances in diabetics, but the evidence is not sufficiently strong to recommend it as a clinical diagnostic tool at this point *(41)*.

Manometry is another useful technique in the assessment of upper gut motility disorders *(42)*. In diabetic gastroparesis there is often absence of normal interdigestive motor cycles in the stomach. This observation might explain the formation of bezoars, as phase III activity plays a role in the evacuation of large (>5 mm) indigestible solids from the stomach *(7)*. However, the most consistent abnormality is antral hypomotility after ingestion of a solid meal. This hypomotility is often characterized by a decreased frequency of phasic pressure waves. In more severe cases, there is also reduced wave amplitude *(43)*.

Other evidence of upper gut dysmotility includes episodes of pylorospasm (prolonged and intense tonic contractions), which were found in 14 out of 24 diabetics with the gastroparesis syndrome *(38)*. Abnormal manometric patterns may not be limited to the stomach. Camilleri and Malagelada *(39)* observed reduced duodeno–jejunal phasic pressure activity (4 out of 14 patients) and nonpropagated bursts of powerful contractions in the proximal small bowel (9 out of 14 patients) (Fig. 4).

Therapy of Gastroparesis

Treatment of diabetic gastroparesis has two facets: one, treatment of autonomic neuropathy and of hyperglycemia that are major pathogenetic substrates; and two, correction of the motor disorder itself *(44)*. Ruboxistaurin appears as a promising disease-modifying therapy for autonomic neuropathy, currently undergoing phase III trials *(45)*. Epalrestat, an aldose reductase inhibitor used in the treatment of diabetic neuropathy has also shown positive effects on the electrogastrogram of patients with diabetic gastroparesis, but electrogastrography is not considered sufficiently reliable to draw firm conclusions *(46)*. Attempts at correcting the motor disorder might include a variety of nutritional, pharmacological, and electrical stimulation and ancillary methods *(44)*. Dietary measures are important and patients with severe feeding problems might even require surgical implantation of a feeding jejunostomy, sometimes complemented by a "venting" gastrostomy that serves to decompress the gastric cavity on demand *(47,48)*.

Prokinetics (metoclopramide, domperidone, cisapride, cinitrapride, and others) constitute the conventional and standard approach to pharmacotherapy. Prokinetic drugs in combination with dietary measures bring symptomatic relief in most patients *(47,49)*. Nevertheless, it should be remembered that diabetic gastropathy improvement in gastric emptying does not equate symptom relief *(50)*. Complementary centrally acting drugs may need to be administered. For instance, some patients with severe nausea and vomiting will require concurrent central antiemetics, except if treated with a prokinetic drug with central antiemetic properties, such as metoclopramide.

Indeed, metoclopramide remains a very useful drug for the treatment of diabetic gastroparesis on account of its dual effect: central antiemetic and gastric prokinetic. However, the risk of dystonic side-effects, prolactin-related side-effects and the more remote, but fearful risk of inducing tardive dyskinesia must be considered *(51)*. Furthermore, despite many published studies, the long-term efficacy and toxicity assessment of metoclopramide remains uncertain because many of the original studies are quite old and substandard in their methodology.

Domperidone is a peripheral D_2 dopamine antagonist that lacks central toxicity effects, although it might still retain some central antinauseating properties on account of the emetic centers in the medulla being partially outside the blood–brain barrier. A comparative trial of domperidone against cisapride in children with diabetes mellitus and gastroparesis concluded that domperidone was more effective *(52)*. Despite its lack of central antiemetic properties, cisapride was until recently a broadly used and apparently effective agent, but has been *de facto* removed from the market because of the risk of inducing cardiac arryhtmia *(32)*. Cinitapride is an analogous drug available in some countries and seemingly safe.

Erithromycin, a motilin receptor agonist, is a highly effective prokinetic agent, particularly when administered as iv boluses in acute flare-ups of gastroparesis. It induces a sweeping gastric peristaltic contraction, which empties retained content into the small bowel. Unfortunately, its mid- and long-term efficacy when given orally has been cast into doubt. In addition, concerns have arisen about recommending sustained antibiotic administration. Newer motilin agonists devoid of antibiotic properties are under development. Two such molecules, KC 11458 and ABT-229 have been subjected to clinical trail, but neither has shown much efficacy in the clinical setting *(53,54)*. Further molecules also with motilin agonist properties are at the preclinical stage.

Other pharmacological approaches are worth considering. Clonidine, an α-2 adrenergic agonist, has been proposed on a clinical basis, but a recent trial against placebo failed to show any meaningful prokinetic effect in a group of patients with diabetic gastroparesis *(55)*. Sildenafil, a phosphodiesterase-5 inhibitor with some positive effects on esophageal spasm has been tried to counteract pyloric spasm in diabetic gastroparesis, but preliminary results are not too encouraging *(56)*. With similar objectives, namely achieving sustained pyloric relaxation, botulinum toxin injection into pyloric muscle through endoscopy has been tried with some success *(57–59)*, but series are small and follow-up quite short. Botox effects are temporary anyway.

Gastric pacing is a relatively new treatment modality which holds promise. Gastric stimulation devices are surgically implanted, first temporarily and, permanently if patients show positive responses. Several series have been published and report substantial improvement in nausea and vomiting in association with improved quality of life *(60,61)*. Interestingly, despite symptomatic improvement, gastric emptying rates are either not accelerated or only modestly accelerated. Nutritional parameters do tend to improve. Hospital admission also decreases *(62,63)*. On balance, gastric pacing is a potential option for patients who fail or cannot tolerate pharmacological treatment. So caution must be exerted before recommending it because evidence in favor of this method is not yet conclusive.

Psychological care of patients with symptomatic diabetic gastroparesis is of utmost importance as many of the symptoms associated with this condition are aggravated by anxiety. In truly desperate situations, subtotal gastrectomy with Roux-en-Y loop anastomosis has been undertaken to relieve intractable vomiting and its metabolic consequences *(64)*.

MID AND LOWER GUT DYSFUNCTION (DIABETIC DIARRHEA AND CONSTIPATION)

Diarrhea or constipation, or both, are among the most common GI complaints encountered in patients with diabetes. These disorders of bowel habit reflect, at least in part, small bowel and colonic dysfunction.

DIARRHEA

Pathogenesis

The pathogenesis of diarrhea in patients with diabetes is poorly understood and probably multifactorial. It may be caused by disturbances directly related to diabetes (primary causes) or to late complications (secondary causes). Among primary causes, visceral neuropathy is a key factor but other factors probably contribute as well. Functional changes such as accelerated transit time and decreased intestinal tone might be associated with enhanced cholinergic and decreased β-adrenergic receptor activities *(65)*. Neuroendocrine peptide dysfuntions might also be involved. El-Salhy and Spangeus *(66)* have shown that in diabetic mice antral VIP and galanin levels are increased, whereas colonic PYY concentrations are decreased. These particular anomalies in enteric peptide profile would favor the development of diarrhea, whereas other anomalies in peptide levels could favor constipation.

Low et al. *(67)* examined the correlation between various GI symptoms attributable to autonomic neuropathy (diarrhea among them) and objective autonomic impairment measured by laboratory tests in patients with type 1 diabetes mellitus. Their findings suggest that both symptoms and autonomic dysfunction are common in diabetes.

However, they could not always establish a causal relation between autonomic dysfunction and the clinical manifestations. Rosa-e-Silva et al. *(68)* observed rapid transit rates in the distal small bowel of patients with type 1 diabetes mellitus with strong correlation with the presence of orthostatic hypotension, suggesting that autonomic neuropathy is the common link between both findings. In patients with a postganglionic sympathetic lesion, Camilleri et al. *(69)* found manometric evidence of intestinal dysmotility in the form of incoordinated bursts of nonpropagated phase III-like activity, although not all of these patients had diarrhea. Among other primary causes of diabetic diarrhea, microangiopathy and functional mucosal abnormalities might also play a role.

Secondary causes of diarrhea in diabetics potentially include bacterial overgrowth abnormalities in bile acid enterohepatic circulation, and exocrine pancreatic insufficiency. The first two might be facilitated by intestinal transit abnormalities that are themselves secondary to intestinal dysmotility. Exocrine pancreatic insufficiency occurs more frequently in diabetics than controls *(70)*, particularly in patients with associated overweight. Exceptionally, pancreatic exocrine insufficiency becomes severe enough to contribute to malabsorption. Abnormal stools and intolerance of dietary fat are symptoms that might suggest this complication in diabetics. The diagnosis might be established simply and noninvasively by measurement of elastase 1 in the stools *(71)*.

Finally, drugs must be considered as a potential pathogenetic factor. For instance, metformine treatment of diabetes is associated with frequent GI side-effects including diarrhea. The latter is not corrected by concomitant odansetron treatment, suggesting that $5HT_3$ receptors are not implicated *(72)*.

Clinical Findings and Evaluation

Diabetic diarrhea was first recognized in 1936 by Bargen et al. *(73)* (Table 2). The diarrhea is watery, often severe, and preceded by abdominal cramps and it occurs particularly at night and may be accompanied by fecal incontinence. Symptoms are intermittent and might last from a few hours to several weeks. During remissions, patients may shift and complain of constipation, resembling the bowel movement alternance characteristic of irritable bowel syndrome. Mild steatorrhea, although not common is compatible with the diabetic diarrhea syndrome, whereas weight loss is unusual. Other signs of autonomic neuropathy may be present concomitantly.

The diagnosis of chronic diabetic diarrhea is essentially one of exclusion. A major problem with this approach remains that some of the main conditions in the differential diagnosis (pancreatic insufficiency, bacterial overgrowth, celiac sprue) can themselves be part of the diabetic diarrhea syndrome. A careful history should be taken to exclude osmotic diarrhea from excessive ingestion of nonabsorbable hexitols (e.g., sorbitol). A 48–72-hour stool collection for weight and fat measurement used to be standard approach, but it is cumbersome and nowadays tends to be bypassed in favor of other tests, as listed in Table 2.

When steatorrhea is found, pancreatic insufficiency should be excluded by performing a pancreatic function test or, if these are not available, by a trial with oral pancreatic enzymes. The degree of steatorrhea relative to diarrhea might sometimes be a useful clue in distinguishing pancreatic insufficiency from that caused by other GI diseases *(74)*. Bacterial overgrowth might be demonstrated by breath tests. Although a positive

Table 2
Evaluation of Chronic Diarrhea in a Patient With Diabetes

Stools: weight, fat, occult blood, examination for ova, parasites, and culture
Colonoscopy (rectal biopsy)
Radiographic studies: plain film of the abdomen; small bowel barium studies; abdominal CT scan
Small bowel biopsy
Small bowel aspirate for giardia and bacteria
Breath tests for malabsorption and bacterial overgrowth
Serum vitamin B_{12} and folate
Pancreatic function tests (elastase 1 in stools, other)
Therapeutic trials with antibiotics, gluten-free diet, pancreatic enzyme supplements

response to antibiotics is suggestive, it is not reliable evidence because diabetic diarrhea often shows spontaneous remissions.

Celiac disease might be associated with diabetes and accompanied by features of more severe malabsorption (considerable steatorrhea, hypoalbuminemia, anemia, abnormal Schilling and xylose test, low serum folate) than is characteristic of diabetic diarrhea. Serological tests for celiac disease are advisable. Small bowel biopsies might be helpful but are not specific for gluten enteropathy because blunting of villi might occur in bacterial overgrowth and other conditions. A favorable clinical and histological response to gluten-free diet is helpful in confirming the diagnosis.

Sometimes, diabetics may also experience abdominal pain because of thoracolumbar diabetic radiculopathy with no evidence of GI pathological findings. A careful history of the typical burning, sharp dermatomal pain, the chronic course, and the electromyogram and thermoregulatory sweat test findings would point to the correct diagnosis of this syndrome.

From a purely clinical standpoint, it is important to recognize the occurrence of pseudodiarrhea (also denominated low volume diarrhea), which in fact represents constipation with impaction of hard stools in the lower colon and rectum. These patients often complain to clinicians of "diarrhea" because they have frequent bowel movements expelling small quantities of liquid residue, which leaks around the impacted solid faeces. There is often associated tenesmus and incontinence. Pseudodiarrhea is in fact constipation, and should be treated as such.

Treatment of Diabetic Diarrhea

A number of treatments have been proposed: antibiotics for bacterial overgrowth, resin cholestyramine, and pancreatic enzyme supplements. Also, antidiarrheal agents such as loperamide, codeine, and anticholinergics have been tried *(75)*. These antidiarrheals may reduce stool frequency, but often do not diminish stool volume. Treatment of severe diabetic diarrhea with octreotide has been reported as quite successful. Octreotide inhibits peptide secretion including serotonin, gastrin, and motilin, and at the same time directly suppresses GI motility *(76)* and improves fluid and electrolyte absorption. Octreotide reduces diabetic diarrhea and its consequences *(77,78)*. Octreotide sc injections may be started at 50 μg twice daily and increased to 100 μg thrice daily as needed. If effective, consideration must be given to using monthly im injections of a long-acting octreotide preparation to make it more comfortable to the patients. Attention must be given to reduce insulin dosage needs on account of inhibition of release of glucagon, growth hormone, and other peptides by octreotide. Potential for hypoglycemic episodes exists.

CONSTIPATION

Pathogenesis

Constipation and the use of laxatives are relatively common in patients with diabetes mellitus *(79)* but the mechanism of constipation remains unclear. Epidemiological studies in community-based practices suggest that physicians should not immediately assume that GI symptoms in patients with diabetes mellitus represent a complication of diabetes mellitus *(80)*. Diabetic autonomic neuropathy may be implicated in some patients, but other factors might also be important. For instance, evacuatory dysfunction is another important factor *(81)*. Jung et al. *(82)* showed in a study involving patients with type 2 diabetes mellitus that those with constipation had longer total colonic transit times than those without constipation. However, there was no difference in colonic transit times between patients with and without cardiovascular autonomic neuropathy. Another study by Ron et al. *(83)* in elderly, frail patients showed a high prevalence of constipation associated with prolonged colonic transit times. However, no significant differences were noted between patients with and without diabetes. Iida et al. *(84)* showed in type 2 diabetics an association between prolonged colonic transit measured by the radiopaque pellet method and autonomic cardiovascular dysfunction. In one study, constipation in type 1 diabetics was found to be associated with the use of calcium channel blockers *(80)*.

Poor glycemic control is probably an important contributory factor *(85)*. Indeed, acute hyperglycemia affects anorectal motor and sensory function *(86)*. The natural history of constipation in diabetics does not seem to predict symptom change over time *(87)*.

Clinical Findings and Evaluation

It is difficult to separate constipation in patients with diabetes from that occurring among the normal population because constipation is such a highly prevalent symptom (Table 3). The depth of diagnostic evaluation in a patient with diabetes complaining of constipation depends on the severity of constipation and on the associated symptoms. Digital examination, testing of stools for occult blood, proctosigmoidoscopy, and barium enema, or better yet, full colonoscopy should be performed to rule out colonic malignancy.

Anorectal manometry might be useful to evaluate the rectoanal inhibitory reflex *(88)*, which is absent in Hirschsprung's disease. Colonic segmental transit time can be derived from the mean segmental transit time of radiopaque markers through right colon, left colon, and rectosigmoid area. These tests should help distinguish between diffuse colonic hypomotility and rectosigmoid dysfunction (outlet obstruction). Unfortunately, the sensitivity and the specificity of these procedures have not been specifically evaluated in diabetics.

Table 3
Evaluation of Colonic and Anorectal Dysfunction in a Patient With Diabetes

Constipation
Digital examination
Stools: occult blood
Barium enema
Colonoscopy (biopsy)
Colonic segmental transit time
Anorectal manometry
Fecal incontinence
24-hour stool weight
Anorectal manometry
Maximum basal sphincter pressure
Maximum "squeeze" sphincter pressure
Rectoanal inhibitory reflex
Tests of continence
Solids: solid sphere
Liquids: rectally infused saline

Treatment of Constipation

Treatment of constipation in diabetics does not differ from those without diabetes. However, besides conventional anticonstipation measures, acarbose has proven valuable in the treatment of diabetics. Because it reduces prolonged colonic transit times in constipated diabetics in addition to its beneficial effect in the control of diabetes *(89)*.

FECAL INCONTINENCE

Pathogenesis

Fecal incontinence is a challenging clinical condition particularly in elderly diabetics. It has been estimated that upto one-fifth of patients with diabetes have fecal incontinence, although prevalences depend on criteria of incontinence applied. The incidence of fecal incontinence in diabetics appears to correlate with duration of the disease *(90)*. Incontinence is probably multifactorial and involves age-related changes, diabetic neuropathy, multimorbidity, and polymedication *(91)*. However, instability of the internal sphincter probably plays a major role in incontinent diabetics *(92)*. Another important cause is fecal impaction *(93)*.

The vast majority of patients with diabetes with fecal incontinence have normal or only moderately increased daily stool volumes, but also exhibit multiple abnormalities of anorectal sensory and motor functions *(94)*. Fecal incontinence might be associated with severe diabetic diarrhea or constitute an apparently independent disorder. Diarrhea might, of course, produce stress on the continence mechanisms that are already impaired.

Clinical Findings and Evaluation

In evaluating fecal incontinence in patients with diabetes it is important to take an accurate history and to assess stool weight. Incontinent diabetics may complain of "diarrhea," eventhough their 24-hour stool weights are within normal limits (Table 3).

Anorectal function can be evaluated by anorectal manometry and tests of continence for solids and liquids. Anorectal manometry gives information about the maximum basal sphincter pressure, the maximum "squeeze" sphincter pressure, and the rectoanal inhibitory reflex (inflation of a balloon in the rectum causes a reflex relaxation of the internal anal sphincter). Continence for solids and liquids can be directly assessed simulating the stress of stools with a solid sphere or with rectally infused saline. Unfortunately, these tests do not appear to be very helpful in making therapeutic decisions. Appropriate treatment of incontinence in diabetics includes optimizing blood sugar control and biofeedback therapy. Surgical intervention should be reserved for cases refractory to medical treatment or for those patients with rectocele or obstetrical injury *(95)*. The clinical outcome of surgical treatment of incontinence is far from uniform and caution is advisable before recommending it.

REFERENCES

1. Chandran M, Chu NV, Edelman SV. Gastrointestinal disturbances in diabetes. *Curr Diab Rep* 2003;3(1):43–48.
2. Perusicova J. Gastrointestinal complications in diabetes mellitus. *Vnitr Lek* 2004;50(5):338–343.
3. Bytzer P, Talley NJ, Leemon M, Young LJ, Jones MP, Horowitz M. Prevalence of gastrointestinal symptoms associated with diabetes mellitus: a population-based survey of 15,000 adults. *Arch Intern Med* 2001;161(16):1989–1996.
4. Annese V, Bassotti G, Caruso N, et al. Gastrointestinal motor dysfunction, symptoms, and neuropathy in noninsulin-dependent (type 2) diabetes mellitus. *J Clin Gastroenterol* 1999;29(2):171–177.
5. Kassander P. Asymptomatic gastric retention in diabetes (gastroparesis diabeticorum). *Ann Int Med* 1958;48:797.
6. Rundles RW. Diabetic neuropathy. General review with report of 125 cases. *Medicine* 1945;24:111.
7. Malagelada JR, Rees WDR, Mazzotta LJ, Go VLW. Gastric motor abnormalities in diabetic and postvagotomy gastroparesis: Effect of metoclopramide and bethanechol. *Gastroenterology* 1980;78:286.
8. Smith B. Neuropathology of the esophagus in diabetes mellitus. *J Neurol Neurosurg Psych* 1974;37:1151.
9. Nishida T, Tsuji S, Tsujii M, et al. Gastroesophageal reflux disease related to diabetes: Analysis of 241 cases with type 2 diabetes mellitus. *J Gastroenterol Hepatol* 2004; 19(3):258–265.
10. Lluch I, Ascaso JF, Mora F, et al. Gastroesophageal reflux in diabetes mellitus. *Am J Gastroenterol* 1999;94(4):919–924.
11. Jackson AL, Rashed H, Cardoso S, et al. Assessment of gastric electrical activity and autonomic function among diabetic and nondiabetic patients with symptoms of gastroesophageal reflux. *Dig Dis Sci* 2000;45(9):1727–1730.
12. Antwi Ch, Krahulec B, Michalko L, Strbova L, Hlinstakova S, Balazovjech I. Does diabetic autonomic neuropathy influence the clinical manifestations of reflux esophagitis? *Bratisl Lek Listy* 2003;104(4–5):139–142.
13. Kinekawa F, Kubo F, Matsuda K, et al. Relationship between esophageal dysfunction and neuropathy in diabetic patients. *Am J Gastroenterol* 2001;96(7):2026–2032.
14. Loo FD, Dodds WJ, Soergel KH, Arndorfer RC, Helm JF, Hogan WJ. Multipeaked esophageal peristaltic pressure waves in patients with diabetic neuropathy. *Gastroenterology* 1985;88:485.

15. Holloway RH, Tippett MD, Horowitz M, Maddox AF, Moten J, Russo A. Relationship between esophageal motility and transit in patients with type I diabetes mellitus. *Am J Gastroenterol* 1999;94(11):3150–3157.
16. Lovecek M, Gryga A, Herman J, Svach I, Duda M. Esophageal dysfunction in a female patient with diabetes mellitus and achalasia. *Bratisl Lek Listy* 2004;105(3):101–103.
17. Clouse RE, Reidel WL, Lustman PJ. Correlation of esophageal motility abnormalities with neuropsychiatric states in diabetics (abstract). *Gastroenterology* 1985;88:1351.
18. Smith DS, Williams CS, Ferris CD. Diagnosis and treatment of chronic gastroparesis and chronic intestinal pseudo-obstruction. *Gastroenterol Clin North Am* 2003;32(2):619–658.
19. Smith DS, Ferris CD. Current concepts in diabetic gastroparesis. *Drugs* 2003;63(13): 1339–1358.
20. Camilleri M. Advances in diabetic gastroparesis. *Rev Gastroenterol Disord* 2002;2(2): 47–56.
21. Migdalis L, Thomaides T, Chairopoulos C, Kalogeropoulou C, Charalabides J, Mantzara F. Changes of gastric emptying rate and gastrin levels are early indicators of autonomic neuropathy in type II diabetic patients. *Clin Auton Res* 2001;11(4):259–263.
22. Owyang C, Hasler WL. Physiology and pathophysiology of the interstitial cells of Cajal: from bench to bedside. VI. Pathogenesis and therapeutic approaches to human gastric dysrhythmias. *Am J Physiol Gastrointest Liver Physiol* 2002;283(1):G8–G15.
23. Horowitz M, O'Donovan D, Jones KL, Feinle C, Rayner CK, Samsom M. Gastric emptying in diabetes: clinical significance and treatment. *Diabete Med* 2002;19(3):177–194.
24. Folwaczny C, Wawarta R, Otto B, Friedrich S, Landgraf R, Riepl RL. Gastric emptying of solid and liquid meals in healthy controls compared with long-term type-1 diabetes mellitus under optimal glucose control. *Exp Clin Endocrinol Diabetes* 2003;111(4): 223–229.
25. Horowitz M, Jones KL, Harding PE, Wishart JM. Relationship between the effects of cisapride on gastric emptying and plasma glucose concentrations in diabetic gastroparesis. *Digestion* 2002;65(1):41–46.
26. De Block CE, De Leeuw IH, Pelckmans PA, Callens D, Maday E, Van Gaal LF. Delayed gastric emptying and gastric autoimmunity in type 1 diabetes. *Diabetes Care* 2002; 25(5):912–917.
27. Azami Y. Diabetes mellitus associated with superior mesenteric artery syndrome: report of two cases. *Int Med* 2001;40(8):736–739.
28. Horowitz M, Su YC, Rayner CK, Jones KL. Gastroparesis: prevalence, clinical significance and treatment. *Can J Gastroenterol* 2001;15(12):805–813.
29. Tomi S, Plazinska M, Zagorowicz E, Ziolkowski B, Muszynski J. Gastric emptying disorders in diabetes mellitus. *Pol Arch Med Wewn* 2002;108(3):879–886.
30. Vinik AI, Maser RE, Mitchell BD, Freeman R. Diabetic autonomic neuropathy. *Diabetes Care* 2003;26(5):1553–1579.
31. Lehmann R, Honegger RA, Feinle C, Fried M, Spinas GA, Schwizer W. Glucose control is not improved by accelerating gastric emptying in patients with type 1 diabetes mellitus and gastroparesis. a pilot study with cisapride as a model drug. *Exp Clin Endocrinol Diabete* 2003;111(5):255–261.
32. Braden B, Enghofer M, Schaub M, Usadel KH, Caspary WF, Lembcke B. Long-term cisapride treatment improves diabetic gastroparesis but not glycaemic control. *Aliment Pharmacol Ther* 2002;16(7):1341–1346.
33. Zahn A, Langhans CD, Hoffner S, et al. Measurement of gastric emptying by 13C-octanoic acid breath test versus scintigraphy in diabetics. *Z Gastroenterol* 2003;41(5):383–390.
34. Kockar MC, Kayahan IK, Bavbek N. Diabetic gastroparesis in association with autonomic neuropathy and microvasculopathy. *Acta Med Okayama* 2002;56(5):237–243.

35. Huszno B, Trofimiuk M, Placzkiewicz E, et al. Co-occurrence of diabetic gastropathy and cardiovascular vegetative neuropathy in patients with diabetes type 1. *Folia Med Cracov* 2001;42(3):105–111.
36. Jones KL, Russo A, Berry MK, Stevens JE, Wishart JM, Horowitz M. A longitudinal study of gastric emptying and upper gastrointestinal symptoms in patients with diabetes mellitus. *Am J Med* 2002;113(6):449–455.
37. James AN, Ryan JP, Crowell MD, Parkman HP. Regional gastric contractility alterations in a diabetic gastroparesis mouse model: effects of cholinergic and serotoninergic stimulation. *Am J Physiol Gastrointest Liver Physiol* 2004;287(3):G612–G619. Epub 2004.
38. Mearin F, Camilleri M, Malagelada JR. Pyloric dysfunction in diabetic gastroparesis. *Gastroenterology* 90:1919–1925, 86.
39. Camilleri M, Malagelada JR. Abnormal intestinal motility in diabetics with the gastroparesis syndrome. *Eur J Clin Invest* 1984;14:420.
40. Darwiche G, Bjorgell O, Thorsson O, Almer LO. Correlation between simultaneous scintigraphic and ultrasonographic measurement of gastric emptying in patients with type 1 diabetes mellitus. *J Ultrasound Med* 2003;22(5):459–466.
41. Lawlor PM, McCullough JA, Byrne PJ, Reynolds JV. Electrogastrography: a non-invasive measurement of gastric function. *Ir J Med Sci* 2001;170(2):126–131.
42. Malagelada JR, Stanghellini V. Manometric evaluation of upper gut symptoms. *Gastroenterology* 1985;88:1223.
43. Malagelada JR, Camilleri M, Stanghellini V. Manometric diagnosis of gastrointestinal motility disorders. Thieme-Stratton, New York, 1986.
44. O'Donovan D, Feinle-Bisset C, Jones K, Horowitz M. Idiopathic and Diabetic Gastroparesis. *Curr Treat Options Gastroenterol* 2003;6(4):299–309.
45. Duby JJ, Campbell RK, Setter SM, White JR, Rasmussen KA. Diabetic neuropathy: an intensive review. *Am J Health Syst Pharm* 2004;61(2):160–173; quiz 175–176.
46. Okamoto H, Nomura M, Nakaya Y, et al. Effects of epalrestat, an aldose reductase inhibitor, on diabetic neuropathy and gastroparesis. *Int Med* 2003;42(8):655–664.
47. Stanciu GO. Gastroparesis and its management. *Rev Med Chir Soc Med Nat Iasi* 2001; 105(3):451–456.
48. Gentilcore D, O'Donovan D, Jones KL, Horowitz M. Nutrition therapy for diabetic gastroparesis. *Curr Diab Rep* 2003;3(5):418–426.
49. Keil R. Prokinetics and diabetes mellitus. *Vnitr Lek* 2004;50(5):358,360–362.
50. Talley NJ. Diabetic gastropathy and prokinetics. *Am J Gastroenterol* 2003;98(2):264–271.
51. Lata PF, Pigarelli DL. Chronic metoclopramide therapy for diabetic gastroparesis. *Ann Pharmacother* 2003;37(1):122–126.
52. Franzese A, Borrelli O, Corrado G, et al. Domperidone is more effective than cisapride in children with diabetic gastroparesis. *Aliment Pharmacol Ther* 2002;16(5):951–957.
53. Russo A, Stevens JE, Giles N, et al. Effect of the motilin agonist KC 11458 on gastric emptying in diabetic gastroparesis. *Aliment Pharmacol Ther* 2004;20(3):333–338.
54. Talley NJ, Verlinden M, Geenen DJ, et al. Effects of a motilin receptor agonist (ABT-229) on upper gastrointestinal symptoms in type 1 diabetes mellitus: a randomised, double blind, placebo controlled trial. *Gut* 2001;49(3):395–401.
55. Huilgol V, Evans J, Hellman RS, Soergel KH. Acute effect of clonidine on gastric emptying in patients with diabetic gastropathy and controls. *Aliment Pharmacol Ther* 2002;16(5):945–950.
56. Dishy V, Cohen Pour M, Feldman L, et al. The effect of sildenafil on gastric emptying in patients with end-stage renal failure and symptoms of gastroparesis. *Clin Pharmacol Ther* 2004;76(3):281–286.

57. Lacy BE, Crowell MD, Schettler-Duncan A, Mathis C, Pasricha PJ. The treatment of diabetic gastroparesis with botulinum toxin injection of the pylorus. *Diabetes Care* 2004;27(10):2341–2347.
58. Lacy BE, Zayat EN, Crowell MD, Schuster MM. Botulinum toxin for the treatment of gastroparesis: a preliminary report. *Am J Gastroenterol* 2002;97(6):1548–1552.
59. Ezzeddine D, Jit R, Katz N, Gopalswamy N, Bhutani MS. Pyloric injection of botulinum toxin for treatment of diabetic gastroparesis. *Gastrointest Endosc* 2002;55(7):920–923.
60. Forster J, Sarosiek I, Delcore R, Lin Z, Raju GS, McCallum RW. Gastric pacing is a new surgical treatment for gastroparesis. *Am J Surg* 2001;182(6):676–681.
61. Abell T, Lou J, Tabbaa M, Batista O, Malinowski S, Al-Juburi A. Gastric electrical stimulation for gastroparesis improves nutritional parameters at short, intermediate, and long-term follow-up. *JPEN J Parenter Enteral Nutr* 2003;27(4):277–281.
62. Forster J, Sarosiek I, Lin Z, et al. Further experience with gastric stimulation to treat drug refractory gastroparesis. *Am J Surg* 2003;186(6):690–695.
63. Lin Z, Forster J, Sarosiek I, McCallum RW. Treatment of diabetic gastroparesis by high-frequency gastric electrical stimulation. *Diabetes Care* 2004;27(5):1071–1076.
64. Watkins PJ, Buxton-Thomas MS, Howard ER. Long-term outcome after gastrectomy for intractable diabetic gastroparesis. *Diabete Med* 2003;20(1):58–63.
65. Anjaneyulu M, Ramarao P. Studies on gastrointestinal tract functional changes in diabetic animals. *Methods Find Exp Clin Pharmacol* 2002;24(2):71–75.
66. El-Salhy M, Spangeus A. Gastric emptying in animal models of human diabetes: correlation to blood glucose level and gut neuroendocrine peptide content. *Ups J Med Sci* 2002;107(2):89–99.
67. Low PA, Benrud-Larson LM, Sletten DM, et al. Autonomic symptoms and diabetic neuropathy: a population-based study. *Diabetes Care* 2004;27(12):2942–2947.
68. Rosa-e-Silva L, Troncon LE, Oliveira RB, Foss MC, Braga FJ, Gallo Junior L. Rapid distal small bowel transit associated with sympathetic denervation in type I diabetes mellitus. *Gut* 1996;39(5):748–756.
69. Camilleri M, Stanghellini V, Sheps SG, Malagelada JR. Gastrointestinal motility disturbances due to postganglionic sympathetic lesions (abstract). *Clin Res* 1984;32:489A.
70. Nunes AC, Pontes JM, Rosa A, Gomes L, Carvalheiro M, Freitas D. Screening for pancreatic exocrine insufficiency in patients with diabetes mellitus. *Am J Gastroenterol* 2003;98(12):2672–2675.
71. Richter ML, Wagner T. Pancreatic exocrine insufficiency in patients with diabetes mellitus. Current state of our knowledge and practical consequences. *Fortschr Med Orig* 2001;119(Suppl 2):77–79.
72. Hoffmann IS, Roa M, Torrico F, Cubeddu LX. Ondansetron and metformin-induced gastrointestinal side effects. *Am J Ther* 2003;10(6):447–451.
73. Bargen JA, Bollman JL, Kepler EJ. The "diarrhea of diabetes" and steatorrhea of pancreatic insufficiency. *Proc Staff Meet Mayo Clin* 1936;11:737.
74. Bo-Linn G, Fordtran JS. Fecal fat concentration in patients with steatorrhea. *Gastroenterology* 1984;87:319.
75. Ogbonnaya K, Arem R. Diabetic diarrhea. *Arch Intern Med* 1990;150:262–267.
76. Farthing M. Effective treatment of diabetic diarrhea with a somatostatin analogue. *Gut* 1992;33:1578–1580.
77. Nakabayashi H, Fujii S, Milwa U, Seta T, Takeda R. Marked improvement of diabetic diarrhea with the somatostatin analogue octreotide. *Arch Int Med* 1994;154:1863–1867.
78. Meyer C, O'Neal DN, Connell W, Alford F, Ward G, Jenkins AJ. Octeotride treatment of severe diabetic diarrhoea. *Int Med J* 2003;33:617–624.
79. Spangeus A, El-Salhy M, Suhr O, Eriksson J, Lithner F. Prevalence of gastrointestinal symptoms in young and middle-aged diabetic patients. *Scand J Gastroenterol* 1999; 34(12):1196–1202.

80. Maleki D, Locke GR 3rd, Camilleri M, et al. Gastrointestinal tract symptoms among persons with diabetes mellitus in the community. *Arch Intern Med* 2000;160(18):2808–2816.
81. Maleki D, Camilleri M, Burton DD, et al. Pilot study of pathophysiology of constipation among community diabetics. *Dig Dis Sci* 1998;43(11):2373–2378.
82. Jung HK, Kim DY, Moon IH, Hong YS. Colonic transit time in diabetic patients—comparison with healthy subjects and the effect of autonomic neuropathy. *Yonsei Med J* 2003;44(2):265–272.
83. Ron Y, Leibovitz A, Monastirski N, Habot B, Segal R. Colonic transit time in diabetic and nondiabetic long-term care patients. *Gerontology* 2002;48(4):250–253.
84. Iida M, Ikeda M, Kishimoto M, et al. Evaluation of gut motility in type II diabetes by the radiopaque marker method. *J Gastroenterol Hepatol* 2000;15(4):381–385.
85. Hammer J, Howell S, Bytzer P, Horowitz M, Talley NJ. Symptom clustering in subjects with and without diabetes mellitus: a population-based study of 15,000 Australian adults. *Am J Gastroenterol* 2003;98(2):391–398.
86. Russo A, Sun WM, Sattawatthamrong Y, et al. Acute hyperglycaemia affects anorectal motor and sensory function in normal subjects. *Gut* 1997;41(4):494–499.
87. Talley NJ, Howell S, Jones MP, Horowitz M. Predictors of turnover of lower gastrointestinal symptoms in diabetes mellitus. *Am J Gastroenterol* 2002;97(12):3087–3094.
88. Martelli H, Devroede G, Arhan P, Duguay C, Dornic C, Faverdin C. Some parameters of large bowel motility in normal man. *Gastroenterology* 1978;75:612.
89. Ron Y, Wainstein J, Leibovitz A, et al. The effect of acarbose on the colonic transit time of elderly long-term care patients with type 2 diabetes mellitus. *J Gerontol A Biol Sci Med Sci* 2002;57(2):M111–M114.
90. Epanomeritakis E, Koutsoumbi P, Tsiaoussis I, et al. Impairment of anorectal function in diabetes mellitus parallels duration of disease. *Dis Colon Rectum* 1999;42(11):1394–1400.
91. Fusgen I, Gruss HJ. Fecal incontinence in elderly diabeteic patients. *Wien Med Wochenschr* 2003;153(17–18):398–401.
92. Sun WM, Katsinelos P, Horowitz M, Read NW. Disturbances in anorectal function in patients with diabetes mellitus and faecal incontinence. *Eur J Gastroenterol Hepatol* 1996;8(10):1007–1012.
93. Stevens TK, Soffer EE, Palmer RM. Fecal incontinence in elderly patients: common, treatable, yet often undiagnosed. *Cleve Clin J Med* 2003;70(5):441–448.
94. Wald A. Incontinence and anorectal dysfunction in patients with diabetes mellitus. *Eur J Gastroenterol Hepatol* 1995;7(8):737–739.
95. Cooper ZR, Rose S. Fecal incontinence: a clinical approach. *Mt Sinai J Med* 2000; 67(2):96–105.

27
Genitourinary Complications

Dan Ziegler and Christian Stief

SUMMARY

Urogenital complications are frequently found in patients with diabetes. In the overwhelming majority, neuropathy and/or angiopathy are the etiologies or most pronounced coetiologies of micturition or sexual dysfunctions. As the impairment of bladder storage and emptying as well as the erectile and ejaculatory dysfunction may have severe organic and psychosocial consequences, their existence (often inapparent to the patient) should be systematically screened for in the routine diabetes clinic. Given hints of existence, comprehensive evaluation of the impaired organ system is mandatory. For treatment, a wide spectrum of various approaches is available and can be individually offered following appropriate diagnosis.

Key Words: Bladder dysfunction; cystopathy; diabetes; erectile dysfunction; female sexual dysfunction; neuropathy.

INTRODUCTION

Disturbances in bladder emptying and/or storage are often asymptomatic to the patient, especially in the beginning of this diabetic complication. In contrast, sexual dysfunctions are readily perceived by the patient. Sexual dysfunctions as erectile or ejaculatory dysfunction and infertility are frequently found in the male diabetic compared with the nondiabetic population. Although these sexual dysfunctions often exert a dramatic negative impact on psychosocial living and self esteem of the patients with diabetes, they remain unacknowledged in many instances. They do not attract medical attention and thereby possible treatment either owing to the shame and embarrassment of the patient or to unawareness or old-fashioned negligence of the problem by the physician. As the impairment of bladder storage and emptying as well as sexual dysfunction may have severe organic and psychosocial consequences, their existence (often in apparent to the patient) should be systematically screened for in the routine diabetes clinic. Given hints of existence, comprehensive evaluation of the impaired organ system is mandatory. For treatment, a wide spectrum of various approaches is available and can be individually offered after appropriate diagnosis *(1)*.

From: *Contemporary Diabetes: Diabetic Neuropathy: Clinical Management, Second Edition*
Edited by: A. Veves and R. Malik © Humana Press Inc., Totowa, NJ

BLADDER DYSFUNCTION

Physiology of Micturition

In the adult, storage capacity of the urinary bladder is 300–600 mL. Until the final volume is reached only a minimal intravesical pressure increase is observed and involuntary spinal reflexes avoid uninhibited contractions. During the filling phase, afferent impulses from the bladder are suppressed both by intraspinal and cerebral mechanisms; furthermore, the sphincter apparatus is activated. When the maximal storage capacity is being reached, afferent impulses transmit this information to the conscience level. Then, efferent motor activity from the pontine micturition center through the nuclei intermediolaterales of the spinal micturition centers at the level of Th 10–L 2 and S 2–4 initiate the micturition. These impulses are transmitted to the secondary cholinergic neuron within the pelvic plexus. Peripherally, micturition is initiated by relaxation of the extrinsic striated sphincteric muscle and contraction of the smooth muscles of the bladder wall. In the absence of relevant anatomical subvesical obstruction, complete bladder emptying occurs in the presence of rather low intravesical pressures *(1)*.

Pathophysiology and Clinical Symptomatology of the Diabetic Bladder

In the rat with experimentally induced diabetes, micturition disturbances start with degeneration of the afferent myelinated fibers *(2)*. Neurogenically mediated bladder contraction is altered in the diabetic rats, which show an increased response to electrical field stimulation and a reduced cholinergic response. However, the purinergic response does not appear to be altered, whereas a residual nonadrenergic–noncholinergic (NANC) component of contractile response of unknown origin is increased *(3)*. Diabetes-induced decrease in the contractility of bladder wall smooth muscle in rabbits has been linked to an increased expression of thin filament proteins, calponin, tropomyosin, and caldesmon, which might alter the contractile and cytoskeletal structure in bladder myocytes. The overexpression of these thin filament associated proteins, which suppresses actin–myosin interaction and actomyosin adenosine triphosphatase, and the enhancement of this suppression by tropomyosin are likely to have an effect on the relationship between force and myosin light chain phosphorylation. Thus, requiring higher levels of phosphorylation in diabetic detrusor compared with that of control. The downstream effects of high glucose (e.g., oxidative stress) appear to modulate the transcriptional regulation of thin filament mediated regulatory proteins in bladder smooth muscle *(4)*.

In man, "diabetic bladder" describes a syndrome of reduced awareness of bladder filling, followed by increased bladder storage capacity and decreased bladder contractility. The reduction of sensation of a filled bladder (caused by the degeneration of the afferent myelinated fibers) is rapidly followed by degeneration of the nonmyelinated efferent fibers resulting with detrusor hypocontractility. This hypocontractility translates clinically into reduced urinary flow, incomplete bladder emptying, recurrent urinary tract infections (UTI) and, as end stage disease, into bladder desensitization and acontractility with overflow incontinence. In contrast to this classical scenario of a diabetic bladder, autonomic neuropathy may cause irritative symptoms as urge, pollakiuria, nocturia, or incontinence in the presence of other urological diseases *(5–7)*.

Bladder Dysfunction in Women With Diabetes

It has been estimated that urinary incontinence may affect nearly 50% of middle aged and older women, leading to significant distress, limitations in daily functioning, and poorer quality of life. Diabetes is associated with an increased risk of incontinence by 30–100%. It has been suggested that interventions that prevent or delay onset of diabetes may also prevent urinary incontinence. In the diabetes prevention program the prevalence of weekly stress incontinence was decreased by the diabetes prevention program intensive lifestyle intervention. Reducing incontinence may be a powerful motivator for women with impaired glucose tolerance to choose lifestyle modification to prevent diabetes *(8)*. Recent large observational studies have identified urge incontinence, an involuntary loss of urine with a feeling of urgency, as increased among women with diabetes, whereas there was no increased risk for stress incontinence, an involuntary loss of urine with physical activity *(8)*. Women with diabetes treated with insulin are at considerably higher risk of urge incontinence than those treated with oral medications or diet *(9)*. However, little is known about how diabetes may contribute to the incidence or severity of urinary incontinence.

Bladder Dysfunction in Men With Diabetes

Lower urinary tract symptoms (LUTS) are common, age-related complaints that are often attributed to benign prostatic hyperplasia (BPH). LUTS and BPH increase rapidly with age starting at about 50 years. Straining, intermittency, postvoid dribbling, and weak stream may signify urethral obstruction from BPH. However, among men with diabetes, similar symptoms may also result from bladder dysfunction because of denervation and poor detrusor contractility. Other complex associations of LUTS and BPH among men with diabetes include symptoms of urgency, frequency, and nocturia that may occur from detrusor overactivity resulting from BPH, and/or microvascular complications associated with diabetes, increasing hyperactivity of the detrusor. Because previous studies have failed to differentiate LUTS from BPH in men with diabetes, the effect of diabetes on the development or presence of LUTS and BPH remains controversial *(8)*.

Recent evidence suggests that LUTS may occur more frequently among men with diabetes, with an estimated 25% to nearly twofold increased risk of LUTS in men with diabetes. Furthermore, among men with BPH, diabetes is associated with more LUTS symptoms compared with men without diabetes *(8)*. Experimental evidence suggests that early alterations in sodium and potassium channels occur in both BPH and diabetes similar to neuropathic models. These changes trigger altered excitability, leading to detrusor overactivity and urinary frequency. With time, impaired contractility because of a myopathy can lead to incomplete emptying. Thus, a combination of several factors with differing time courses lead to LUTS and known urodynamic findings, making discerning an etiology and distinguishing classic diabetic cystopathy from neural plasticity accompanying obstruction because of BPH problematic *(8)*.

Diagnostic Approach to Micturition Disturbances

In 40–80% of urologically asymptomatic patients with diabetes, abnormal findings were obtained in a detailed urodynamic work up. Many of these patients were aware of their abnormal micturition patterns only in structured questioning. However, these often asymptomatic micturition disturbances may have deleterious consequences for the upper urinary tract with significant renal impairment or even end stage renal disease. This low incidence of symptoms in the presence of possible severe consequences necessitates the inclusion of specific questions regarding micturition patterns in the yearly routine diabetic check up. Here, frequency, sensation of incomplete bladder emptying, UTI, urge symptoms, dysuria, nocturia, incontinence and necessity to use abdominal strain to empty the bladder should be specifically addressed. In unclear situations, a micturition protocol for three consecutive days and nights may be helpful. A urinary lab completes the routine urinary bladder function check *(1)*.

Given anamnestic hints for micturition disorders or recurrent UTI, a noninvasive urological work up consisting a uroflometry and a postvoid ultrasound of the bladder should be initiated. A full urological work up with formal urodynamics and radiological imaging of the urinary tract is needed in the presence of recurrent UTI or abnormal noninvasive findings. Endoscopic diagnostic procedures will be instituted according to the findings of the aforementioned diagnostics. Depending on the therapeutic option planned, further and mostly highly specialized diagnostic procedures are needed, for example, putting "temporary wires" as time-confined percutaneous testing of the effect of neurostimulation or instruction of self-catheterization before surgical construction of a catheterizable neobladder (*see* specific procedures) *(10)*.

Therapeutic Options for Micturition Disturbances

The need for treatment of micturition disorders is determined by the subjective and objective severeness of the impairment, by its etiology, its urological (nondiabetic) comorbidities, its secondary negative impact on the upper urinary tract as well as by the intellectual and manual capacities of the patient. Although autonomic neuropathy will most likely be a reason for voiding dysfunctions in a patient with diabetes, other cofactors or coetiologies such as hormone deficiency, obstructive prostatic hyperplasia, or urethral and meatal stenosis may play an important role and must be taken into account when treatment options are considered and discussed with the patient. To determine these individual variables, the aforementioned rationalized urological approach is mandatory before treatment. The majority of diabetic voiding dysfunctions can be safely managed by conservative approaches. However, close follow-up of the patient might be necessary for early detection of treatment failures and avoidance of secondary complications *(1)*.

Treatment of a *large capacity bladder* might start with regular voiding intervals (during daytime, three hourly intervals are often appropriate). Furthermore, the patient is advised to take his time to void and to try to relax his pelvic floor during micturition. An hypo- or even acontractile bladder may benefit from pharmacotherapy with parasympathomimetics. In the presence of a mild-to-moderate infravesical prostatic obstruction, an α-blocking drug can be additionally prescribed. If recurrent UTIs are observed inspite of these therapies and residual postvoid urine is significantly more than 100 mL, either clean intermitted self-catheterization (4–5 times daily) should be started or a suprapubic catheter be put. Surgical reduction of the bladder's capacity has not been very successful in the past; the ability of neuromodulation or -neurostimulation to restore bladder emptying in these patients (in the presence of autonomic neuropathy) also seems very limited *(10–13)*.

Anatomical *infravesical obstruction* is mostly seen in elderly male patients, although urethral strictures are a frequent cause of recurrent UTI in females. In case of a significant bladder outlet obstruction by BPH, ablative procedures (transurethral resection, laser evaporization, thermoablation, open surgery) should be recommended. Urethral or meatal strictures warrant endoscopic or formal repair *(14)*.

Stress *incontinence* by a descensus of the pelvic floor and insufficiency of the sphincteric mechanisms is a frequent finding in elderly women with diabetes. Depending on the severity of symptoms and the individual's preference, various approaches may be chosen. In mild-to-moderate cases, conservative options as functional rehabilitation by regular pelvic floor exercises, local or systemic hormonal replacement, or vaginal electrostimulation result in good therapeutic responses. However, these treatment modalities require regular application and good patient's motivation. The principle of the surgical correction for stress incontinence is elevation of the pelvic floor by various procedures. Here, success rates of minimally invasive sling procedures (Raz, Stamey) are at approximately 50% (or less than that figure) after 5 years, whereas formal surgical repair (fascial sling, Burch) attains rates of 80% dryness after 5 years. Implantation of an artificial sphincter for correction of urinary stress incontinence in an elderly diabetic should be critically discussed and remain a last resort if all other approaches failed as it is accompanied by an increased rate of prosthesis infection compared with the nondiabetic *(1)*.

Pollakiuria, dysuria, *urge*, or incontinence symptoms may be caused by neurogenic bladder hyperreflexia in the patient with diabetes. Compared with stress incontinence, most of these symptoms respond well to conservative treatment. The mainstay of pharmacotherapy are antimuscarinic or "spasmolytic" (direct smooth muscle relaxant) agents; however, as these pharmacological approaches exert none or only very limited bladder selectivity, their individual effectivity is often limited. Nonpharmacological approaches for the urge symptom complex consist vaginal electrostimulation as well as neuromodulation (electrical stimulation of sacral nerves) *(1)*.

ERECTILE DYSFUNCTION

Epidemiology

Erectile dysfunction (ED), defined as the consistent or recurrent inability of a man to attain and/or maintain a penile erection sufficient for sexual activity *(15)*, is one of the most common sexual dysfunctions in men. ED is more common with advancing age, and since the aged population will increase, its prevalence will continue to rise *(16)*. Diabetes mellitus is the most frequent organic cause for ED, the onset of which starts about 15 years earlier in the diabetic than in the nondiabetic population. In the Massachusetts Male Aging Study (MMAS), the age-adjusted prevalence of minimal, moderate, or complete ED was 17, 25, and 10% among 1238 men without diabetes and 8, 30, and 25% among 52 treated men with diabetes, respectively *(17)*. Thus, although the number of diabetic subjects in the MMAS was low, this population based study showed an increased prevalence particularly of complete ED among men with diabetes. In the Cologne Male Survey *(18)* the prevalence of ED was threefold increased, reaching 60% among men with diabetes compared with only 19% in the general population. The presence of diabetes was associated with an increased odds ratio for ED by 3.95 (2.98–5.23). The prevalence of ED in the younger age groups (40–60 years) with diabetes was as high as in the older groups without diabetes (60–80 years). Thus, in presence of diabetes the development of ED starts around 20 years earlier than in the nondiabetic population. The crude incidence rate of ED in the MMAS was 26 cases/1000 man-years in 847 men aged 40–69 without ED at baseline who were followed for an average of 8.8 years *(19)*. Population projections for men in this age group suggest an estimate of 617.715 new cases of ED per year for the United States. The age adjusted risk of ED was higher for men with lower education, diabetes, heart disease, and hypertension. The incidence rate of ED in men with diabetes was twofold increased, with 50 cases/1000 man-years. In a population based study from southern Wisconsin the prevalence of ED among 365 patients with type 1 diabetes increased with increasing age from 1.1% in those aged 21–30 years to 47.1% in those 43 years of age or older and with increasing duration of diabetes *(20)*. In a study from Italy including 9868 men with diabetes, 45.5% of those aged more than 59 years reported ED. Risk factors and clinical correlates included the following (OR [95% CI]): autonomic neuropathy (5.0 [3.9–6.4]), diabetic foot (4 [2.9–5.5]), peripheral neuropathy (3.3 [2.9–3.8]), peripheral arterial disease (2.8 [2.4–3.3]), nephropathy (2.3 [1.9–2.8]), poor glycemic control (2.3 [2–2.6]), retinopathy (2.2 [2.0–2.4]), hypertension (2.1 [1.6–2.9]), and diabetes duration (2 [1.8–2.2]) *(21)*. In another survey from Italy the combination of diabetes and hypertension was the major risk factor for ED, giving an OR (95% CI) of 8.1 (1.2–55) as compared with diabetes without hypertension at 4.6 (1.6–13.7), hypertension without diabetes at 1.4 (0.7–3.2), current smoking at 1.7 (1.2–2.4), and exsmoking at 1.6 (1.1–2.3) *(22)*. However, even when neuropathic complications are present, psychiatric illness such as generalized anxiety disorder or depression may be important contributors to ED in men with diabetes *(23)*. Thus, a psychogenic component must not be overlooked in many patients.

Physiology and Pathophysiology

Penile erection is a neurovascular event modulated by psychological factors and hormonal status depending on appropriate trabecular smooth muscle and arterial relaxation in the corpus cavernosum. On sexual stimulation, nerve impulses cause the release of cholinergic and NANC neurotransmitters that mediate erectile function by relaxing the smooth muscle of the corpus cavernosum. A principal neural mediator of erection is nitric oxide (NO), which activates guanil cyclase to form intracellular cyclic guanosine monophosphate (GMP), a potent second messenger for smooth muscle relaxation (Fig. 1). Cyclic GMP in turn activates a specific protein kinase, which phosphorylates certain proteins and ion channels, resulting in a drop of cytosolic calcium concentrations and relaxation of the smooth muscle. During the return to the flaccid state, cyclic GMP is hydrolyzed GMP by phosphodiesterase (PDE) type 5 *(2,9)*. In the corpus cavernosum four PDE isoforms have been identified (types 2–5), but PDE 5 is the predominant isoform, whereas the others do not appear to have an important role in erection *(24)*.

The pathogenesis of ED in diabetes is thought to be multifactorial as it may be linked to neuropathy, accelerated atherosclerosis, and alterations in the corporal erectile tissue. Such alterations may include smooth muscle degeneration, abnormal collagen deposition, and endothelial cell dysfunction *(25)*. If irreversible, these corporal degenerative changes can limit the success of any pharmacotherapy. Advanced glycation end products

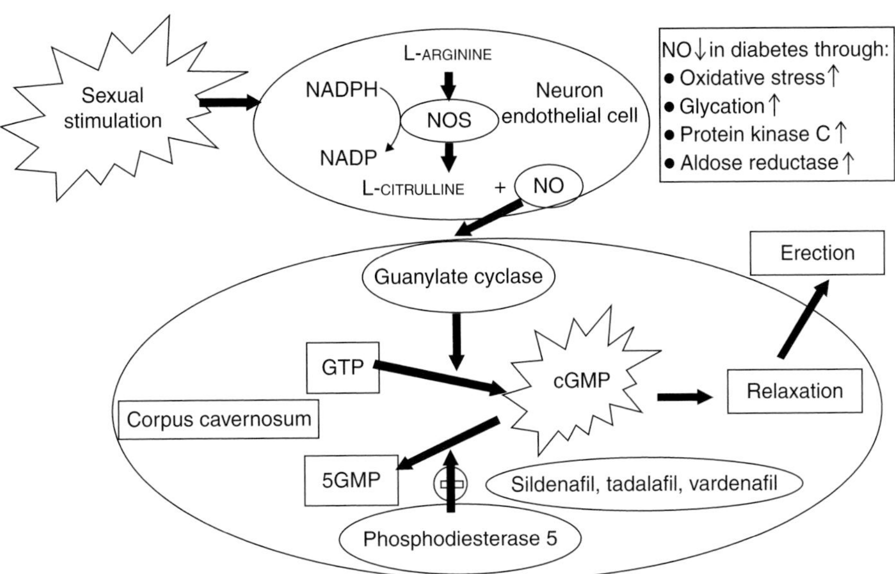

Fig. 1. Mechanisms of erection mediated by cavernosal smooth muscle relaxation including the generation of nitric oxide by nitric oxide synthase, which is impaired in diabetes. ROS, reactive oxygen species; PKC, protein kinase C; AR, aldose reductase.

have been shown to quench NO and to be elevated in human diabetic penile tissue. It has been hypothesized that advanced glycation end products may mediate ED through upregulation of inducible nitric oxide synthase and downregulation of endothelial NOS (eNOS) *(26)*. Furthermore, protein kinase C activation by diabetes may reduce NOS activity *(27)*.

In vivo studies of isolated corpus cavernosum tissue from men with diabetes have shown functional impairment in neurogenic and endothelium-dependent relaxation of corpus cavernosum smooth muscle *(28)*. In diabetic rats endothelium-dependent NO mediated relaxation to acetylcholine and NANC stimulation are reduced by 40% after 4–8 weeks *(29)*. These alterations were prevented by administration of the antioxidant α-lipoic acid, suggesting an involvement of increased oxidative stress. In contrast, endothelium-independent relaxation to the NO donor sodium nitroprusside is not impaired by diabetes *(29)*. Increased penile endothelial and total NOS activity was found after 2–3 months in diabetic rats *(30)*. However, after 4–8 months reduced penile total (endothelial and neuronal) NOS activity and neuronal NOS levels were observed in type 1 and type 2 diabetic rats *(31)*. Thus, diabetes-induced changes in NOS activity may be biphasic, with an initial increase followed by a decrease. Because RhoA/Rho-kinase may suppress eNOS, RhoA/Rho-kinase could contribute to diabetes-related erectile dysfunction and downregulation of eNOS. Colocalization of Rho-kinase and eNOS protein is present in the endothelium of the corpus cavernosum. Diabetic rats transfected with an adeno-associated virus encoding the dominant-negative RhoA mutant (AAVTCMV19NRhoA) had a reduction in RhoA/Rho-kinase and MYPT-1 phosphorylation at a time when cavernosal eNOS protein, constitutive NOS activity, and cGMP levels were restored to levels found in control rats. AAVT19NRhoA gene transfer

Table 1
Practical Three-Step Algorithm for Diagnosis of Erectile Dysfunction

Step 1:	General sexual history
	Clinical examination; relevant laboratory parameters
	Information about treatment options
Step 2:	Therapeutic trial with PDE5 inhibitor
Step 3:	Intracavernous pharmacotesting: color Doppler or duplex ultrasound of penile arteries

improved erectile responses in the diabetic rats to values similar to controls. Thus, activation of the RhoA/Rho-kinase pathway may represent one important mechanism for the down-regulation of penile eNOS in diabetes, implying that inhibition of RhoA/Rho-kinase improves eNOS protein content and activity and thereby restores erectile function in diabetes *(32)*.

Diagnosis

A good clinical history and physical examination are the basis of assessment. It is important to establish the nature of the erectile problem and to distinguish it from other forms of sexual difficulty, such as penile curvature or premature ejaculation. An interview with the partner is advisable and will confirm the problem, but might also reveal other causes of the difficulties, for example, vaginal dryness. The relative importance of psychological and organic factors may be determined from the history. Drugs which may be associated with ED include tranquillizers (phenothiazines, benzodiazepines), antidepressants (tricyclics, selective serotonin reuptake inhibitors), and antihypertensives (β-blockers, vasodilators, central sympathomimetics, ganglion blockers, diuretics, ACE inhibitors) *(33)*. In most patients sophisticated investigation is not indicated. A three-step diagnostic approach is shown in Table 1. A detailed history is most important, and for many patients examination can be limited to the regular monitoring of diabetes and its risk factors and complications as well as examination of the genitalia. Patients should be informed about the advantages and disadvantages of each treatment and given advice on treatment outcome and ease of use *(34)*.

Management

A stepwise therapeutic approach for ED is shown in Table 2. An algorithm for treatment of ED has recently been suggested by the second international consultation on erectile and sexual dysfunctions (*15*; Fig. 2). The initial management should be to advise the patient to reduce possible risk factors and to optimize glycemic control. However, no studies are available to show that improvement in glycemic control will exert a favorable effect on ED. In fact, a recent study could not demonstrate an effect of intensive diabetes therapy maintained for 2 years on ED in men with type 2 diabetes *(35)*. Healthy lifestyle factors are associated with maintenance of erectile function in men. A controlled study recently evaluated the effect of weight loss and increased physical activity on erectile and endothelial functions in obese men. Men randomly assigned to the intervention group received detailed advice about how to achieve a loss of 10% or more in their total body weight by reducing caloric intake and increasing their level of physical activity. Men in the control group were given general information about healthy food

Table 2
Stepwise Algorithm for Treatment of Erectile Dysfunction

General management	Control of risk factors and diabetes; sexual counseling	
Pharmacological treatment	*First line therapy*	*Dose range*
	Sildenafil (Viagra)	50–100 mg
	Vardenafil (Levitra)	10–20 mg
	Tadalafil (Cialis)	10–20 mg
	Oral therapy inappropriate	
	Transurethral alprostadil (MUSE)	500–1000 μg
	Intracavernosal injection therapy:	
	Alprostadil (Caverject®)	5–20 μg
	Papaverine/phentolamine (Androskat)	
	Thymoxamine (Erecnos)	10–20 mg
	VIP/Phentolamine (Invicorp)	
	Papaverine/phentolamine/alprostadil (Trimix)	
Surgery and mechanical treatments	*Pharmacological therapy inappropriate*	
	Vacuum devices	
	Arterial/venous surgery	
	Penile prostheses	

choices and exercise. After 2 years the mean international index of erectile function (IIEF) score improved in the intervention group from 13.9 to 17 points, but not in the control group. In multivariate analyses, changes in body-mass index, physical activity, and C-reactive protein were independently associated with changes in IIEF score. Thus, lifestyle changes are associated with improvement in sexual function in obese men with ED *(36)*.

Even if the cause is organic, almost all men with ED will be affected psychologically. Sexual counseling is an important aspect of any treatment, and it is preferable to also involve the partner.

Oral Agents

Most men consider this to be the treatment of choice. The oral treatment options and their mechanisms of action are summarized in Table 3.

Central Initiators

Yohimbine. Yohimbine was the first drug officially listed for this indication. Yohimbine acts through central α-2-receptor blockade and thus, increases the centrally initiated efferences of the erectogenic axis. Although, its effectivity is often debated because of insufficient historic data, it showed a significant effect in a recent double blind prospective study compared with placebo. Its side effect profile is benign including palpitations, tremor, hypertension, and anxiety. The proerectile effect usually starts after about 2 weeks *(37)*. In a meta-analysis yohimbine has been found to be more effective than placebo for all types of ED combined, but the effect was most prominent in nonorganic ED *(38)*. Because of its marginal effect on organic ED, yohimbine cannot be generally recommended for treatment of ED in men with diabetes.

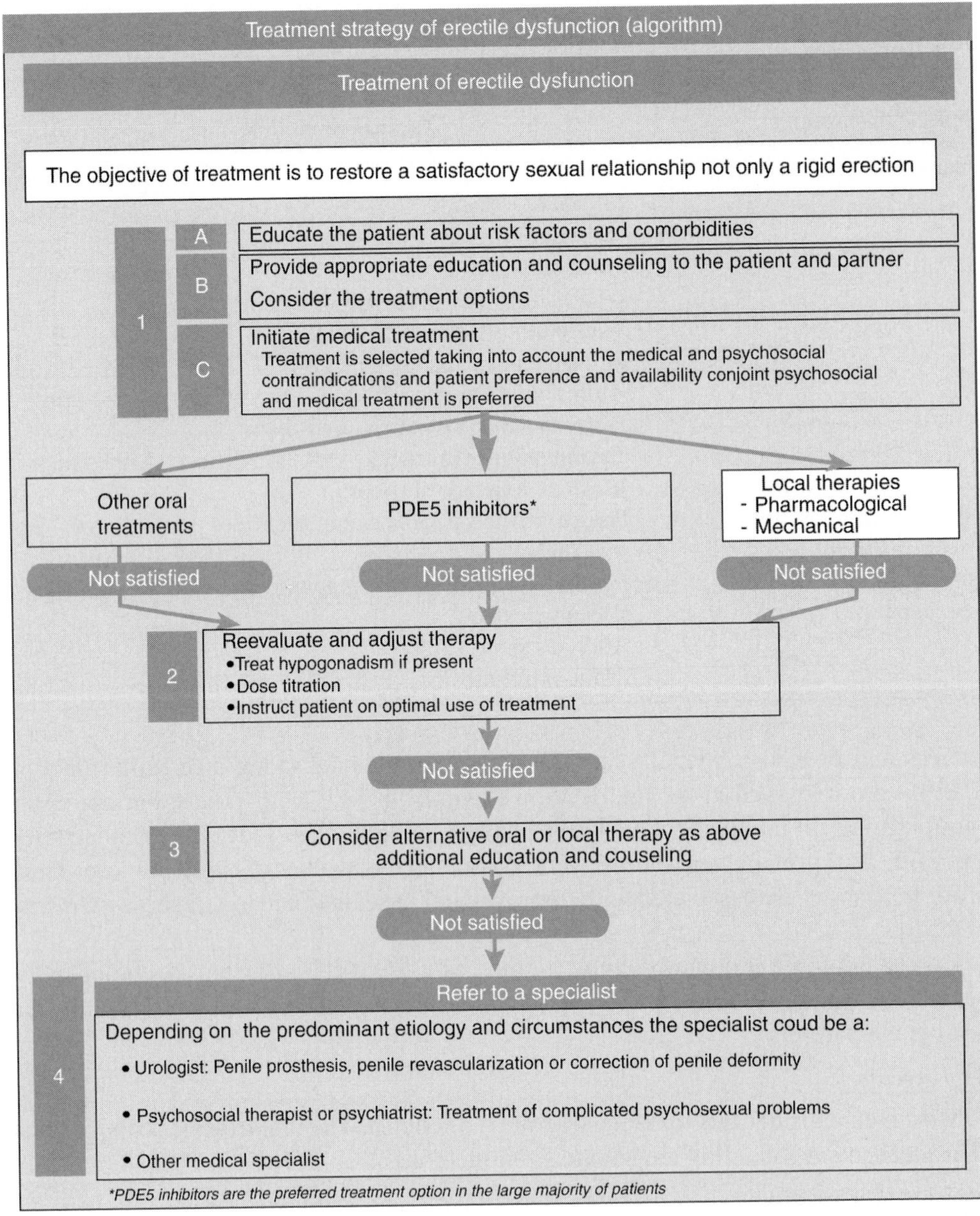

Fig. 2. Algorithm for treatment of erectile dysfunction *(15)*.

Apomorphine. Apomorphine is a potent emetic agent that acts through central dopaminergic (D1 or D2) receptors as well as central m-, d-, and k-receptors. In the hypothalamus, it increases the centrally initiated efferences of the erectogenic axis thus, improving the erectile response in a patient with erectile failure *(39)*. In large multicenter studies, a proerectile effect with full erections was observed after sublingual doses of 2, 4, and 6 mg apomorphine with an acceptable and dose-dependent rate of nausea side effects. A dose-dependent efficacy (defined as erections allowing intercourse/attempts) of 48–66% vs 37% for Placebo was observed. Similarly, side effects were also

Table 3
Agents for Oral Treatment of Erectile Dysfunction

Central mechanism of action
- Yohimbine (α_2 adrenergic antagonist)
- Apomorphine (dopamine receptor agonist)

Peripheral mechanism of action
- Phentolamine (nonselective adrenergic antagonist)
- Phosphodiesterase isoenzyme type 5 inhibitors:
  - Sildenafil
  - Vardenafil
  - Tadalafil

strongly dose-dependent: Nausea was seen in 0.4–17% (vs 0.2–0.4% for Placebo), hypotension in 0.7–4.8 and syncope in 0.7–2.1%. These side effects tended to disappear in frequency and intensity with increasing use of the medication in an individual patient. There was no effect of apomorphine on mood and desire *(40,41)*.

A 4-week multicenter, cross-over, placebo-controlled trial using the sublingual formulation of apomorphine (Uprima®) evaluated 90 patients with diabetes on the 4 mg dose and 86 patients on the 5 mg dose. The percent of attempts resulting in an erection firm enough for intercourse (primary end point) were 14.5 and 24.6% for placebo and 4 mg, respectively ($p = 0.02$) and 27.2 and 34.1% for placebo and 5 mg, respectively ($p = 0.18$). In the posthoc combined analysis the corresponding rates were 20.4 and 28.9%, respectively ($p = 0.009$). Thus, no dose response could be demonstrated in this trial. The FDA concluded from these data that even though the 4 mg dose and the combined analysis showed statistical significance, the clinical significance is questionable because of the relatively modest benefits noted over placebo *(42)*. Indeed, the number needed to treat for the 4 mg dose treatment based on the aforementioned results is relatively high, i.e., 10 patients need to be treated in order to achieve an erection firm enough for intercourse in 1 of these patients. The rates of nausea, the most prominent adverse effect of apomorphine, were 21.2, 12.9, and 1% for 4 mg, 5 mg, and placebo, respectively. The corresponding rates of vomiting were 6.7, 1, and 0%, respectively. Moreover, three syncopal events and three episodes of significant hypotension were reported in patients taking apomorphine *(42)*.

PERIPHERAL CONDITIONERS

Phosphodiesterase 5 Inhibitors

Sildenafil (Viagra®). To understand the mode of action of Sildenafil, a drug believed to act predominantly through PDE 5-inhibition, the basic physiology is briefly explained. The cAMP and cGMP are synthesized from the corresponding nucleoside triphosphates by their respective membrane bound or soluble adenylate or guanylate cyclases. cAMP and cGMP are inactivated by PDE and by hydrolytic cleavage of the 3′-ribose-phosphate bond (*see* Fig. 1). Because the distribution and functional role of PDE isoenzymes varies in different tissues, selective inhibitors have the potential to exert at least partially specific tissue effects. Currently, more than 40 PDE-isoenzymes and -isoforms are known *(43)*. The functional assays revealed a predominant functional role for PDE3 and 5 *(44)*. There was no difference in PDE-expression in patients with diabetes compared with patients without diabetes with erectile dysfunction.

Sildenafil acts as conditioner on the cavernous smooth muscle side by blocking PDE5. It is the first effective oral drug that has been approved for the treatment of ED and is generally regarded as a first-line treatment of ED of various causes including diabetes. Sildenafil is taken 60 minutes before anticipated sexual activity and its effects last approximately 4 hours. The drug is available in three doses (25, 50, or 100 mg). It does not stimulate the sexual desire and provoke an erection as such, but enhances the continued relaxation of the cavernous smooth muscle initiated by the release of endogenous nitric oxide with an improved quality of erection (Fig. 1).

In a controlled, flexible-dose US multicenter trial including a mixed group of 268 men with type 1 and type 2 diabetes the rates of those with improved erections after 12 weeks of treatment with 25–100 mg sildenafil were 56% as compared with 10% in the placebo group *(45)*. In a 12-week European multicenter trial including 219 men with type 2 diabetes the response rate was even higher achieving 64.6% on sildenafil vs 10.5% on placebo *(46)*. The estimated percent of intercourse attempts that were successful significantly improved from baseline to end of treatment in patients receiving sildenafil (14.4–58.8%) compared with those receiving placebo (13.2–14.4%). Three quarters of the patients required the 100 mg sildenafil dose. The response rates were independent of the baseline HbA1c levels and number of chronic complications, thus suggesting that sildenafil is effective in improving ED even in cases with poor glycemic control and in presence of angiopathy and neuropathy. In a combined analysis of 11 controlled trials of sildenafil (25–100 mg) the percents of the maximum score for the six questions in the erectile function domain of the IIEF were 6% among 69 type 1 and 60.8% among 399 men with type 1 diabetes on sildenafil as compared with 39.3% among 452 men with diabetes on placebo *(47)*.

Side effects consist mainly of headache (18%), facial flushing (15%), and dyspepsia (2%). A mild and transient disturbance of color vision and also increased sensitivity to light or blurred vision has been found in 4.5% of men with diabetes *(46)*. Concerns have been expressed regarding an increased number of deaths associated with sildenafil as compared with other treatments for ED *(48)*. However, after an average follow-up of 6 months the prescription event monitoring study including 5601 sildenafil users from England showed an expected mortality rate of 28.9/1000 per year for ischaemic heart disease/myocardial infarctions. The comparison rate in the general population of England in 1998 was 73.9/1000 per year *(49)*, whereas the prevalence of diabetes in the cohort was 15%, which is similar to the rate of 16% included in the clinical trials of sildenafil, but higher than the rate of 3.3% of men with diabetes. Although, these results are reassuring, further follow-up of this study and other pharmacoepidemiological research is needed for confirmation. In men with severe stenosis of at least one coronary artery, acute administration of sildenafil (100 mg) did not result in adverse haemodynamic effects on coronary blood flow or vascular resistance, but coronary flow reserve was improved *(50)*.

Apart from its effect on ED, favorable effects of sildenafil have recently been reported in pilot studies of various disorders including primary pulmonary hypertension, achalasia, and endothelial dysfunction. The endothelium modulates the actual and the demand vascular tone, the antithrombotic and antiadhesive properties of the vessel wall, vascular wall architecture, and vascular permeability. Endothelial dysfunction is regarded as an early key event in the development of atherosclerosis, which is accelerated in diabetes. It has recently been demonstrated that erectile and endothelial dysfunction are associated in patients with type 2 diabetes. Plasma concentrations of markers for endothelial dysfunction such as, soluble thrombomodulin, P-selectin, and intercellular cell adhesion molecules-1 were significantly elevated in patients with type 2 diabetes with ED compared with those without ED and were inversely related to the IIEF *(51)*. Endothelium-dependent flow-mediated dilatation induced by 5 minutes occlusion of the brachial artery measured by ultrasound imaging is a reliable index of endothelial function that is impaired in patients with diabetes. In a recent controlled crossover trial acute (25 mg) and chronic (25 mg per day for 2 weeks) administration of sildenafil (25 mg) improved endothelial function as compared with placebo in patients with type 2 diabetes, suggesting that PDE-5 inhibition may exert favorable cardiovascular effects *(52)*. Thus, similarly, in patients with heart failure who frequently show endothelial dysfunction, the latter was improved after single-dose administration of 25 and 50 mg sildenafil, respectively *(53)*. These findings require further confirmation in larger studies.

According to the recommendations of the American Heart Association sildenafil is contraindicated in men taking nitrates because of the risk of hypotension and those with severe cardiovascular disease. Before sildenafil is prescribed, treadmill testing may be indicated in men with heart disease to assess the risk of cardiac ischemia during sexual intercourse. Initial monitoring of blood pressure after the administration of sildenafil may be indicated in men with congestive heart disease who have borderline low blood pressure and low volume status and men being treated with complicated, multidrug antihypertensive regimens *(54)*.

Because sildenafil treatment is costly and ED is not a life-threatening illness, the appropriateness of insurance coverage for sildenafil has been questioned. However, recent cost-effectiveness studies using cost per quality-adjusted life-year gained as outcome measures have shown that sildenafil treatment compared favorably with intracavernosal injection therapy *(55)* or with accepted therapies for other medical conditions *(56)*.

Because some men do not respond to sildenafil treatment, attempts have been undertaken to characterize these nonresponders. A recent penile biopsy study identified severe vascular lesions and atrophy of cavernous smooth muscle to represent the main factors that determined the lack in response to 100 mg sildenafil in men with ED aged from 28 to 74 years. The age, diabetes, and low testosterone level were not related to the response failures *(57)*.

Tadalafil (Cialis®). In a 12-week multicenter trial including 216 men with diabetes (type 2: 91%), but excluding sildenafil nonresponders, the rates of men with improved erections were 64% with 20 mg tadalafil, 56% with 10 mg tadalafil, and 25% on placebo *(58)*. Both tadalafil 10 mg and 20 mg were superior to placebo in improving penetration ability (IIEF question 3) and ability to maintain an erection during intercourse. Thus, although nonresponders to sildenafil were excluded, the effect of tadalafil was not superior to that of sildenafil. Treatment-related adverse events (>5%) on 20 mg, 10 mg, and placebo were dyspepsia (8.3, 11, and 0%) and headache (6.9, 8.2, and 1.4%). Despite more severe baseline erectile dysfunction in men with diabetes as compared with the men without diabetes with ED, tadalafil was efficacious and well tolerated. As reported for other PDE type 5 inhibitors, the response to tadalafil was slightly

Parameter	Vardenafil (20 mg)	Sildenafil (100 mg)	Tadalafil (20 mg)
T_{max} (min)	40	70	120 (30–720)
$T_{1/2}$ (h)	4–4.8	3.8	17.5

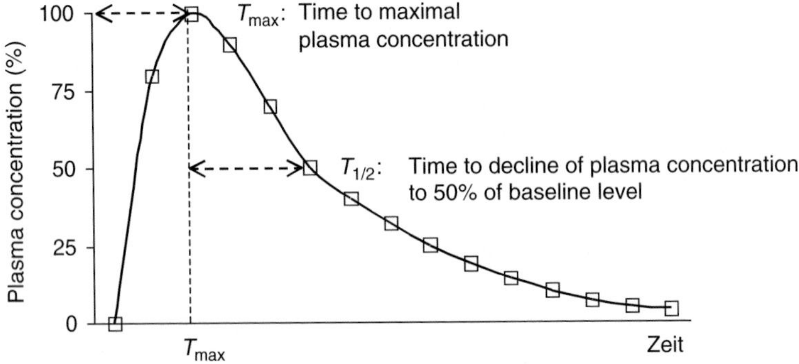

Fig. 3. Pharmacokinetics of PDE 5 inhibitors.

lower in men with diabetes than in men without diabetes *(59)*. The pharmacokinetic profile of tadalafil differs from that of sildenafil and vardenafil in that it has a much longer half-life (Fig. 3). This means that the effect of tadalafil might last for more than 24 h or even longer, whereas the duration of action for the other two drugs is around 4–5 hours. Such a longer "window of opportunity" may be preferable by some men, but similarly possible side effects may also be prolonged.

Vardenafil (Levitra®). In a large 12-week multicenter trial including 439 men with diabetes (type 2: 88%) that excluded sildenafil nonresponders, the rates of men with improved erections were 72% with 20 mg vardenafil, 57% with 10 mg vardenafil, and 13% on placebo *(60a)*. Both vardenafil 10 mg and 20 mg were superior to placebo in improving the IIEF erectile function domain score (questions 1–5, 15). In a recent study including 302 men with type 1 diabetes vardenafil given in a flexible dose of 5–20 mg effectively improved erectile function regardless of the level of glycemic control and as well as tolerated *(60b)*. Similar to tadalafil, despite the exclusion of nonresponders to sildenafil the effect of vardenafil was comparable to that reported previously for sildenafil. Treatment-related adverse events (>5%) on 20 mg, 10 mg, and placebo were headache (10, 9, and 2%), flushing (10, 9, and <1%), and headache (6, 3, and 0%).

Phentolamine (Vasomax®). The nonselective α-blocking agent phentolamine was evaluated for a possible beneficial effect on the erectile behavior. In prospective, randomized, double blind studies, a beneficial effect of orally administered fast-resolving phentolamine on the erectile capacity of men with erectile dysfunction was shown. These beneficial effects were more pronounced in elderly men. The side effect profile of this drug introduced decades ago for other indications seems to be safe with stuffy nose and some hypotension being the most frequent complaints. However, published data are minimal so that a thorough evaluation is not possible for the moment *(61)*.

Vacuum Devices

These have the merit of being noninvasive and may be effective in all men. They create a vacuum around the penis and blood is drawn into the corporal spaces. A band is slipped off the plastic cylinder around the base of the penis to maintain penile tumescence without rigidity in the crura. The disadvantages are that they require some degree of dexterity in handling them, and some time spent in application of the device. They should only be used for 30 minutes at a time, and require the willing cooperation of the partner. There are few side effects although there is some degree of discomfort and the penis feels cold. Ejaculation is usually blocked and some men feel this makes orgasm less satisfactory. Bruising can occur in 10–15% of men. Vacuum devices are particularly useful in older men in stable relationships and when other treatment options are ineffective. They may also be used to augment the result of pharmacotherapy. Some men find that the constrictive ring is a useful aid in itself for maintaining the erection without the use of a vacuum device *(33)*. However, the long-term drop-out rates among users of vacuum constriction devices are relatively high. A recent study showed an overall drop-out rate of more than 3 years for the ErecAid® system of 65%, i.e., 100% in men with mild ED, 56% in those with moderate ED, and 70% in those with complete ED. The main reasons for stopping its use were that the device was ineffective (57%), too cumbersome (24%), and too painful (20%) *(62)*.

Transurethral Alprostadil

Alprostadil was first licensed for the treatment of erectile dysfunction by intracavernous injection. Alprostadil, the synthetic preparation of the naturally occurring prostaglandin E1 acts by initiating the erection. In contrast to sildenafil it initiates the relaxation of cavernous smooth muscle to bring about erection. This drug has been incorporated into a pellet that can be given by intraurethral application medical urethral system for erection (MUSE). Patients need to be instructed in the use of MUSE which is introduced into the urethra with a disposable applicator. The patient first passes urine to act as a lubricant to facilitate the passage of the applicator and the absorption of the drug. Absorption of the drug is also facilitated by the patient rolling his penis between the palms of his hands. Some patients find that a constrictive ring around the base of the penis enhances the efficacy. The erection takes about 10 minutes to develop and the dose range varies between 125 and 1000 μg although the majority of patients require 500 or 1000 μg. The use of MUSE is contraindicated without a condom when the partner is pregnant or likely to conceive *(33)*.

In the US and European multicenter trials about 65% of men with different causes of ED who tried MUSE had erections sufficient for intercourse during in-clinic testing *(63,64)*. About half of the treatments at home were successful, but the drop-out rate after 15 months was 75%, the main reason being lack of efficacy *(64)*. The most common side effects are penile pain (30%), urethral burning (12%), or minor urethral bleeding (5%) *(65)*. Systemic side effects (such as hypotension or even syncope) were usually uncommon but helped to highlight the role of the physician in administering the first supervised dose. Disappointing results have been reported in a study conducted in a urology practice setting, in which an adequate rigidity score was achieved in only 13 and 30% of the patients using 500 and 1000 μg, respectively. Pain, discomfort, or burning in the penis were observed in 18%, but orthostatic hypotension (defined as a decrease in systolic/diastolic blood pressure by

20/10 mmHg or orthostatic symptoms) was present in 41% of the patients. The discontinuation rate was very high, achieving 81% after 2–3 months *(66)*.

Intracavernosal Injection Therapy

Intracavernosal therapy requires some specialist knowledge and the ability to treat priapism should it occur. Many specialists used to regard this as the standard treatment and use it for both diagnostic and therapeutic reasons although its role as first line therapy has been replaced by less invasive treatment modalities. Patients need to be taught how to perform selfinjection and the dose needs to be chosen carefully to avoid prolonged erections or priapism. Some patients find it helpful to use one of the many autoinjector devices available. The erection occurs after 10 minutes and may be enhanced by sexual stimulation. The incidence of complications varies with the different pharmacological agents. Some pain is not uncommon but long-term problems are limited to priapism or penile fibrosis.

Alprostadil is the most widely used agent *(67,68)*. It is effective in more than 80% of patients with different aetiologies of ED and has a low incidence of side effects. In a recent comparative study of intracavernosal vs intraurethral administration of alprostadil the rates of erections sufficient for sexual intercourse were 82.5 vs 53.0%, respectively *(68)*. Patient and partner satisfaction was higher with intracavernosal injection, and more patients preferred this therapy. Penile pain occurs in 15–50% of patients but is often not troublesome. The dose range is 5–20 μg but some physicians will increase it further or use a combination with papaverine and phentolamine. Priapism occurs in about 1% of patients. The cumulative incidence of penile fibrosis was 11.7% after a period of 4 years, and the risk of irreversible fibrotic alterations was 5% *(69)*. About half of the cases with fibrosis resolved spontaneously. Other less frequently used agents include thymoxamine (moxisylyte hydrocholoride [Erecnos®]), papaverine/phentolamine mixtures (Androskat®), papaverine/phentolamine/alprostadil mixtures (Trimix®), and VIP/Phentolamine (Invicorp®).

Penile Prostheses and Surgery

This type of treatment is carried out only after careful patient selection and a trial of the less invasive options. There are a number of different devices ranging from the simple malleable prosthesis to more complex hydraulic prostheses. The choice of prosthesis is very much dependent on the wishes of the patient and is often cost-related. A prosthesis does not restore a normal erection but makes the penis rigid enough for sexual intercourse. The hydraulic prostheses have the advantage of flaccidity and are now mechanically reliable with revision rates less than 5% per annum. Infection remains a major complication in approximately 3–5% of cases with different causes of ED and usually leads to removal of the device *(33)*. Arterial reconstruction is associated with complication rates of more than 30% and remains an experimental procedure which cannot be generally recommended to patients with diabetes with ED.

OTHER SEXUAL PROBLEMS IN MEN WITH DIABETES

Diminished or absent testicular pain has been described as an early sign of autonomic neuropathy. Retrograde ejaculation from the prostatic urethra into the bladder might occur occasionally and follows loss of sympathetic innervation of the internal sphincter, which normally contracts during ejaculation. Complete loss of ejaculation probably indicates widespread pelvic sympathetic involvement and, like retrograde ejaculation, causes infertility, which may be treated by insemination *(70)*.

FEMALE SEXUAL DYSFUNCTION

Female sexual dysfunctions (FSD) include persistent or recurrent disorders of sexual interest/desire, disorders of subjective and genital arousal, orgasm disorder, pain and difficulty with attempted or completed intercourse. The scientific knowledge on sexual dysfunction in women with diabetes is rudimentary. Sexual dysfunction was observed in 27% of women with type 1 diabetes. FSD was not related to age, BMI, HbA1c, duration of diabetes, and diabetic complications. However, FSD was related to depression and the quality of the partner relationship *(71)*. Recently, the prevalence of FSD in premenopausal women with the metabolic syndrome was compared with the general female population. Women with the metabolic syndrome had reduced mean full female sexual function index score, reduced satisfaction rate, and higher circulating levels of C-reactive protein (CRP). There was an inverse relation between CRP levels and female sexual function index score *(72)*.

Problems affecting sexuality in women with diabetes are fatigue, changes in perimenstrual blood glucose control, vaginitis, decreased sexual desire, decreased vaginal lubrication, and an increased time to reach orgasm. Even minor episodes of depression, which is twice more frequent than in men can result in a loss of libido. To which degree these symptoms are related to autonomic neuropathy has also been examined in a few studies, the results of which are at variance *(73)*. The examination for a women with diabetes with sexual dysfunction should include the duration of symptoms, psychological state, concommitant, medications, presence of vaginitis, cystitis and other infections, frequency of intercourse, blood pressure, BMI, retinal status, pelvic examination, presence of discharge, and glycemic control *(74)*.

REFERENCES

1. Stief CG, Ziegler D. Diabetic autonomic neuropathy. Urogenital system, In *Textbook of diabetic neuropathy* (Gries FA, Cameron NE, Low PA, Ziegler D, eds.), Thieme, Stuttgart, New York, 2003;262–274.
2. Paro M, Prashar A, Prosdocimi M, Cherian PV, Fiori MG, Sima, AAF. Urinary bladder dyfunction in the BB/W diabetic rat. *J Urol* 1994;151:781–786.
3. Liu G, Daneshgari F. Alterations in neurogenically mediated contractile responses of urinary bladder in rats with diabetes. *Am J Physiol Renal Physiol* 2005;288:F1220–F1226.
4. Mannikarottu AS, Changolkar AK, Disanto ME, Wein AJ, Chacko S. Over expression of smooth muscle thin filament associated proteins in the bladder wall of diabetics. *J Urol* 2005;174:360–364.
5. Ellenberg M. Development of urinary bladder dysfunction in diabetes mellitus. *Ann Int Med* 1980;92:321–323.
6. Kaplan SA, Blavas TeAE, Urodynamic findings in patients with diabetic cystopathy. *J Urol* 1995;153:342–344.
7. Starer P, Libow L. Cystometric evaluation of bladder dysfunction in elderly diabetic patients. *Arch Intern Med* 1990;150:810–816.
8. Brown JS, Wessells H, Chancellor MB, et al. Urologic complications of diabetes. *Diabetes Care* 2005;28:177–185.
9. Jackson RA, Vittinghoff E, Kanaya AM, et al. Aging and Body Composition (Health ABC) Research Group: Urinary incontinence in elderly women: finding from the Health, Aging, and Body Composition Study. *Obstet Gynecol* 2004;104:301–307.

10. Thon WF, und Stief CG. Blasenfunktionsstörungen als urologische Diabetes-Komplikation. *Der Kassenarzt* 1996;23:40–48.
11. Thon WF, und Grünewald V. Neurostimulation. *Curr Opin Urol* 1993;3:295–302.
12. Grünewald V, Thon WF, Jonas U. Neuromodulation bei neurogener Blasenfunktionsstörung, In Neurogene Blasenfunktionsstörungen (herausgeg von Stöhrer M, Madersbacher H, und Palmtag H, eds.), Springer, Heidelberg 1996, pp. 163–175.
13. Thon WF. Elektrostimulation der sakralen Spinalnerven bei Blasenfunktionsstörungen. *Med Welt* 1994;45:195–203.
14. Eri LM, Tveter KJ. Alpha blockade in the treatment of symptomatic benign prostatic hyperplasia. *J Urol* 1995;154:923–934.
15. Lue TF, Giuliano F, Montorsi F, et al. Summary of the recommendations on sexual dysfunctions in men. *J Sex Med* 2004;1:6–23.
16. Wagner G, Saenz de, Tejada I. Update on male erectile dysfunction. *Br Med J* 1998;316: 678–682.
17. Feldman HA, Goldstein I, Hatzichristou DG, Krane RJ, McKinlay JB. Impotence and its medical and psychosocial correlates: results of the Massachusetts male ageing study. *J Urol* 1994;151:54–61.
18. Braun M, Wassmer G, Klotz T, Reifenrath B, Mathers M, Engelmann U. Epidemiology of erectile dysfunction: results of the "Cologne Male Survey." *Int J Impot Res* 2000;12:305–311.
19. Johannes CB, Araujo AB, Feldman HA, Derby CA, Kleinman KP, McKinlay JB. Incidence of erectile dysfunction in men 40 to 69 years old: longitudinal results from the Massachusetts male aging study. *J Urol* 2000;163:460–463.
20. Klein R, Klein BE, Lee KE, Moss SE, Cruickshanks KJ. Prevalence of self-reported erectile dysfunction in people with long-term IDDM. *Diabetes Care* 1996;19:135–141.
21. Fedele D, Coscelli C, Santeusanio F, et al. Erectile dysfunction in diabetic subjects in Italy. *Diabetes Care* 1998;21:1973–1977.
22. Parazzini F, Menchini FF, Bortolotti A, et al. Frequency and determinants of erectile dysfunction in Italy. *Eur Urol* 2000;37:43–49.
23. Lustman PJ, Clouse RE. Relationship of psychiatric illness to impotence in men with diabetes. *Diabetes Care* 1990;13:893–895.
24. Lue TF. Erectile dysfunction. *N Engl J Med* 2000;342:1802–1813.
25. Saenz de Tejada I, Goldstein I. Diabetic penile neuropathy. *Urol Clin North Am* 1988;15:17–22.
26. Seftel AD, Vaziri ND, Ni Z, et al. Advanced glycation end products in human penis: elevation in diabetic tissue, site of deposition, and possible effect through iNOS or eNOS. *Urology* 1997;50:1016–1026.
27. Hirata K, Kuroda R, Sakoda T, et al. Inhibition of endothelial nitric oxide synthase activity by protein kinase C. *Hypertension* 1995;25:180–185.
28. Saenz de, Tejada I, Goldstein I, Azadzoi K, Krane RJ, Cohen RA. Impaired neurogenic and endothelium-mediated relaxation of penile smooth muscle from diabetic men with impotence. *N Engl J Med* 1989;320:1025–1030.
29. Keegan A, Cotter MA, Cameron NE. Effects of diabetes and treatment with the antioxidant α-lipoic acid on endothelial and neurogenic responses of corpus cavernosum in rats. *Diabetologia* 1999;42:343–350.
30. Elabbady AA, Gagnon C, Hassouna MM, Begin LR, Elhilali MM. Diabets mellitus increases nitric oxide synthase in penises but not in major pelvic ganglia of rats. *Br J Urol* 1995;76:196–202.
31. Vernet D, Cai L, Garban H, et al. Reduction of penile nitric oxide synthase in diabetic BB/WORdp (type I) and BBZ/WORdp (type II) rats with erectile dysfunction. *Endocrinology* 1995;136:5709–5717.

32. Bivalacqua TJ, Champion HC, Usta MF, et al. RhoA/Rho-kinase suppresses endothelial nitric oxide synthase in the penis: a mechanism for diabetes-associated erectile dysfunction. *Proc Natl Acad Sci USA* 2004;101:9121–9126.
33. American Urological Association. Management of Erectile Dysfunction ('05/updated'06), http://www.auanet.org/guidelines/main_reports/edmgmt/chapter1.pdf.
34. Ralph D, McNicholas T. UK management guidelines for erectile dysfunction. *BMJ* 2000;321:499–503.
35. Azad N, Emanuele NV, Abraira C, et al. The effects of intensive glycemic control on neuropathy in the VA Cooperative Study on Type II diabetes mellitus. *J Diabetes Complications* 2000;13:307–313.
36. Esposito K, Giugliano F, Di Palo C, et al. Effect of lifestyle changes on erectile dysfunction in obese men: a randomized controlled trial. *JAMA* 2004;291:2978–2984.
37. Vogt HJ, Brandl P, Kockott G, et al. Double-blind, placebo-controlled safety and efficacy trial with yohimbine hydrochloride in the treatment of nonorganic erectile dysfunction. *Int J Impot Res* 1997;9(3):155–161.
38. Ernst E, Pittler MH. Yohimbine for erectile dysfunction: a systematic review and meta-analysis of randomized clinical trials. *J Urol* 1998;159:433–436.
39. Rampin O, Bernabe J, Guilano F. Spinal control of penile erection. *World J Urol* 1997;15:2–13.
40. Padma-Nathan H, Auerbach S, Lewis R, Lewand M, et al. Efficacy and safety of Apomorphin vs placebo for male erectile dysfunction. *J Urol* 1999;161:821.
41. Lewis R, Agre K, Rudd D. Efficacy of Apomorphin vs Placebo for erectile dysfunction in patients with hypertension. *J Urol* 1999;161:822.
42. Reproductive Health Drugs Advisory Committee. Urology Subcommittee. www.fda.gov/ohrms/dockets/ac/00/transcripts/36021.rtf.
43. Küthe A, Wiedentoth A, Stief C, Mägert H, Forssmann W, Jonas U. Identification of 13 PDE isoforms in human cavernous tissue. *Eur Urol* 1999;35:404.
44. Taher A, Stief CG, Raida M, Jonas U, Forssmann WG. Cyclic nucleotide phosphodiesterase activity in human cavernous smooth muscle and the effect of various selective inhibitors. *Int J Impotence Res* 1992;4(Suppl 2):P11.
45. Rendell MS, Rajfer J, Wicker PA, Smith MD. Sildenafil for treatment of erectile dysfunction in men with diabetes: a randomized controlled trial. Sildenafil Diabetes Study Group. *JAMA* 1999;281:421–426.
46. Boulton AJM, Selam J-L, Sweeney M, Ziegler D. Sildenafil citrate for the treatment of erectile dysfunction in men with type II diabetes mellitus. *Diabetologia* 2001;44:1296–1301.
47. Sellam R, Ziegler D, Boulton AJM. Sildenafil citrate is effective and well tolerated for the treatment of erectile dysfunction in men with Type 1 or Type 2 diabetes mellitus. *Diabetologia* 2000;43(Suppl 1):A253.
48. Mitka M. Some men who take Viagra die—Why? *JAMA* 2000;283:590–593.
49. Shakir SAW, Wilton LV, Boshier A, Layton D, Heeley E. Cardiovascular events in users of sildenafil: results from first phase of prescription event monitoring in England. *Br Med J* 2001;322:651–652.
50. Herrmann HC, Chang G, Klugherz BD, Mahoney PD. Hemodynamic effects of sildenafil in men with severe coronary artery disease. *N Engl J Med* 2000;342:1622–1626.
51. De Angelis L, Marfella MA, Siniscalchi M, et al. Erectile and endothelial dysfunction in Type II diabetes: a possible link. *Diabetologia* 2001;44:1155–1160.
52. Desouza C, Parulkar A, Lumpkin D, Akers D, Fonseca VA. Acute and prolonged effects of sildenafil on brachial artery flow-mediated dilatation in type 2 diabetes. *Diabetes Care* 2002;25:1336–1339.
53. Katz SD, Balidemaj K, Homma S, Wu H, Wang J, Maybaum S. Acute type 5 phosphodiesterase inhibition with Sildenafil enhances Flow mediated vasodilation in patients with chronic heart failure. *J Am Coll Cardiol* 2000;36:845–851.

54. Cheitlin MD, Hutter AM, Brindis RG, et al. Use of sildenafil (Viagra) in patients with cardiovascular disease. *Circulation* 1999;99:168–177.
55. Stolk EA, Busschbach JJ, Caffa M, Meuleman EJ, Rutten FF. Cost utility analysis of sildenafil compared with papaverine-phentolamine injections. *BMJ* 2000;320:1165–1168.
56. Smith KJ, Roberts MS. The cost-effectiveness of sildenafil. *Ann Intern Med* 2000;132: 933–937.
57. Wespes E, Rammal A, Garbar C. Sildenafil non-responders: haemodynamic and morphometric studies. *Eur Urol* 2005;48:136–139.
58. Saenz de, Tejada I, Anglin G, Knight JR, Emmick JT. Effects of tadalafil on erectile dysfunction in men with diabetes. *Diabetes Care* 2002;25:2159–2164.
59. Fonseca V, Seftel A, Denne J, Fredlund P. Impact of diabetes mellitus on the severity of erectile dysfunction and response to treatment: analysis of data from tadalafil clinical trials. *Diabetologia* 2004;47:1914–1923.
60a. Goldstein I, Young JM, Fischer J, et al. Vardenafil, a new phosphodiesterase type 5 inhibitor, in the treatment of erectile dysfunction in men with diabetes: a multicenter double-blind placebo-controlled fixed-dose study. *Diabetes Care* 2003;26:777–783.
60b. Ziegler D, Merfort F, van Ahlen H, Yassin A, Reblin T, Neureither M. Efficacy and safety of flexible-dose vardenafil in men with type 1 diabetes and erectile dysfunction. *J Sex Med* 2006;3:883–891.
61. Becker AJ, Stief CG, Machtens S, Schultheiss D, Truss MC, Jonas U. Oral phentolamine as treatment for erectile dysfunction. *J Urol* 1998;159:1214–1216.
62. Dutta TC, Eid JF. Vacuum constriction devices for erectile dysfunction: a long-term, prospective study of patients with mild, moderate, and severe dysfunction. *Urology* 1999; 54:891–893.
63. Padma-Nathan H, Hellstrom WJ, Kaiser FE, et al. Treatment of men with erectile dysfunction with transurethral alprostadil. Medicated Urethral System for Erection (MUSE) Study Group. *N Engl J Med* 1997;336:1–7.
64. Porst H. Transurethrale Alprostadilapplikation mit MUSE™ (medicated urethral system for erection). *Urologe* [A] 1998;37:410–416.
65. Spivack AP, Peterson CA, Cowley C, et al. Long-term safety profile of transurethral alprostadil for the treatment of erectile dysfunction. *J Urol* 1997;157(Supp l):203.
66. Fulgham PF, Cochran JS, Denman JL, et al. Disappointing initial results with transurethral alprostadil for erectile dysfunction in a urology practice setting. *J Urol* 1998;160:2041–2046.
67. Linet OI, Ogrinc FG. Efficacy and safety of intracavernosal alprostadil in men with erectile dysfunction. The Alprostadil Study Group. *N Engl J Med* 1996;334:873–877.
68. Shabsigh R, Padma-Nathan H, Gittleman M, McMurray J, Kaufman J, Goldstein I. Intracavernous alprostadil alfadex is more efficacious, better tolerated, and preferred over intraurethral alprostadil plus optional actis: a comparative, randomized, crossover, multicenter study. *Urology* 2000;55:109–113.
69. Porst H, Buvat J, Meuleman EJH, Michal V, Wagner G. Final results of a prospective multicenter study with self-injection therapy with PGE_1 after 4 years of follow-up. *Int J Impot Res* 1996;6:151:D118.
70. Ewing DJ, Clarke BF. Diabetic autonomic neuropathy: present insights and future prospects. *Diabetes Care* 1986;9:648–665.
71. Enzlin P, Mathieu C, Van Den Bruel A, Vanderschueren D, Demyttenaere K. Prevalence and predictors of sexual dysfunction in patients with type 1 diabetes. *Diabetes Care* 2003;26:409–414.
72. Esposito K, Ciotola M, Marfella R, Di Tommaso D, Cobellis L, Giugliano D. The metabolic syndrome: a cause of sexual dysfunction in women. *Int J Impot Res* 2005;17:224–226.
73. Enzlin P, Mathieu C, Vanderschueren D, Demyttenaere K. Diabetes mellitus and female sexuality: a review of 25 years' research. *Diabetes Med* 1998;15:809–815.
74. Jovanovic L. Sex and the woman with diabetes: desire versus dysfunction. *IDF Bull* 1998;43:23–28.

28
Management of Diabetic Foot Complications

Thomas E. Lyons

SUMMARY

Diabetic foot complications are the result of an interplay between impaired wound healing, peripheral vascular disease and neuropathy. The peripheral neuropathy seen with diabetes mellitus affects sensory, motor and autonomic neurons and results in increased susceptibility to pathology. The most common problem is the presence of wounds that are difficult to heal. Therefore, the prevention of the formation of these wounds is of paramount importance in patients who are identified as being at risk for forming these wounds. Treatment involves a multidisciplinary approach and requires adequate perfusion, proper wound care, and appropriate protection of the wound from pressure or offloading. Neuroosteoarthropathy or Charcot's disease of the foot is also common in diabetic neuropathic patients. The main underlying cause is neuropathy which often results in the musculoskeletal disruption of the architecture of the foot and leads to severe deformity. Management of this condition is a challenge and failure may result in limb loss. The present chapter will review the pathophysiology of diabetic foot problems and the currently established therapeutic approaches.

Key Words: Foot complications; neuropathic ulcerations; charcot wounds.

INTRODUCTION

Complications involving the foot are common in patients with diabetes mellitus. Manifestations of these complications range from the simple to more complex entities, which are limb or even life threatening. The treatment of these complications ranges from simple office-based interventions to prolonged hospitalizations. Foot pathology remains the leading diabetic complication requiring hospitalization *(1)*. The incidence of diabetes in the general population is expected to rise as well as the prevalence of diabetic foot complications is likely to increase. The costs of these complications are owing not only to the medical costs, but also because of costs of lost productivity. For example, in 2002, the medical costs for treating patients with diabetes mellitus was 92 billion. An additional 40 billion could be attributable to lost productivity. The number of people diagnosed with diabetes mellitus is expected to increase as will the cost of treatment. It is projected that the costs of treatment will increase to approximately 160 billion by 2010 and near 200 billion by 2020 *(2)*.

From: *Contemporary Diabetes: Diabetic Neuropathy: Clinical Management, Second Edition*
Edited by: A. Veves and R. Malik © Humana Press Inc., Totowa, NJ

Diabetic foot complications therefore represent a major public health challenge of growing proportions.

Relatively recently, risk factors and causal pathways leading to diabetic foot problems have been identified. The importance of the major risk factors for the development of diabetic foot ulcers, which include peripheral neuropathy, peripheral vascular disease, and high foot pressures is well known. These, along with other factors result in the development of diabetic foot complications, which will be discussed later in the chapter. It is hoped that better appreciation of the pathogenesis of diabetic foot complications will afford us effective and successful preventative strategies aimed at limb salvage.

EPIDEMIOLOGY

Two of the most significant diabetic foot complications are foot ulcers and lower extremity amputations. These two entities are responsible for the substantial utilization of medical efforts and healthcare resources, in addition to contributing to significant morbidity and mortality in the patient with diabetes. Foot ulcers result from a number of etiological factors, and are wounds that are associated with delayed healing. These etiological factors arise from pathophysiological changes in the diabetic state, anatomical deformities in the diabetic foot, and environmental influences. Annually, 2% of all patients with diabetes will develop a foot ulcer *(3)*, whereas 15% will ulcerate during a lifetime *(3,4)*. The prevalence of diabetic foot ulcers has been reported to range from 5.3% to 10.5% *(3,5–7)*. This variation in range may be because of the lack of awareness and appropriate preventative care on the part of both patient and provider. Furthermore, this wide variation may be because of the fact that most studies select only patients with diabetes who are at risk for diabetic foot complications for inclusion in evaluation of ulcer formation. Nonetheless, the aforementioned figures illustrate the chronicity of the problem of ulcerations in patients with diabetes.

The cost of diabetic foot complications vary considerably, probably depending on the problem, its severity, its outcome, and extent of intervention required. The majority of the costs are attributed to inpatient expenditures *(8)*. The cost of treating an ulceration without surgical intervention approaches several thousand dollars, whereas those ulcers that are ultimately treated with an amputation can cost many times higher *(9)*.

Foot ulcerations precede 85% of amputations and so the relationship between ulcers and lower extremity amputations is obvious *(10,11)*. Alarmingly, 15% of all foot ulcers will ultimately require amputation, indeed the major risk factor for amputation is ulceration representing the major risk factor for amputation. Ultimately 15% of all ulcerations may evolve an amputation at some level *(3)*. Other risk factors for amputation include greater duration of diabetes, peripheral vascular disease, peripheral neuropathy, poor glycemic control, prior history of foot ulcers, previous foot surgery and amputation, retinopathy, and nephropathy *(12–17)*.

In the United States, approximately 50% of all amputations are performed on patients with diabetes *(18)*, which is about 60% of total amputation *(19)*. Amputation rates have also been shown to vary with both gender and ethnicity. Being male, African American, or Hispanic has been associated with higher risk for amputation *(20,21)*. Lack of access to education and routine preventative care may be the underlying reason for this increase. When programs designed to prevent and promote awareness of diabetic foot complications were instituted in high-risk populations, the rate of amputations was decreased by nearly 50% *(22,23)*.

In the early 1990's, there were approximately 60,000 lower extremity amputations in the diabetic population performed per year with an estimated expense of USD 30,000–60,000 per case *(24)*. The incidence of lower extremity amputations continues to escalate despite greater awareness levels and promotion of preventative care. Since 1990, the rate of lower extremity amputation in patients with diabetes has increased and 82,000 amputations were performed from 2000 to 2001 *(25)*.

As the data illustrates, diabetic foot complications can place an overwhelming burden on patients, their families, and healthcare professionals. The total cost of diabetic foot complications in the United States has been estimated to approach 4 billion annually, as extrapolated from the costs of ulcer care and amputations *(26)*. Continued efforts to identify high-risk patients, ensure adequate availability of preventative care, and prompt treatment remain the best means of reducing the destructive consequences of amputations and death.

DIABETIC FOOT ULCERATION

The Pathway to Foot Ulceration

The risk factors for diabetic foot ulceration can be categorized into three distinct groups: pathophysiological, anatomic deformities, and environmental influences. The pathophysiological changes, which occur at the biomolecular level lead to changes that result in the development of peripheral sensory neuropathy, peripheral vascular disease, and a compromised immune system with alteration in wound healing capabilities. The second group with anatomic deformities are largely the result of motor neuropathy and in some cases Charcot neuroarthropathy. Finally, external or environmental influences in the form of acute or chronic trauma often precipitates the initiation of ulceration with initial soft tissue injury.

It is important to note that most of these risk factors do not act independently to produce foot ulceration. Instead, it is usually a combination of these risk factors that triggers a pathway leading to ulceration. Such risk factors can consist of a number of component causes, such as peripheral neuropathy, foot trauma, foot deformity, lower limb ischemia, foot edema, and callus formation. However, some risk factors seem to be more important in causing ulcerations. A critical triad of neuropathy, minor foot trauma, and foot deformity was found in more than 63% of foot ulcers in one study *(27)*. As shown in Fig. 1, in the vast majority of diabetic foot ulceration, the first major component is the development of sensory neuropathy that causes pain insensitivity *(11)*. The next component is the development of trauma, usually related to the high foot pressures that develop under the foot during walking. The trauma caused by the elevated foot pressures seen during normal walking are often the result of the changes in foot structure that occur as a result of the motor component of peripheral neuropathy. The third major component is the impaired wound healing, related to altered immune response, reduced blood supply at the wound area and abnormal expression of growth factors and other cytokines that are involved in the healing process. It is usually the combination of

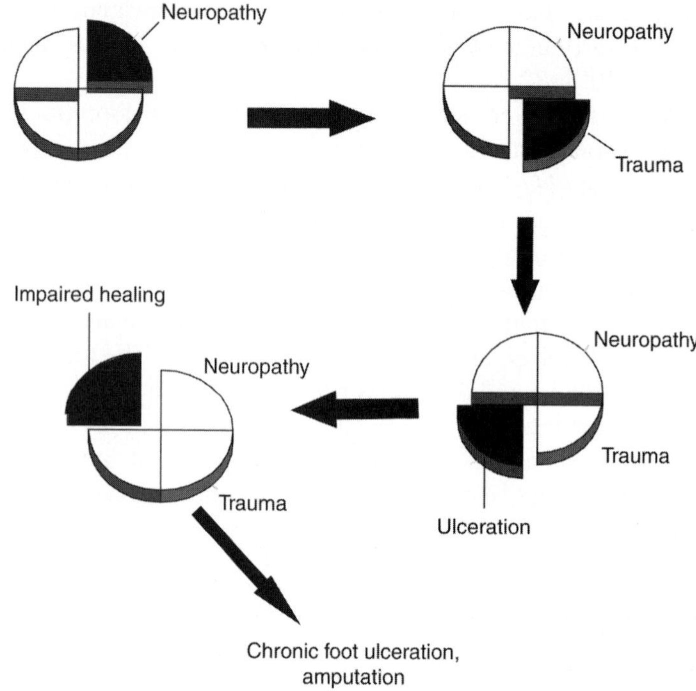

Fig. 1. The pathway to foot ulceration. Sensory neuropathy, associated with pain insensitivity is the first component of the pathway. However, the development of ulceration also requires the existence of trauma, usually, related to the plantar tissue stress and injury that results from the development of high foot pressures during walking. The presence of the third component, impaired wound healing because of reduced blood flow in the ulcer area and aberrant expression of growth factors and cytokines, prevents the wound closure and leads to the development of chronic ulceration and, in some cases, amputation. (Modified from ref. *10*.)

these three major components that lead to the development of chronic ulceration and amputation in cases where these progress to a limb or life threatening situation.

Peripheral Sensory Neuropathy

Reported in approximately 30–50% of all diabetic patients peripheral sensory neuropathy has been found to be the most common and sensitive predictor for foot ulceration in a patient with diabetes *(28,29)*. In a study that specifically studied casual pathways of diabetic foot ulceration, the presence of neuropathy was reported in 78% of cases *(27)*. The presence of peripheral sensory neuropathy initiates a series of events that eventually results in foot ulceration. A foot with impaired sensation provides little or no feedback to higher centers that cause a patient to continue to walk with little or no change in gait. This means that others with normal sensation would have the feedback to stop ambulating or at least alter their gait to allow the affected traumatized area to heal. With an inability to detect the pain signals that warn of impending tissue trauma, the insensate foot is exposed to continued increased pressures that hastens tissue damage leading to ulceration. This combination of increased forces coupled with impaired protective sensation are the key elements for ulcer genesis.

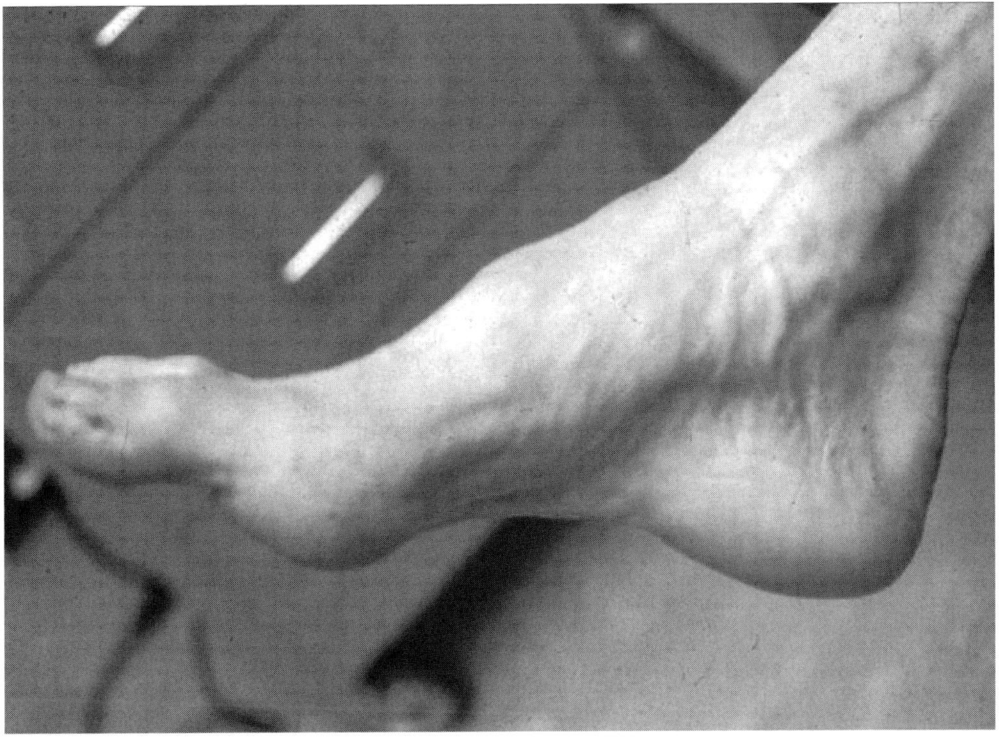

Fig. 2. Changes related to motor neuropathy (minor foot). There is extensive wasting of the intrinsic muscles of the foot that results to clawing of the toes and prominence of the metatarsal heads.

Autonomic and Motor Neuropathy

Autonomic neuropathy is common in patients with long-standing diabetes. In the lower extremity, autonomic neuropathy might result arteriovenous shunting, resulting in the small arteries dilating *(30)*. The resultant distension of the foot veins is not diminished even with foot elevation. Consequently, a neuropathic edema recalcitrant to diuretic therapy is observed. In addition to swelling, the neuropathic foot is also noted to be warm as a result of arterio–venous shunting *(31)*. Autonomic neuropathy might decrease the activity of normally innervated skin appendages, such as sweat glands of the feet. The result is that the skin can become dry and less elastic. Dry, stiff skin cracks more easily forming splits or fissures notably around the heel rim and plantar medial aspect of the first metatarsophalangeal (MTP) especially during the dryer months. These cracks or fissures can become infected, resulting in a local cellulitis or they may even result in small longitudinal ulcerations that potentially can become infected *(32)*.

Motor neuropathy in the foot causes weakness and wasting of the small intrinsic muscles, classically termed the "intrinsic minus" foot (Fig. 2). This leads to muscular imbalance with a characteristic clawing of the toes and plantarflexion of the metatarsal heads. Why? it seems that the intrinsic muscles of the foot act to stabilize and hold the phalanges of the toes straight as the long flexors and extensor tendons acting through their insertions into the distal phalanx pull the toes "up" into dorsiflexion as if "taking the foot off the gas pedal" or "down" into plantarflexion as if "stepping on the gas pedal." As the long flexors and extensors pull at the tips of the toes, the toes must be held straight and rigid. If the intrinsic muscles are unable to do this, the toes contract back into a hammertoe and ride up onto the metatarsal head forcing it into the weight-bearing surface with greater force. In addition, as the toes contract back into hammertoes, the fat pad plantar to the metatarsal heads shifts anteriorly. The soft tissue plantar to the metatarsophalangeal joints is not able to disperse the forces in this area as well as the plantar fat pad. Very often the atrophied intrinsics mean there is less bulk in the arch, which translates into less soft tissue bulk in the arch that is able to bear weight. The overall result of the changes in the foot because of motor neuropathy is a foot with a high arch, prominent metatarsal heads with very little plantar cushion, and hammertoes that are driving the metatarsal heads into the weight-bearing surface. The prominences at the plantar metatarsal head level and the digital level serve as areas of focal pressures with possible irritation from footwear. In the setting of sensory neuropathy, these areas of increased pressure brought about by the changes of motor neuropathy are at risk for ulceration.

Peak Plantar Pressures

Diabetic ulcers can occur on any part of the foot, but are clinically observed most frequently on the plantar surfaces. The predilection of diabetic foot ulcers to the plantar surfaces is related to the trauma that develops in these areas because of the increased peak plantar pressures during walking *(33)*. Under normal conditions, the foot has the ability to distribute high forces that are applied on the plantar surface, especially on the ball of the foot, and therefore avoid the development of high foot pressures. This ability is greatly impaired in diabetes and is mainly because of the changes in the foot that are related to motor neuropathy that were described earlier and limited joint mobility (LJM) (*see* next section on joint mobility). As a result of this, the pressures under certain areas of the diabetic foot can be considerably high and lead to tissue injury even after walking short distances. As previously mentioned, in the presence of sensory neuropathy, the patient is unaware of warning signs of this injury, such as pain, and continues to walk until tissue integrity is compromised and foot ulceration occurs.

Numerous studies have shown that foot pressures are high in diabetic neuropathic patients *(34–37)*. The high pressures tend to aggregate in the forefoot area or sites with bony prominence in the case of patients with Charcot neuroarthropathy. Usually, most ulcers develop under these areas of high foot pressures, but the development of ulceration in other foot areas can also occur. The development of high foot pressures starts in the early stages of diabetic neuropathy, even in the subclinical phase of the disease. One of the first steps is the transfer of high peak pressures from the heel area to the forefoot area, in the absence of any clinically detectable neuropathy *(36)*. As neuropathy worsens and the clawing of the toes develops, there is further transfer of peak pressures from the toes to the forefoot area. In cases of severe neuropathy, the forefoot pressures are greatly elevated and the ratio between forefoot to rear foot pressures is increased as it would be expected. A forefoot to rearfoot ratio more than two was found to be more specific in identifying patients at risk for ulceration *(38)*.

There are ample data to suggest that elevated foot pressures might predict a site of foot ulceration *(34,35,39,40)*, but foot pressure measurements are characterized by a comparatively low sensitivity and are therefore not recommended as a primary screening tool

(33). Nonetheless, they do have a reasonable specificity and can be used in selected cases as a guide for the provision of proper foot wear that attenuates high pressures and therefore, decreases the risk of foot ulceration *(41)*.

Limited Joint Mobility

Restriction of joint mobility is well documented in diabetes and is related mainly to collagen glycosylation that results in thickening of the periarticular structures, such as tendons, ligaments, and joint capsules *(42,43)*. At the foot level, all joints might be involved though the subtalar and metatarsalphalangeal joints carry with them significant implications. The subtalar joint plays a major role in flattening of the arch or pronation. This is a shock absorbing mechanism of the foot, as the flattening of the arch reduces and attenuates ground reactive forces. LJM affecting the subtalar joint results in a foot that flattens out minimally or not at all. Consequently, LJM impairs the ability of the foot to adapt to the ground surface and absorb the shock that develops when the heel makes contact with the ground during walking. As a result of this, high foot pressures develop, mainly in the forefoot area, and are considered to be an additional factor in the development of foot ulceration *(37,44–46)*. LJM also appears to vary along racial lines as compared with black patients, other patients have significantly less joint mobility *(47)*.

Collagen glycosylation is also implicated in decreasing the resiliency of the Achilles tendon in patients with diabetes. Decreased motion of the Achilles tendon creates an equinus deformity with a further shift of plantar forces to the forefoot region *(48)*. Surgical lengthening of the Achilles tendon has been found to effectively distribute plantar pressures more uniformly, decreasing the peak forces at the metatarsal region *(49)*. But, surgical lengthening of the Achilles tendon does not restore plantar forefoot pressures to normal. This suggests that other structures may be involved to some extent. The plantar fascia itself might thicken and increase its resistance to tensile force rendering the arch of the foot less ability to undergo pronation *(50)*. These results might further increase pressures under the metatarsal heads. The increased thickness of the plantar fascia also affects motion at the MTP's. It has attachments from the plantar aspect of the calcaneus to the base of the toes. If the plantar fascia becomes thick and tight, it then correlates with decreased motion of the MTP's as a closed plantar fascia will restrict motion of the toes. Therefore, glycolsylation of collagen might also affect the mobility of the MTP's, which might increase pressures at sites related to motion of the MTP's. An example of this is the hallus interphalangeal joint (HIPJ), which is often the site of plantar ulcerations in cases of reduced mobility of the first MTP. When there is reduced dorsiflexion, i.e., reduced motion of pulling the great toe toward the knee, the HIPJ must hyperextend in terminal stance and a great deal of pressure is placed on the plantar aspect of the HIPJ predisposing to ulceration.

Peripheral Vascular Disease

Macrocirculation

Peripheral vascular disease is sometimes seen in patients with diabetes and pedal ulceration. It might be present in approximately 30% of cases *(27)*. Impaired blood supply no doubt is a risk factor although not a major factor. It becomes a major factor after an ulceration has formed and becomes a major risk factor for amputation. Both microcirculatory and macrocirculatory changes occur in patients with diabetes with peripheral vascular disease. Macrocirculatory disease in the patient with diabetes is identical to the atherosclerotic changes found in nondiabetics. Microcirculatory disease, on the other hand, is unique to the patient with diabetes.

Microcirculation

Changes in the microcirculation in the foot of a patient with diabetes significantly impairs the ability of wound healing. Whereas, there are no occlusive lesions in the diabetic microcirculation, structural changes occur most notably by thickening of the basement membrane. However, this does not result in narrowing of the capillary lumen *(51)*, but instead decreases the elastic properties of the capillary vessel walls and therefore, limits vasodilatation capacity. The basement membrane thickening might also impair the normal exchange of nutrients and cellular migration, decreasing the ability of the diabetic foot to fight infection *(52)*. Despite these structural changes, it is the functional changes that are the most important. More specifically, during the last decade it has been realized that these changes are related mainly to the dysfunction of the endothelial cell and vascular smooth muscle cell of the arterioles, and the impairment of the nerve-axon reflex.

The single layer thick endothelium forms the luminal surface of all blood vessels. Normally, the endothelium synthesizes and releases vasoactive substances including vasodilators, such as nitric oxide, prostacyclin, and endothelium-derived hyperpolarizing factor and vasoconstrictors, such as endothelin, and prostaglandins that are vital in maintaining vascular tone and regulating blood flow *(53)*. These vasomodulators primarily act at the vascular smooth muscle cells that are adjacent to the endothelial cells. The atherosclerotic changes seen in large vessels disease, such as monocyte migration or foam cell formation are not evident in those changes seen with the microcirculation. In addition, endothelial cells participate in angiogenesis, an important factor of the wound healing process.

Recent work during the last decade has shown that both the endothelium-dependent vasodilation and the independent one (that reflects the function of the vascular smooth muscle cell function) are impaired not only in diabetes, but also in the prediabetic stage as well (Fig. 3) *(54)*. Furthermore, even in healthy subjects the microcirculation vasodilatory capacity at the foot level is reduced when it is compared with the forearm level. Thus, the additional reduction in vasodilation that is caused by diabetes can be critical for the skin and other foot tissues, as it restricts the maximal blood flow to levels that cannot sustain normal wound healing *(55)*. Studies in our unit have shown that the endothelium-dependent vasodilation is equally impaired in diabetic neuropathic patients without large vessel disease and adequate arterial blood flow and in patients with obstructive arterial disease requiring bypass operation. The endothelium-dependent vasodilation was also impaired in both groups, but was more pronounced in patients with large vessel disease *(56,57)*.

Another important factor that affects the neuropathic foot microcirculation is the impairment of the nerve-axon reflex. Under normal conditions, stimulation of the C-nociceptive fibers leads to retrograde stimulation of adjacent fibers, which secrete a number of vasomodulators, such as substance P, calcitonin gene related peptide (GCRP), histamine, and so on, that produce vasodilation (also known as Lewis triple flare

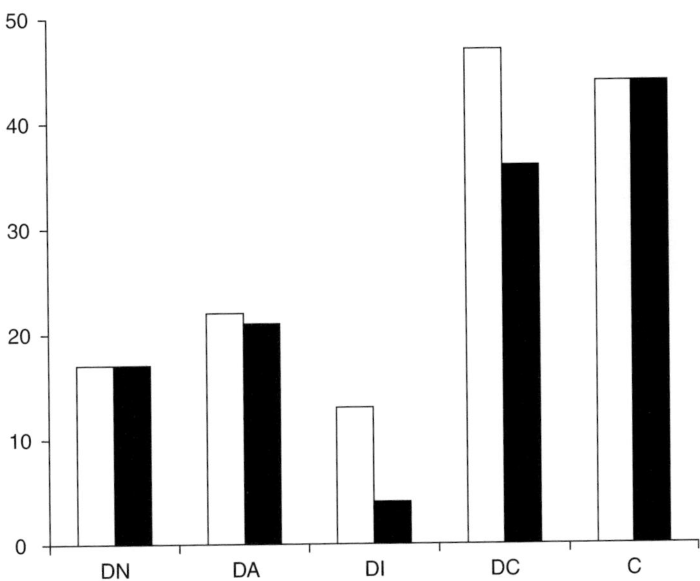

Fig. 3. The vasodilatory response to the iontophoresis of acetylcholine (hatched bars) and sodium nitroprusside (black bars) at the foot level. The response to acetylcholine (endothelium dependent vasodilation) was equally reduced in the diabetic neuropathic patients with a history of foot ulceration (DN group), the patients with both neuropathy and peripheral vascular disease (DI), and the patients with Charcot neuroarthropathy (DA) when compared with nonneuropathic diabetic patients (D) and healthy controls (C), $p < 0.0001$. The response to sodium nitroprusside (endothelium independent vasodilation) was more pronounced in the DI group and also, reduced in the DN and DA groups compared with D and C groups, $p < 0.0001$. These results indicate that both the endothelial cell and vascular smooth muscle cell of the skin microcirculation are impaired in the neuropathic diabetic foot (from ref. *50*).

response) (Fig. 4). This response is equal to one-third of the maximal vasodilatory capacity and is responsible for the hyperemia that is observed in areas that are close to injury.

As it would be expected, the nerve-axon-reflex-related vasodilation is almost absent in diabetic naturopathic patients. This response remains absent even after successful bypass surgery to the pedal arteries that establishes satisfactory blood flow in the foot large vessels *(58)*. This is probably the main reason that hyperemia, a major sign of inflammation, is absent in patients with diabetes with infection of the foot. Thus, even the presence of neuropathy alone can lead to impaired blood flow under conditions of stress *(59–61)*.

At the molecular level, the reduction of endothelium-dependent vasodilation seems to be related to the reduced expression of endothelial nitric oxide synthase, by the endothelial cells of the microvasculature that is located in the skin of neuropathic foot *(54)*. Whether this reduction is also related to the development of neuropathy is not clear. However, the expression of endothelial nitric oxide synthase by endothelial cells at the forearm level is not affected by diabetes. Other mechanisms that contribute to the observed functional changes include reduced poly(ADP-ribose) polymerase activity and increased nitrotyrosine formation *(57)*.

Despite the lack of complete understanding of the involved mechanisms, the main understanding from work that was conducted during the last decade is that the microcirculation

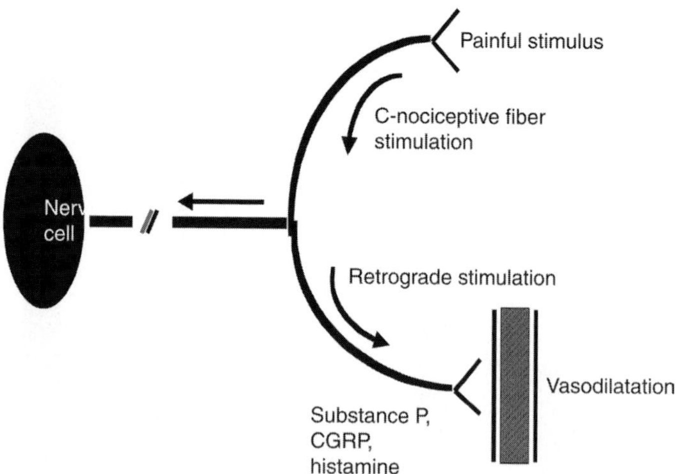

Fig. 4. The nerve axon reflex. Stimulation of the C-nociceptive fibers causes retrograde stimulation of adjacent fibers that release active vasodilators such as histamine, substance P, and calcitonin gene-related peptide. The final result is hyperemia during injury or inflammation. Because of the presence of peripheral neuropathy, this response (also known in physiology as Lewis triple flare response) is absent in diabetic patients.

of diabetic neuropathic foot fails to maximally vasodilate under conditions of stress. Thus, even in the absence of any peripheral disease and in the presence of adequate blood flow in the large vessels, the skin blood flow is impaired when injury occurs and this is one of the major factors that are related to impaired wound healing. Therefore, the neuropathic diabetic foot should be considered functionally ischemic regardless of the presence or absence of vascular disease. In addition, lack of hyperemia should not be interpreted as lack of inflammation or infection.

Impaired Wound Healing

As shown in Fig. 1, impaired wound healing is a major factor that contributes to the development of chronic foot ulceration and amputation. Initially, it was thought that failure to heal a diabetic ulcer was related to continuous walking on the injured foot, mainly because of the pain insensitivity, and the existence of peripheral arterial disease. However, it is currently realized that two other major factors contribute to this impairment, namely the functional changes in the microcirculation and changes in cellular activity, and the expression of the various growth factors and cytokines that are normally involved in tissue repair and wound healing.

The normal wound healing process entails a complex interplay between connective tissue formation, cellular activity, and growth factor activation. All three of these physiological processes are altered in the diabetic state and contribute to the poor healing of diabetic foot ulcers. Collagen, the most abundant protein in connective tissue, is an integral component of dermis, bones, tendons, and ligaments. Collagen synthesis and degradation in wound repair are complex processes that continue at the wound site long after the injury. The resulting scar tissue following wound repair never fully regains the tensile strength of the original intact skin. Instead, scar collagen retains only 70–80%

tensile strength of the original collagen *(62)*. The balance between collagen synthesis and degradation in wound repair is tenuous, and disease states such as diabetes can shift the balance to one side, disrupting the wound healing process.

The normal inflammatory stage of wound repair involves an orchestrated interaction of resident cells, such as epithelial cells, fibroblasts, dendritic cells, and endothelial cells with biochemical activity *(62)*. In addition to these resident cells, platelets, neutrophils, T-cells, natural killer cells, and macrophages are recruited to the wound site. These cells migrate to the injury site to mediate the inflammation, coagulation, and angiogenesis processes occurring in the wound healing process.

Growth factors influence the wound healing process through inhibitory or stimulatory effect on the local wound environment. Growth factors, such as growth platelet-derived growth factor (PDGF), basic fibroblast growth factor, and vascular endothelial growth factor have all been found in wound fluid. These growth factors are known to be integral in the chemotaxis, migration, stimulation, and proliferation of cells and matrix substances necessary for wound healing. Therefore, the altered secretion or absence of these growth factors in diabetic foot ulcers can potentially impair wound healing. Recent investigation of the role these growth factors play in wound healing appears to support this hypothesis *(63)*.

In diabetes, there are major abnormalities in all the above mechanisms. Thus, collagen synthesis markedly decreased, at both the collagen peptide production level as well as the post-translational modification of collagen degradation *(42)*. In addition, hyperglycemia can potentially mitigate the cellular activity in the inflammatory process. More specifically, the morphological characteristics of macrophages are transformed in such a manner that it impairs their function *(64)*. Furthermore, inhibition of skin keratinocyte proliferation in the presence of increased cellular differentiation leads to an imbalance in keratinocyte production, an essential step in the wound healing process *(65)*. Finally, the expression of various growth factors, such as PDGF and vascular endothelial growth factor is reduced, whereas the expression of matrix metalloproteinases is increased. The upgraded expression of the matrix metalloproteinases's results in increased proteolytic activity and inactivation of the growth factors that are necessary for proper wound healing.

The final result of the aforementioned changes is that that diabetic ulcers are "stuck" in the inflammatory phase of the wound healing process. Under normal circumstances, during this phase that lasts for only 2–3 days, the wound is cleaned of any bacteria and is covered by an eschar that is devoid of any tensile strength. The inflammatory phase is followed by the proliferative phase that is characterized by angiogenesis, expression of numerous growth factors, cell migration, collagen production, and results in complete wound closure. It is currently believed that aberrant expression of growth factors and cytokines is the main reason that the diabetic foot ulcer fails to progress to the proliferative phase and remains in a chronic inflammatory state. Further understanding of this process will help in the development of new treatments in the future *(66,67)*.

Additional Risk Factors

Other risk factors for the development of diabetic foot ulcers include long duration of diabetes, earlier foot ulcer, and earlier amputation. Duration of diabetes for more than 20 years has been found to increase the risk of ulceration sixfold when compared with patients with a history of diabetes of less than 9 years *(68)*. A number of studies have demonstrated that a previous history of ulceration or amputation significantly increases the likelihood of a subsequent ulcer *(6,69)*. Previous surgical intervention including partial amputation may destabilize the foot and the process might accelerate in the intrinsic minus foot. It is also believed that a unilateral amputation might cause additional stress on the contralateral limb.

CLINICAL EXAMINATION AND SCREENING TECHNIQUES TO IDENTIFY THE PATIENT AT RISK OF FOOT ULCERATION

It is well-known that prevention remains the best means of averting the potentially devastating results of diabetic foot complications. It has been estimated that up to 80% of diabetic foot ulcers are preventable *(70)*. Accordingly, routine clinical examination to identify those patients at risk for ulceration has been advocated *(71)*. This involves a simple but thorough history and clinical examination consisting of a basic examination of the foot to include vascular, neurological, dermatological, and musculoskeletal examination.

Clinical evaluation of a patient with diabetes should begin with a thorough history to determine if a patient has a history of previous ulceration or amputation. A past history of ulceration or amputation increases the risk for future ulceration, infection, and amputation. Up to 60% of patients with diabetes with a history of a foot ulcer will develop another ulcer within a year following wound healing *(72)*. Three possible explanations for this have been proposed.

1. The risk factors that were necessary to cause the previous ulceration are in most cases still present;
2. The skin and soft tissue on the site of earlier ulceration may not have the same properties after healing has occurred in this area as compared with before the ulcer was present. Therefore, the skin and soft tissue might be altered and more prone to subsequent breakdown; and
3. Areas of previous amputation may leave a residual deformity that by themselves are areas of increased pressure that might be prone to ulceration. Additionally, any previous surgical interventions might alter pedal biomechanics, resulting in imbalances where areas of high pressure develop, which may subsequently ulcerate.

Other aspects of the history should include a history of symptoms of neuropathy. For example, numbness, tingling, burning, hypersensitivity, cold sensations, or any other altered sensations in the feet or legs should be noted. Painful symptoms, such as sharp shooting or aching pains should also be noted. Obviously, it should be emphasized that the absence of neuropathic symptoms is not to be equated with the absence of neuropathy and that a large number of patients develop neuropathic ulceration without ever having or noticing any symptoms.

The clinical examination begins with the vascular assessment. Peripheral vascular disease is the cause in approximately 25% of foot ulcers and might contribute to the inability of an ulcer to heal *(73)*. Vascular assessment includes a brief history for the existence of claudication. Clinical examination for the palpation of all lower extremity pulses and the presence or absence of hair should be carried out. The skin should be inspected for texture, turgor, color, and temperature. The absence of hair growth and skin atrophy are clues to impaired circulation. The absence of palpable foot pulses or

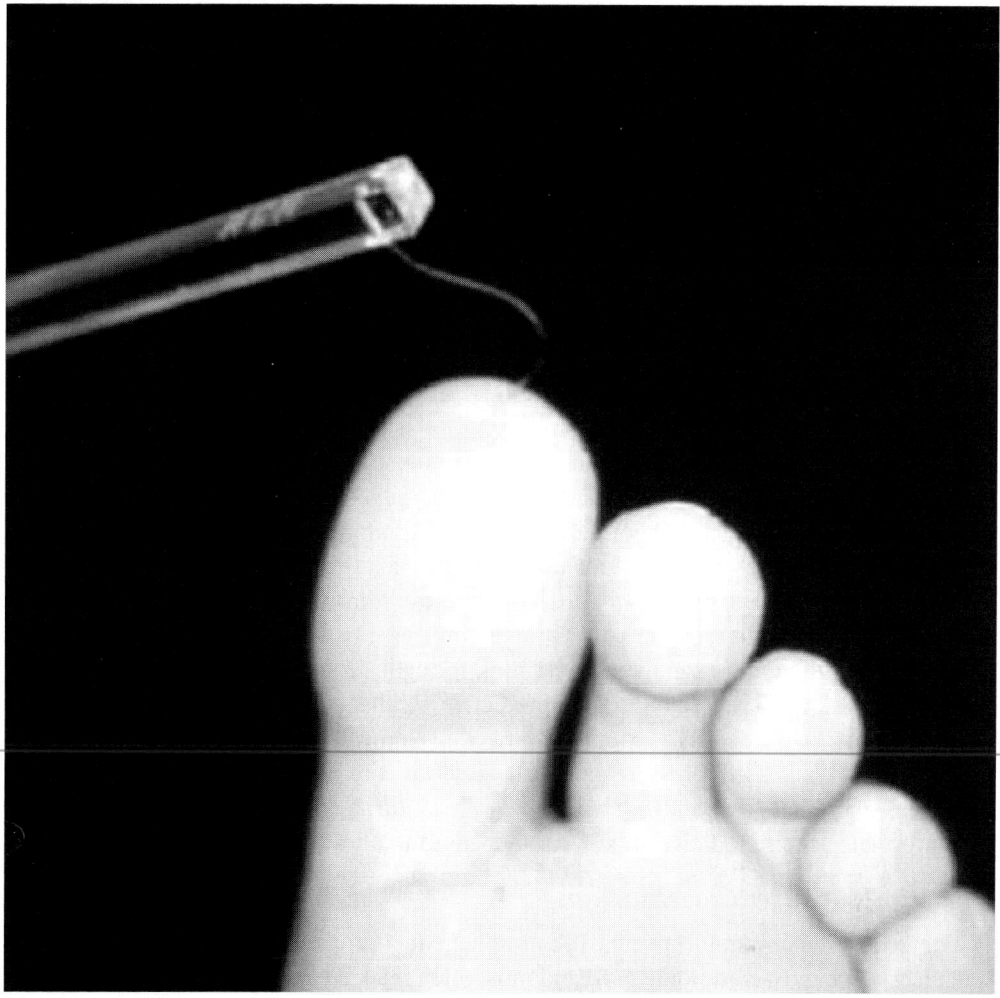

Fig. 5. The 5.07 Semmes–Weinstein Monofilament. The filaments is flexed when 10 gr of pressure is applied on the skin. Failure to feel a 5.07 strongly indicates that the patient is at risk of developing foot ulceration.

the existence of a nonhealing ulceration should prompt noninvasive vascular examination along with consultation with a vascular surgeon.

The next step in the clinical examination involves neurological testing to evaluate for the presence of neuropathy. The perception of pain, touch, and vibration can be easily tested using simple standard equipment, such as a pin prick, cotton or wool, and a tuning fork. The main feature the clinician should look for is a sensory level below which all the earlier mentioned modalities are reduced. The examination should be completed by testing the ability of the patient to feel a 5.07 Semmes–Weinstein monofilament (SWM) at the very least at the pulp of toes 1, 3, and 5 as well as the corresponding metatarsophalangeal joints (Fig. 5). Additional sites include two sites on the plantar aspect of the midfoot, one site on the plantar aspect of the heel, and one on the dorsum of the midfoot. Inability to feel the 5.07 SWM and/or the presence of a sensory level can identify 99% of all patients with diabetes who are at risk of foot ulceration *(74,75)*. These are simple, quick techniques with inexpensive equipment and should be performed at least once a year in all patients with diabetes. Patients with a sensory level or abnormality Semmes–Weinstien monofilament testing may be at risk of ulceration and should be provided preventive care *(70,75,76)*.

Vibration pressure threshold (VPT) is another effective technique to identify patients at risk of ulceration. VPT is commonly measured with a hand-held biothesiometer device that applies voltage in the range of 0–50 Volts (V). The test is performed by placing the vibrating stylus on the pulp of the great toe or the malleolus. Failure to detect a value of 25 V is considered indicative of a foot at risk for ulceration *(28)*. When compared with SWM testing, the sensitivity of VPT approaches only 79% and it requires more sophisticated and expensive equipment. Accordingly, it cannot be recommended as the technique of choice *(74,75)*.

Clinical examination concludes with a thorough musculoskeletal examination to appreciate and understand the overall structure and dynamics of the foot being evaluated. An inspection for the presence of foot deformities and limitation of joint mobility is carried out. Both these entities increase foot pressures that lead to ulceration. Osseous prominences can be observed secondary to Charcot neuroarthropathy, motor neuropathy, and common foot deformities, such as hallux abductovalgus, hallux limitus/rigidus, and hammertoes. In addition, the examiner should look for callus formation. In the past, the presence of calluses was speculated to be a protective mechanism with debridement of these lesions not recommended. However, it is now well-known that most calluses are actually focal areas of increased pressure and can serve as sites of potential ulceration *(77)*. Any areas of erythema secondary to shoe wear irritation should be protected with padding or appropriate accommodative shoe wear dispensed to alleviate the pressure.

Diabetic Foot Ulcer Classification

There have been numerous classification schemes proposed for describing diabetic foot ulcers. The most commonly used and most often referred to is the Wagner system *(78)*. The Wagner system classifies diabetic foot ulcers into five distinct grades, based on anatomical location and depth. Wagner grade 0 describes a pre- or postulcerative lesion. Grade 0 ulcerations are healed sites of ulcerations although risk factors for ulcer development, such as calluses and foot deformities are present. Wagner grade 1 ulcerations are superficial, full thickness ulcers with penetration past the epidermis. Grade 1 lesions are often indicative of the presence of peripheral sensory neuropathy, and usually another risk factor for ulceration. Continued weight-bearing on grade 1 ulcerations will result in progression past the dermis with involvement of deeper structures, such as tendons, ligaments, joint capsules, and neurovascular structures. These are grade 2 ulcerations. Grade 2 lesions do not probe to bone and osteomyelitis is not present. Wagner grade 3 ulcerations are characterized by the presence of deep infection with or without bone involvement and are usually the result of grade 2 ulcerations, which have worsened because of inadequate or lack of effective treatment. Other factors include lesions with rapidly forming tissue necrosis or puncture wounds. Wagner grade 4 ulcers present with partial gangrene of the foot. Grade 4 ulcers typically are associated with peripheral vascular disease. Infection is also present and necessitates aggressive management by a limb salvage team in order to limit tissue loss. Partial amputation in patients with these ulcerations is not uncommon. Grade 5 ulcers are characterized by extensive necrosis and gangrene of the foot, which is usually best addressed with aggressive treatment and amputation.

The Wagner classification system for diabetic foot ulcers is popular, but has its drawbacks. The first three grades provide an understanding as to the depth. However, there is no indication as to the status of the patients perfusion or the presence of infection. The patient's perfusion status and the presence of infection are key points in ulcer evaluation. Grades 4 and 5 ulcerations are severe, hence that aggressive debridement and minor or major amputation are often necessary. Essentially, these conditions are so severe that the aggressive treatment necessary means that the conditions are only very temporary. That and the fact that they are not as common are reasons that grades 4 and 5 are rarely used. Because of these shortcomings, other classification systems have been proposed including one described by Lavery, et al. *(79)* that aims to be more inclusive of all types of neuropathic foot lesions in addition to providing predictors of outcomes and response to therapy. This classification system mirrors the Wagner classification, but instead incorporates the presence or absence of infection and/or ischemia within each grade *(80)*. This classification scheme has the added benefit of correlating expected outcomes with increasing stage and grade. The factors determining increasing grade are depth and presence or absence of infection and ischemia. These newer classifications are more inclusive, but more difficult to remember and use in the clinical setting. Because of this, efforts have been made to devise a new system. For purposes of describing ulcerations by clinicians of various specialties who may not be aware of complex ulcer classifications, it is easier to just remember the three factors important in accurately describing foot ulcerations: depth, presence or absence of infection, and the patient's vascular status. These three factors will allow a clinician to effectively articulate the status of a patient with an ulceration.

Treatment Principles of Foot Ulceration

Treatment of diabetic foot ulcers varies greatly depending on the severity of the ulceration as well as the presence of ischemia. However, basic key points of treatment for full thickness ulcers are effective debridement, offloading of pressure, treatment of infection, and local wound care. In addition, a greater understanding of the pathophysiology of wound healing has led to advanced wound care products demonstrating promise in accelerating wound healing.

Debridement

The goal of wound debridement is the complete removal of all necrotic, dysvascular, and nonviable tissue in order to achieve a red, granular wound bed. Sharp surgical debridement using sharp instruments, such as a scalpel blade is ideal *(81)* (Fig. 6). Using this technique all nonviable tissue are removed until a healthy bleeding ulcer bed is produced with saucerization of the wound edges. Ulcerations with redundant hyperkeratotic rim should be aggressively debrided to remove this hyperkeratotic tissue. This will help to reduce pressure on the wound when the patient ambulates. It will also facilitate better visualization of the wound for a more thorough evaluation. The bacterial

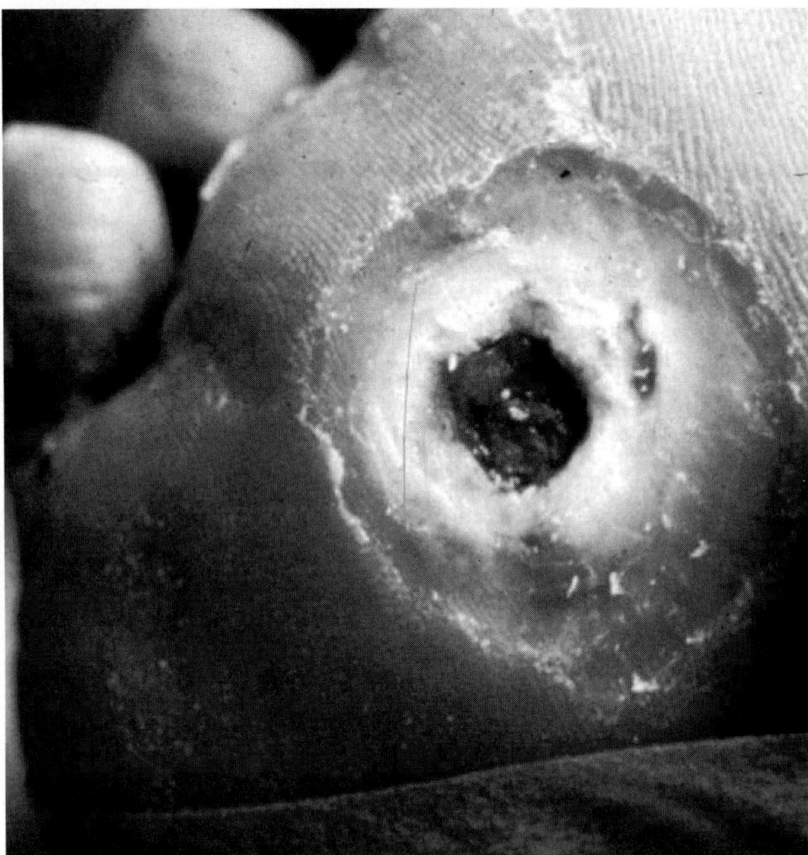

Fig. 6. A grade 2 ulcer after surgical debridement. Adequate debridement is achieved when all exuberant callous tissue and necrotic tissue have been removed and a clean granular base is revealed.

load at the ulcer site can also be reduced by debriding an ulceration aggressively. This procedure can be performed in the office setting except in the rare cases when extensive debridement is required or sensation to the foot is not intact and the use of the operating room might be required. In addition, in the event that ischemia is suspected, aggressive debridement should be delayed until vascular examination and revascularization are achieved.

Other debridement techniques are also available, but none has gained universal acceptance. Autolytic debridement refers the body's own mechanism of removing devitalized tissue. This process is primarily undertaken by macrophages, which release proteolytic enzymes to degrade nonviable tissue *(82)*. However, this method requires adequate arterial perfusion as well as wound hydration and can be slow and tedious. It often involves the use of occlusive dressings left in place for 2–3 days. Enzymatic debridement involves the use of topical agents with the ability to degrade necrotic tissue using proteolytic enzymes. These agents are typically applied to a wound under an occlusive dressing. Indications for use are limited and are generally, indicated to slowly soften large eschars or debride decubitus ulcerations in sensate limbs. Drawbacks to this form of debridement include the lengthy process and considerable expense of these agents *(83)*. Finally, mechanical debridement gently loosens and removes slough from the wound bed. The simplest form of this technique is the commonly applied wet-to-dry saline gauze. The moist gauze dries on the wound. Upon removal of the dried gauze, the adhered tissue will be removed with the dressing. The material that is removed is very superficial tissue. Where this is an inexpensive and relatively easy technique, it can remove both viable and nonviable tissue and cause pain in the sensate foot. Caution must be exerted in using this type of dressing to a wound with a granulating base that only requires epithelialization to close. This type of dressing might remove epithelial tissue with each dressing change and therefore, should not be used in this situation as opposed to a adherent dressing, which is more ideal.

Pressure Offloading

Reduction of pressures is essential in the healing of plantar foot ulcers. As discussed previously, ulcerations occur in high pressure areas of the insensate foot. There are a number of methods used for the reduction of foot pressures, with varying success rates. The most popular methods include total contact casting, half shoes, short leg walkers, and felted foam dressings.

Total contact casting has been considered the most effective means of offloading diabetic foot ulcers as measured by wound healing rate *(84)*. Described by Paul Brand, total contact casting involves the use of a well-molded minimally padded plaster cast to distribute pressures evenly to the entire limb. It allows for patient mobility during treatment and has been found to help control edema linked to impairment of healing *(85)* while maintaining the forced patient compliance because of the inability to remove the apparatus. Disadvantages include the considerable skill and time required for application, the possibility of secondary skin lesions because of cast irritation, and the inability to assess the wound daily. Patients also complain of the total contact cast making sleeping and showering difficult.

Because of the considerable disadvantages associated with the total contact cast, few clinicians use it as the technique of choice in regular clinical practice. Instead, commercially available off the shelf devices, such as the half shoe and prefabricated short leg walker are more commonly used. Both these devices are relatively inexpensive, easy to use, and readily accepted by the patient. However, pressure reduction is significantly less compared with total contact casting and patient compliance cannot be assured because of the removable nature of the devices *(86)*.

Felted foam dressings are accommodative offloading devices fashioned from a felt-foam pad with an aperture corresponding to the ulceration for customized pressure relief. The pad is attached to the patients skin with a pliable adhesive, preventing migration of the pad, and thereby ensuring a degree of patient compliance (Fig. 7). Wound care and wound assessment can be performed through the aperture or window that is created for access to the wound. The felted foam is often used in conjunction with a surgical shoe or half-shoe and must be changed every 10–14 days to ensure integrity of the dressing. Felted foam dressings in combination with a surgical shoe or half-shoe were found to be more effective in pressure reduction when compared with a short leg walker or a half-shoe alone *(87)*.

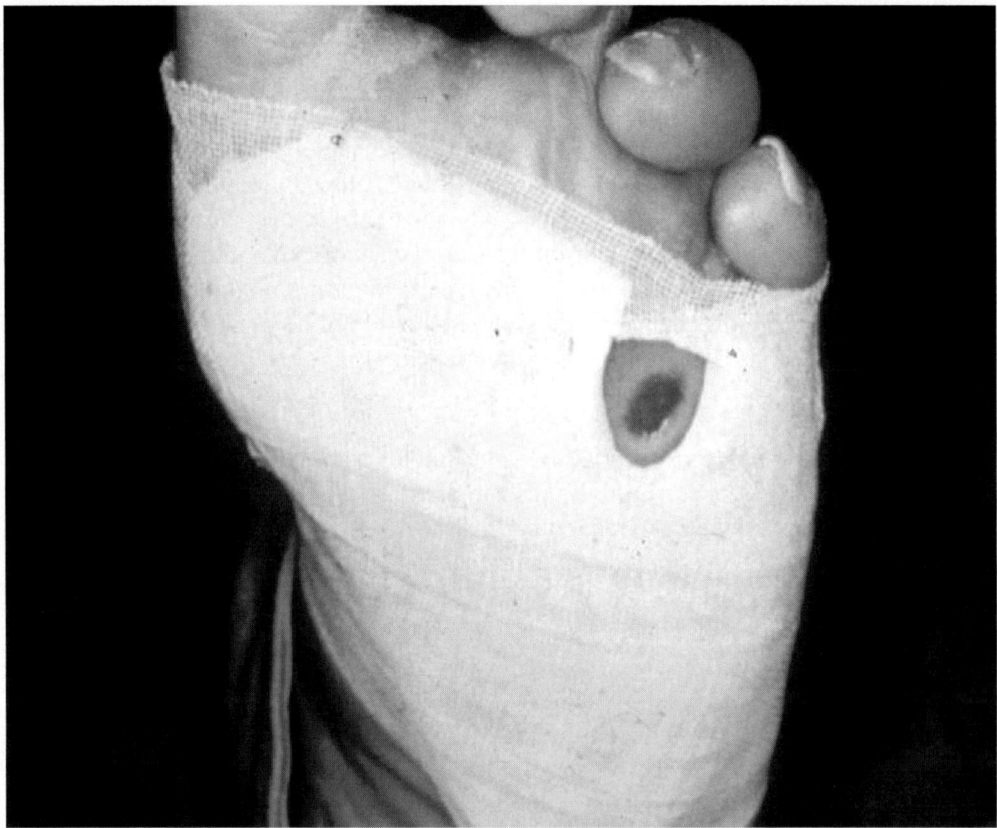

Fig. 7. The felted foam dressing is an effective pressure offloading modality for patients with Wagner 1 and 2 foot ulcers. The felted foam can stay in place for 1 week whereas wound care and wound assessment can be performed through the aperture portion.

Treatment of Infection

Bacteria colonize ulcerations and these ulcerations may serve as a portal of entry resulting in the development of an infection. Diagnosis of infection is primarily based on clinical appearance, relying on clinical signs such as erythema, edema, pain, tenderness, and warmth. Care must be taken to diagnose and treat infections sufficiently as mild cellulitis can rapidly progress to a limb threatening infection if left untreated. Indeed the spectrum of infections might range from the local cellulites to severe, limb threatening deep abscesses with osteomyelitis. Additional clinical information may be obtained with cultures, radiographs, and more advanced imaging techniques. When clinical infection of an ulcer is suspected, cultures of the wound will aid in directing subsequent antibiotic therapy. Empirical antibiotic therapy should be started for cases of infection, with revision of therapy pending culture results.

Radiographical imaging of the infected foot can demonstrate increased density and thickening of the subcutaneous fat along with blurring of the usually visible fat planes *(88)*. Presence of osseous changes, such as periosteal reaction, cortical bone destruction, and focal osteopenia might suggest a diagnosis of osteomyelitis. However, these

Table 1
Selected Antibiotic Regimens for Initial Empiric Therapy of Foot Infections in Patients With Diabetes Mellitus[a]

Infection	Antimicrobial regimen[b]
Non Limb threatening	Cephalexin 500 mg p.o. q 6 hour
	Clindamycin 300 mg p.o. q 8 hour
	Amoxicillin-clavulanate (875/125 mg) one q 12 hour
	Dicloxacillin 500 mg p.o. q 6 hour
	Levofloxacin 500–750 mg p.o. q day
Limb threatening	Ceftriaxone[c] 1 gm iv daily + clindamycin 450–600 mg iv q 8 hour
	Ciprofloxacin 400 mg iv q 12 hour + clindamycin 450–600 mg iv q 8 hour
	Ampicillin/sulbactam 3 g iv q 6 hour
	Ticarcillin/clavulanate 3.1 g iv q 4–6 hour
	Piperacillin/tazobactam 3.375 g iv q 4 hour or 4.5 g iv q 6 hour
	Fluoroquinolone[d] iv + metronidazole 500 mg iv q 6 hour
Life threatening	Imipenem cilastatin 500 mg iv q 6 hour
	Piperacillin/tazobactam 4.5 g iv q 6 hour + gentamicin[e] 1.5 mg/kg iv q 8 hour
	Vancomycin 1 g iv q 12 hour + gentamicin + metronidazole

[a]From ref. *89*.
[b]Doses for patients with normal renal function.
[c]An alternative is cefotaxime 2 g iv q 8 hour.
[d]Fluoroquinolone with increased activity against gram positive cocci, for example, levofloxacin 500–750 mg iv q day.
[e]Can be given as single daily dose 5.1 mg/kg per day.
p. o., orally; q, every.

changes only become evident after osteomyelitis has been present for 10–14 days and require up to 50% bone loss before becoming recognizable *(89)*. Advanced imaging techniques, such as magnetic resonance imaging and computed tomography may aid in the accurate diagnosis of osteomyelitis as well as demonstrate abscess formations.

Treatment of infection involves debridement of all necrotic tissue with aggressive, adequate drainage along with antibiotic therapy. Antibiotic selection should take into account the likely causative organisms, whereas bearing in mind the potential toxicity of the agents. In the diabetic foot, the bacteria most likely responsible for minor, non-limb threatening infections such as a cellulitis are *Staphylococcus* and *Streptococci*. Whereas more severe, deeper, and limb-threatening infections are generally the consequence of a polymicrobial infection *(90)*. Empirical antibiotic selection should be based on the suspected bacterial pathogens along with modifications to address anticipated resistant pathogens that might have been present during earlier episodes of infection. Antibiotic selection should minimize toxicity and be cost effective. Broad spectrum antimicrobial therapy should be initiated empirically with reassessment following the results of culture data. The main antibiotic regimens for initial empiric therapy that are used in our unit is shown in Table 1 *(91)*.

The duration of antimicrobial therapy for severe soft tissue infections of the foot is based on response to the antibiotics and wound care. Two weeks of therapy is the usual guideline, however, recalcitrant infections might require longer courses. Even if the ulcer has not fully healed, antibiotics can be discontinued when evidence of infection has resolved. Continuation of antibiotics beyond this duration has not demonstrated any effect on wound healing *(92,93)*.

Wound Care

The effective use of dressings is essential to ensure the optimal management of diabetic foot ulcers. In recent years, the concept of a clean, moist, wound-healing environment has been widely accepted. Benefits to this approach include prevention of tissue dehydration and cell death, acceleration of angiogenesis, and facilitating the interaction of growth factors with the target cells *(94)*. In addition, patients have reported less discomfort with moist wound dressings. The notion that a moist wound environment increases the risk of developing an infection appears to be unfounded. There are a multitude of wound care products available in the market that promote moist wound healing, however, wet-to-dry normal saline gauze remains the standard of care.

Advanced Wound Care Products

Advanced wound care products have been developed in response to an improved understanding of the impaired wound healing integral in the diabetic foot ulcer. A greater understanding of wound pathophysiology with deficiencies, such as decreased growth factors production and altered cellular inactivity have led to the development of products that address these deficiencies. These include recombinant platelet-derived growth factor and biological skin substitutes.

Recombinant human PDGF-BB (becaplermin) is the only growth factor to date approved by the US Food and Drug Administration for the treatment of diabetic foot ulcers. PDGF-B is a potent mitogen and chemotactic agent for connective tissue and stromal cells and may act to increase the wound vascularization by stimulating endothelial cell proliferation, movement, and tube formation. Levels of PDGF have been shown to be lower in chronic wounds *(95)*. Becaplermin as it is known, is formulated as a gel to help maintain proper moisture balance. It was found to increase both the incidence of complete wound closure and decreased the time to achieve complete wound healing *(96)*.

Biological skin substitutes, also known as living skin equivalents (LSE), are commercially available. The LSEs are produced through tissue-engineering technology. Available for epidermal, dermal, and composite (epidermal and dermal) wounds, LSEs offer distinct advantages compared with traditional skin grafting as their use is noninvasive, does not require anesthesia, can be performed in an outpatient setting, and avoids potential donor site complications, such as infection and scarring *(97)*. Two LSEs were approved for use in diabetic foot ulcers, Dermagraft (Advanced Tissue Sciences Inc, La Jolla, CA) and Apligraf (Novartis Pharmaceutical Corp., Basel). Dermagraft consists of neonatal dermal fibroblasts cultured in vitro onto a bioabsorbable polyglactin mesh, producing a living, metabolically active tissue containing the normal dermal matrix proteins and cytokines. Dermagraft has been shown to incorporate quickly into the wound with good vascularization and with no adverse side-effects *(98,99)*. In a prospective randomized multicenter study, Dermagraft-treated ulcers were shown to compare favorably with more complete and rapid healing. Along with the added benefit of a reduction in the ulcer recurrence rate compared with conventional therapy *(100)*. Dermagraft has since been discontinued.

Apligraf is considered a composite graft, containing both epidermal and dermal components. The outer layer consists of allogenic human keratinocytes constructed with an inner dermal layer consisting of human fibroblasts on type 1 collagen dispersed in a protein matrix. Apligraf histologically resembles human skin, but it does not contain structures, such as blood vessels, hair follicles, or sweat glands. Interestingly, Apligraf acts like human skin, producing all the cytokines and growth factors produced by normal skin during the wound healing process *(101)*. In diabetic foot ulcers, Apligraf was shown to significantly increase the wound healing rate as well as decreasing the median time to complete wound closure *(102,103)*. Ulcer recurrence rate was similar in both Apligraf-treated ulcers and standard treatment groups *(103)*.

The exact mechanism of action of Dermagraft and Apligraf is not completely understood. It is believed that improved wound healing is because of filling of the wound with extracellular matrix proteins and with the subsequent induction, and expression of growth factors and cytokines necessary for wound healing. Additionally, the matrix components might further facilitate the recruitment of cells to the wound to enhance wound healing.

Although, advanced wound care products can increase the rate of complete wound healing, they carry the disadvantage of being very expensive, to the extent that their use is prohibited in some societies with limited resources. However, even in prosperous societies their use is not recommended in all patients as they carry a heavy economic cost. Therefore, they are not considered a first line agent. The current consensus is that they should be utilized only in cases that are likely to fail standard care. The identification of such patients is therefore very important as it can help individual patients heal their ulcers, whereas at the same time do not impose an economical burden on the society.

Observing the changes in wound area during a 4-week period, whereas intensive standard care is administered, is the best currently available method to identify the patients who do not respond to standard care and are more likely to benefit by advanced care wound products (Fig. 8). The wound area is calculated by measuring the maximal width and length of the ulcer. Patients who fail to reduce the wound area by 50% during this period are unlikely to achieve complete wound closure in the next few months and should be selected for additional advanced treatment *(104)*. Therefore, patients who exceed the 50% reduction should be expected to heal in a reasonable period of time and should continue to receive standard care. However, in those patients where ulcer area reduction slows to less than 50%, their progress must be monitored carefully as a change in their wound care may need to be considered.

Treatment by Ulcer Severity

Treatment of the diabetic foot ulcer requires a thorough assessment of factors such as size, depth, location, and presence/absence of infection or ischemia. The location of the ulcer is a clue to the etiology of the wound and offloading measures necessary to minimize motion at the ulcer site. Size will help in determining the length of time required for wound healing. Depth is very important in determining the proximity of adjacent structures. The presence of infection should be addressed with appropriate antibiotic therapy or surgical incision and drainage when required. Ischemic ulcers demand revascularization techniques in order for wound healing to proceed.

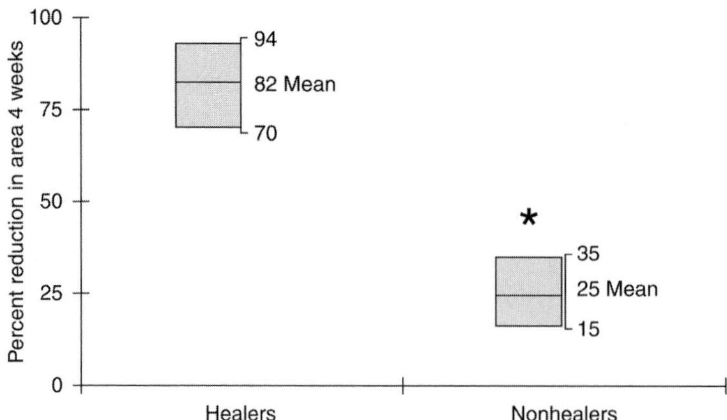

Fig. 8. Mean percent ulcer area reduction during the first 4 weeks of a prospective study that followed up a large number of patients for a 12-week period. Patients who completely healed their ulcer during the 12-week period of the study are characterized as Healers and those who failed to heal their ulcer as nonhealers. The ulcer area was measured by multiplying the length by the width of the ulcer. During the first 4 weeks of the study, the Healers had a mean percent ulcer area reduction of 82% (95% CI 70-94) significantly higher to that of the nonhealers who had a 25% reduction (95% CI 15-35, $p < 0.001$). The midpoint between the percentage area reduction from baseline at 4 weeks in patients healed against those not healed at 12 weeks was 53%. Subjects with an ulcer area reduction above the 4-week median had a 12-week healing rate of 58%, whereas those less than that had a healing rate of only 9% ($p < 0.01$). Thus, patients who fail to reduce their ulcer area half over a 4-week period should be considered as to be unlikely to heal and the use of advanced wound care products may be justifiable (from ref. *100*).

The treatment of ulcers based on grade, as delineated by the Wagner classification, will be presented here. It is important to note that as a general rule, Wagner grades 0 and 1 and the vast majority of grade 2 ulcers are largely managed on an outpatient basis whereas Wagner grades 3, 4, and 5 might require hospitalization. Table 2 describes the management of specific Wagner classified foot ulcers based on treatment rendered and medical personnel involved.

Wagner Grade 0

As mentioned earlier, all patients identified as being at risk of developing foot ulceration should be classified as grade 0. The management of the grade 0 foot consists primarily of patient education and regular foot care in an effort to prevent the development of foot ulceration. The patients should be informed of the risks associated with the neuropathic foot along with the early signs and symptoms of infection. In addition, the need of regular foot care by a specialist and the avoidance of certain dangerous self-care interventions should be emphasized. Daily inspection of the foot by the patient or a member of his close environment is critical. Diabetic literature with simple and easily understood guidelines is available worldwide by various sources and all patients should have access to this information.

Regular visits for podiatric care should be part of the patients healthcare management. Clinical inspection of the feet should be performed with evaluation of vascular perfusion to the foot. Hyperkeratotic lesions, such as corns and calluses should be

Table 2
Principles of Treatment and Medical Personnel Involved in Diabetic Foot Ulcers Based on the Wagner Classification

	Principles of treatment	Provider involved
Wagner 0	Patient education, outpatient routine preventative foot care, and protective shoewear	Diabetes educator, podiatrist, pedorthotist
Wagner 1	Outpatient ulcer care with debridement and offloading	Podiatrist
Wagner 2	Outpatient ulcer care with debridement, offloading and wound care. Treatment of infection as warranted	Podiatrist
Wagner 3	Outpatient/inpatient ulcer care consisting of bedside or surgical debridement with offloading and wound care. Treatment of infection as necessary	Podiatrist, surgeon, infectious disease
Wagner 4	Inpatient care consisting of surgical debridement and antibiotic therapy. Revascularization might be required with possible amputation	Podiatrist, vascular surgeon, infectious disease, orthopedic surgeon
Wagner 5	Inpatient care consisting of revascularization if possible and probable amputation	Vascular surgeon, orthopedic surgeon, rehabilitation therapy

debrided at these visits. Shoes and socks should be evaluated to determine if they are adequate. Extra-depth diabetic shoes and custom-molded inserts both serve to protect osseous prominences and also effectively reduce plantar foot pressures *(105)*. High foot pressures often present on the plantar aspect of the forefoot can also be reduced with the use of padded socks *(106)*.

Wagner Grade 1

A Grade 1 ulceration is defined as one that has penetrated beyond the epidermis. The presence of sensory neuropathy and at least one other risk factor is common. The ulcer should be evaluated for size, depth, location, and any signs of infection. The presence of drainage, as well as the type of drainage should be noted. The treatment of a Wagner grade 1 ulcer includes debridement of all nonviable tissue, local wound care, offloading of pressures, and antibiotic therapy if infection is poresent. Sharp debridement of the ulcer should be performed as previously discussed in this chapter. Following debridement, the foot must be off-loaded to minimize pressure and motion at the site of ulceration although, the patient continues to ambulate. Patients must also be counseled to limit ambulation and to use crutches if necessary. The authors commonly use the felted foam dressing for offloading. This method is easy to perform, relatively inexpensive, and reproducible. Wound care can be performed through a window in the felted foam dressing.

Ulcerations that recur might warrant surgical correction of any underlying structural deformity. Surgical procedures, such as digital arthroplasties, metatarsal osteotomies, metatarsal head resections, and mid- and hindfoot exostectomies, have all proved useful in the prevention of recurrent ulcerations *(107–111)*.

Wagner Grade 2

Grade 2 is a full thickness ulcer that penetrates beyond the dermis with involvement of deeper structures, such as tendons, ligaments, or joint capsules. The management of such ulcers is usually based on an outpatient basis although hospitalization can be considered in deep wounds that expose tendons and complications such as peripheral vascular disease, and infection is suspected.

Outpatient care for the full thickness ulcer that has anon-infected granulating basis is similar to the grade 1 ulceration described earlier. Broad spectrum antibiotics might be added in case infection is suspected and dressing changes might be performed more often in cases of heavy exudates. Advanced wound care products may be considered for patients who are not exhibiting a satisfactory progress using the previously described criteria. Patients with grade 2 ulcerations treated as outpatients if necessary must be directed to aggressively offload the foot using crutches. With deeper structures in such close proximity, optimal patient compliance is necessary to avoid furthermore complications, such as cellulitis, abscess formation, and osteomyelitis.

Involvement of deep structures to the base of the ulcer should be managed with aggressive debridement, complete bed rest, empiric use of broad-spectrum antibiotics, and occasionally hospitalization *(112)*. The foot may require surgical debridement in order to remove all necrotic and nonviable tissue that may impede granulation tissue. Debridement should be carried out until there is evidence of healthy, red, granulation tissue to the base. Additionally, all sinus tracts should be explored and drained. Intraoperative deep cultures should be taken for identification of the pathogen responsible for infection.

In the event that vascular insufficiency is suspected, incision and drainage of the infected foot should not be delayed. Adequate drainage of the infected foot is paramount to limb salvage. Delaying of surgical drainage may lead to furthermore tissue loss as well as potential limb loss *(113)*. Instead, vascular consultation should be initiated as soon as possible, even if it occurs after surgical drainage.

Wagner Grade 3

Grade 3 ulcerations are characterized by the presence of deep infection with bone involvement and abscess collections. Grade 3 ulcers are usually the result of grade 2 ulcers that fail to respond, aggressive bacterial infections, or puncture wounds, resulting in direct inoculation of bone. Because of the depth of these ulcers and the presence of purulent collections and bone infection, these ulcers require hospitalization with adequate drainage of all infection and debridement of all infected bone. Prolonged antibiotic therapy might be required.

Adequate drainage of infection is key in managing grade 3 ulcerations. All sinus tracts must be explored and all necrotic and nonviable tissue debrided. In cases of severe infection, open amputations of digits or rays might be required to prevent the spread of infection. Once the infection has cleared and granulation of the wound bed observed, thought can be given to coverage of the wound. In instances where soft tissue coverage is adequate, delayed primary closure can be undertaken. However, more often than not in these extensive wounds, significant soft tissue defects might be present, requiring osseous remodeling in addition to tissue flaps or skin grafts to provide wound coverage *(114)*. No single technique can be applied universally as each case is unique. Instead, a flexible approach will maximize limb salvage.

Wagner Grade 4

Grade 4 ulcerations demonstrate partial foot gangrene. These ulcers are usually complicated by ischemia, osteomyelitis, and sepsis. A team approach is required in order to minimize the extent of tissue loss and prevent amputation. Consultations with vascular surgeons, podiatrists, infectious disease specialists, and plastic surgeons are essential for limb salvage. The primary goal in the management of these ulcers is to limit the extent of tissue loss.

Gangrenous changes can result from minor trauma in the face of severe arterial insufficiency or when overwhelming infection results in occlusion of digital arterial branches *(11,115)*. Initial treatment of gangrene secondary to severe arterial insufficiency should begin with vascular assessment and when possible should be followed by revascularization *(113)*. In severe infections resulting in local ischemia, aggressive drainage along with appropriate antibiotic therapy should be instituted to limit tissue loss.

Wagner Grade 5

Grade 5 ulcerations demonstrate extensive necrosis of the entire foot as a direct result of arterial insufficiency. Primary amputation is the only treatment for extensive gangrene. However, vascular assessment and revascularization should always be attempted to allow for amputation at the most distal level of the foot.

CHARCOT NEUROARTHROPATHY

Charcot neuroarthropathy is a noninfectious progression of joint destruction characterized by pathological fractures and joint dislocations. Although it was initially described by Musgrave in 1704, its name was attributed to J.M. Charcot in 1868 *(116)*. The disease involves joint destruction of accompanying common diseases that manifest with peripheral neuropathy, such as leprosy, tertiary syphilis, chronic alcoholism, and spina bifida *(117)*. Diabetes mellitus is currently the primary cause of Charcot neuroarthropathy.

Etiology

The exact etiology of Charcot neuroarthropathy remains unclear. There are two leading theories: the neurotraumatic (German) theory, and the neurovascular (French) theory. The neurotraumatic theory proposed that repeated microtrauma on neuropathic joints results in the eventual joint destruction *(118)*. Repetitive minor stresses on insensate joints produce intracapsular effusions, ligamentous laxity, and joint instability. With continued use of the foot, degeneration of the joints continues, often resulting in severe joint dislocation, fractures, and deformity mostly because of arch collapse.

In contrast, the neurovascular theory suggested that the main factor is the autonomic neuropathy-related hyperemia that causes excessive bone resorption and leads to weakening of the bone *(119)*. The hyperemic bone resorption thus allows for increased risk of fractures with joint dislocation and destruction evident in Charcot joints. This theory corresponds to the clinical observation that Charcot neuroarthropathy occurs most commonly in patients with palpable pedal pulses *(120)*. Further support to this hypothesis is provided by studies in the unit that have shown that the nonspecific hyperemic response to skin heating is increased in patients with neuroarthropathy, when compared with patient with diabetes with equally severe neuropathy *(54)*. The current consensus is that the process of Charcot neuroarthropathy is secondary to a combination of both the neurovascular and neurotraumatic theories.

Clinical Findings

Regardless of the exact etiology, the Charcot foot usually presents as a warm, non-painful, swelling of the foot. Usually, there is no evidence of an open wound and an infectious process, although often suspected it can be excluded based on lack of clinical findings to support infection. Occasionally, patients may describe a precedent history of minor trauma; however, this is frequently so trivial that the patient is unable to recall the incident. Trauma in the form of foot surgery can also be another precipitating factor. The Charcot neuroarthropathy can occur in either the ipsilateral or contralateral limb following foot surgery. This phenomenon can be attributed to the likely alteration in weight-bearing forces in joints of the foot, triggering the changes in Charcot joint.

Initial evaluation of Charcot neuroarthropathy requires a thorough clinical and radiographical examination of the foot. Clinical examination reveals a warm, edematous foot often with evidence of crepitus with joint range of motion of the affected joint. Joint laxity is often present. Most commonly, pain is absent or significantly less than expected from the clinical presentation. Radiographical findings may reveal a spectrum of findings from subtle subluxation to frank dislocation with osseous debris and fragmentation. The most common site affected in the foot is the tarsometatarsal joint *(121)*. The extent of fragmentation and joint destruction is variable and most often related to the particular joints affected and the degree of ambulation before the diagnosis. Advanced imaging techniques, such as CT scans and magnetic resonance imaging are rarely necessary to make the diagnosis of Charcot joint especially in advanced cases and instead may be more useful in preoperative surgical planning in certain cases.

There are three identifiable clinical phases of Charcot neuroarthropathy: acute, coalescence, and remodeling. The acute phase is characterized by clinical findings of edema, erythema, localized warmth, and joint crepitus with range of motion examination. The coalescence phase begins when skin temperature normalizes and joint crepitus diminishes. With a period of duration lasting from months to years, the remodeling phase is characterized by joint stabilization and remodeling.

Resolution of Charcot neuroarthropathy can result in a deformed foot with obvious bony prominences susceptible to ulceration (Fig. 9) *(122)*. If diagnosed early and sufficient immobilization is rendered, the possibility of joint collapse with resulting osseous prominences may be mitigated. However, in instances of misdiagnosis or inadequate immobilization, a "rocker-bottom" type foot can result, with gross deformities of the involved joint and prominent areas to the plantar aspect of the foot. These prominent areas often on the plantar aspect of the midfoot are prone to increased pressure and ulceration.

Treatment

The treatment of choice for acute Charcot foot is complete immobilization and non-weight-bearing. Immobilization can be achieved with casts, splints or braces, and non-weight-bearing aid with the use of crutches, walkers, or wheelchairs. Failure to adequately immobilize the foot might result in furthermore fragmentation of bone with progression of

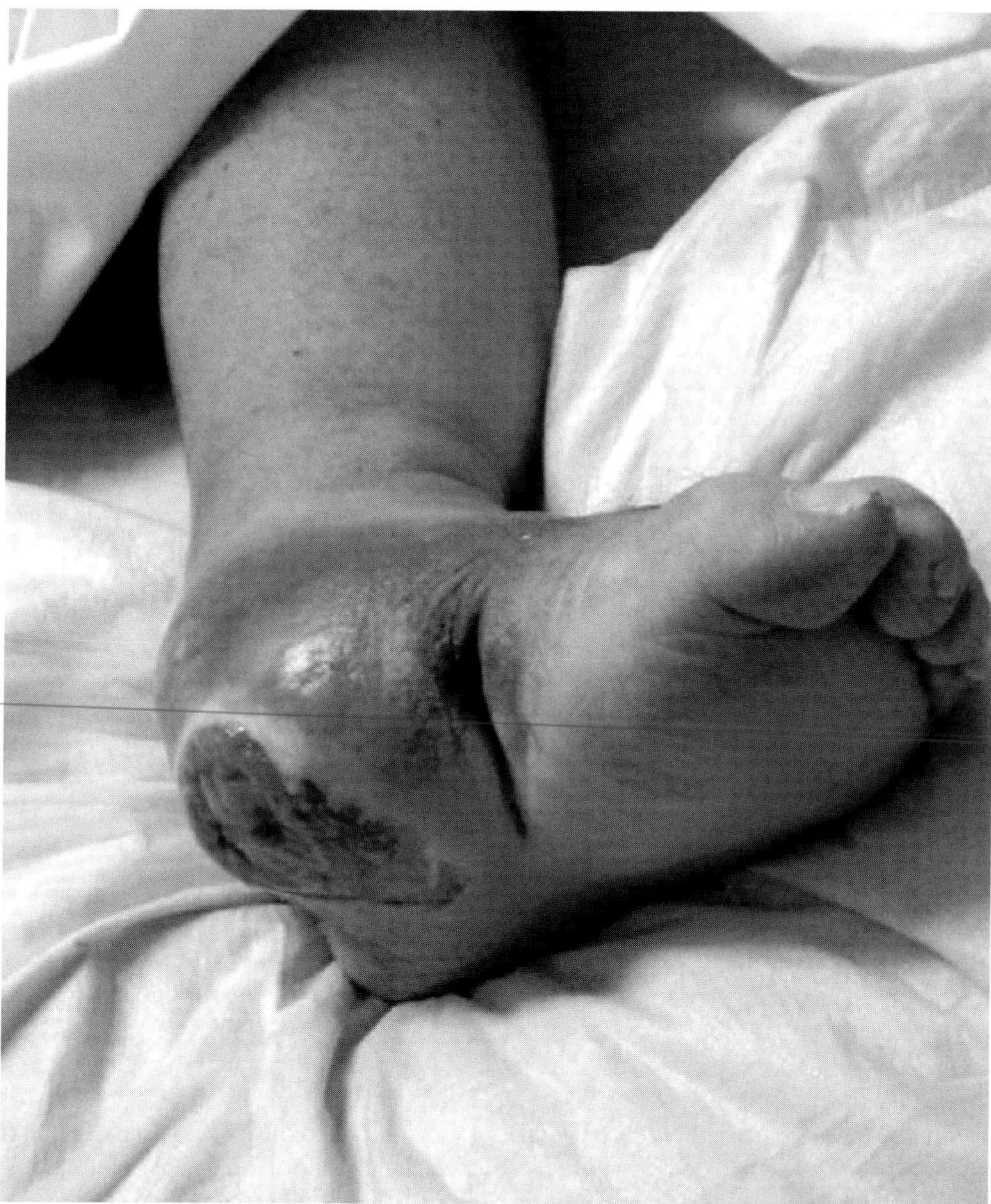

Fig. 9. *(Continued)*

the joint deformity, resulting in a nonplantigrade foot. The ultimate goal of immobilization therapy is to allow for the foot to coalesce in a shape that will allow for eventual ambulation.

Immobilization and nonweight-bearing should continue until the acute phase of Charcot has ended and the coalescence phase commenced. The duration of immobilization varies from 8 to 32 weeks *(123,124)*. The decision to begin weight-bearing may be best made by clinical parameters such as foot temperature (should be the same with the contralateral limb) and resolution of erythema and edema, rather than an arbitrary time period. Serial radiographs may also aid in the decision making process. Evidence

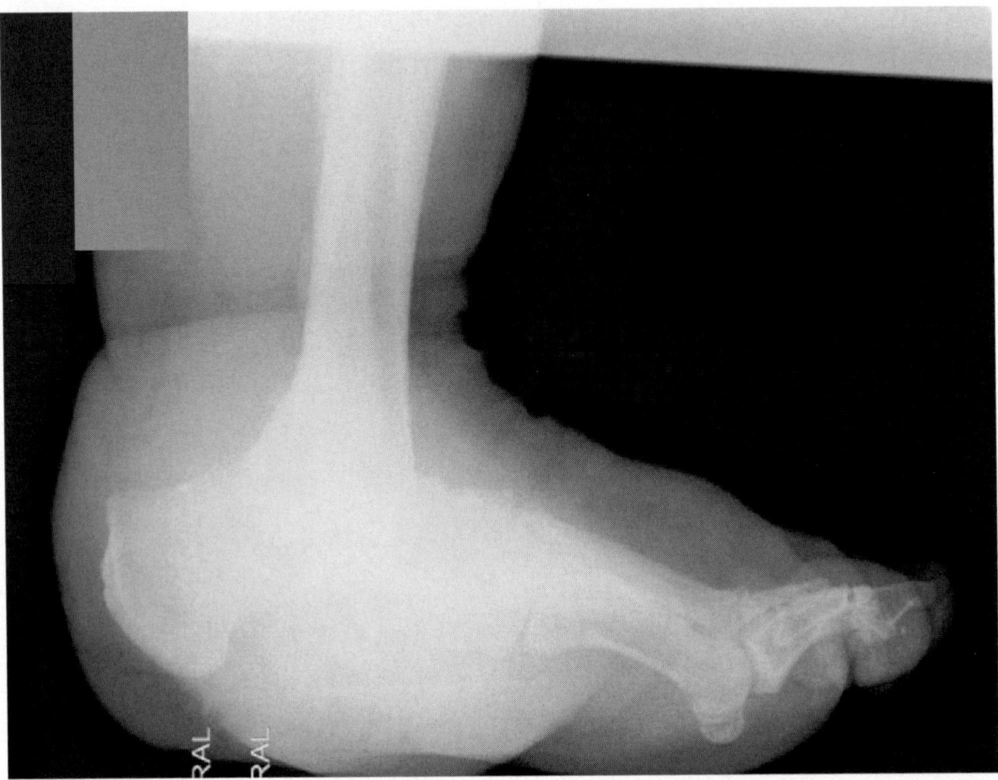

Fig. 9. (A) Midfoot Charcot neuroarthropathy in a patient with diabetes with severe peripheral neuropathy. Severe foot deformity has resulted to an area where high pressures have been applied during walking leading to extensive ulceration. **(B)** X-ray from the same patient shows extensive destruction of the midfoot joints.

of osseous consolidation, union of fractures, and reduction in soft tissue edema are radiographical clues that coalescence has begun.

Once weight-bearing is deemed safe, return to ambulation should be performed in a gradual manner. Typically, weight-bearing is begun allowing only 15–20 pounds of weight on the affected limb, with 10 pound increments added on a weekly basis. Should symptoms of the acute phase, such as edema, erythema, and warmth appear, immobilization and nonweight-bearing should be resumed until resolution of these symptoms occur. As weight-bearing progresses, the patient is eventually allowed to fully ambulate short distances without the use of assistive devices.

In recent years, increased attention has been given to surgical reconstruction of the severely deformed Charcot foot. In cases where immobilization and nonweight-bearing have failed to prevent extensive joint dislocation, a rocker-bottom type foot with osseous prominences can be the end result. This type of foot is highly susceptible to ulceration. Therefore, arthrodesis of the involved joints might provide a stable platform for ambulation in addition to preventing future ulcerations. However, patients undergoing joint fusions will require extended periods of postoperative immobilization and nonweight-bearing, and therefore, should be screened carefully. Arthrodesis in patients who are identified early before advanced bone destruction occurs is gaining especially in compliant patients *(125)*.

REFERENCES

1. Sanders LJ. Diabetes mellitus: prevention of amputation. *J Am Podiatr Med Assoc* 1994;84(7):322–328.
2. Hogan P, Dall T, Nikolov P. Economic costs of diabetes in the US in 2002. *Diabetes Care* 2003;26(3):917–932.
3. Ramsey SD, Newton K, Blough D, et al. Incidence, outcomes, and cost of foot ulcers in patients with diabetes. *Diabetes Care* 1999;22:382–387.
4. Palumbo PJ, Melton LJ. Peripheral vascular disease and diabetes, in *Diabetes in America* (Harris MI, Hamman RF, eds.), Govt. Printing Office, Washington, DC, US, 1985, pp. XV1– XV21.
5. Borssen B, Bergenheim T, Lithner F. The epidemiology of foot lesions in diabetic patients aged 15–50 years. *Diabet Med* 1999;7:438–444.
6. Kumar S, Asche HA, Fernando DJ. The prevalence of foot ulceration and its correlates in type 2 diabetic patients: a population-based study. *Diabet Med* 1994;11:480–484.
7. Moss SE, Klein R, Klein BE. The prevalence and incidence of lower extremity amputation in a diabetic population. *Arch Int Med* 1992;152:610–616.
8. Harrington C, Zagari MJ, Corea J, Klitenic J. A cost analysis of diabetic lower extremity lcers. *Diabetes Care* 2000;23:1333–1338.
9. Apelqvist J, Ragnarson-Tennvall G, Persson U, Larson J. Diabetic foot ulcers in a multidisciplinary setting: an economic analysis of primary healing and healing with amputation. *J Int Med* 1994;235:463–471.
10. Reiber GE, Boyko E, Smith DG. Lower extremity ulcers and amputations in individuals with diabetes, in *Diabetes in America* (Boyko EJ, Reiber GE, Bennett PH, eds.), Govt. Printing Office, Washington, DC, US, 1995, pp. 409–427.
11. Pecoraro RE, Reiber GE, Burgess EM. Pathways to diabetic limb amputation: basis for prevention. *Diabetes Care* 1990;13:513–521.
12. Reiber GE, Pecorraro RE, Koepsell TD. Risk factors for amputation in patients with diabetes mellitus: a case-control study. *Ann Int Med* 1992;117:97–105.
13. Lehto S, Pyorala K, Ronnemaa T, Laakso M. Risk factors predicting lower extremity amputations in Patients with NIDDM. *Diabetes Care* 1996;19:607–612.
14. Nelson RG, Gohdes DM, Everhart JE, et al. Lower extremity amputations in NIDDM: 12 year follow-up study in Pima Indians. *Diabetes Care* 1988;11:8–16.
15. Sittonen OL, Niskanen LK, Laakso M, Tiitonen J, Pyorala K. Lower extremity amputations in diabetic and nondiabetic patients. *Diabetes Care* 1988;11:8–16.
16. Resnick HE, Valsania P, Phillips CL. Diabetes mellitus and nontraumatic lower extremity amputation in black and white Americans: The National Health and Nutrition Examination Survey epidemiologic follow-up study, 1971–1992. *Arch Int Med* 1999;159:2470–2475.
17. Wrobel JS, Mayfield JA, Reiber GE. Geographic variation of lower-extremity major amputation in individuals with and without diabetes in the Medicare population. *Diabetes Care* 2001;24:1–5.
18. Most RS, Sinnock P. The epidemiology of lower extremity amputations in diabetic individuals. *Diabetes Care* 1983;6:87–91.
19. National Institute of Diabetes and Digestive and Kidney Diseases. National Diabetes Statistics fact sheet: general information and national estimates on diabetes in the United States, 2003. Bethesda, MD: US Department of Health and Human Services, National

Institutes of Health, 2003. Rev. ed. Bethesda, MD: US Department of Health and Human Services, National Institutes of Health, 2004.
20. Flegal KM, Ezzati TM, Harris M, et al. Prevalence of diabetes in Mexican Americans, Cubans and Puerto Ricans from the Hispanic Health and Nutrition Examination Survey, 1982-1984. *Diabetes Care* 1991;14:628–638.
21. Roseman JM. Diabetes in black Americans, in *Diabetes in America*, Govt. Printing Office, Washington, DC, US, 1985.
22. Edmonds ME, Blundell MP, Morris ME, Thomas EM, Cotton LT, Watkins PJ. Improved survival of the diabetic foot: the role of a specialized foot clinic. *J Med* 1986;60:763–771.
23. Lippmann HI. Must loss of a limb be a consequence of diabetes mellitus? *Diabetes Care* 1979;2:432–436.
24. Reiber GE. Diabetic foot care: guidelines and financial implications. *Diabetes Care* 1992;15:29–31.
25. Centers for Disease Control and Prevention. National diabetes fact sheet: general information and national estimates on diabetes in the United States, 2002. Atlanta, GA: US Department of Health and Human Services, Centers for Disease Control and Prevention, 2003.
26. Bakker K, Rauwerda JA, Schaper NC. *Diabetes Metab Res Rev* 2000;16(Suppl 1):S1.
27. Reiber GE, Vileikyte L, Boyko EJ, et al. Causal pathways for incident lower-extremity ulcers in patients with diabetes from two settings. *Diabetes Care* 1999;22:157–162.
28. Young MJ, Breddy JL, Veves A, Boulton AJ. The prediction of diabetic neuropathic foot ulceration using vibration perception thresholds. A prospective study. *Diabetes Care* 1994; 17:557–560.
29. Adler AI, Boyko EJ, Ahroni JH, Stensel V, Forsberg RC, Smith DG. Risk factors for diabetic peripheral sensory neuropathy. Results of the Seattle prospective diabetic foot study. *Diabetes Care* 1997;96:223–228.
30. Ward JD, Simms JM, Knight G, Boulton AJ, Sandler DA. Venous distension in the diabetic neuropathic foot. *J R Soc Med* 1983;76:1011–1014.
31. Boulton AJ, Scarpello JH, Ward JD. Venous oxygenation in the diabetic neuropathic foot: Evidence of arteriovenous shunting? *Diabetologia* 1982;22:6–8.
32. Tegner R. The effect of skin temperature on vibratory sensitivity in polyneuropathy. *J Neurol Neurosurg Psychiatr* 1985;48:176–178.
33. Boulton AJ, Hardisty CA, Betts RP, et al. Dynamic foot pressure and other studies as diagnostic and management aids in diabetic neuropathy. *Diabetes Care* 1983;1:26–33.
34. Stokes IA, Furis IB, Hutton WC. The neuropathic ulcer and loads on the foot in diabetic patients. *Acta Orthop Scand* 1975;46:839–847.
35. Ctercteko G, Dhanendran M, Hutton WC, et al. Vertical forces acting on the feet of diabetic patients with neuropathic ulceration. *Br J Surg* 1981;68:608–614.
36. Veves A, Fernando DJ, Walewski P, et al. A study of plantar pressures in a diabetic clinic population. *Foot* 1991;2:89–92.
37. Fernando DJ, Masson EA, Veves A, Boulton AJ. Relationship of limited joint mobility to abnormal foot pressures and diabetic foot ulceration. *Diabetes Care* 1991;14(1):8–11.
38. Caselli A, Pham HT, Giurini JM, Armstrong DG, Veves A. The forefoot/rearfoot plantar pressure ratio is increased in severe diabetic neuropathy and can predict foot ulceration. *Diabetes Care* 2002;25:1066–1071.
39. Veves A, Murray HJ, Young MJ, et al. The risk of foot ulceration in diabetic patients with high foot pressure: a prospective study. *Diabetologia* 1992;35:660–663.
40. Kelly PJ, Coventry MB. Neurotrophic ulcers of the feet: review of 47 cases. *JAMA* 1958; 168:388.
41. Sarnow MR, Veves A, Giurini JM, et al. In-shoe foot pressure measurements in diabetic patients with at-risk feet and in healthy subjects. *Diabetes Care* 1994;17:1002–1006.

42. Crisp AJ, Heathcote JG. Connective tissue abnormalities in diabetes mellitus. *J R Coll Phys* 1984;18:132–141.
43. Vlassara H, Brownlee M, Cerami A. Nonenzymatic glycosylation: rose in the pathogenesis of diabetic complications. *Clin Chem* 1986;32:B37–B41.
44. Delbridge L, Perry P, Marr S, et al. Limited joint mobility in the diabetic foot: relationship to neuropathic ulceration. *Diabet Med* 1988;5:333–337.
45. Mueller MJ, Diamond JE, Delitto A, Sinacore DR. Insensitivity, limited joint mobility, and plantar ulcers in patients with diabetes mellitus. *Phys Ther* 1989;69:453–462.
46. Birke JA, Franks BD, Foto JG. First ray joint limitation, pressure, and ulceration of the first metatarsal head in diabetes mellitus. *Foot Ankle* 1995;16:277–284.
47. Veves A, Sarnow MR, Giurini JM, et al. Differences in joint mobility and foot pressures between black and white diabetic patients. *Diabet Med* 1995;12:585–589.
48. Grant WP, Sullivan R, Soenshine DE, et al. Electron microscopic investigation of the effects of diabetes mellitus on the Achilles tendon. *J Foot Ankle Surg* 1997;36:272–278.
49. Armstrong DG, Stacpoole-Shea S, Nguyen HC, Harkless LB. Lengthening of the Achilles tendon in diabetic patients who are at high risk for ulceration of the foot. *J Bone Joint Surg* 1999;81A:535–538.
50. D'Ambrogi E, Giurato L, D'Agostino MA, et al. Contribution of plantar fascia to the increased forefoot pressures in diabetic patients. *Diabetes Care* 2003;26(5):1525–1529.
51. Parving HH, Viberti GC, Keen H, Christiansen JS, Lassen NA. Hemodynamic factors in the genesis of diabetic microangiopathy. *Metabolism* 1983;32:943–949.
52. Rayman G, Williams SA, Spencer PD, et al. Impaired microvascular hyperaemic response to minor skin trauma in type I diabetes. *BMJ* 1986;292:1295–1298.
53. Vane JR, Anggard EE, Botting RM. Regulatory functions of the vascular endothelium. *N Engl J Med* 1990;323:27–36.
54. Veves A, Akbari, CM, Primavera J, et al. Endothelial dysfunction and the expression of endothelial nitric oxide synthetase in diabetic neuropathy, vascular disease, and foot ulceration. *Diabetes* 1998;47:457–463.
55. Arora S, Smakowski P, Frykberg RG, Freeman R, LoGerfo FW, Veves A. Differences in foot and forearm skin microcirculation in diabetic patients with and without neuropathy. *Diabetes Care* 1998;21:1339–1344.
56. Caballero AE, Arora S, Saouaf R, et al. Microvascular and macrovascular reactivity is reduced in subjects at risk for type 2 diabetes. *Diabetes* 1999;48:1856–1862.
57. Szabo C, Zanchi A, Komjati K, et al. Poly (ADP-Ribose) polymerase is activated in subjects at risk of developing type 2 diabetes and is associated with impaired vascular reactivity. *Circulation* 2002;106:2680–2686.
58. Arora S, Pomposelli F, LoGerfo FW, Veves A. Cutaneous microcirculation in the neuropathic diabetic foot improves significantly but not completely after successful lower extremity revascularization. *J Vasc Surg* 2002;35:501–505.
59. Caselli A, Rich J, Hanane T, Uccioli L, Veves A. Role of C-nociceptive fibers in the nerve axon reflex-related vasodilation in diabetes. *Neurol* 2003;60:297–300.
60. Hamdy O, Abou-Elenin K, LoGerfo FW, Horton ES, Veves A. Contribution of nerve-axon reflex-related vasodilation to the total skin vasodilation in diabetic patients with and without neuropathy. *Diabetes Care* 2001;24:344–349.
61. Parkhouse N, LeQueen PM. Impaired neurogenic vascular response in patients with diabetes and neuropathic foot lesions. *N Engl J Med* 1988;318:1306–1309.
62. Schilling JA. Wound healing. *Physiol Rev* 1968;48:374–423.
63. Cooper DM, Yu EZ, Hennesey P, et al. Determination of endogenous cytokines in chronic wounds. *Ann Surg* 1994;219:688–692.
64. Zykova SN, Jenssen TG, Berdal M, et al. Altered cytokine and nitric oxide secretion in vitro by macrophages from diabetic type II-like db/db mice. *Diabetes* 2000;40:1451–1458.

65. Spravchikov N, Sizyakov G, Gartsbein M, et al. Glucose effects on skin keratinocytes. *Diabetes* 2001;50:1627–1635.
66. Jude EB, Boulton AJ, Ferguson MW, Appleton I. The role of nitric oxide synthase isoforms and arginase in the pathogenesis of diabetic foot ulcers: possible modulatory effects by transforming growth factor beta 1. *Diabetologia* 1999;42:748–757.
67. Loots MA, Lamme EN, Zeegelaar J, Mekkes JR, Bos JD, Middelkoop E. Differences in Cellular infiltrate and extracellular matrix of chronic diabetic and venous ulcers versus acute wounds. *J Invest Dermatol* 1998;111:850–857.
68. Rith-Najarian SJ, Stolusky T, Gohdes DM. Identifying diabetic patients at high risk for lower-extremity amputation in a primary health care setting. *Diabetes Care* 1992;22:1036–1042.
69. Boyko E, Ahroni JH, Stensel V, et al. A prospective study of risk factors for diabetic foot ulcer: the Seattle Diabetic Foot Study. *Diabetes Care* 1999;22:1036–1042.
70. Mayfield JA, Reiber GE, Sanders LJ, et al. Preventative foot care in people with diabetes. *Diabetes Care* 1998;21:2161–2177.
71. Boulton AJ, Gries FA, Jervell J. Guidelines for the diagnosis and outpatient management of diabetic periperal neuropathy. *Diabet Med* 1998;15:508–514.
72. Helm PA, Walker SC, Pulliam GF. Recurrence of neuropathic ulcerations following healing in a total contact cast. *Arch Phys Med Rehabil* 1991;72:967–970.
73. Thompson FJ, Veves A, Ashe H, et al. A team approach to diabetic foot care-the Manchester experience. *Foot* 1991;1:75–82.
74. Kumar S, Fernando DJ, Veves A, Knowles EA, Young MJ, Boulton AJ. Semmes-Weinstein monofilaments: a simple, effective and inexpensive screening device for identifying diabetic patients at risk of foot ulceration. *Diabetes Res Clin Pract* 1991;13:63–67.
75. Pham H, Armstrong DG, Harvey C, Harkless LB, Giurini JM, Veves A. Screening techniques to identify people at high risk for diabetic foot ulceration. *Diabetes Care* 2000;23:606–611.
76. McNeely MJ, Boyko E, Ahroni JH. The independent contributions of diabetic neuropathy and vasculopathy in foot ulceration: how great are the risks? *Diabetes Care* 1995;18:216–219.
77. Young MJ, Cavanagh PR, Thomas G, Johnson MM, Murray H, Boulton AJ. The effect of callus removal on dynamic plantar pressures in diabetic patients. *Diabetic Med* 1992;9:55–57.
78. Wagner FW. The dysvascular foot: a system for diagnosis and treatment. *Foot Ankle* 1981;2:64.
79. Lavery LA, Armstrong DG, Harkless LB. Classification of diabetic foot wounds. *J Foot Ankle Surg* 1996;36:528–531.
80. Armstrong DG, Lavery L, Harkless LB. Validation of a diabetic wound classification system. *Diabet Med* 1998;21:855–859.
81. Steed DL, Donohoe D, Wbster MW, Lindsley L. Diabetic Ulcer Study Group. Effect of extensive debridement and treatment on the healing of diabetic foot ulcers. *J Am Coll Surg* 1996;183:61–64.
82. Clark RAF. Mechanisms of cutaneous wound repair, in *Hematology in General Medicine* (Fitzpatrick TB, et al., eds.), McGraw-Hill, New York, 1993.
83. Bale S. A guide to wound debridement. *J Wound Care* 1997;6:179–182.
84. Armstrong DG, Nguyen HC, Lavery LA, et al. Offloading the diabetic foot wound: A randomized clinical trial. *Diabetes Care* 2001;24:1019–1022.
85. Mueller MJ, Diamond JE, Sinacore DR, et al. Total contact casting in treatment of diabetic plantar ulcers. *Diabetes Care* 1989;12:364–387.
86. Lavery LA, Vela SA, Lavery DC, et al. Reducting dynamic foot pressures in high-risk diabetics with foot ulcerations: A comparison of treatments. *Diabetes Care* 1996;19:818–821.

87. Birke JA, Fred B, Krieger LA, Sliman K. The effectiveness of an accommodative dressing in offloading pressure over areas of previous metatarsal head ulceration. *Wounds* 2003;15:33–39.
88. Cheung Y, Hochman M, Brophy DP. Radiographic Changes in the Diabetic Foot. in *The Diabetic Foot* (Veves A, Giurini JM, Logerfo FW, eds.), Humana Press, Totowa, NJ, 2002, pp. 179–205.
89. Bonakdar-Pour A, Gaines VD. The radiology of osteomyelitis. *Orthop Clin North Am* 1983;14:21–37.
90. Lipsky BA, Pecoraro RE, Wheat LJ. The diabetic foot: soft tissue and bone infection. *Infect Dis Clin North Am* 1990;4:409–432.
91. Karchmer AW. Microbiology and treatment of diabetic foot infections, in *The Diabetic Foot. Medical and Surgical Management* (Veves A, Giurini JM, LoGerfo FW, eds.), Humana Press, Totowa, NJ, 2002, pp. 207–220.
92. Lipsky BA, Pecoraro RE, Larson SA, Hanley ME, Ahroni JH. Outpatient management of uncomplicated lower-extremity infections in diabetic patients. *Arch Int Med* 1990;150:790–797.
93. Jones EW, Edwards R, Finch R, Jaffcoate WJ. A microbiologic study of diabetic foot lesions. *Diabet Med* 1984;2:213–215.
94. Field FK, Kerstein MD. Overview of wound healing in a moist environment. *Am J of Surg* 1994;167(1A):2S–6S.
95. Cooper DM, Yu EZ, Hennesey P, et al. Determination of endogenous cytokines in chronic wounds. *Ann Surg* 1994;219:688–692.
96. Wieman TJ, Smiell JM, Su Y. Efficacy and safety of a topical gel formulation of recombinant human platelet-derived growth factor-BB (Becaplermin) in patients with chronic neuropathic diabetic ulcers. *Diabetes Care* 1998;21:822–827.
97. Muhart M, McFalls S, Kirsner RS, et al. Behavior of tissue-engineered skin. *Arch Dermatol* 1999;135:913–918.
98. Hansbrough JF, Dore C, Hansbrough WB. Clinical trials of a living dermal tissue replacement placed beneath meshed, split-thickness skin grafts on excised burn wounds. *J Burn Care Rehabil* 1992;13:519–529.
99. Cooper ML, Hansbrough JF, Spielvogel RL, et al. In vivo optimization of a living dermal substitute employing cultured human fibroblasts on a biodegradable polyglycolic acid or polyglactin mesh. *Biomaterials* 1991;12:243–248.
100. Gentzkow GD, Iwasaki SD, Hershon KS, et al. Use of Dermagraft, a cultured human dermis, to treat diabetic foot ulcers. *Diabetes Care* 1996;19:350–354.
101. Eaglstein WH, Iriondo M, Laszio K. A composite skin substitute (Graftskin) for surgical wounds: a clinical experience. *Dermat Surg* 1995;21:839–834.
102. Brem H, Balledux J, Bloom T, Kerstein M, Hollier L. Healing of diabetic foot ulcers and pressure ulcers with human skin equivalent. *Arch Surg* 2000;135:627–634.
103. Veves A, Falanga V, Armstrong DG, Sabolinski ML. Graftskin, a human skin equivalent, is effective in the management of noninfected neuropathic diabetic foot ulcers. *Diabetes Care* 2001;24:290–295.
104. Sheehan P, Jones P, Caselli A, Giurini JM, Veves A. Percent change in wound area of diabetic foot ulcers over a 4-week period is a robust predictor of complete healing in a 12-week prospective trial. *Plasti Reconstr Surg* 2006;(7 Suppl):2395–2445.
105. Chanteleau E, Kushner T, Spraul M. How effective is cushioned therapeutic footwear in protecting diabetic feet. *Diabet Med* 1990;7:355–359.
106. Veves A, Masson EA, Fernando DJ, Boulton AJ. Use of experimental padded hosiery to reduce abnormal foot pressures in diabetic neuropathy. *Diabetes Care* 1989;12: 653–655.
107. Gudas CJ. Prophylactic surgery in the diabetic foot. *Clin Podiatr Med Surg* 1987;4: 445–458.

108. Tillo TH, Giurini JM, Habershaw GM, Chrzan JS, Rowbotham JL. Review of metatarsal osteotomies for the treatment of neuropathic ulcerations. *J Am Podiatr Med Assoc* 1990; 80:211–217.
109. Giurini JM, Basile P, Chrzan JS, Habershaw GM, Rosenblum BI. Panmetatarsal head resection: a viable alternative to the transmetatarsal amputation. *J Am Podiatr Med Assoc* 1993;83:101–107.
110. Giurini JM, Rosenblum BI. The role of foot surgery in patients with diabetes. *Clin Podiatr Med Surg* 1995;12:119–127.
111. Rosenblum BI, Giurini JM, Chrzan JS, Habershaw GM. Preventing loss of the great toe with the hallux interphalangeal joint arthroplasty. *J Foot Ankle Surg* 1994;33:557–560.
112. Gibbons GW. The diabetic foot: amputations and drainage of infection. *J Vasc Surg* 1987; 5:791–793.
113. Taylor LM, Porter JM. The clinical course of diabetic patients who require emergent foot surgery because of infection or ischemia. *J Vasc Surg* 1987;6:454–459.
114. Attinger CE. Use of soft tissue techniques for the salvage of the diabetic foot, in *Medical and Surgical Management of the Diabetic Foot* (Kominsky SJ, ed.), Mosby-Year Book, Boston, 1994.
115. Edmonds M, Foster A, Oreenhill M, et al. Acute septic vasculitis not diabetic micro antiopathy leads to digital necrosis in the neuropathic foot. *Diabet Med* 1992;9(Suppl l):P85.
116. Charcot JM. Sur quelques arthropathies qui paraissent dependre d'une lesion du cerveau ou de la moelle epiniere. *Arch Physiol Norm Pathol* 1868;1:61.
117. Sanders LJ, Frykberg RG. Diabetic neuropathic osteoarthropathy: Charcot Foto, in *The High Risk Foot in Diabetes Mellitus* (Frykberg RG, ed.), Churchill Livingsto ne, New York, 1991, pp. 297–338.
118. Delano PJ. The pathogenesis of Charcot's joint. *AJR* 1946;(56)2:189–200.
119. Edmonds ME, Roberts VC, Watkins PJ. Blood flow in the diabetic neuropathic foot. *Diabetologia* 1982;22:9–15.
120. Edelman SV, Kosofsky EM, Paul RA, et al. Neuro-osteoarthropathy (Charcot's joint) in diabetes mellitus following revascularization surgery: three case reports and a review of the literature. *Arch Int Med* 1987;147:1504–1508.
121. Sinha S, Munichoodappa C, Kozak GP. Neuroarthropathy (Charcot joints) in diabetes mellitus: clinical study of 101 cases. *Medicine* 1972;52:191–210.
122. Sanders LJ, Frykberg RG. Diabetic neuropathic osteoarthropathy: Charcot Foot, in *The High Risk Foot in Diabetes Mellitus* (Frykberg RG, ed.), Churchill Livingsto ne, New York, 1991, pp. 297–338.
123. Giurini JM, Chrzan JS, Gibbons GW, Habershaw GH. Charcot's disease in diabetic patients. *Postgrad Med* 1991;89:163–169.
124. Frykberg RG. Charcot Changes in the Diabetic Foot, in *The Diabetic Foot* (Veves A, Giurini JM, LoGerfo FW, eds.), Humana Press, Totawa, 2002, pp. 221–246.
125. Simon S, Tejwani S, Wilson D, et al. Arthrodesis as an alternative to nonoperative management of charcot arthropathy of the diabetic foot. *JBJS* 2000;82A:939–950.

Index

O

P

Q

R

S

T

U

V